Internal Medicine
Diagnosis and Therapy

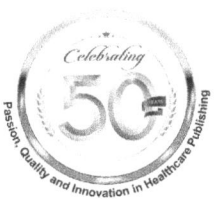

Internal Medicine Diagnosis and Therapy

2nd Edition

(Late) M Gabriel Khan
MD FRCP (London) FACC FRCPC MB BCh (Queen's Belfast)
Former Associate Professor
Department of Medicine and
Division of Cardiology
University of Ottawa
The Ottawa Hospital
Ottawa, Ontario, Canada

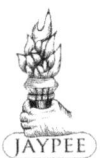

JAYPEE BROTHERS MEDICAL PUBLISHERS
The Health Sciences Publisher
New Delhi | London

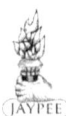 **Jaypee Brothers Medical Publishers (P) Ltd.**

Headquarters
Jaypee Brothers Medical Publishers (P) Ltd.
4838/24, Ansari Road, Daryaganj
New Delhi 110 002, India
Phone: +91-11-43574357
Fax: +91-11-43574314
Email: jaypee@jaypeebrothers.com

Overseas Office
JP Medical Ltd.
83, Victoria Street, London
SW1H 0HW (UK)
Phone: +44 20 3170 8910
Fax: +44 (0)20 3008 6180
E-mail: info@jpmedpub.com

Website: www.jaypeebrothers.com
Website: www.jaypeedigital.com

© 2020, Jaypee Brothers Medical Publishers

The views and opinions expressed in this book are solely those of the original contributor(s)/author(s) and do not necessarily represent those of editor(s) of the book.

All rights reserved. No part of this publication may be reproduced, stored or transmitted in any form or by any means, electronic, mechanical, photocopying, recording or otherwise, without the prior permission in writing of the publishers.

All brand names and product names used in this book are trade names, service marks, trademarks or registered trademarks of their respective owners. The publisher is not associated with any product or vendor mentioned in this book.

Medical knowledge and practice change constantly. This book is designed to provide accurate, authoritative information about the subject matter in question. However, readers are advised to check the most current information available on procedures included and check information from the manufacturer of each product to be administered, to verify the recommended dose, formula, method and duration of administration, adverse effects and contraindications. It is the responsibility of the practitioner to take all appropriate safety precautions. Neither the publisher nor the author(s)/editor(s) assume any liability for any injury and/or damage to persons or property arising from or related to use of material in this book.

This book is sold on the understanding that the publisher is not engaged in providing professional medical services. If such advice or services are required, the services of a competent medical professional should be sought.

Every effort has been made where necessary to contact holders of copyright to obtain permission to reproduce copyright material. If any have been inadvertently overlooked, the publisher will be pleased to make the necessary arrangements at the first opportunity. The **CD/DVD-ROM** (if any) provided in the sealed envelope with this book is complimentary and free of cost. **Not meant for sale.**

Inquiries for bulk sales may be solicited at: jaypee@jaypeebrothers.com

Internal Medicine: Diagnosis and Therapy

First Edition: 1994

Section Edition: **2020**

ISBN: 978-93-5270-670-9

Preface

The aim of this book is to provide internists, family physicians, general practitioners, and doctors in the field with an accurate and up-to-date source of easily retrievable information on how to diagnose and treat medical diseases and conditions frequently encountered in office practice. In order to accomplish this objective, we strived to provide:
- Accuracy
- Up-to-date information and depth of coverage in areas of internal medicine relevant to hospital and office practice
- Clarity of writing with an emphasis on practical information
- Succinctness.

The publisher recognizes that to reach the intended audience, the following are also essential requirements:
- The format and printing style hold the key
- Readers find it a nuisance perusing a compressed text
- People, including doctors do not have the time to read even e-version
- A well-spaced and bulleted format is necessary, so that the material can be easily understood. Thus, maximum text is presented in bulleted format.

There are a few other books that deal mainly with therapeutics and are aimed at students and interns. Our book is aimed at practitioners, internists, family physicians, general practitioners, etc.
- Accurate diagnosis and relevant pathophysiology are essential to evolve adequate therapy, and in our text, these areas are well covered. This is one of the first medium-sized books to cover all of internal medicine, giving practical straightforward advice.
- By deleting anatomy, dermatology, oncology, physiology, pathology, microbiology, preventive medicine, genetics, embryology, and other topics found in large volume internal medicine textbooks, a powerful practical book on internal medicine can emerge. The tersely written bulleted style allows the text to accommodate a wealth of relevant practical clinical information on diagnosis and therapeutics that should appeal to our audience.
- My recent novel discovery is described in the book. Annually 1 million die in India from heart attack, stroke, and peripheral vascular disease. Glucose does not cause atheroma; high cholesterol and low-density lipoprotein cholesterol (LDL-C) do; but I have found a culprit that occurs in more than 50% of diabetics.

- Sitosterol blood elevation climbs to high levels in genetic familial sitosterolemia and causes severe atheroma and early death (age 15–25); but even level of 5–10 mg/dL is likely dangerous as is a cholesterol or LDL level of 5–7 mmol/L. This chapter gives a new therapy for diabetes.
- I provided 14 cardiology chapters, also syncope and pulmonary embolism, updated the internal medicine chapters from the 1st edition.

M Gabriel Khan

Acknowledgments

We are thankful to Shri Jitendar P Vij (Group Chairman), Mr Ankit Vij (Managing Director), Ms Chetna Malhotra Vohra (Associate Director—Content Strategy), Ms Nedup Denka Bhutia (Development Editor) and the team of M/s Jaypee Brothers Medical Publishers (P) Ltd, New Delhi, India, for giving a go-ahead at the very beginning and helping us in every way possible to bring out this book.

Contents

1. **Hypertension** 1
   - Primary Hypertension   *1*
   - Hypertension in Elderly   *23*
   - Accelerated, Resistant, or Malignant Hypertension   *24*
   - Hypertensive Emergencies   *25*
   - Hypertension in Pregnancy   *31*
   - Secondary Hypertension   *35*
2. **Angina** 43
   - Classification   *43*
   - Stable Angina   *44*
   - Unstable Angina   *63*
3. **Acute Myocardial Infarction** 65
   - Pathophysiologic Implications   *65*
   - Diagnosis   *69*
   - Public Education and Physician Interaction   *77*
   - Risk Stratification   *78*
   - Therapy   *79*
4. **Sitosterolemia** 97
   - An Overview   *98*
   - Ezetimibe: A New Drug for Diabetics   *100*
   - Foods with High-sitosterol Content   *102*
   - Sitosterol in Nondiabetic Patients   *102*
5. **Heart Failure** 105
   - Diagnostic Hallmarks   *105*
   - Causes   *110*
   - Precipitating Factors   *111*
   - Pathophysiology   *111*
   - Compensatory Adjustments   *113*
   - Therapy: Nonspecific   *114*
   - Drug-combination Choice   *115*
6. **Arrhythmias** 129
   - Supraventricular Arrhythmias   *134*
   - Management of Ventricular Premature Beats and Ventricular Tachycardia   *148*

7. **Pericarditis/Cardiac Tamponade** 163
   - Pericarditis   *163*
   - Cardiac Tamponade   *167*
   - Constrictive Pericarditis   *169*

8. **Valvular Heart Disease and Rheumatic Fever** 174
   - Aortic Stenosis   *174*
   - Aortic Regurgitation   *181*
   - Mitral Stenosis   *187*
   - Mitral Regurgitation   *196*
   - Mitral Valve Prolapse   *198*
   - Rheumatic Fever   *205*

9. **Dyslipidemia and Sitosterolemia** 207
   - Atheroma   *207*
   - Primary Dyslipidemia   *210*
   - Secondary Dyslipidemia   *212*
   - Sitosterol   *214*
   - Triglycerides   *216*
   - Dietary Management   *216*
   - Drug Therapy   *221*
   - New Drug Class and New Therapies   *230*
   - Management of Elevated Serum Triglycerides   *233*

10. **Infective Endocarditis** 237
    - Diagnosis   *237*
    - Investigations   *238*
    - Therapy   *241*

11. **Cardiac Arrest** 249
    - Causes   *250*
    - Cardiopulmonary Resuscitation Studies   *252*
    - Management of Ventricular Fibrillation   *253*
    - Drug Therapy   *254*
    - Bradyarrhythmias: Asystole or Electromechanical Dissociation   *257*
    - Percutaneous Coronary Intervention   *259*

12. **Cardiomyopathy** 261
    - Hypertrophic Cardiomyopathy   *261*
    - Dilated Cardiomyopathy   *271*
    - Restrictive Cardiomyopathy   *273*
    - Specific Heart Muscle Disease   *275*

13.	**Syncope**	278
	• History and Physical Examination *281*	
	• Causes *283*	
	• Electrophysiologic Study *287*	
	• Head-up Tilt Testing *288*	
	• Pacing *288*	
14.	**Bronchodilators: Asthma–COPD**	289
	• Bronchodilators *289*	
	• Asthma *299*	
	• Chronic Obstructive Pulmonary Disease *309*	
15.	**Pneumonias**	320
	• Community-acquired Pneumonia *320*	
	• Typical Pneumonias *326*	
	• Atypical Pneumonias *329*	
	• Empiric (Initial) Therapy *333*	
	• Nosocomial Pneumonia *335*	
	• Anaerobic Pleuropulmonary Infections *340*	
16.	**Pulmonary Embolism**	367
	• Diagnosis *367*	
	• Management *375*	
17.	**Pleural Diseases: Pleural Effusions**	377
	• Physiology of Pleural Fluid Formation *377*	
	• Approach to Patients with Pleural Effusion *378*	
	• Transudative Pleural Effusions *383*	
	• Exudative Pleural Effusions *385*	
	• Malignant Pleural Effusions *390*	
	• Parapneumonic Effusions and Bacterial Infections of the Pleural Space *393*	
18.	**Gastrointestinal Diseases**	400
	• Irritable Bowel Syndrome *400*	
	• Peptic Ulcer Disease *402*	
	• Hydrogen Potassium Atpase (Proton Pump) Inhibitors *405*	
	• Malabsorption Syndromes *410*	
	• Inflammatory Bowel Disease *411*	
	• Gallstones *420*	
	• Pancreatitis *421*	
	• Gastrointestinal Bleeding *424*	

- Upper Gastrointestinal Bleeding 426
- Lower Gastrointestinal Bleeding 428

19. Liver Diseases ... 430
- Cirrhosis 430
- Hepatobiliary Manifestations of AIDS 439
- Liver Abscess 444
- Cholecystitis 445

20. Neurologic Disorders ... 447
- Coma 447
- Epilepsy 449
- Drug-related Seizures 450
- Febrile Seizures 452
- Status Epilepticus 453
- Wernicke's Encephalopathy 455
- Neuroleptic Malignant Syndrome 456
- Migraine 458
- Dizziness Vertigo 461
- Transient Ischemic Attacks 462
- Stroke 464
- Parkinson's Disease 468
- Myasthenia Gravis 470
- Acute Polyneuropathy 472
- Acute Spinal Cord Compression 474
- Infections of the Central Nervous System 475
- Review Article 487

21. Renal Diseases ... 489
- Acute Renal Failure 489
- Chronic Renal Failure 495
- Glomerular Disease 501
- Renal Stones 508
- Scleroderma (Systemic Sclerosis) 509

22. Hematologic Disorders ... 511
- Anemia 511
- Microcytic Hypochromic Anemia 511
- Normocytic Normochromic Anemias 514
- Secondary Anemia 518
- Anemia with Marrow Disruption 519

- Immunohemolytic Anemia *522*
- Thalassemia *525*
- Porphyria *526*
- Macrocytic (Megaloblastic) Anemia *527*
- Folic Acid Deficiency *528*
- Vitamin B_{12} Deficiency *529*
- Disorders of Hemostasis *530*
- Functional Platelet Disorders *535*
- Inherited Coagulation Defects *536*
- Acquired Coagulation Factor Deficiencies *540*
- Thrombotic Disorders *542*
- Platelet Disorders: Thrombocytopenia and Thrombopathy *543*
- Problems with Leukocytes and Their Management *546*
- Myeloproliferative Disorders *555*
- Other Myeloproliferative Syndromes *558*
- Paraproteinemia *558*

23. **Rheumatic Disorders** 563
    - Diagnosis *563*
    - Investigations *569*
    - Pharmacology and the Rheumatic Diseases *570*
    - Osteoarthritis *573*
    - Nonarticular Rheumatic Disorders *575*
    - Monoarticular Arthritis *581*
    - Pauciarticular Arthritis *587*
    - Rheumatoid Diseases *595*
    - Systemic Lupus Erythematosus *601*
    - Antiphospholipid Syndrome *603*
    - Mixed Connective Tissue Disease *603*
    - Necrotizing Vasculitis *606*
    - Giant Cell Arteritis *609*

24. **Sodium, Potassium, and Calcium Disturbances** 611
    - Hyponatremia *611*
    - Hypokalemia *615*
    - Hyperkalemia *616*
    - Hypercalcemia *619*

25. **Type 2 Diabetes Mellitus** 625
    - A Major Error Made by the Medical Profession Over 70 Years *625*

- New A1c Recommendations 625
- Diagnosis 626
- Types 627
- Impaired Glucose Tolerance 628
- Hypersitosterolemia 628
- Acute Complications of Diabetes 628
- Chronic Complications of Diabetes 633
- Management of Diabetes Mellitus 642

26. Endocrine Disorders ... 652
- Thyroid Diseases 652
- Adrenal Diseases 663
- Anterior Pituitary Diseases 669
- Posterior Pituitary Disorders 673

27. Miscellaneous Disorders ... 678
- Amyloid 678
- Atrial Myxoma 680
- Brugada Syndrome 680
- Chagas Disease 684
- Ehlers–Danlos Syndrome 686
- Hemochromatosis 686
- Lyme Carditis 688
- Marfan Syndrome 690
- Turner Syndrome 692
- Kawasaki Syndrome 693
- Takayasu Arteritis 694

28. Superior Quality Electrocardiograms Produced by Electrode Placements ... 700

Index ... 707

CHAPTER 1

Hypertension

INTRODUCTION

Systolic blood pressure (BP) constantly greater than 140 mm Hg in patients less than age 65 and greater than or equal to 160 mm Hg in patients more than age 65 is significant and requires aggressive control, especially in patients with coronary heart disease (CHD), congestive heart failure (CHF), cardiomegaly, renal dysfunction, diabetes, or a strong family history of cardiovascular events.

PRIMARY HYPERTENSION

- In about 95% of hypertensive adults aged 20–70, no identifiable cause can be determined. Their hypertension should be defined as primary, idiopathic, or essential. In approximately 5% of cases, a secondary cause for hypertension is present.
- Information obtained from the patient's history, physical examination/response to previous drug therapy, complete blood count (CBC), urinalysis, serum creatinine, albumin–creatinine ratio (ACR), blood urea nitrogen or BUN, electrolytes particularly serum potassium (K), total and low-density lipoprotein cholesterol (LDL-C), electrocardiogram, (ECG), and chest X-ray should give clues that might initiate further investigation to identify the presence of secondary hypertension.

Nondrug Therapy

Nondrug therapy should be rigorously tried in all patients with mild hypertension prior to drug therapy.
- Weight ↓ virtually always results in a lowering of BP; small group sessions organized by weight loss clinics have the greatest success
- Low sodium (Na) diet. A 2-g Na diet is sufficient, and compliance is feasible. Table 1.1 lists foods with their comparative Na content.
- Cessation of smoking
- Avoidance of alcohol or ↓ in alcohol intake
- Removal of stress and/or learning to deal with stress
- Relaxation and exercise.

Table 1.1: List of foods with comparative sodium (Na) content.

Food	Portion	Sodium (in mg)
Bouillon	1 cube	900
Bacon back	1 slice	500
Bacon side (fried crisp)	1 slice	75
Beef (lean, cooked)	3 oz (90 g)	60
Garlic salt	1 teaspoon (15 mL)	2,000
Garlic powder	1 teaspoon	2
Ham cured	3 oz (90 g)	1,000
Ham fresh cooked	3 oz	100
Ketchup	1 tablespoon	150
Milk pudding instant whole	1 cup (250 mL)	1,000
Meat tenderized regular	1 teaspoon	2,000
Meat tenderized low Na	1 teaspoon	2
Olive green	1	100
Pickle dill	Large (10 × 4½ cm)	1,900
Peanuts dry roasted	1 cup	1,000
Peanuts dry roasted (unsalted)	1 cup	10
Wieners	1 (50 g)	500
Canned foods		
Carrots	4 oz	400
Carrots raw		40
Corn whole kernel	1 cup	400
Corn frozen	1 cup	10
Corn beef cooked	4 oz	1000
Crab	3 oz	900
Peas cooked green	1 cup	5
Shrimp	3 oz	2,000
Salmon salt added	3 oz	500
Salmon no salt added	3 oz	50
Soups (majority)	1 cup (250 mL)	1,000
Sauerkraut	1 cup (250 mL)	1,800
Salad dressing		
Blue cheese	15 mL	160
French regular	15 mL	200
Italian	15 mL	110
Oil and vinegar	15 mL	1
Thousand Island	15 mL	90

Contd...

Contd...

Food	Portion	Sodium (in mg)
Fast food		
Chopped steak	one portion	1,000
Fried chicken	3 piece dinner	2,000
Fish and chips	one portion	1,000
Hamburger	double	1,000
Roast beef sandwich	One	1,000
Pizza	one medium	1,000

Normal diet contains 1,000–3,000 mg sodium.
Most packages that contain constituents to make gravies are high in salt.

These measures may result in adequate control of hypertension in less than 33% of patients with mild hypertension.

Drug Therapy

Annually worldwide 1 million die within 72 hours from cardiogenic shock. For the millions of individuals at cardiac risk, it is advisable to maintain a systolic BP greater than 130 mm Hg and not less than 120 mm Hg to ameliorate cardiogenic shock. The American College of Cardiology (ACC), American Heart Association (AHA) hypertension experts formulated nonsensical guidelines (2017) that state: normal systolic BP is less than 130 mm Hg. I emphasize that a level of approximately 110–120 might suffice for individuals without risk but is certainly dangerous for those with moderate or high risk for cardiovascular events.

- Blood pressure 145–160 mm Hg: Strive for monotherapy in the treatment of mild systolic hypertension whenever possible. The ideal choice is a drug that is effective for 24 hours when given once daily and that produces few or no adverse effects.
- Although there are more than 1 billion hypertensives who require treatment, there are only four groups of drugs to treat them: diuretics, β-blockers, angiotensin-converting enzyme (ACE) inhibitors, or angiotensin receptor blockers (ARBs), calcium (Ca) antagonists, and several replicas.
- One of the four drugs stipulated above is chosen based on characteristics of the individual—such as age, race, and concomitant disease—to manage mild systolic hypertension BP 140–160 mm Hg.
- Diastolic hypertension always requires two or more drugs to gain control.
- Each of the four classes of first-step drugs has unique pharmacologic properties that can be tailored to the hemodynamic, neurohormonal, and volume-related factors as well as the concomitant diseases that may exist in certain subsets of hypertensive patients.

Flowchart 1.1: Suggested drug choices for hypertensive patients not of African origin with mild-to-moderate hypertension (systolic blood pressure = 140–180 mm Hg).

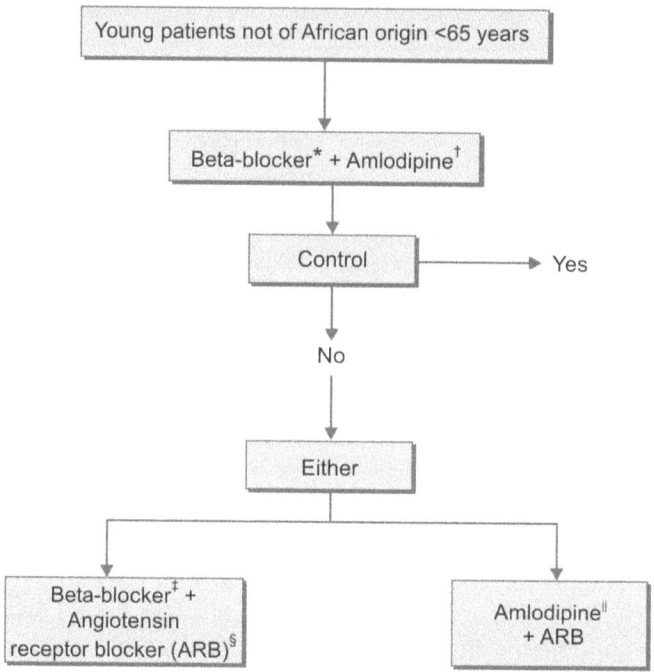

*,‡If mild hypertension, try one drug but low dose; monotherapy may succeed in approximately 45%. Then small doses of both drugs: timolol 5 mg, propranolol LA 80–240 mg; bisoprolol 5–10 mg (if cardioselective necessary) are best beta-blocker choice, propranolol and calcium antagonists only in nonsmokers. Atenolol not recommended.
§Angiotensin receptor blocker is as effective as ACE inhibitor and preferred to avoid angioedema, rare death (particularly in Africans and probably East Indians), ER visit or cough. Best choice is losartan, 25–50 mg, avoid valsartan, as it interacts with beta-blockers. Avoid telmisartan.
‖Calcium antagonist, amlodipine best choice, used in most large randomized controlled trials (RCTs). Safest dihydropyridine calcium antagonist; avoid verapamil due to risk of HF, and bradycardia; all made worse if added to beta-blocker.
†Combinations allow smaller doses of drug; fewer side effects; amlodipine + timolol (β1 and β2 drug strongly recommended if family history of myocardial infarction (MI) or diabetic.

- Combinations are often needed for BP greater than 160 systolic in individuals to age 75; (Flowcharts 1.1 to 1.4).
- Patients less than age 70 respond best to β-blockers or ACE inhibitors, but β-blockers have the advantage of providing some cardioprotection depending on the β-blocker used and the presence or absence of smoking. Effectiveness of propranolol and Ca antagonists is blunted by cigarette smoking.

Beta-blocker choice: timolol, bisoprolol, metoprolol, propranolol in nonsmokers are recommended. Beta-blockers are the only drugs that prevent sudden cardiac death (Table 1.2).

Flowchart 1.2: Suggested drug choices for hypertensive patients of African origin with mild-to-moderate systolic hypertension (blood pressure = 145–180 mm Hg).

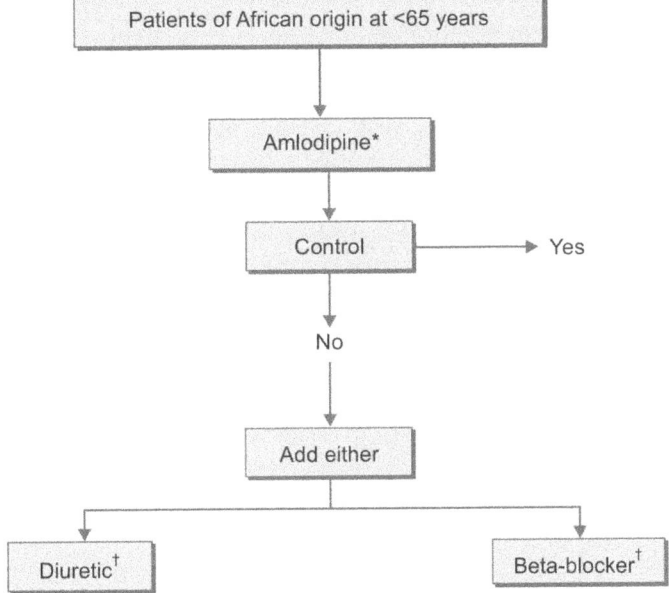

*Good response to monotherapy expected more than 70%. Diltiazem long-acting controlled release is also recommended. Verapamil not advisable.
†Combinations allow smaller doses of drug; fewer side effects; amlodipine + timolol (β1 and β2 drug strongly recommended if family history of myocardial infarction (MI) or diabetic; see Chapter 17). Timolol can prevent sudden deaths or nonfatal infarcts in smokers and nonsmokers bisoprolol 5–10 mg/day is a proven antihypertensive drug for most patients with mild hypertension and is needed if chronic obstructive pulmonary disease (COPD).

- Atenolol must not be used because it is the most widely used but the most ineffective β-blocker (Khan 2003, 2017).
- A drug that works in one patient may fail in the second.
- Patients more than age 70 and blacks with low-renin essential hypertension respond best to diuretics or Ca antagonists, but β-blockers and ACE inhibitors are effective in greater than 50% of blacks and the elderly and may be suitable for use in these patients.
- Calcium antagonists are effective at all ages and in all grades of primary and secondary hypertension. It is a must for emergency reduction of severe hypertension because the other three drugs are mild acting and takes days to significantly reduce high levels.
- Amlodipine or nifedipine must be used if hypertension is severe BP greater than 180 mm Hg despite adequate diuretic therapy.
- In females with a high risk for osteoporosis, diuretics are first choice as they are the only antihypertensive agents that ↑ bone mass. The SHEP has confirmed a salutary effect of low-dose chlorthalidone with or

6 Internal Medicine: Diagnosis and Therapy

Flowchart 1.3: Suggested drug choices for hypertensive patients older than age 64, with mild to moderate hypertension (systolic blood pressure = 145–180 mm Hg any ethnicity).

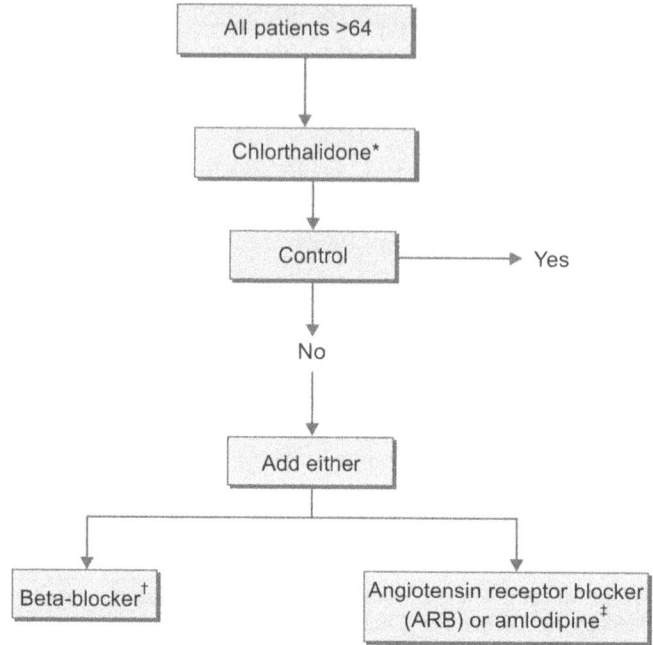

*12.5 mg/day; much more effective than other thiazides. Proven 100% the best drug in the soundly run large ALLHAT, shown to be safer and as effective as ACE inhibitor or amlodipine; but may cause significant hypokalemia. If serum potassium falls to less than 3.5 mmol/L, add amiloride to prevent this.
Chlorthalidone or hydrochlorothiazide 12.5 mg/day + amiloride to conserve potassium and assist thiazide diuresis; assess renal function and serum potassium.
†If not controlled replace diuretic with amlodipine.
‡ACE inhibitor not recommended as risk of angioedema particularly in individuals of African origin; ARB of choice is losartan 25–50 mg/day; avoid telmisartan (see text for TRANSCEND and PRoFESS study failures). Calcium antagonist not recommended if known or probable left ventricular dysfunction as may cause heart failure (HF). ALLHAT—the amlodipine group had a 32.5% higher risk of HF (p <0.001) with a 6-year absolute risk difference of 2.5% and a 35% higher risk of hospitalized/fatal HF (p <0.001). Risk is higher for nifedipine other dihydropyridines and diltiazem and much higher for verapamil. Use amlodipine or nifedipine only if other agents fail to control BP, and in the absence of left ventricular dysfunction. Amlodipine is often necessary for severe hypertension at a dose of 5–7.5 mg/day; edema of legs can be a bothersome adverse effect.

  without added β-blocker therapy on cardiovascular and cerebrovascular mortality in patients aged 65–86 who have isolated systolic hypertension.
- The thiazide diuretic chlorthalidone confers lower risk for pelvic and hip fractures than other antihypertensive drugs, according to a secondary analysis from the randomized ALLHAT trial. (They certainly increase bone mass and significantly prevent fractures. Falls and fractures are common in the elderly.)

Flowchart 1.4: Suggested drug choices for hypertensive patients with prior heart failure, or probable LV dysfunction, old MI, atrial fibrillation or other heart disease.

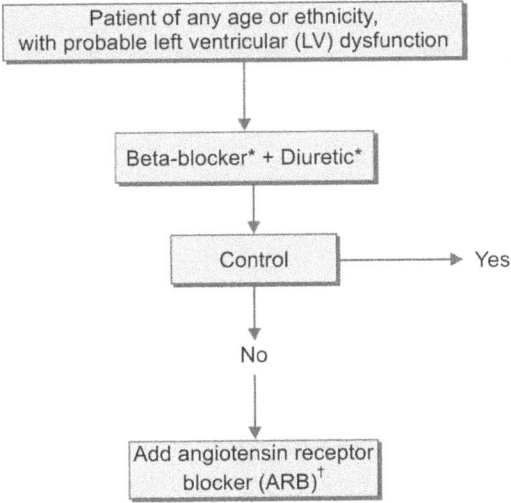

*Small dose either drug: timolol 2.5–5 mg twice daily or propranolol in nonsmokers 120–240 mg/day; β1 and β2 drugs more cardioprotective than cardioselective.
Bisoprolol 5–10 mg also advisable for most patients and for chronic obstructive pulmonary disease (COPD).
†ACE inhibitor not recommended as risk of angioedema particularly in individuals of African or Indian origin.
ARB of choice is losartan 25–50 mg/day; avoid telmisartan (see text for TRANSCEND and PRoFESS study failures). Calcium antagonist not recommended as may cause heart failure.

Table 1.2: Beta-blockers drugs currently available that prevent sudden cardiac death.

	Control	Drug	% Decrease
Propranolol			
Total sudden death*	78	60	23
5 am–11 am	31	11	64
Total deaths	188/1460	138/1456	26
Timolol†			
Total sudden death	95	47	50
Instant, within seconds	38	11	71
Total deaths	117/718	67/670	42
Metoprolol#			
Total sudden death	21	9	57##
Total deaths	31/147	25/154	19##

Contd...

Contd...

	Control	Drug	% Decrease
MERIT-HF^			
Total sudden death	132	79	40.2
Total deaths	217/2001	145/1990	33.2
Bisoprolol‡			
Total sudden death	83	48	42.2
Total deaths	228/1320	156/1327	31.6

[Only four beta-blockers of the 12 available definitely prevent sudden cardiac death; they all gain high brain concentration. Atenolol and sotalol gain poor brain concentration and are ineffective; atenolol use should be curtailed.]
*BHAT study, AM sudden death (Peters et al. 1989) follow-up 25 months, propranolol 120–240 mg daily.
†Timolol Norwegian MI study; mean duration 17 months follow-up: 10 mg twice daily. A superior drug rarely used; beta-blockers are not all alike.
#Metoprolol: A very small study of only approximately 150 patients in each group followed for 3 years.
##"This reduction in cardiac mortality did not reach statistical significance, as was to be expected from our sample size" (Olsson et al. 1985).
^In MERIT-HF, there were fewer sudden deaths in the metoprolol CR/XL group than in the placebo group [79 vs 132, 0.59 (0.45–0.78); p = 0.0002] and deaths from worsening heart failure [30 vs 58, 0.51 (0.33–0.79); p = 0.0023].
‡Bisoprolol in CIBIS; significant decrease in deaths and sudden death.
Carvedilol did not prevent sudden death in two large RCTs; total mortality in RCT was not significantly reduced in post MI patients.
Source: Reproduced with permission from Khan MG. Practical Cardiology. New Delhi, India: Jaypee Brothers Medical Publishers (P) Ltd.; 2018. p. 312.

- Age less than 70 or in the elderly: A β-blocker plus a Ca antagonist amlodipine or nifedipine extended release; a β-blocker plus a small dose of a thiazide diuretic; or a β-blocker plus an ACE inhibitor, although their effects are not always complimentary, the latter two agents are cardioprotective. If a diuretic agent is used and hypokalemia is observed, add amiloride.
- *Spironolactone* is not recommended although some believe the drug is indicated for resistant hypertension. Triamterene may cause renal calculi. Amiloride is the only diuretic agent that has salutary antiarrhythmic properties and replaces spironolactone that causes hormonal adverse effects. Spironolactone is not indicated for hypertension and withdrawn in the United Kingdom (1990).
- Nifedipine has more negative inotropic action than amlodipine and poses a higher risk for precipitating CHF.
- Coronary heart disease: In patients with CHD or in those who are at high risk for CHD events, a β-blocker plus amlodipine is advisable.

- Alpha blockers (e g doxazosin) are contraindicated because they cause CHF and may rupture aneurysms because they increase cardiac ejection velocity.

Beta-blockers

These agents are as effective as other agents in the young and the elderly with mild hypertension. They are the only agents that may prevent sudden cardiac death (*see* Table 1.2).

The notion that β-blockers are not effective or harmful or cause genuine diabetes is false. Nonetheless this is a notion held by many experts who write guidelines (UK and USA)
- See later discussion; indication in the elderly

A Medical Research Council (MRC) Working Party confirmed that 25% of patients were lost to follow-up and more than half the patients were not taking the therapy assigned by the end of the study.
- This misleading finding nevertheless led to a published editorial by Messerli et al. (1998) entitled "Are β-blockers efficacious as first-line therapy for hypertension in the elderly?" These analysts concluded that β-blockers should not be first-line therapy for elderly hypertensives. This advice has spread worldwide.

A small dose of a β-blocking drug, e.g. bisoprolol 2.5–5 mg (not atenolol), is successfully administered for the commonly occurring atrial fibrillation of the elderly or for angina or post-myocardial infarction (MI) and should be just as safe for the elderly hypertensive whose BP must not be aggressively lowered by an ACE inhibitor or Ca antagonist resulting in falls.
- Atenolol is a most ineffective, but is the most used β-blocker in randomized controlled trials (RCTs) performed in hypertensive patients from 1984 to 2012. A meta-analysis by Lindholm et al. concluded with a statement placed on the front cover of the Lancet:

  Beta-blockers should not remain first choice in the treatment of primary hypertension. In 14 studies analyzed by Lindholm et al., atenolol was the β-blocker used; in four small trials, mixtures of atenolol, metoprolol, and pindolol were used.

  The Lindholm meta-analysis 24 caused much stir and reduced β-blocker prescriptions for hypertension. In a Lancet letter, Cruickshank (2006) stated that by lumping together all randomized hypertension trials involving β-blockers, Lars Lindholm and colleagues have arrived at misleading conclusions, but letters in journals are perused by few readers.

Reasons for atenolol's poor efficacy: Lipid-soluble β-blockers (bisoprolol, metoprolol, propranolol, and timolol) have all been proven in large RCTs to significantly decrease fatal and nonfatal MI, and sudden cardiac death (*see* Table 1.2). They all attain high brain concentration block sympathetic discharge in the hypothalamus better than water-soluble agents, atenolol and sotalol. Timolol in the Norwegian trial caused an astounding 71% reduction in sudden cardiac deaths. The lipophilic agents are metabolized in the liver and obtain high brain concentration, which may confer some adverse effects. Increased brain concentration and ↑ of central vagal tone confers greater cardiac protection.

Äblad et al. in a rabbit model showed that although metoprolol (lipophilic) and atenolol (hydrophilic) caused equal β-blockade, only metoprolol caused a reduction in cardiac death. Metoprolol but not atenolol caused a significant increase in RR interval variation and thus a favorable alteration in sympathetic tone. Most important, increased brain concentration and elevation of central vagal tone confers cardiovascular protection.

Pyeritz emphasized that β-blocker therapy currently remains the "standard of care", and all patients should receive treatment, regardless of the presence or absence of aortic dilatation. "Atenolol administered twice daily is currently the drug of choice of many practitioners because it has long half-life and is relatively cardioselective, with fewer central nervous system (CNS) and other side effects." Lacro et al. indicated that that an NIH RCT of subjects with Marfan syndrome comparing atenolol and losartan should provide some answers. This was completed in 2014 and presented at the AHA. Results for both drugs were similar.

Atenolol is said to cause less adverse effects than other β-blockers, and we partially agree because the drug was commonly used in our cardiac clinics from 1984 to 1998. Use was discontinued from 2003. Both lower adverse central effects and less salutary effects are observed because of the low brain concentration causing more placebo effects.

It must be emphasized that atenolol does not provide a full 24-hour action. Neutel et al. indicated that bisoprolol reduced ambulatory systolic and diastolic pressures by 43% and 49%, respectively, more than atenolol during early morning hours. The drug fails to quell early morning catecholamine surge, a time at which there is an increased risk of ischemia and sudden death. It is not surprising, therefore, that atenolol is only partially cardiovascular disease (CVD) protective, and showed relative poor performance compared with ACE inhibitor and Ca antagonists and diuretics in RCTs of hypertension. The drug was never tested in a long-term post-MI, or heart failure RCT, and there is no proof that it can prevent sudden cardiac death (*see* Table 1.2).

Atenolol is not recommended because of poor efficacy:
- Provided that salutary effects are not nullified by cigarette smoking. Äblad et al. in a rabbit model showed that while both metoprolol (lipophilic) and atenolol (hydrophilic) caused equal β-blockade, only metoprolol caused a ↓ in sudden cardiac death. Metoprolol, but not atenolol, caused a significant ↑ in RR interval variation that indicates an

in parasympathetic tone. Only the β-blockers with lipophilic properties—Bisoprolol, metoprolol, timolol and propranolol—in nonsmokers have been shown in clinical trials to prevent sudden cardiac death. It is important for the physician to select an appropriate β-blocker with the understanding that β-blockers are not all alike.
- Statements in editorials such as "β-blockers do not reduce cardiac mortality in hypertensives" must be considered erroneous because β-blockers possess subtle differences that are clinically important. It is not surprising that cardiac mortality was not reduced by propranolol in smokers in the large hypertension clinical trials of the 1980s. Thus, meta-analyses do not reflect the maximum cardioprotective effects of β-blocking agents.
- The protective cardiovascular effects of hepatic-metabolized β-blockers such as propranolol and penbutolol are blunted by cigarette smoking.
- *Timolol, metoprolol, and bisoprolol have been shown to be effective in preventing cardiac deaths in smokers and nonsmokers.*, patients who insist on smoking ↑ their risk of sudden death and other CHD events, and in this large group of patients, the choice of a β-blocker is important.

Beta-blockers with more than moderate intrinsic sympathomimetic activity (ISA) are not recommended because they may blunt the cardioprotective lifesaving potential.

Beta-blockers are considered first-choice therapy for the management of hypertension in several subsets of patients in whom no contraindications to β-blockade exist.

Indications: They include:
- Patients less than age 70
- Beta-blockers are first choice in patients with CHD manifested by angina, silent ischemia, and following MI
- First choice in patients with arrhythmias
- Patients with left ventricular hypertrophy (LVH) are at high risk for sudden death; β-blockers are the only cardioactive agents that have been proven to prevent sudden cardiac death (*see* Table 1.2)
- Patients with increased adrenergic activity, including the younger age group, who often have high plasma norepinephrine levels, and patients with hyperkinetic heart syndrome, alcohol withdrawal hypertension, or the hyperdynamic β-adrenergic circulatory state, with labile or elevated BP and palpitations
- Orthostatic hypertension, with an exaggerated ↑ in diastolic pressure on standing, usually indicates increased adrenergic tone; β-blockers have a salutary effect in this subset.
- Patients prone to postural hypotension may benefit since these agents, unlike all other antihypertensives, do not usually ↓ systemic vascular resistance.
- First choice for patients with aneurysms

- In females more than age 55, β-blockers are a rational choice because the incidence of myocardial rupture is high in hypertensive women who sustain a first infarction. Beta-blockers protect sufficiently from myocardial rupture to warrant their use in patients considered at risk. The combination of a β-blocking agent and a low-dose diuretic is advisable if prevention of osteoporosis also requires therapeutic consideration.

Beta-blockers are indicated in the elderly over age 75. There is still no clear consensus regarding the mechanisms by which β-blocking drugs cause a ↓ in BP. An interplay of mechanisms appears to be responsible. Negative chronotropic and inotropic effects lead to a ↓ in cardiac output and some ↓ in BP. Antagonism of sympathetically mediated renin ralease and ↓ in plasma renin have a role. Added mechanisms include CNS effects, ↓ in norepinephrine release, ↓ in plasma volume and venomotor tone, resetting of baroreceptor levels, and inhibition of the catecholamine pressor response to stress. Strongly indicated in the elderly more than age 75.

The MRC Working Party (1992) investigators confirmed that 25% of patients were lost to follow-up and more than half the patients were not taking the therapy assigned by the end of the study. This blunderbuss study nevertheless led to a published editorial by Messerli et al. (1998) entitled "Are β-blockers efficacious as first-line therapy for hypertension in the elderly?" These analysts concluded that β-blockers should not be first-line therapy for elderly hypertensives. This incorrect advice has spread worldwide.

Contraindications:
- Congestive heart failure
- Asthma, severe chronic obstructive pulmonary disease (COPD), allergic rhinitis
- Severe peripheral vascular disease (PVD)
- Heart block, sick sinus syndrome
- Diabetics prone to hypoglycemia—however, if β-blocker therapy is needed in patients with stable or mild diabetes, a cardioselective agent such as metoprolol is preferred.

Adverse effects: These include precipitation of CHF in patients with poor LV systolic function [ejection fraction (EF) <30%]. Symptomatic bradycardia is bothersome in less than 10% of treated patients, bronchospasm may be precipitated in asthmatics and patients with COPD. Dizziness, weakness, fatigue, vivid dreams, rarely depression, and very rarely psychosis and loss of hearing may occur.

Impotence occurs in less than 2% of patients. Based on studies utilizing greater than 39,000 patients, 0.4% reported impotence. The incidence is much less than observed with the use of diuretics and is not greater than that reported for ACE inhibitors or Ca antagonists. Raynaud's phenomenon and worsening of intermittent claudication are bothersome features of β-blocker therapy. A few cases of exacerbation of psoriasis have been reported. Labetalol is a β-blocker with alpha1-blocking activity and has two major adverse effects not observed with pure β-blocking agents: (1) postural hypotension is not uncommon, and (2) life-threatening hepatic necrosis has been observed.

Caution: Avoid abrupt cessation of β-blocker therapy in patients with CHD because angina may worsen. If necessary, discontinue β-blockers gradually over 2–3 weeks and instruct the patient to refrain from moderate exertion. Rarely, rebound hypertension is precipitated.

Interactions:
- With hepatic-metabolized β-blockers are observed when drugs, such as cimetidine or chlorpheniramine, which ↓ hepatic blood flow, are used concomitantly.
- Hypertensive crisis can occur with cough and cold remedies containing phenylpropanolamine.
- An increased risk for anaphylactoid reaction from contrast media and immunotherapy in patients on β-blockers has been reported.

Diuretics

These economical, one-a-day drugs can be recommended as first line in selected patients. The SHEP confirms the salutary effects of low-dose diuretic therapy. In the SHEP, chlorthalidone, 12.5-mg alone or in combination with β-blocker resulted in a significant ↓ in the risk of stroke, MI, and left ventricular failure (LVF). The exact mechanism of action by which diuretics produce a ↓ in BP is unknown. A ↓ in vascular volume, negative Na balance, and long-term arteriolar dilation occurs.

Chlorthalidone, a 6.25-mg dose, appears to suffice in individuals of Indian origin; if 12.5 mg is needed add amiloride to conserve potassium and enhance action.

Indications: Small-dose diuretic therapy is particularly useful in the following categories of patients:
- More than age 65 (*see* SHEP and HYVET trials)
- Blacks, who usually have low renin hypertension
- Concomitant CHF or renal dysfunction
- Particularly females more than age 45, who may be at risk for osteoporosis. Diuretics are the only antihypertensive drugs that have been shown to ↑ bone mineral density and to ↓ the risk of hip fractures in both women and men.
- As second-line agent to enhance the BP-lowering effect of β-blockers, ACE inhibitors, vasodilators, and/or centrally acting drugs.

Disadvantages:
- Hypokalemia occurs in less than 25% of patients treated with 25-mg of hydrochlorothiazide (HCTZ) or an equivalent dose of another thiazide daily. This occurrence is dose related. A 25- or 50-mg dose of HCTZ is expected to cause a ↓ in serum K of about 0.3–0.6 mEq/L, respectively, in susceptible individuals. Patients given a thiazide should be screened in 2 months and then q 6 months for hypokalemia. If hypokalemia develops, it is advisable to change to a K-sparing diuretic (Moduretic or Dyazide) after correction of the K deletion.
- Patients who show hypokalemia despite K supplements or K-sparing diuretics are best treated by replacing the diuretic with an ACE inhibitor.

Adverse effects: Impotence, weakness, and fatigue; the incidence of impotence is greater than that observed with the use of β-blockers. Hyponatremia may develop over a period of weeks or years in some susceptible individuals; electrolyte imbalance and hypomagnesemia; gout; rarely, thrombocytopenia, agranulocytosis, and pancreatitis.
- Thiazide appears in breast milk, crosses the placental barrier, and can cause decreased placental perfusion, fetal or neonatal thrombocytopenia, jaundice, and acute pancreatitis. Avoid during pregnancy and lactation.

Interactions: They occur with oral anticoagulants and steroids; an in serum lithium levels may occur; nonsteroidal anti-inflammatory drugs (NSAIDs), including aspirin, interfere with the diuretic effect of furosemide.

Bendrofluazide: Supplied—tablets; 2.5 mg, 5 mg. Dosage—2.5–5 mg qd.
Hydrochlorothiazide: Supplied—tablets; 25 mg. Dosage—commence with 12.5 mg; then, if needed, 25 mg, once daily but potassium may fall; thus, amiloride 5 mg may be added. Alternate-day therapy may suffice in some patients with mild hypertension.

Potassium-sparing Diuretics

- Amiloride 2.5–5 mg daily if needed to prevent hypokalemia
- Spironolactone is not recommended.
- *Triamterene* (HCTZ 25 mg and triamterene 50 mg, a K-sparing diuretic) is not recommended; triamterene may cause kidney stone.

Contraindications to the use of K-sparing diuretics include renal failure, concomitant use of ACE inhibitors and/or K supplements; with renal calculi avoid triamterene.

Other Diuretics

Indapamide: It is chemically related to chlorthalidone but has an added mild vasodilator effect, which is not related to diuretic action. The incidence

of hypokalemia is similar to that of thiazides, but indapamide produced no disturbances in blood lipid, blood glucose, or insulin levels in hypertensive patients administered 2.5 mg qd for 1 year.
- Because approximately 60% of indapamide is excreted by the kidney, the drug should not be administered to patients with mild renal dysfunction.
- Dosing interval does not require adjustment, but periodic evaluation of serum K and creatinine is advised.
- *Supplied*: tablet; 2.5 mg. *Dosage*: 1 tablet each morning. A dose greater than 2.5 mg qd is not advisable.

Furosemide (Frusemide, UK): This powerful loop diuretic is less effective than thiazides in mild hypertension. However, thiazides, with the exception of metolazone, lose their natriuretic effect when the glomerular filtration rate (GFR) falls below 25 mL/h while loop diuretics retain their effectiveness.
- Furosemide is not advised for the treatment of hypertension except when there is concomitant CHF or severe renal dysfunction.

Angiotensin-converting Enzyme Inhibitors

These agents have provided a major advance in the management of hypertension. They are useful first-line agents (Table 1.3). These inhibitors of ACE prevent the conversion of angiotensin I to the potent vasoconstrictor, angiotensin II. This action causes arteriolar dilation and a $\downarrow$ in total systemic vascular resistance as well as diminished sympathetic activity causing vasodilation (but HR does not $\uparrow$ as occurs with other vasodilators) and a $\downarrow$ in aldosterone secretion. The $\downarrow$ in aldosterone secretion causes both Na excretion and K retention. The pharmacologic profile and dosages of ACE inhibitors are given in Table 1.4.

Indications:
- ACE inhibitors are most effective in patients with high-renin hypertension and especially in Caucasians less than age 65, but are effective in the elderly.
- Hypertensives with left ventricular (LV) dysfunction or CHF
- Diabetics with hypertension of all grades. Importantly, mild hypertension (systolic 140–160 mm Hg, diastolic 90–95 mm Hg) in diabetics must be aggressively treated, preferably with an ACE inhibitor
- Patients with renal dysfunction: ACE inhibitors appear to preserve nephron life (see contraindication solitary kidney and/or critical renal artery stenosis).

Contraindications:
- Renal artery stenosis of a solitary kidney or severe bilateral renal artery stenosis
- Severe anemia

Table 1.3: Daily dosage of antihypertensive drugs.

Drugs	Doses Initial	Usual maintenance	Maximum*
ACE inhibitors			
Captopril (Capoten)	12.5–25	50–100	150
Enalapril (Vasotec)	2.5–5	10–20	40
Lisinopril (Prinivil, Zestril)	2.5–5	10–20	40
Benazepril (Lotensin)	5	5–30	40
Fosinopril (Monopril) 10 mg	5–10	10–30	40
Perindopril	1–2	2–6	8
Quinapril (Accupril)	2.5–5	5–30	40
Ramipril (Altace)	1.25–2.5	2.5–5	20
Alpha-Adrenergic Antagonists			
Prazosin (Minipress)	1 (0.5, UK)	5–15	20
Terazosin (Hytrin)	1	2–10	15
Calcium Antagonists			
Amlodipine (Norvasc)	2.5–5	5–10	10
Diltiazem‡ 60, 90, 120 mg	90	180–240	360
Cardizem CD	180	180–240	300
Cardizem SR 90, 120 mg	90	180–360	360
Adizem SR (UK) 120 mg	120	120–360	360
Nifedipine			
Nifedipine Extended Release:			
Adalat CC, Procardia XL,	30	60–90	120
Adalat XL(C) 30, 60, 90 mg			
Adalat PA 10 mg (C)	20–40	40–80	120
Adalat Retard 10 mg (UK)			
Adalat Retard 20 mg (UK)	20–40	60–80	80
Verapamil 80, 120 mg, 40, 80, 120, 160 mg (UK)	160	160–360	480

Contd...

Contd...

Drugs	Doses		
	Initial	Usual maintenance	Maximum*
Calan SR 120, 180, 240 mg	120	120–360	480
Isoptin SR 120, 180, 240 mg	120	120–360	480
Verelan 120, 240 mg			
Nicardipine 20, 30 mg	40	40–60	90
Cardene			
Nitrendipine	5	5–20	40
Baypress			
Felodipine			
Plendil 5, 10 mg	5	5–10	15
Isradipine 2.5, 5 mg	2.5–5	5–10	30
DynaCirc			
Central Acting			
Clonidine (Catapress)	0.1	0.2–0.8	1
Guanabenz (Wytensin)	4	8	16
Guanfacine (Tenex)	1	1	3
Methyldopa (Aldomet)	250–500	500–1000	1500
Beta Blockers			
Acebutolol (Sectral, Monitan)	200–400	400–800	1000
Atenolol (Tenormin)	25–50	50–100	100
Labetalol (Trandate, Normodyne)	100–400	500–1000	1200
Metoprolol (Toprol XL, Lopressor, Betaloc)	50	50–200	300
Nadolol (Corgard)	40–80	40–160	160
Penbutolol (Levatol)	20	20–40	80
Pindolol (Visken)	7.5–15	10–15	30
Proprandolol (Inderal)	40–120	160–240	240
Inderal LA	80	80–240	240
Sotalol (Sotacor, C, UK)	80	160	240

Contd...

Contd...

	Doses		
Drugs	Initial	Usual maintenance	Maximum*
Timolol (Blocadren)	5–10	10–20	40
Diuretics			
Bendroflumethiazide	2.5	2.5	5
Bendrofluazide (UK)	2.5	2.5–5	5
Benzthiazide	12.5	2.5	50
Chlorothiazide	125	250	500
Chlorthalidone	12.5	25	50
Hydrochlorothiazide	12.5–25	25–50	50
Hydroflumethiazide	12.5–25	25–50	50
Indapamide	2.5	2.5	2.5
Methylclothiazide	2.5	2.5	5
Metolazone	1.25	2.5	10
Polythiazide	2	2	4
Quinethazone	25	25	50
Trichlormethiazide	1	2	4
Bumetanide	0.5	1–5	10
Furosemide (Frusemide, UK)	40	40–160	240

*In clinical practice, a dose less than the manufacturer's maximum is advised and reduces the incidence of adverse effects.
†See Table 1.4
‡Not appropriate for the elderly or those with renal or hepatic impairment (British National Formulary, 1992)
C = Canada
UK = United Kingdom
Note: All drugs are available in the United States, except where labeled "C" or "UK."

- Urticaria, angioedema
- Aortic stenosis
- Hypertrophic and restrictive cardiomyopathy; hypertensive, hypertrophic "cardiomyopathy" of the elderly with impaired ventricular relaxation
- Severe carotid artery stenosis
- Hypertensive patients with concomitant unstable angina
- Uric acid renal calculi
- Pregnancy and breastfeeding
- Porphyria
- Relative contraindications include patients with collagen vascular diseases or concomitant use of immunosuppressives, since neutropenia

Table 1.4: The pharmacological profile and dosages of ACE inhibitors.

	Captopril	Enalapril	Lisinopril	Ramipril
USA and Canada	Capoten	Vasotec	Prinivil, Zestril	Altace
UK	Capoten	Innovace	Carace, Zestril	Tritace
Europe	Lopril, Lopirin	Xanef, Renitec	Carace, Zestril	Tritace
Pro-drug	No	Yes	No	Partial
Action				
apparent (hours)	1/2	2–4	2–4	3–6
peak effect (hours)	1–2	5	4–8	3–6
duration (hours)	8–12	12–24	24–30	24–48
Half-life (hours)	2–3	11	13	14–30
Metabolism	Partly hepatic	Hepatic	None	Partial
Elimination	Renal	Renal	Renal	Renal
SH group	Yes	No	No	No
Approved use USA**	Hypertension	Hypertension	Hypertension	Hypertension
Heart failure	Yes	Yes	No	No
Equivalent dose	100 mg	20 mg	20 mg	10 mg
Initial dose	12.5 mg	2.5 mg	2.5 mg	1.25–2.5 mg
Total daily dose				
Hypertension	50–150 mg	5–40 mg	5–40 mg	2.5–20 mg
heart failure	25–100 mg	5–20 mg		
Dose frequency*	2–3 daily	1–2 daily	1 daily	1 daily
Supplied	12.5, 25, 50, 100 mg	2.5, 5, 10, 20 mg	5, 10, 20, 40 mg 2.5 UK; 5, 10, 20, 40 mg	1.25, 2.5, 5, 10 mg

*Increase dosing interval with renal failure
**Also approved for hypertension: Benazepril (Lotensin) Fosinopril (Monopril); Quinapril (Accupril): *see* Table 1.3 and text.

and rare agranulocytosis observed with ACE inhibitors appear to occur mainly in this subset of patients.

Adverse effects: Hyperkalemia in patients with renal failure, pruritus and rash in about 10% of patients, and loss of taste in approximately 7% of patients. A rare but important adverse effect is angioedema of the face, mouth, or larynx, which may occur in approximately 0.5% of treated patients and can be fatal. Rarely, mouth ulcers, neurologic dysfunction, gastrointestinal (GI) disturbances, and proteinuria occur in about 1% of patients with preexisting renal disease. Neutropenia and agranulocytosis are rare and occur mainly in patients with serious intercurrent illness, particularly immunologic disturbances, altered immune response, or collagen vascular disease. Cough occurs in about 10% of treated patients, and wheezing, myalgia, muscle cramps, hair loss, impotence or decreased libido, hepatitis or occurrence of antinuclear antibodies, and pemphigus occasionally occur.

Interactions: Interactions with lithium, allopurinol, acebutolol, hydralazine, NSAIDs, procainamide, pindolol, steroids, tocainide, immunosuppressives, and other drugs that alter immune response. Drugs that ↑ serum K levels have been emphasized.

Captopril: *Supplied*—tablets; 12.5 mg, 25 mg, 50 mg, 100 mg. *Dosage*—commence with 12.5 mg bid, 1/2 hour before meals; ↑ over days or weeks to 25-75 mg bid, which is the dose required by the majority of patients. The maximum suggested dose is 150 mg qd in severe hypertension. Serious side effects are more common in patients given a daily dose of greater than or equal to 200 mg. Increase the dose interval in renal failure. Decrease the initial dose to 6.25 mg in the elderly or if a diuretic is used concomitantly.

Captopril 100 mg = approximately 20 mg enalapril, 20 mg lisinopril, 20 mg ramipril, 5 mg alacepril, 35 mg pentopril.

Enalapril: *Supplied*—tablets; 2.5 mg, 5 mg, 10 mg, 20 mg. *Dosage*—2.5-5 mg qd; ↑ over days to months to 10-30 mg qd in one or two divided doses with or without food. Maximum 40 mg qd or less often in renal failure. In the elderly or in patients receiving a diuretic, begin with a dose of 2.5 mg qd.

Cilazapril: *Supplied*—tablets; 1 mg, 2.5 mg, 5 mg. *Dosage*—1-2.5 mg qd; maximum 5 mg qd.

Lisinopril: *Supplied*—tablets; 2.5 mg (UK), 5 mg, 10 mg, 20 mg, 40 mg. *Dosage*—2.5 mg once daily; ↑ to 10-30 mg; maximum 40 mg qd or less often in renal failure. Discontinue diuretic for 2-3 days prior to commencing lisinopril and resume later if required.

Benazepril: *Supplied*—5 mg, 10 mg, 20 mg, 40 mg. *Dosage*—5 mg; ↑ as needed to usual maintenance 5-30 mg; maximum suggested 40 mg. Commence with 2.5 mg in the elderly or if a diuretic is given concomitantly. Not affected by food or antacids or antibiotics; some hepatic elimination occurs.

Fosinopril: *Supplied*—tablets; 10 mg, 20 mg. *Dosage*—5-10 mg once daily; ↑ slowly, if required, to 20 mg and with assessment of renal function; maximum 40 mg qd with or without food but avoid taking within 2 hours of antacids. Initial dose 2.5 mg in the elderly or in patients receiving a diuretic. Fosinopril is the only phosphinic acid class of the ACE inhibitors; the carboxylic acid class includes benazepril, enalapril, lisinopril, quinapril, and ramipril; captopril is the only sulfhydryl agent. Monopril has an advantage of compensatory hepatic elimination in patients with renal failure and minimizes accumulation in patients with renal insufficiency.

Perindopril: *Supplied*—tablets 2 mg. *Dosage*—2 mg qd; ↑ if required, after monitoring BP, to 4–8 mg qd. Discontinue diuretic 3 days prior and resume later, if needed.

In the PROGRESS trial perindopril reduced BP in less than 42% of subjects; indapamide was needed in greater than 55%

Only patients on combination therapy had stroke reduction. Only the subgroup receiving both perindopril and indapamide had reduced stroke recurrence; the study design did not include a subgroup randomized to indapamide alone

Quinapril: *Supplied*—tablets; 5 mg; 10 mg, 20 mg, 40 mg. *Dosage*—5 mg once daily; usual maintenance 20–40 mg qd. Reduce the initial dose to 2.5 mg qd in the elderly, renal dysfunction, or with diuretic use. *Interaction*—tetracyclines.

Ramipril: *Supplied*—capsules; 1.25 mg, 2.5 mg, 5 mg, 10 mg. *Dosage*—1.25 mg once daily; ↑ if needed, to 2.5–5 mg and with assessment of renal function; maximum 20 mg qd.

Caution: Angioedema is a life-threatening condition more common in individuals of African descent. ARBs must not be substituted as they do cause angioedema albeit rarely.

Angiotensin Receptor Blockers

These agents are not all alike and caution is required.

The safety of the ARB olmesartan is questionable after two ongoing trials among patients with type 2 diabetes suggested increased risk for cardiovascular death with the drug. The US Food and Drug Administration (FDA) issued a warning July 3, 2013 that olmesartan medoxomil may cause sprue-like enteropathy several months to years after initiation of treatment.

Angiotensin receptor blockers appear to be associated with a modestly increased risk for cancer, according to a meta-analysis published in the Lancet Oncology, Telmisartan was commonly used (Nissen made the comment). Should we be concerned about all ARBs or a single drug, telmisartan?

Miceli and colleagues conducted a retrospective, observational, cohort study of prospectively collected data on 10,023 consecutive patients undergoing isolated isolated coronary artery bypass grafting (CABG) to May 2008. Of these, 3,052 patients receiving preoperative ACE inhibitor were matched to a control group by propensity score analysis. Preoperative ACE inhibitor therapy was associated with a doubling in the risk of death (1.3% vs 0.7%; p = 0.013). In a multivariate analysis, preoperative ACE inhibitor treatment was an independent predictor of mortality (p = 0.04), postoperative renal dysfunction (PRD) (p = 0.0002), use of inotropic drugs (p <0.0001), and atrial fibrillation (p <0.0001). Preoperative treatment with ACE inhibitor is associated with an increased risk of mortality, use of inotropic support, PRD, and new onset of postoperative atrial fibrillation.

Telmisartan is said to be as effective as ramipril [ONTARGET] yet when tested in a large soundly run RCT, PRoFESS the drug failed:
- Subjects were randomized to receive telmisartan 80 mg/day (n = 2,954) or placebo (n = 2,972). At 56 months follow-up the drug failed to decrease recurrent stroke. Therapy with telmisartan initiated soon after an ischemic stroke and continued for 2.5 years did not significantly lower the rate of recurrent stroke, major cardiovascular events, or diabetes.

Even the composite outcome of cardiovascular death, MI, stroke, or hospitalization for heart failure was not statistically significantly different from the placebo group, p = 0·216.

TRANSCEND investigators studied the effects of telmisartan on cardiovascular events in high-risk patients intolerant to ACE inhibitors. Participants were randomly assigned to ramipril 10 mg a day (n = 8,576), telmisartan 80 mg a day (n = 8,542), or to a combination of both drugs (n = 8,502]. Therapy for 56 months, with telmisartan although shown in ONTARGET to be equivalent to ramipril, failed to decrease total mortality and had no significant effect on the primary outcome and hospitalizations for heart failure.

Calcium Antagonists

The BP-lowering effects of Ca antagonists are due to peripheral arteriolar dilation. Normally, Ca enters the cells through slow Ca channels and binds to the regulatory protein troponin, removing the inhibitory action of tropomyosin, which in the presence of adenosine triphosphate, allows interaction between myosin and actin, resulting in contraction of the muscle cell. Ca antagonists inhibit Ca entry into cells by blocking voltage-dependent Ca channels, thereby inhibiting contractility of vascular smooth muscle and producing vasodilation.

Adverse effects: The approved long-acting preparations for hypertension—amlodipine (Norvasc), nifedipine extended release, and verapamil SR—produce pedal edema, mild facial flushing, dizziness, headaches, leg cramps, gastroesophageal reflux, and rarely sexual dysfunction in much the same frequency. Minor side effects include gingival hypertrophy, blurred vision, muscle cramps, and burning in the gums. Rare side effects include depression, psychosis, and worsening of renal failure. Diltiazem may cause mild elevation in liver function tests and rarely acute hepatic injury. Care is required in patients with severe hepatic dysfunction, and dosage, especially of diltiazem and verapamil, must be reduced to avoid toxicity. Ca antagonists should be avoided in pregnancy and by lactating mothers. Nifedipine has been used with salutary effects during the last trimester of

Table 1.5: Calcium antagonists—drug interactions.				
	Digoxin Level	Quinidine	Amiodarone	Beta Blocker
Nifedipine	No change	No change or ↓	No change	Safe
Diltiazem	40% ↑	↑	Sinus arrest	Caution*
Verapamil	50–75% ↑	↑	Contraindicated	Contraindicated*

*See text

pregnancy as short-term therapy for the control of accelerated hypertension of preeclampsia. Further studies are required to document safety of long-term therapy.

Contraindications: Moderate or severe aortic stenosis. Diltiazem and verapamil are contraindicated with sick sinus syndrome, arrhythmia, bradycardia, heart block, LV dysfunction, or EF less than 40%.

Interactions: See Table 1.5.

Amlodipine: *Supplied*—tablets; 5 mg, 10 mg. *Dosage*—5 mg once daily; ↑ if needed to 10 mg. In the elderly, hepatic impairment or as added therapy initial dose 2.5 mg qd. Because amlodipine is extensively metabolized by the liver and half-life is 56 hours in hepatic dysfunction, caution is necessary in these patients. Once-daily amlodipine provides gradual onset of action and steady plasma levels over 24 hours with minimal peak-to-trough effects. This agent has been safely administered to patients with Class II-III CHF and may be used in hypertensives with mild or moderate LV dysfunction with close follow-up, especially if other agents are contraindicated. The drug has a role in hypertensives with concomitant angina and/or LV dysfunction. FDA-approved for both hypertension and angina.

Diltiazem: Controlled or sustained release (*Supplied*—90 mg, 120 mg. *Dosage*—60 mg bid; ↑ if needed to 120–360 mg qd.)
Non slow release tablets are not advisable.

Nifedipine (extended release): *Dosage*—30 mg once daily; ↑ if needed to maximum 60 mg once daily; avoid 90 mg.

Nitrendipine: *Supplied*—tablets; 10 mg. *Dosage*—5-10 mg once or bid; ↑ as needed to 20 mg once or twice daily.

Nicardipine: *Supplied*—capsules; 20 mg, 30 mg. *Dosage*—20 mg tid; maximum 30 mg tid.

HYPERTENSION IN ELDERLY

- Guidelines for the management of isolated systolic hypertension in patients aged 65–85 have been clarified by the results of the SHEP, and the SHEP indicates a threefold and twofold ↑ in the risk of stroke and

CHD in elderly hypertensive patients with systolic BPs greater than 180 mm Hg. The treated patients in the SHEP showed a 36% ↓ in risk of stroke (p = 0.0003), a 27% ↓ in CHD event rates, and a 54% ↓ in risk of LV failure.
- The SHEP results indicate that it is advisable to treat all patients aged 65–85 who have isolated systolic hypertension constantly greater than 180 mm Hg. In patients with systolic BP in the range 180–240 mm Hg, a 20% to maximum 25% ↓ in systolic pressure is recommended, based on the results of the SHEP.
- *HYVET trial proved diuretic effective.*
- A double-blind RCT of 3,845 hypertensive patients 80 years of age or older.

Stepped-care therapy began with indapamide with addition of perindopril as needed. At 2 years, the trial was halted because active treatment, as compared with placebo, was associated with a 21% reduction in the relative risk of death from any cause, a 64% reduction in the relative risk of heart failure, and a 30% reduction in the relative risk of stroke (Beckett et al. 2008).
- Beta-blocker small dose is strongly advised.

ACCELERATED, RESISTANT, OR MALIGNANT HYPERTENSION

In patients with moderate or severe essential or secondary hypertension treated with antihypertensive agents, acceleration and refractoriness of hypertension may occur because of:
- Poor compliance
- Increased salt intake in salt-sensitive individuals
- Rebound from discontinuation of centrally acting drugs, clonidine, guanfacine, methyldopa, and, rarely, β-blockers or Ca antagonists
- Drug interactions: Phenylpropanolamine combined with β-blockers. NSAIDs ↓ the natriuretic action of diuretics and the BP-lowering effect of ACE inhibitors and β-blocker; acetylsalicylic acid or other NSAIDs may interfere with the diuretic effect of loop diuretics
- Renal failure: In this situation, thiazides are rendered ineffective and BP may ↑
- Hyperaldosteronism.

Treated or untreated patients may present with severe hypertension that is difficult to control, including the rare presentation with malignant hypertension and diastolic BP greater than 140 mm Hg with or without end-organ damage. The presence of papilledema is not essential for the diagnosis of malignant hypertension.

In about 15% of cases with severe resistant hypertension, a secondary cause is present. Renal artery stenosis is an important cause in both young and older patients. Atherosclerotic occlusion of the renal artery may suddenly worsen, thus causing accelerated hypertension.

Pheochromocytoma and other causes of secondary hypertension must be excluded. See Secondary Hypertension, later in chapter.

Therapy

In most cases of severe hypertension with diastolic BP greater than 115 mm Hg, combination drug therapy is necessary. Renal failure causes resistance to thiazide diuretics, and high doses of furosemide combined with other agents may be required. Provided that CHF or other contraindications to β-blockade are absent, β-blockers are useful in most patients who have severe hypertension, regardless of the underlying cause. All antihypertensive agents, with the exception of β-blockers, cause a ↓ in systemic vascular resistance and fortunately have different sites of action. Therefore, they may be combined in these difficult scenarios.

HYPERTENSIVE EMERGENCIES

Hypertensive crisis: It is usually subclassified into either hypertensive emergency or urgency.

Hypertensive urgencies: They refer to other situations in which it is advisable to reduce markedly elevated BP within a day or two, rather than within minutes using oral drugs. These situations include:
- *Upper level of stage 3 hypertension*: BP commonly systolic greater than 220 mm Hg, diastolic greater than 120 mm Hg; decrease to 180/100 mm Hg preferably with oral medications.
- Nifedipine capsules if available 10 mg immediately. Do not use extended, controlled use formulation as slow acting.
  Amlodipine 5 mg may be tried.

If needed hydralazine intravenous (IV) infusion, or slow bolus is advisable, is indicated for hypertensive urgencies particularly if the condition is associated with renal failure or preeclampsia.

The recommended test dose is 10 mg followed in 30 minutes by an IV infusion of 10–20 mg/h, depending on the response. A maintenance dose of 5–10 mg/h is recommended with continuous monitoring of heart rate and BP. Oral hydralazine is commenced within 24 hours, 100–200 mg daily. If there is no contraindication to β-blockers, propranolol is given IV 1–4 mg and then orally 120–240 mg daily in addition (or the equivalent dose of another β-blocker). Furosemide 40 mg IV followed by oral HCTZ or furosemide greatly improves.

Hypertensive emergency is defined as a severe sudden elevation in BP, generally diastolic greater than 120–130 mm Hg; some clinicians add: and/or systolic BP greater than 220 mm Hg. The systolic pressures should reflect a knowledge of previous BPs, such as a rise within days from 160–170 to greater than 220 mm Hg systolic; the rate of rise of BP in relation to previous BP is more important than the absolute BP. Most important, the sudden excessive elevation in BP should be associated with *acute* organ damage or dysfunction, which confers an immediate threat to the integrity of the cardiovascular system and to life.

In aortic dissection or acute pulmonary edema, a BP of 200/110 mm Hg must be reduced. Conditions associated with emergencies are given in Table 1.6.

Types of hypertensive emergencies include:
- Accelerated malignant hypertension
- Acute coronary insufficiency
- Acute pulmonary edema (LVF)
- Acute renal dysfunction
- Aortic dissection
- Catecholamine crisis
- Eclampsia
- Hypertensive encephalopathy
- Subarachnoid hemorrhage
- Perioperative hypertension.

Emergencies require reduction in BP within minutes by IV therapy.

For hypertensive emergencies, the goal is to produce an immediate but modest reduction in BP. The objective, in most patients, is to achieve no greater than a 20% reduction from baseline of the mean arterial pressure or to reduce the diastolic BP to 110 mm Hg and no less than 100 mm Hg over a period of several minutes to several hours depending on the clinical situation. The BP is maintained at this level for a further 12-24 hours, at which time oral therapy should be instituted and a decision made as to the necessity for further lowering of BP. These guidelines do not apply in patients with aortic dissection, in whom BP must be reduced to a much lower level along with the use of a β-blocking agent to decrease the rate of rise of aortic pressure.

Caution is necessary: nitroprusside and labetalol have caused precipitous reductions in BP in some patients, resulting in cerebral and myocardial ischemia and/or MI.

Labetalol: Dosage—20-80 mg bolus over at least 1 minute, repeat after 5 minutes, then every 10-15 minutes if needed to maximum 200 mg; IV infusion: 0.5-2 mg/min

Nitroprusside: Start the infusion at the lower dose range (0.5-1 µg/kg/min) and adjust in increments of 0.2 µg/kg/min, usually every 5 minutes until the desired BP reduction is obtained. The average dose is 3 µg/kg/min (range, 0.5-8 µg/kg/min). A lower initial dose of 300 ng/kg/min has been used.

Hypertension 27

Table 1.6: Treatment of hypertensive emergencies associated with complications.

Agent	Heart failure	Encephalopathy	Cerebral hemorrhage	Other CVA	Renal failure	PHEO	Dissecting aneurysm	Pre-eclampsia
Nitroprusside	1	1	1	1	CI	2	1	CI
Nitroglycerin	1 or 2	—	—	—	—	—	—	—
Nifedipine	*2†	3*	CI	CI	1 or 2	3	CI	2 or 3 +
Diazoxide	CI	2	CI	3	1	CI	CI	CI
Labetalol	CI	2 or 3	1* or 2	1* or 2	1 or 2	AT	2*	2 or 3 +
Propranolol**	CI	4 or AT	4 or AT	4 or AT	2 or AT	AT***	1 AT	3 or AT
Trimethaphan	CI	—	—	—	—	—	2	CI
Hydralazine	CI	CI	4	4	2 or AT	CI	CI	1
Furosemide	AT always	4 or AT	—	—	AT always	CI	CI	CI
Methyldopa	4	4 or AT	4	4	3	CI	—	1 or 2
Captopril	1, 2 or AT	—	—	—	—	—	CI	CI
Phentolamine	—	—	—	—	—	1	—	CI

1 = first choice
2 and 3 = second and third choice
4 = rare use or if other drugs unavailable
AT = added therapy, provides reduction in dosages of combined drugs reduces adverse effects, ensures oral agent commenced early
CI = contraindicated
† = CI in myocardial ischemia
+ = Not approved by the FDA
* = if nitroprusside unavailable, give oral 10 mg nifedipine capsule see dagger
** = or other beat blocker
*** = atenolol or other betai, selective drug used if severe tachyarrhythmia
— = not recommended
Caution: The goal is to produce an immediate but only modest and preferably titrated reduction in blood pressure

Control of Blood Pressure

Diastolic BP consistently greater than 140 mm Hg with evidence of target organ damage—e.g. retinal hemorrhages, papilledema, acute pulmonary edema, decreased renal function, cerebrovascular accident, or hypertensive encephalopathy—requires immediate but carefully monitored, modest ↓ of BP. A 20-25% ↓ from baseline diastolic and/or systolic BP avoids relative hypotension and is sufficient to produce salutary effects.

- In dissecting aneurysm, BP may be markedly elevated or remain modestly elevated in the range of 160-190 mm Hg systolic, diastolic 90-100 mm Hg, and is considered a special hypertensive emergency, as BP must be promptly lowered within minutes. This is usually achieved by using nitroprusside; a β-blocker is also necessary to ↓ the rate of rise of aortic pressure and to prevent further dissection.
- In patients with cerebrovascular accident, caution is required because elevations in BP may fluctuate, being triggered by cerebral irritation, and it is essential to carefully monitor the BP for a few hours to confirm that the diastolic pressure is constantly elevated. The need for lowering the BP should be carefully considered and, if deemed necessary, the slow controlled titrated lowering of BP with the use of either nitroprusside or labetalol is used, depending on the cause of hypertension, underlying disease process, and complication. There is some evidence that nitroprusside increases intracranial pressure, but clinically the drug is effective.
- Labetalol is a reasonable alternative, provided that precautions for the use of a β-blocking drug are enforced. Labetalol causes postural hypotension, and the patient must remain in bed. Also, the BP-lowering effect may occasionally last 1-12 hours whereas the hypotensive effect of nitroprusside dissipates within minutes of cessation of the infusion.
- Pulmonary edema due to severe hypertension can be controlled with oral nifedipine and furosemide. If myocardial ischemia is suspected, nifedipine is contraindicated and nitroglycerin IV infusion is advisable (see Table 1.6). The combination of IV nitroglycerin and furosemide should suffice, but if pressure remains markedly elevated, nitroprusside is indicated. Labetalol is contraindicated with CHF; captopril could be used in this situation.
- Renal failure is usually associated with volume overload, and furosemide 80-160 mg IV should be administered. Oral nifedipine also has a role, and in this subset, sublingual nifedipine has been used widely and successfully. The oral preparation, however, lowers BP as quickly as sublingual administration and is the preferred route. Failure of nifedipine therapy should prompt the use of labetalol IV infusion as well as continuation of oral nifedipine capsules to wean the patient off labetalol as quickly as possible.

Drug Therapy

- *Nitroprusside*: Nitroprusside infusion reduces BP to any desired level and is the treatment of choice for hypertensive emergencies that require the lowering of BP, except when nitroprusside is contraindicated. Caution is needed in patients with inadequate cerebral circulation *Dosage*: 50 mg sodium nitroprusside in 100 mL 5% dextrose water is a convenient solution for use with a nitroprusside infusion pump. See Table 1.7 for the appropriate rate of infusion based on the weight of the patient.

Table 1.7: Nitroprusside infusion pump chart [Nitroprusside 50 mg (1 vial) in 100 mL (500 mg/L)].

	Weight (kg)						
	40	50	60	70	80	90	100
Dosage (μg/kg/min)	Rate (mL/hr)						
0.2	1	1	1	2	2	2	2
0.5	2	3	4	4	5	5	6
0.8	4	5	6	7	8	9	10
1.0	5	6	7	8	10	11	12
1.2	6	7	9	10	12	13	14
1.5	7	9	11	13	14	16	18
1.8	9	11	13	15	17	19	22
2.0	10	12	14	17	19	22	24
2.2	11	13	16	18	21	24	26
2.5	12	15	18	21	24	27	30
2.8	13	17	20	23	27	30	34
3.0	14	18	22	25	29	32	36
3.2	15	19	23	27	31	35	38
3.5	17	21	25	29	34	38	42
3.8	18	23	27	32	36	41	46
4.0	19	24	29	34	38	43	48
4.5	22	27	32	38	43	49	54
5.0	24	30	36	42	48	54	60
6.0	29	36	43	50	58	65	72

The above rates apply only for a 500 mg/l concentration of nitroprusside. If a different concentration must be used, appropriate adjustments in rates should be made. Start at 0.2 μg/kg/min. Increase slowly. Average dose 3 (μg/kg/min). Usual dose range 0.5–5.0 μg/kg/min.
Source: Khan MG. Hypertension. In: Cardiac Drug Therapy, 3rd edition. London: W.B. Saunders; 1992.

Wrap the infusion bottle in aluminum foil or other opaque material to protect it from light. The solution must be used within 4 hours. Start the infusion at 0.5 µg/kg/minute and ↑ by 0.2 µg/kg/minute q 5 minutes until the desired BP is obtained. *Dosage range*: 0.5–6 µg/kg/minute. It is important to begin oral antihypertensive agents as soon as possible so that the patient can be weaned off nitroprusside.

Contraindications: Pregnancy, severe anemia, and severe hepatic dysfunction because cyanide poisoning may occur; if renal disease is present and the use of nitroprusside is extended for greater than 2 days, thiocyanate may accumulate.

- *Nifedipine:* It administered as capsules is a most useful agent in the management of hypertensive emergencies and is of special value in patients with hypertensive encephalopathy and renal failure. Nifedipine is contraindicated in the management of cerebrovascular accidents, including hemorrhage, and in patients with myocardial ischemia because in these situations a slow, careful titration is needed to avoid a rapid ↓ in BP which may precipitate cerebral or myocardial ischemia. *Dosage*—10-mg capsule q 2–4 hours for 4–8 doses, along with furosemide if volume hypertension or renal failure is present.
- Sublingual nifedipine is effective but no longer recommended; may cause cerebral infarction, myocardial ischemia, and MI have been precipitated. Importantly, nifedipine 10-mg capsule, used orally, causes BP lowering that is of the same magnitude and acts as rapidly as the sublingual approach. Thus, oral administration is the method of choice

  Contraindications: Myocardial ischemia. Abrupt, uncontrolled ↓ in BP may lead to ischemia and infarction.
- *Labetalol*: This alpha β-blocker is indicated for the management of hypertensive emergencies caused by renal failure, clonidine withdrawal, and dissecting aneurysm, although in the latter situation a combination of nitroprusside and a β-blocker is preferable. *Dosage*—IV infusion of 2 mg/min, 20–160 mg/h under close and continuous supervision. The patient must be recumbent during and for 4 hours following the infusion. Hypotensive effects may last 1–12 hours after cessation of the infusion. Alternatively, give bolus injections 20 mg over 1 minute repeated after 5 minutes, if necessary, to a maximum of 200 mg. Excessive bradycardia can be controlled with IV atropine, 0.6–2 mg, in divided doses.
- *Hydralazine*: This vasodilator has a role when nitroprusside, nifedipine, and labetalol are not available. The drug is particularly useful for hypertensive emergencies associated with renal failure and in pregnancy. *Dosage*—a 10-mg test dose is followed in 30 minutes by IV infusion of 10–20 mg/h; maintenance dose is 5–10 mg/h. The addition of furosemide and a β-blocker to hydralazine greatly enhances antihypertensive effects, and the latter agent prevents tachycardia.

- *Nitroglycerin*: It is useful in hypertensive states associated with myocardial ischemia, CHF, MI, and following CABS or other vascular reconstructive surgery and during cardiac catheterization. *Dosage—see* Infusion Pump Chart, Table 1.7.

HYPERTENSION IN PREGNANCY

- Hypertension in pregnancy is present if the BP taken greater than or equal to 6 hours apart is greater than 140/90 mm Hg or if there is an above the baseline of 30 mm Hg systolic or 15 mm Hg diastolic. A mean arterial pressure greater than 90 mm Hg (systolic pressure + twice the diastolic ÷ by 3) causes a twofold ↑ in perinatal mortality.
- Blood pressure should be estimated with patient sitting or semireclined, because the BP may be lower in the recumbent position.
- Beta-blockers, methyldopa, and hydralazine have all been successfully used in the management of hypertension from the 16th week to delivery and for hypertensive complications during pregnancy. Reduced birth weight, neonatal bradycardia, and hypoglycemia have been reported with β-blockers. However, recent results using β-blockers have shown better control of BP and less effect on the fetus than observed with methyldopa or hydralazine.
- Caution is necessary to avoid using antihypertensive agents during the first and early half of the second trimester of pregnancy to prevent the rare possibility of inducing congenital malformations. Early pregnancy is fortunately associated with vasodilation, which protects from hypertension.

The antihypertensive agents methyldopa, β-blockers, and hydralazine are considered relatively safe for chronic use from the 16th week to delivery. Agents suitable for short-term use during the third trimester if no alternative exists include:

- Thiazide diuretics are contraindicated.
- Nifedipine 10–20 mg bid for hypertensive emergencies during the last trimester if other agents are not effective, are contraindicated, or cause serious adverse effects. Nifedipine should be avoided during labor because Ca antagonists may cause cessation of uterine contractions. Diltiazem and verapamil are contraindicated in pregnancy and during lactation. These agents must not be used concomitantly with magnesium sulfate because severe hypotension may occur.

Drugs contraindicated: Nitroprusside (there is a risk of cyanide toxicity and fetal death) and ACE inhibitors (these agents may cause skull defects and oligohydramnios or may disturb fetal and neonatal renal function and BP control).

Beta-blockers: They have advantages over methyldopa for prolonged treatment of chronic hypertension during the last trimester.

- These agents do not usually cause orthostatic hypotension, somnolence, or significant depression. Also, methyldopa must be taken two or three times daily as opposed to β-blockers, which are given once daily.
- The most common β-blockers used during pregnancy are *labetalol, atenolol,* and *pindolol.* Atenolol caused no fetal adverse effects in 120 pregnant women; neonates showed a minor incidence of transient bradycardia not requiring therapy, and a 1-year follow-up gave results similar to those observed with methyldopa, with no differences in development or growth indices (Reynolds et al. 1984). In another study, 4 years follow-up revealed all normal infants (Olofsson et al. 1986).

Chronic atenolol therapy does not increase the incidence of neonatal respiratory distress syndrome. In one study, no child in the actively treated group required ventilation, as opposed to seven infants in the control group requiring ventilation for the respiratory distress syndrome (Rubin et al. 1983).

- Other studies with atenolol have found significantly lower infant birth and placental weights compared with the nontreatment arm (Churchill and Beevers 1999), and the concern appears to be unique to atenolol used for long-term but not for short-term treatment.

Adverse effects of β-blockers used during pregnancy include: fetal or neonatal bradycardia; premature or prolonged labor; delayed spontaneous breathing in the newborn, mainly observed with IV use; and rarely neonatal hypoglycemia.

Intrauterine growth retardation is often mentioned with the use of atenolol, and low infant birth weight may occur with long-term treatment.

20 mg/h titrated slowly with continuous BP monitoring; the dose is doubled every 30 min if needed to 40 mg, maximum 160 mg/h. The combination with IV hydralazine allows lower doses of both agents with fewer side effects.

Labetalol is a β-adrenergic blocking agent with alpha1-blocking properties, and thus it causes vasodilation.

The latter effect may result in orthostatic hypotension.

Labetalol is as effective as methyldopa in controlling hypertension during pregnancy.

- The drug is extremely useful in the acute short-term management of severe resistant hypertension just before labor or during delivery. Avoid in asthmatics. Some state that labetalol is generally safer and preferable to atenolol (Churchill and Beevers 1999).

Adverse effects include about a 27% incidence of intrauterine growth retardation. The pregnant woman may experience perioral numbness, tingling, and itching of the scalp, and rarely a lupus-like illness, a lichenoid rash; a rare association is retroplacental hemorrhage (Lindheimer and Katz 1985).

- *A rare but life-threatening complication is acute hepatic necrosis* (Clarke et al. 1990).

- These serious side effects are not caused by other β-adrenergic blockers.
- Labetalol use should be confined to hypertensive emergencies.
- The drug has a role given intravenously in the management of severe resistant hypertension (diastolic BP >110 mm Hg) associated with preeclampsia occurring just before or during delivery. Labetalol given intravenously appears to be more effective than IV hydralazine or methyldopa. The BP-lowering effect is more predictable, and the drug causes less tachycardia and appears to cause less fetal distress than hydralazine.

Drug name: Hydralazine.
Supplied: 25 mg.
Dosage: 25 mg twice daily, increasing to three times daily; maximum 100 mg daily before the addition of a β-blocking drug.

For hypertensive crisis: IV bolus 5-10 mg.

Hydralazine:
- A pure arteriolar vasodilator and has been used extensively for acute control of severe hypertension in the third trimester of pregnancy.
- The drug is teratogenic in animals.
- Safety for chronic use is not as secure as that observed with methyldopa or β-blockers.
- The drug causes reflex tachycardia and sodium and water retention, which may necessitate the use of a diuretic or a β-blocker to blunt tachycardia as well as to enhance the antihypertensive effect.

The drug has a role in the short-term management of severe hypertension during late pregnancy unresponsive to methyldopa or β-blockers. Acute lowering of BP is necessary in severe preeclampsia to prevent cerebral hemorrhage, the main cause of the increase in maternal mortality seen in preeclampsia. The drug is very useful when a modest dose is combined with a low dose of a β-blocking drug, such as atenolol 50 mg daily, or as an adjunct to methyldopa; combination therapy prevents tachycardia and headaches caused by hydralazine.

Blood pressure greater than 110 mm Hg associated with preeclampsia occurring just before or during delivery. Intravenous labetalol is more effective than IV hydralazine or methyldopa. The BP-lowering effect is more predictable and it causes less tachycardia and appears to cause less fetal distress than hydralazine.

Dosage: 25 mg twice daily, increasing to three times daily; maximum 100 mg daily before the addition of a β-blocking drug.

For hypertensive crisis: IV bolus 5-10 mg.

Propranolol: Dosage—20-40 mg tid; ↑ propranolol is the only β-blocker advised during lactation because concentration in breast milk is less than that of other β-blockers.

Labetalol: Dosage—100-200 mg bid; maximum 800 mg qd is effective. The drug has been implicated in causing retroplacental hemorrhage. Postural hypotension, perioral numbness, itching of the scalp, positive ANA, and Lupus-like syndrome have been observed. Acute hepatic necrosis is a rare but life-threatening complication. Thus, labetalol must not be considered just another β-blocking drug.

Methyldopa: *Dosage*—125-250 mg bid; ↑ the dose only after several reassessments over two or three visits; maximum suggested 500 mg bid.

In a study of 117 methyldopa-treated women, 1 (0.9%) fetal death occurred and 9 (7.2%) fetal deaths occurred in the control group of 125 women. No significant differences were noted at 7-year follow-up of children born to women in both groups.

If BP control is urgently needed prior to delivery, methyldopa is preferred to β-adrenergic blockers. The addition of hydralazine may be required if methyldopa is not sufficiently effective.

Thiazide diuretics are relatively contraindicated since they ↓ placental blood flow, causing low birth weight.

Hypertensive Crisis of Pregnancy

Severe hypertension of pregnancy, especially near term or during labor, associated with diastolic pressures greater than 105 mm Hg may require urgent treatment with the following agents and/or combinations.

Hydralazine (Apresoline): *Dosage*—5 mg IV over 10-20 minutes, then 5-10 mg q 20-30 minutes, or, after the first bolus, given by IV infusion 5 mg/h, ↑ to 10 mg, maximum 15 mg/h, with continuous evaluation of HR and BP and fetal monitoring; fetal distress may occur. In the United Kingdom, the drug is initially given by the above method or by IV infusion; 200-300 µg/minute; maintenance usually 50-150 µg/minute.

Methyldopa: *Dosage*—500 mg orally causes BP ↓ within 6 hours. IV 250-500 mg in 100 mL 5% dextrose in water, over 30 minutes to 1 hour, q 6 hours.

Magnesium sulfate is extremely useful in patients with preeclampsia to prevent convulsions. *Dosage*—4 g diluted in 100-200 mL IV solution infused over 20 minutes, then 2 g/h with careful monitoring of BP and urinary output. The drug is continued during labor and for greater than 24-hour postpartum. Combination therapy utilizing the vasodilator action of hydralazine, the central action of methyldopa, and enhancement by magnesium sulfate usually produces salutary effects with less adverse effects than observed with high doses of a single agent. Magnesium sulfate has only mild antihypertensive effects and is not considered an antihypertensive agent. The major benefit of this drug is to prevent seizures associated with preeclampsia. *Caution*: Magnesium sulfate must not be used concomitantly with nifedipine because severe hypotension may be precipitated; magnesium sulfate should be avoided in patients with renal failure.

SECONDARY HYPERTENSION

Causes of secondary hypertension and their approximate incidence include:
- Renal parenchymal disease   3%
- Renovascular disease   1%
- Cushing's syndrome   0.1%
- Pheochromocytoma   0.1%
- Primary hyperaldosteronism   >0.2%
- Coarctation   0.1%
- Estrogens   0.4%
- Alcohol   ≥0.2%

Renal Parenchymal Disease

The history and physical and laboratory screening indicate the type and duration of the underlying disease. Screening includes assessment for:
- Presence and type of urinary casts
- Degree of proteinuria and anemia
- Level of serum creatinine, urea or BUN, serum Ca, phosphate, and albumin.

Common underlying diseases: Chronic glomerulonephritis, diabetic nephropathy, collagen vascular disease, polycystic kidney, chronic pyelonephritis, interstitial renal disease.

An ↑ in total peripheral resistance, hypervolemia, increased total body Na stores, and a high cardiac output contribute to the hypertension of renal failure.

Therapy

Furosemide: As emphasized under the section on diuretics, above, thiazides lose their natriuretic effect in patients with GFR less than 25 mL/h or serum creatinine greater than 2.3 mg/dL (203 μmol/L). *Dosage*: Furosemide 80–240 mg qd or bumetanide 5–10 mg qd may be expected to produce sufficient natriuresis, which is best reflected in the degree of weight loss. Rarely, less than 500 mg furosemide or 240 mg plus 5 mg metolazone may be required.

Beta-blockers: These agents combined with diuretics are effective in reducing BP in patients with chronic renal failure. Atenolol, nadolol, and sotalol are excreted by the kidney; their dosing interval should be increased, and the total daily dose may have to be reduced in chronic renal failure. Propranolol and metoprolol are actively metabolized, do not require dose adjustment, and are preferred for the management of hypertension with renal failure.

Calcium antagonists: Nifedipine has had extensive trials and been proven effective in reducing total peripheral resistance, which is usually markedly increased in patients with chronic renal failure. Nifedipine and diltiazem are metabolized, and dosages may not require alteration. However, a few cases of patients with renal failure reportedly showed deterioration with nifedipine and diltiazem; recovery of function occurs upon discontinuing the Ca antagonist. Verapamil may accumulate with renal failure and is not advisable. Nifedipine has commonly replaced hydralazine in the combination β-blocker plus diuretic plus vasodilator, but hydralazine may be added to the combination because the mechanism of vasodilation is different and the effect is additive.

Hydralazine: When Ca antagonists are contraindicated or produce adverse effects, hydralazine has a role in lowering total peripheral resistance and BP and has proven effective in patients with severe hypertension associated with renal failure. *Dosage*: 25–100 mg bid. The dosage interval for hydralazine should be increased with chronic renal failure, with creatinine clearance less than 25 mL/minute.

Renovascular Hypertension

Diagnostic considerations in renovascular hypertension include:
- Age of onset (age <30 or >50)
- Sudden onset of malignant, accelerated, or resistant hypertension accompanied by renal bruit
- Sharp rise in serum creatinine after the use of an ACE inhibitor, which is indicative of significant renal artery stenosis.
- Digital subtraction angiography is preferred to renal arteriography.

    Drug management includes the judicious use of combination therapy.
- Beta-blocker, thiazide (furosemide if renal failure is present), and amiloride if K conservation is necessary.
- ACE inhibitors are contraindicated in patients with severe bilateral renal artery stenosis or stenosis of a solitary kidney since in these patients renal circulation is dependent on high levels of angiotensin II. Thus, a sharp ↓ in renal blood flow may occur, and renal failure may ensue with the loss of a solitary kidney.
- Angioplasty and surgery are equally effective and superior to drug therapy in patients in whom renal artery stenosis is due to fibrous dysplasia and hypertension is present for less than 3 years with normal renal function. Angioplasty has a role in patients who are poor surgical candidates. Restenosis post angioplasty frequently occurs, but a second dilation may be rewarding. In patients with unilateral renal artery stenosis, elevation of serum creatinine indicates that nephrosclerosis is present in the contralateral kidney, and a salutary effect of angioplasty or revascularization is unlikely.
- Surgery appears to be somewhat more effective than angioplasty for atherosclerotic renovascular disease. Either therapy is advisable for atherosclerotic occlusion in younger patients with unilateral renal

artery disease, especially when hypertension is difficult to control with antihypertensive agents. A serum creatinine level greater than 1.4 mg/dL (124 µmol/L) and the presence of CHD increases the surgical mortality rate.

Pheochromocytoma

Less than 0.1% of patients with moderate to severe diastolic hypertension are expected to have a pheochromocytoma.
- Approximately 10% of these tumors of the adrenal medulla are bilateral
- 10% are malignant
- 10% are outside the adrenals
- 10% are familial
- Patients with familial or bilateral pheochromocytomas may be part of the Type II multiple endocrine neoplasia syndrome and should be screened for medullary carcinoma of the thyroid and hyperparathyroidism.

Diagnostic Hallmarks

- Severe headaches and profuse sweating
- Palpitations and tremor
- Pallor due to vasoconstriction
- Paroxysmal or diastolic hypertension; severe ↑ of BP with induction of anesthesia, surgery, or use of histamine, phenothiazines, or tricyclic antidepressants
- Postural hypotension
- Weight loss.

The catecholamine metabolic pathway involves conversion of tyrosine to normetanephrine and metanephrine (Flowchart 1.5).

The following investigations are usually diagnostic:

Flowchart 1.5: Catecholamine metabolic pathway.

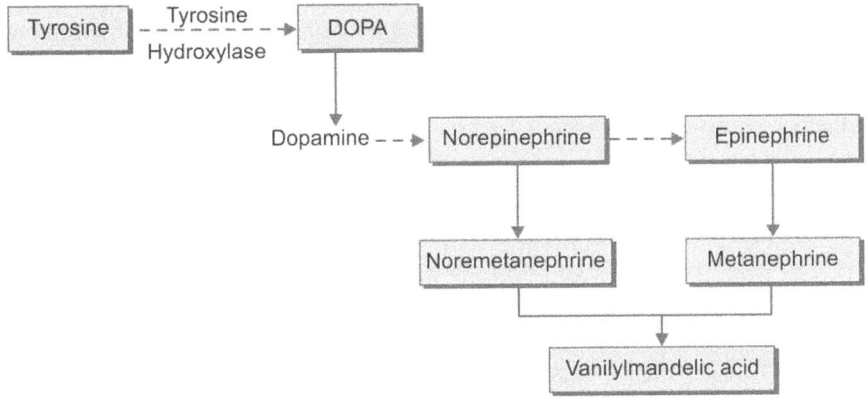

- Elevated 24-hour urine total metanephrine is the most reliable urinary screening test
- Free catecholamines and VMA are often elevated, but interference with urinary screening occurs with phenothiazines, chloral hydrate, and other drugs. Beta-blockers, thiazides, Ca antagonists, and ACE inhibitors, however, cause no interference. A special diet and avoidance of several drugs for greater than 3 days are necessary for accurate VMA results
- An in plasma catecholamines: An assessment is carried out with a heparin lock in an arm vein; the patient is sedated with 1 mg of sublingual lorazepam (Ativan) and is allowed to lie quietly for 20 minutes. Blood is then drawn for epinephrine and norepinephrine levels
- Elevated dopamine serum level is estimated on the same blood sample taken for epinephrine because dopamine may be the only chemical produced by some malignant pheochromocytomas. Plasma catecholamines may be mildly elevated with stress and essential hypertension, diuretics, prazosin, and other alpha1 blockers, hydralazine, labetalol, and Ca antagonists. A computed tomography (CT) scan may reveal a tumor. Iodine-131 metaiodobenzylguanidine (I-131 MIBG) enters chromaffin tissue and a MIBG scan helps identify extra adrenal tumors.

Therapy

Phentolamine (Regitine; Rogitine, Canada and UK): Hypertensive crisis may require the use of phentolamine prior to the administration of phenoxybenzamine. *Dosage*: An infusion of 10–20 µg/kg/min or 5–60 mg over 10–30 min at a rate of 0.1–2 mg/min. The drug has a rapid onset of action and lasts only 10–20 minutes. *Caution*: Deaths due to arrhythmia and acute MI have been reported, and β-blockade may be required. If β-blockers are used, care is required in patients who are considered at high risk for precipitation of CHF.

Nitroprusside: When used to ↓ BP during a crisis, nitroprusside is effective, but complicating tachyarrhythmias may cause problems with management, and β-blockade should not be used without adequate alpha blockade. (*see* Infusion Pump Chart, Table 1.7.)

Phenoxybenzamine (Dibenzyline): Oral therapy with this nonselective alpha blocker is commenced once the BP is under control or if the BP is not severely elevated after control with phentolamine or other agent. *Dosage*: 1–2 mg/kg qd in two or three divided doses, usually 10 mg q 8–12 hours. Increase q 3 or 4 days by 10 mg to a maximum 50 mg tid. Phenoxybenzamine therapy is usually required for control of BP over a period of 1–2 weeks prior to surgery. The drug is contraindicated in CHF.

Nifedipine: This agent, used universally for the management of all grades of hypertension, may be used in the emergency setting, with temporary beneficial results expected in some patients. It may occasionally avoid the use of nitroprusside (*see* Table 1.7).

Patients with pheochromocytoma are hypovolemic, and alpha blockade causes vasodilation. Thus, a marked ↓ in BP may occur, causing severe postural hypotension. Increase in salt intake and vigorous saline infusion are usually required during the 1-2 weeks prior to surgery to prevent severe postural hypotension, but careful monitoring is required to prevent the precipitation of CHF. Postoperative hypotension may be avoided by discontinuing phenoxybenzamine several days prior to surgery.

Beta-blockers: These agents must not be used prior to adequate alpha blockade because unopposed stimulation of alpha receptors can cause a severe ↑ in BP. Beta-blockade may be required after 1 week of alpha blockage if catecholamine-induced arrhythmias require control. A beta-1 selective drug such as atenolol is preferable to propranolol.

Metyrosine (Metirosine, UK) (alpha-methyl-L-tyrosine) (Demser): This agent is an inhibitor of tyrosine hydroxylase (see Flowchart 1.5) and, hence, the synthesis of catecholamines. Metyrosine reduces catecholamine production by about 70% and has a role in the preoperative management of pheochromocytomas as an alternative to phenoxybenzamine. The drug is particularly useful for the management of inoperable tumors. *Dosage*: 250 mg qid; ↑ daily by 250 mg to reach a maximum of 4 g qd. *Adverse effects*: Severe diarrhea, sedation, extra pyramidal symptoms, and hypersensitive reactions.

Surgery: A transabdominal incision is advisable to allow a search of all abdominal chromaffin tissue. Enflurane is considered the safest anesthetic agent as it does not stimulate catecholamine release or sensitize the myocardium to catecholamines. Management of fluid blood volumes necessitates the use of a Swan–Ganz catheter. Elevated BP is controlled with nitroprusside or nitroglycerin, especially in patients where the occurrence of CHF is predictable. Postoperative hypotension and CHF present a greater hazard with the use of alpha blockers and P blockade than with the use of nitroprusside or nitroglycerin.

A surgical cure is expected in 80% of patients. Approximately 10% of patients have a recurrence, and patients should be screened annually for 5 years. The 5-year survival is about 95% for patients with benign tumors and 45% for patients with malignant tumors.

Primary hyperaldosteronism:
- This is usually caused by hyperplasia.
- Of the adrenal cortex, ultrasound and CT of the adrenals are needed tests.

- The serum K falls to low levels less than 3 mmol/L (mEq/L).
- Treatment is excision of the adrenal; but amiloride 5–10 mg/day or spironolactone 50–100 mg/day should curb the symptoms and control the elevated BP until surgery is completed.

Coarctation of the Aorta

Hypertension in the arms with weak, absent, or delayed femoral pulses is a hallmark. After the age of 10, chest X-ray shows notching of the fourth to eighth ribs bilaterally or unilaterally and right sided if the coarctation is proximal to the left subclavian.

Therapy

Drug therapy is often required in the adult prior to surgical correction. Coarctation of the aorta causes activation of the renin angiotensin aldosterone system; thus, ACE inhibitors are first-line agents. All patients should be screened for septal defects, polycystic kidneys, and berry aneurysms; the latter not uncommonly causes the patient's demise.

Surgical repair may not be curative. Postoperative hypertension may be a problem requiring antihypertensive therapy. Aortic dissection may occur distal or proximal to the site of surgical repair. Also, restenosis may require balloon angioplasty, and close follow-up is essential.

Two risk factors have been identified for premature death after surgery:
1. Age at the time of surgical correction: The younger the patient, the better the outcome.
2. Hypertension, both preoperative and postoperative, carries a guarded prognosis.

BIBLIOGRAPHY

1. Äblad B, Bjurö T, Björkman JA, et al. Role of central nervous beta-adrenoceptors in the prevention of ventricular fibrillation through augmentation of cardiac vagal tone. J Am Coll Cardiol. 1991;17(Suppl):165.
2. ALLHAT Collaborative Research Group. Major cardiovascular events in hypertensive patients randomized to doxazosin vs chlorthalidone: the antihypertensive and lipid-lowering treatment to prevent heart attack trial (ALLHAT). JAMA. 2000;283:1967-75.
3. ALLHAT Officers and Coordinators for the ALLHAT Collaborative Research Group. Major outcomes in high-risk hypertensive patients randomized to angiotensin-converting enzyme inhibitor or calcium channel blocker vs. diuretic: the Antihypertensive and Lipid-Lowering Treatment to Prevent Heart Attack Trial (ALLHAT). JAMA. 2002;288:2981-97.
4. Beckett NS, Peters R, Fletcher AE et al. Treatment of hypertension in patients 80 years of age or older. N Engl J Med. 2008;358:1887-98.

5. Beta-Blocker Heart Attack Trial Research Group. A randomized trial of propranolol in patients with acute myocardial infarction. I. Mortality results. JAMA. 1982;247:1707-14.
6. Dargie HJ. Effect of carvedilol on outcome after myocardial infarction in patients with left-ventricular dysfunction: the CAPRICORN randomised trial. Lancet. 2001;357:1385-90.
7. Deary AJ, Schumann AL, Murfet H, et al. Double-blind, placebo-controlled crossover comparison of five classes of antihypertensive drugs. J Hypertens. 2002;20:771-7.
8. Dickerson JE, Hingorani AD, Ashby MJ, et al. Optimisation of antihypertensive treatment by crossover rotation of four major classes. Lancet. 1999;353:2008-13.
9. Heerspink HL, de Zeeuw D. Composite renal endpoints: was ACCOMPLISH accomplished? Lancet. 2010;375(9721):1140-2.
10. Khan MG. Hypertension. In: Khan MG (Ed). Heart Disease Diagnosis and Therapy. New York: Springer; 2018.
11. Khan MG. Hypertension. In: Khan MG (Ed). Practical Cardiology. New Delhi, India: Jaypee Brothers Medical Publishers (P) Ltd.; 2018.
12. Khan MG. Hypertension. In: Khan MG, Bartlett JG, Chopra S, Topol EJ (Eds). Medical Diagnosis and Therapy, 1st edition. Pennsylvania: Lea and Febiger; 1994.
13. Khan MG. Practical Cardiology. New Delhi, India: Jaypee Brothers Medical Publishers (P) Ltd.; 2018.
14. Kokkinos P, Chrysohoou C, Panagiotakos D, et al. Beta-blockade mitigates exercise blood pressure in hypertensive male patients. J Am Coll Cardiol. 2006;47:794-8.
15. Lacro RV, Dietz HC, Wruck LM, et al. Rationale and design of a randomized clinical trial of beta-blocker therapy (atenolol) versus angiotensin II receptor blocker therapy (losartan) in individuals with Marfan syndrome. Am Heart J. 2007;154:624-31.
16. Medical Research Council trial of treatment of hypertension in older adults: principal results. MRC Working Party. BMJ. 1992;304:405-12.
17. Messerli FH, Grossman E, Goldbourt U. Are beta-blockers efficacious as first-line therapy for hypertension in the elderly? A systematic review. JAMA. 1998;279(23):1903-7.
18. Morley-Smith AC, Lyon AR, Stressing the importance of cardiac assessment in pheochromocytoma. J Am Coll Cardiol. 2016;67(20):2375-7.
19. Norwegian Multicenter Study Group. Timolol-induced reduction in mortality and reinfarction in patients surviving acute myocardial infarction. N Engl J Med. 1981;304:801-7.
20. ONTARGET Investigators, Yusuf S, Teo KK, et al. Telmisartan, ramipril, or both in patients at high risk for vascular events. N Engl J Med. 2008;358:1547-59.
21. Packer M, Fowler MB, Roecker EB, et al. Effect of carvedilol on the morbidity of patients with severe chronic heart failure: results of the Carvedilol Prospective Randomized Cumulative Survival (COPERNICUS) study. Circulation. 2002;106:2194-9.
22. Packer M, O'Connor CM, Ghali JK, et al. Effect of amlodipine on morbidity and mortality in severe chronic heart failure. Prospective Randomized Amlodipine Survival Evaluation Study Group. N Engl J Med. 1996;335:1107-14.

23. Peters RW, Muller JE, Goldstein S, et al. Propranolol and the morning increase in the frequency of sudden cardiac deaths (BHAT Study). Am J Cardiol. 1989;63:1518-20.
24. Pitt B. The role of beta-adrenergic blocking agents in preventing sudden cardiac death. Circulation. 1992;85(1 Suppl):):I107-11.
25. PROGRESS Collaborative Group. Randomized trial of a perindopril-based blood pressure-lowering regimen among 6,105 individuals with previous stroke or transient ischaemic attack. Lancet. 2001;358:1033-41.
26. SHEP Cooperative Study Group. Prevention of stroke by antihypertensive drug treatment in older persons with isolated systolic hypertension. Final results of the Systolic Hypertension in the Elderly Program (SHEP). SHEP Cooperative Research Group. JAMA. 1991;265:3255-64.
27. Slater EE, Merrill DD, Guess HA, et al. Clinical profile of angioedema associated with angiotensin-converting enzyme inhibition. JAMA. 1988;260:967-70.
28. Telmisartan Randomised AssessmeNt Study in ACE iNtolerant subjects with cardiovascular Disease (TRANSCEND) Investigators, Yusuf S, Teo K, et al. Effects of the angiotensin-receptor blocker telmisartan on cardiovascular events in high-risk patients intolerant to angiotensin-converting enzyme inhibitors: a randomised controlled trial. Lancet. 2008;372:1174-83.
29. Wood SM, Mann RD, Rawlins MD. Angio-oedema and urticaria associated with angiotensin-converting enzyme inhibitors. Br Med J. 1987;294:91-2.
30. Yusuf S, Diener HC, Sacco RL, et al. Telmisartan to prevent recurrent stroke and cardiovascular events. N Engl J Med. 2008;359:1225-37.

CHAPTER 2

Angina

INTRODUCTION

Diagnosis of angina is based on a careful relevant history. The pain of angina has certain distinctive characteristics:
- A *retrosternal discomfort* precipitated by a particular activity, especially walking quickly up an incline or against the wind. Pain or discomfort disappears within 1-5 minutes of stopping the precipitating activity, in keeping with the concept of oxygen (O_2) supply versus myocardial demand. Discomfort may start in the lower, middle, or upper substernal area, the lower jaw, or the arm.
- *Discomfort is a tightness*, constriction, squeezing, heaviness, pressure, strangulation, burning, nausea, or an indigestion-like feeling of gradual onset that disappears at rest, except with unstable anginal syndromes. Occasionally, the pain is described as sharp and, at times, discomfort is replaced by shortness of breath on exertion.
The intensity of pain ranges from a mere discomfort grade 1 out of 10 to 5 out of 10; the mild discomfort is often described by patients as not really a pain but an uncomfortable feeling in the chest.
- *Area of pain* is usually at least the size of a clenched fist, often occupying most of the central chest area. The patient uses two or more fingers, the entire palm of the hand, or the fist to indicate the pain site. A finger or pencil point area of pain is rarely caused by myocardial ischemia.
- *Relief of pain* in an individual with stable angina always occurs within minutes of cessation of the precipitating exertional or emotional activity. Relief with sublingual nitroglycerin occurs promptly within 1-2 minutes.

CLASSIFICATION

- *Stable angina*: No change in the past 60 days in frequency, duration, or precipitating causes. Pain duration less than 10 minutes. In greater than 90% of patients, stable angina is caused by a greater than 70% obstruction in one or more coronary artery. In less than 10% of individuals, a lesser degree of atheromatous obstruction, coronary artery spasm, or small vessel disease is present.

The Canadian cardiovascular classification grading of angina is widely used to differentiate mild, moderate, or severe stable angina.
- Class 1 angina: Pain is precipitated only by moderate usually prolonged exertion.
- Class 2 angina: Pain on moderate effort, e.g. precipitated by walking uphill or by walking briskly for more than 3 blocks on the level in the cold, against a wind, or provoked by emotional stress. There is "slight limitation of ordinary activity".
- Class 3 angina: Marked limitation of ordinary activity; pain occurs on mild exertion, usually restricting daily chores. Unable to walk 2 blocks on the level at comfortable temperatures and at a normal pace.
- Class 4 angina: Chest discomfort on almost any physical activity, e.g. dressing, shaving, walking less than 100 feet indoors. Pain may be present at rest, a change in pain pattern and precipitating factors may be unstable angina.
- *Unstable angina*

STABLE ANGINA

Pathophysiology

Myocardial ischemia is a dynamic process. It is now clear that three, not two, determinants play a major role in the pathogenesis of myocardial ischemia, which may manifest as the chest pain of angina or remain painless as with silent ischemia.

The three determinants of myocardial ischemia are:
1. Concentric or eccentric coronary atheroma causing greater than about 70% stenosis; concentric plaques are observed mainly with stable angina and there is a tendency for them to be eccentric in patients with frequent rest pain and in those with unstable angina.
2. Increased myocardial O_2 demand.
3. Release of catecholamines occurring at the onset of angina and during the episode in the vast majority of patients with stable angina. Release of catecholamines may actually initiate ischemia, which stimulates further catecholamine release, and a vicious circle perpetuates the O_2 lack (Flowchart 2.1).

When angina is manifest, more than or equal to one coronary artery is expected to show a greater than 70% stenosis on angiography. The obstructive plaque of atheroma is often focal and usually occurs in the proximal portion of a coronary artery; this combination of proximal and focal lesions dictates the success of angioplasty and bypass surgery. In less than 10% of individuals, and especially in diabetics, multifocal longer segmental or diffuse disease exists in the distal coronary tree.
- An obstructive lesion in the left anterior descending (LAD) artery prior to the septal or first diagonal branch is considered proximal and

Flowchart 2.1: Pathophysiology of angina.

```
                    ↑ Exceptional or emotional activity
                                    │
                                    ▼
                              ↑ Catecholamine
         (Vicious circle)        release
    ┌──────────────────────────────┤
    │                              │
    │   Coronary stenosis          │
    │        │                     │
    │   ↓ Coronary blood ← ↓ Diastolic filling ← ↑ Heart rate
    │        flow              period                │
    │                                                │
    │                          ↑ Force and velocity, cardiac
    │                                  contraction
    │                              ↑ Blood pressure
    │                                    │
    │                                    ▼
    │   ┌──────────────────────┐   ┌──────────────────────┐
    │   │ ↓ Myocardial oxygen  │ ← │ ↑ Myocardial oxygen  │
    │   │        supply        │   │       demand         │
    │   └──────────────────────┘   └──────────────────────┘
    │              │
    │              ▼
    │      Myocardial ischemia
    └──────────
```

↑ = Increase
↓ = Decrease

highly significant because it can jeopardize greater than 50% of the left ventricular (LV) myocardium. LAD lesions after the first diagonal affect only about 20% of the myocardium. In approximately 85% and 15% of individuals, the right coronary or left circumflex artery supplies the posterior diaphragmatic portion of the interventricular septum and the diaphragmatic surface of the left ventricle, respectively, and is referred to as the dominant artery. The term "dominant" does not imply a more important artery but does have some clinical bearing on decision making in the management of angina.

- A 25% decrease (↓) in the outer radius of a normal coronary artery results in about a 60% ↓ in a cross-sectional area. However, in an

artery with 75% stenosis, a 10% ↓ in the outer radius would produce a complete occlusion.
- During periods of exercise or exertion, catecholamine release causes an increase (↑) in heart rate (HR), an ↑ in the velocity and force of myocardial contraction producing an elevation in blood pressure (BP), and an ↑ in myocardial O_2 demand. In the presence of significant coronary artery stenosis, an O_2 deficit may occur. Myocardial ischemia increases catecholamine release, resulting in an additional ↑ in HR and BP, with further O_2 lack, and the vicious circle ensues. Importantly, the coronaries fill during the diastolic period, which is shortened during tachycardia.
- Pharmacologic agents that inhibit the initiation or interrupt the dynamic process described above provide rational therapy for myocardial ischemia. It is, therefore, not surprising that β-adrenergic blocking drugs produce salutary effects in the majority of patients with stable angina and represent first-choice oral medications for the management of angina.
- In contrast to the β-blocking drugs, dihydropyridine calcium (Ca) antagonists, when used alone, tend to ↑ HR and, along with other Ca antagonists, do not inhibit the cardiovascular actions of catecholamines. Nitrates also ↑ HR.
- An important consideration in relation to coronary artery spasm is that ischemia from this cause also triggers catecholamine release and worsening of angina. However, coronary artery spasm is a rare cause of myocardial ischemia manifest as stable angina.

Investigative Evaluation

- Patients with the same clinical symptoms may have very different prognoses depending on coronary anatomy; 1-, 2-, or 3-vessel or left main stenoses; and on LV function.
- The failure to predict outcomes based on the clinical presentation often necessitates evaluation with exercise stress testing and echocardiography. Thallium scintigraphy is required in some. It is necessary to evaluate the coronary reserve and degree of proximal stenosis. The goal of initial investigations is to stratify the risk so that those at higher risk can progress to angiography early.
- Lipid levels: Low-density lipoprotein cholesterol (LDL-C) triglycerides, high-density lipoprotein (HDL), fasting glucose and estimated glomerular filtration rate (eGFR) with the patient fasting 12–14 hours.
- The hemoglobin (Hb) is necessary to exclude the rare occurrence of angina precipitated by anemia in patients with atheromatous coronary stenosis. Renal function, approximately assessed by the serum creatinine, is relevant to the choice and dosage of medications.

Electrocardiograms

- Electrocardiograms (ECGs) are expected to be normal in greater than 66% of patients with stable angina, except in individuals with previous myocardial infarction (MI) or concomitant hypertension. However, even a normal record makes a valuable baseline with which to compare future tracings.

Examples of ECG ischemic changes are given in Figures 2.1–2.5.

Minor ST segment depression less than or equal to 1 mm is not an uncommon finding in normal individuals. Consider ST segment changes to be nonspecific if the following prevails:

- ST depression less than or equal to 1 mm in the absence of typical symptoms of unstable angina, including rest pain greater than or equal to 20 minutes (Fig. 2.4)
- Accompanied by baseline drift
- With or without T wave inversion
- Commonly associated with low, flat, or slightly inverted T waves.

Nonspecific ST-T wave changes can be caused by a number of conditions, such as the following:

- Improper electrode contact
- Ischemia (must be considered; the ECG must be interpreted in regard to the clinical findings)
- Electrolyte abnormalities
- Arrhythmias
- Myocarditis
- Pericarditis, constrictive pericarditis
- Intraventricular conduction defects
- Cardiomyopathy
- Pulmonary embolism
- Drink of cold water
- Hyperventilation
- Drug use, including ethanol abuse
- Digoxin
- Subarachnoid hemorrhage or cerebral hemorrhage.

Exercise Stress Testing

This is important in assessing the coronary reserve and in formulating strategies for other therapeutic interventions, especially in patients with Class 1 and 2 angina. It is also useful in assessing the effect of medical therapy. However, the test is not useful in evaluating atypical chest pain, especially in women. The test is contraindicated in patients with aortic stenosis, and obstructive cardiomyopathy.

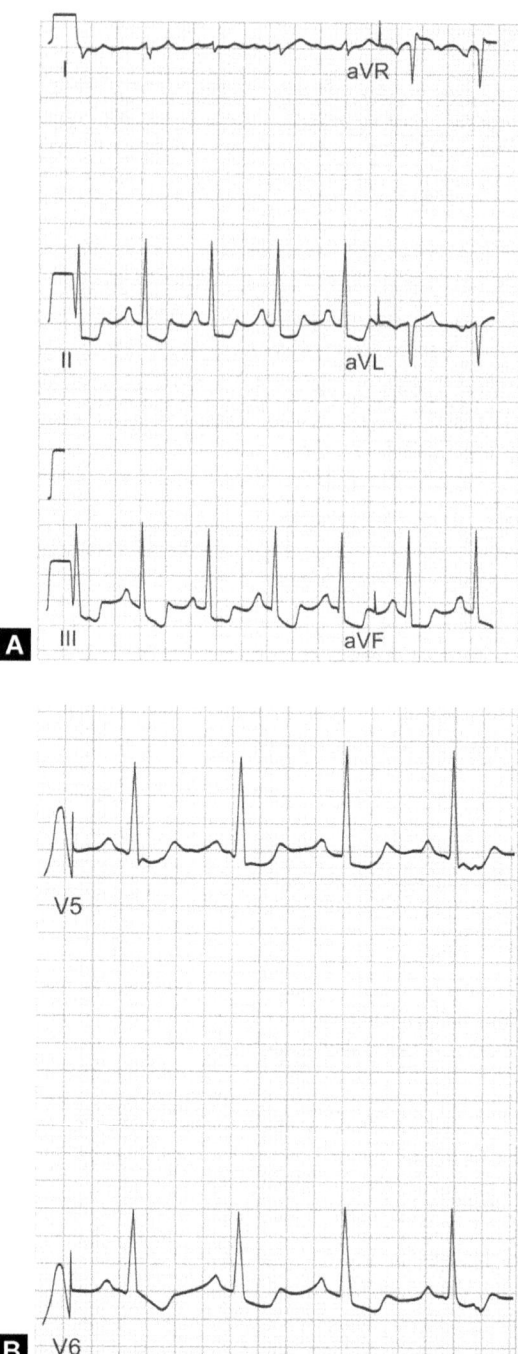

Figs. 2.1A and B: Flat (horizontal) and downsloping ST segment depression greater than 1 mm in a patient with proven angina and obstructive coronary artery disease. (A) Limb leads; (B) Limb leads V5 and V6.

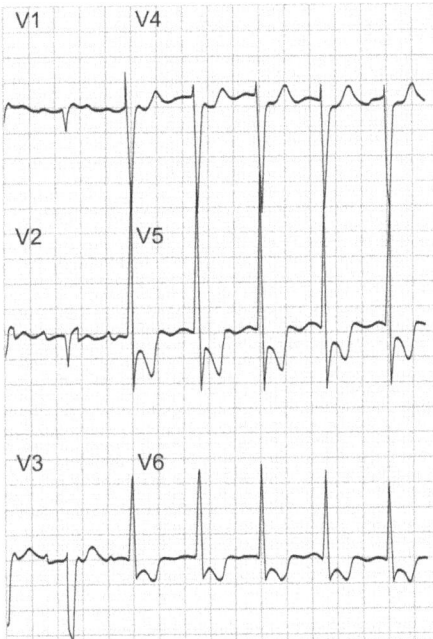

Fig. 2.2: V leads of a patient with severe angina and LV hypertrophy. Note increased voltage and marked ST segment depression in V4 through V6.

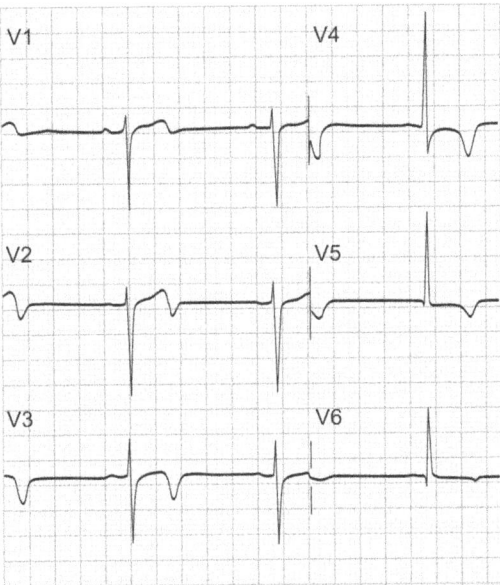

Fig. 2.3: V leads in a patient with unstable angina. ST-T segment abnormalities seen in V1 through V4. The tracing was taken when the patient was pain free. Note the "hitched up" ST segment in V2 and V3 with deep T inversion: The pattern is typical of significant proximal LAD coronary artery stenosis.

50 *Internal Medicine: Diagnosis and Therapy*

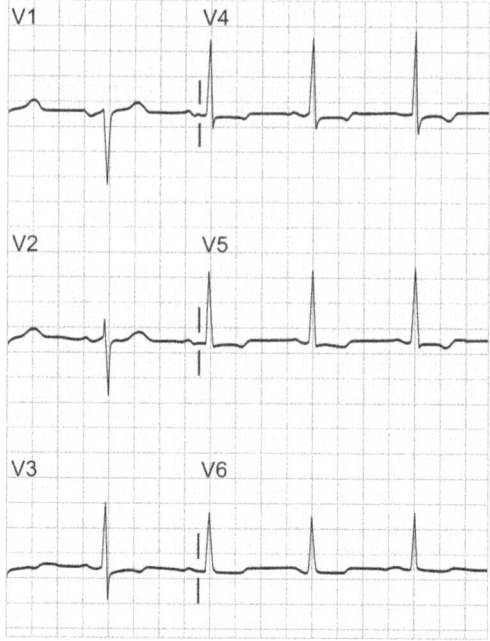

Fig. 2.4: V leads in a patient with no history of heart disease. ST segment is flat in V4 through V6 with minimal T wave inversion; similar findings were observed in leads I and aVL: the anterolateral ST-T wave abnormalities are nonspecific; note that ischemia cannot be excluded. Abnormal ECG.

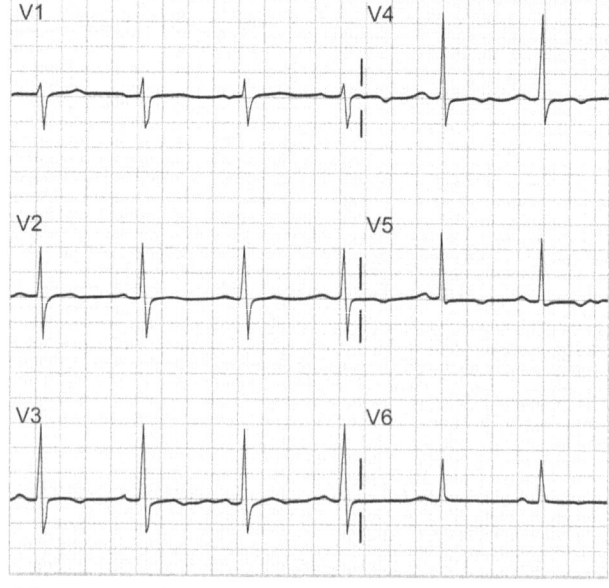

Fig. 2.5: The ST segment is borderline flat but not depressed and is associated with minimal T wave inversion in leads V3 through V6; similar findings were present in leads I and aVL: nonspecific ST-T wave changes. Borderline ECG.

- Patients less than age 60 with angina who can complete greater than 6 minutes of a Bruce protocol treadmill exercise test, achieving greater than 85% of maximal HR without chest pain or ischemia changes, can usually be managed with medical therapy. Patients who can tolerate greater than 9 minutes of a Bruce protocol appear to have a good prognosis. In this subset, if medical therapy is judged by physician and patient to be yielding adequate control of symptoms, coronary angiography is usually not required.
- A positive exercise stress test is indicated by 2:1 mm flat or downsloping ST segment depression, 80 milliseconds after the J point occurring in three consecutive beats. A strongly positive test is indicated by ST segment depression within the first 3 minutes of exercise, downsloping ST segment depression of 2:2 mm, persisting for greater than 4 minutes on cessation of exercise or occurring at low workload: HR less than 120/minute, systolic pressure less than 130 mm Hg, i.e. a low rate-pressure product. Patients in this category have a poor prognosis and are expected to have a large area of myocardium involved by the ischemic process. Patients with strongly positive tests, ischemia occurring prior to 6 minutes, and/or hypotension during exercise have a high probability of having multivessel or left main stem disease and are, therefore, at significant risk. Computed tomography coronary angiogram (CTCA) is useful in many. Coronary angiography is warranted with consideration for coronary angioplasty, percutaneous coronary intervention (PCI), stenting or coronary artery bypass surgery (CABS).

Radionuclide Scintigraphy

Radionuclide perfusing the myocardium is removed by myocardial cells.
- A positive test, a cold spot on the scan, absent radioisotope uptake with filling in later views, indicate ischemic myocardium.
- The test is generally performed in conjunction with an exercise test and is useful in patients with LV hypertrophy and atypical chest pain in which conventional exercise stress testing gives a high rate of false positives. The validity of the test depends on achieving a reasonably high rate-pressure product during the preliminary stress period.
- It has several limitations. Proper methodology is necessary: Image artifacts are common and can lead to false-positive interpretation; false-positive results may occur because of overlying breast shadows, while right ventricular blood pool may attenuate inferoposterior myocardial activity; myocardial apical thinning causes a local ↓ in thallium activity that can be mistaken for ischemic disease; left bundle branch block (LBBB) may produce a false-positive scan. Most of these difficulties are of importance in relation to fixed defects, reversibility being a strong indicator of myocardium at risk. Negative scans may occur with significant lesions in the circumflex or diagonal branches of the LAD.

Widespread disease with global ↓ in uptake will also, paradoxically, yield a negative result.
- In a study of 411 patients that used clinical variables, diabetes, sex, age, and typical angina pattern, 46% of patients were correctly classified into low- or high-risk groups, the latter with documented three-vessel, or left main disease. Thallium imaging resulted in only 3% of the patients being reclassified regarding their risk for severe coronary artery disease (CAD) at a cost of $20,550.
- Dipyridamole or adenosine thallium scintigraphy is a useful investigation in patients with Class 2 angina with the absence of pain at rest who are unable to exercise because of arthritis or peripheral vascular disease (PVD). Patients with Class 3 angina require coronary angiographic assessment. Dipyridamole thallium scintigraphy is contraindicated in patients with unstable angina, postinfarction angina, and non-Q wave infarction; within 3 months of infarction, these patients require coronary angiography. Also, dipyridamole scintigraphy is contraindicated in patients with asthma and chronic obstructive pulmonary disease (COPD).
- Persantine nuclear myocardial perfusion studies are useful in those who cannot exercise on a treadmill or bike, but are not accurate in patients treated with β-blockers because these agents prevent coronary steal caused by dipyridamole. Beta-blockers should be stopped 24–48 hours prior to the test; this is sometimes hazardous.
- Most important, individuals with a negative persantine scan have had documented infarctions within 6 months of the test results.
- Echocardiography may be required in some patients to assess LV systolic function. Stress echocardiography has a role in selected patients.
- Computed tomography coronary angiography for selected patients is useful if available. Invasive coronary angiography is reserved for patients showing poor response to optimal medical therapy.
- In high-risk patients, currently coronary computed tomographic angiography (CCTA) is not advisable because invasive coronary angiograms are needed in this subset.
- Women appear to derive more prognostic information from a CCTA (Pagidipati et al. 2016).
- Williams et al. (2016) conducted a prospective, multicenter, randomized controlled trial (RCT): 4,146 patients were randomized to receive standard care or standard care plus CCTA.

Conclusion: In patients with suspected angina due to CAD, CCTA leads to more appropriate use of invasive angiography and alterations in preventive therapies that were associated with a halving of fatal and nonfatal MI.
- From the median time for preventive therapy initiation (50 days), fatal and nonfatal MI were halved in patients allocated to CCTA compared with those assigned to standard care (Williams et al. 2016).

Therapy

- The COURAGE investigators (2015) did not find a difference in survival between an initial strategy of PCI plus medical therapy and medical therapy alone in patients with stable ischemic heart disease (IHD). *General control of risk factors necessary first steps*:
- Weight, cessation of smoking, removal or avoidance of stress
- Increase mild exercise, better diet
- Control of hypertension with suitable agents
- Serum cholesterol less than 170 mg/dL (4.4 mmol/L), LDL less than 100 mg/dL (2.5 mmol/L) for moderate risk and less than 70 mg/dL = 1.8 mmol/L for high risk, include diabetics (see Chapter 9)
- If LDL-C is not available, use total cholesterol less than 4.4 for moderate risk; less than 4 for highest risk include diabetics.

Drug Therapy

Statins

- The lowering of LDL-C to less than 70 mg/dL (1.8 mmol/L): (conversion; mmol/L × 38.5) is of paramount importance in the treatment of patients with angina. Aggressive control of LDL-C to less than 50 mg/dL (1.3 mmol/L) in patients at high risk: angina postinfarction or diabetics, has been shown to be effective in decreasing reinfarction and death. In these high-risk patients, the addition of an appropriate β-blocker: timolol or propranolol (nonsmokers) is necessary.
- If needed, the statin is combined with 10 mg of ezetimibe to reach the LDL-C goal and to ameliorate atheroma plaque; this combination is particularly necessary in diabetics to normalize elevated blood sitosterol (Khan 2017).

Ezetimibe

We strongly advise ezetimibe for the majority of diabetics, if facilities are available to assess sitosterol blood levels. If elevated greater than 4.5 mg/L (normal 0–4.9 mg/L), ezetimibe is strongly indicated because sitosterol causes atheroma and MI and levels must be maintained less than 3.5 mg/L (Khan 2018).

Patients suitable for medical management usually have the following characteristics:
- Stable angina functional Class 1 and 2, with good family history and nondiabetic.
- Good effort tolerance, negative or weakly positive treadmill exercise test, e.g. beyond 6 minutes of the Bruce protocol. Patients who are unable

to exercise because of intermittent claudication or arthritis cannot be graded as Class 1 and 2.
- Good ventricular function, from echocardiogram greater than 40%.

Aspirin

Aspirin is added to prevent coronary thrombosis, which causes heart attacks.
- Aspirin soft chew, noncoated 80–81 mg daily after a meal is strongly recommended.
- Enteric-coated aspirin is not effective in more than 33% of patients because of poor absorption but if gastric upset with soft chew, then keep soft aspirin for emergency use and take enteric-coated 81 mg daily.
- Chewable, soft aspirin 160–240 mg to be taken if chest pain persists despite adequate use of nitrolingual spray or tablet 0.3 mg; maximum 0.4 mg.
- Kapoor (2008) emphasized in a brief letter that it is important to take note of recent reports of incomplete suppression of platelet aggregation with enteric-coated aspirin as shown by Cox et al. (2006) and Maree et al. (2005). In a randomized, open-label, crossover study of healthy volunteers, incomplete thromboxane (TX) B2 inhibition was found to occur in 8% of the aspirin group and 54.3% of the enteric-coated aspirin group ($p = 0.0004$) (Cox et al. 2006).
- In another study of 131 stable cardiovascular patients treated with enteric-coated aspirin (75 mg/day), 44% of patients failed to attain optimal inhibition of serum TX, indicating suboptimal inhibition of platelet cyclooxygenase-1 (COX-1) activity, and those with an incomplete aspirin response were more likely to demonstrate platelet aggregation to arachidonic acid (21% vs 3%; $p = 0.004$) (Maree et al. 2005).
- In patients who are allergic or intolerant to the use of aspirin, clopidogrel bisulfate is recommended.

Beta-blockers First Choice

Most patients with stable angina Class 1 and 2 are managed with sublingual nitroglycerin and a one-a-day β-blocker. The rationale for a β-blocking drug as a first-choice oral agent is discussed shortly:
- Failure to achieve about a 75% symptomatic relief with an adequate dose of a β-blocker (Table 2.1) might result in the addition of a second agent or the patient may learn to cope with mild angina that quickly disappears on cessation of a precipitating activity. Either a Ca antagonist or a nitrate is considered second choice. If a β-blocker is being used, then amlodipine 5 mg or nifedipine extended release 30 mg to maximum 60 mg qd is advisable.
- If a β-blocker is contraindicated but verapamil is not, then verapamil should be used as it is the most effective Ca antagonist, but is not used

Table 2.1: Dosage of beta-blockers for angina.

Beta-blocker	Initial dose (mg daily)	Maintenance (mg daily)
Metoprolol (tartrate)	50–100 twice daily	100 mg twice daily
Controlled release (succinate)	50 mg once daily	100–200 mg once daily
Propranolol	80–120 mg	80–160 mg
Timolol	5 mg bid	10 mg bid

Table 2.2: Oral and transdermal nitrate preparations and dosage.

Nitrate	Dosage	
Isosorbide dinitrate	Initial	15 mg at 700, 1400 hours
Sustained release	Maintenance	40 mg at 700, 1400 hours
Isosorbide mononitrate	Initial	10 mg at 700, 1400 hours
	Maintenance	20 mg at 700, 1400 hours
	Initial	20–30 mg at 700 hours
Sustained release	Maintenance	40–60 mg at 700 hours
Nitroglycerin (oral tablets) (glyceryl trinitrate oral tablets in the UK)	Initial	1.3 mg at 700, 1400 hours
Nitroglycerin (buccal tablets)	Initial	1 mg
	Maintenance	1 mg, 2 mg, or 3 mg at 700, 1400 hours
Nitrolingual spray 0.4 mg		
Phasic-release nitroglycerin patch: e.g. Transderm-nitro 0.4 mg, 0.6 mg/hour	1 patch	700 hours, remove at 1900 hours

if LV dysfunction, or prior congestive heart failure (CHF). The rationale for this approach is discussed under Ca antagonists and combination therapy. If a nitrate is selected as second line, a sustained release preparation is selected and given once daily or, at most, bid. Preparations and suggested timing of dosing of nitrates are shown in Table 2.2.
- If symptoms remain bothersome, triple therapy with a β-blocker, Ca antagonist, and nitrate is warranted, but this action should prompt consideration for coronary angiography and interventional therapy.

Beta-blockers effects
- Release of catecholamines plays a major role in the initiation and perpetuation of myocardial ischemia in patients with atheromatous coronary stenosis (Flowchart 2.1). Beta-blockers can inhibit the initiation of ischemia, interrupt the dynamic process, and provide rational and effective therapy as well as prolong life.

- Sudden death prevention; β-blockers are the only drugs that prevent sudden cardiac death (Table 2.3).
- Beta-blockers are competitive inhibitors of catecholamines (which they structurally resemble) at β-adrenergic receptors. Their action depends on the ratio of drug to catecholamine concentration at β-adrenoceptor sites. Beta-receptors are part of the adenylyl cyclase system situated in the cell membrane. The ventricle contains β1 and β2 adrenergic receptors in the proportion 70:30. Beta2 predominate in the lung. Adenylyl cyclase in the presence of the stimulatory form of the G protein converts adenosine triphosphate to cyclic adenosine monophosphate (cyclic AMP), the intracellular messenger of β stimulation.

Beta-blockade results in:
- Decrease in HR. Cardiac work is reduced and the increased diastolic interval allows for improved diastolic coronary perfusion especially during exercise.
- Decrease in velocity of cardiac contraction further reduces myocardial O_2 demand, which is particularly important during exertional activities.
- Decrease in cardiac output results in a ↓ in systolic BP and causes a ↓ in the rate-pressure product and a ↓ in myocardial O_2 requirement. These effects are not observed with other antianginal agents.
- A ↓ in ejection velocity reduces hyperdynamic shearing forces imposed on the arterial wall; this might be important at the site of atheroma. Thus, it is possible that β-blockers may ↓ the incidence of plaque rupture and thus protect from fatal or nonfatal MI. These agents ↓ the incidence of myocardial rupture.
- Partial inhibition of exercise-related catecholamines that might initiate vasoconstriction in segments of coronary arteries where atheroma impairs the relaxing effect of the endothelium.
- Increase in ventricular fibrillation (VF) threshold and, thus, a ↓ in the incidence of VF, which may be responsible for the high mortality during the early hours of acute MI and also in VF occurring in other ischemic situations. Beta-blockers are of proven value in the prevention of sudden death in the post-infarction patient.
- A ↓ in early morning platelet aggregation and other salutary effects induced by a ↓ in catecholamine surges may eliminate the early morning peak of transient ischemic periods and ↓ the incidence of early morning mortality and sudden death from MI. Beta-blockers have been shown to ↓ the incidence of sudden death in cardiac patients. This observation has not been documented for any other cardiac medication, including aspirin.
- A ↓ in phase 4 diastolic depolarization is important in suppressing arrhythmias induced by catecholamines, which ↑ diastolic depolarization. This action is opposite to that of digoxin. Thus, β-blockers are useful in the management of digoxin toxicity.

Table 2.3: Total deaths and sudden deaths in beta-blocker randomized control trials of postmyocardial infarction and heart failure patients.

	Control	Drug	% Decrease
Propranolol			
Total sudden deaths*	78	60	23
5 am–11 am	31	11	64
Total deaths	188/1460	138/1456	26
Timolol†			
Total sudden deaths	95	47	50
Instant, within seconds	38	11	71
Total deaths	117/718	67/670	42
Metoprolol#			
Total sudden deaths	21	9	57##
Total deaths	31/147	25/154	19##
MERIT-HF^			
Total sudden deaths	132	79	40.2
Total deaths	217/2001	145/1990	33.2
Bisoprolol‡			
Total sudden deaths	83	48	42.2
Total deaths	228/1320	156/1327	31.6

[Only four beta-blockers of the 12 available definitely prevent sudden cardiac death; they all gain high brain concentration. Atenolol and sotalol gain poor brain concentration and are ineffective; atenolol use should be curtailed.]
*BHAT study, AM sudden death (Peters et al. 1989) follow-up 25 months, propranolol 120–240 mg daily.
†Timolol Norwegian MI study; mean duration 17 months follow-up: 10 mg twice daily. A superior drug rarely used; beta-blockers are not all alike.
#Metoprolol: A very small study of only approximately 150 patients in each group followed for 3 years.
##"This reduction in cardiac mortality did not reach statistical significance, as was to be expected from our sample size" (Olsson et al. 1985).
^In MERIT-HF, there were fewer sudden deaths in the metoprolol CR/XL group than in the placebo group [79 vs 132, 0.59 (0.45–0.78); p = 0.0002] and deaths from worsening heart failure [30 vs 58, 0.51 (0.33–0.79); p = 0.0023].
‡Bisoprolol in CIBIS; significant decrease in deaths and sudden deaths.
Carvedilol did not prevent sudden death in two large RCTs; total mortality in RCT was not significantly reduced in post-MI patients.
Source: Reproduced with permission from Khan MG. Practical Cardiology. New Delhi: Jaypee Brothers Medical Publishers (P) Ltd.; 2018. pp. 312.

- Decreased impulse traffic through the A-V node results in slowing of the ventricular response in atrial fibrillation (AF) or in the termination of peak systolic velocity (PSV).
- Direct blood flow from the epicardial vessels to subendocardial ischemic areas. In contrast, dipyridamole, a vasodilator used in the management of angina in the early 1960s, is now used to dilate epicardial vessels and produce a "steal". Experimental evidence suggests that some Ca antagonists may also direct coronary blood flow from the subendocardium to dilated epicardial vessels. Nitrates appear to have an effect similar to Ca antagonists.

The above-mentioned points have established β-blocking drugs as first-line oral agents in the management of stable angina and indicate the rationale for the algorithmic approach to drug therapy for stable angina.

Choice: Related to subtle differences.
- Beta-blockers with partial agonist activity, such as pindolol, should be avoided in patients with IHD since cardioprotection is not achieved. Acebutolol has only weak agonist activity and one study has shown a beneficial effect and may be used if other β-blockers cause bradycardia less than 48/minute.
- Do not use hepatic-metabolized β-blockers, propranolol, in smokers who would not quit, as the salutary effects of these agents are blunted by cigarette smoking.
- Maximum protection appears to occur with proven agents: timolol, bisoprolol and metoprolol in smokers and in nonsmokers, propranolol mainly in nonsmokers (Table 2.3).
- *Cautions*: Do not use in asthmatics, severe COPD or CHF. Bisoprolol or metoprolol can be used in stable COPD patients.
- The subtle differences in available β-blockers may provide the solution for the apparent lack of protection of some β-blockers. Lipophilic agents that achieve brain concentration may actuate more effective protection from the brain–heart interaction that appears to be involved in the genesis of sudden death in some subsets.

Not recommended drugs:
- *Atenolol* is widely prescribed but is poorly effective because it does not gain sufficient brain concentration that is needed for cardioprotection, and should not be used in clinical trials as done (1985–2009). I rendered the drug obsolete in 2007 cardiac drug therapy.
- *Nadolol* is renally excreted and is not advisable, as poorly effective.
- *Sotalol* is hydrophilic and is not recommended; may cause torsades, malignant arrhythmia.
- *Acebutolol* and pindolol not advisable as stimulant (ISA).

Nitrates

The mononitrates are unaffected by the liver; whereas isosorbide dinitrate undergoes extensive hepatic metabolism. Mononitrates, on entering the walls of veins and arteries, combine with sulfhydryl groups with the formation of nitric oxide, which activates guanylate cyclase to produce cyclic guanosine monophosphate which, in turn, brings about relaxation of vascular smooth muscle at the doses commonly used, with maximal dilation of veins and minimal dilation of arteries. The profound venous dilation causes ↓ in preload and, at high-nitrate dosage, a modest ↓ in afterload occurs. Sulfhydryl groups become depleted by continued exposure to nitrates and tolerance develops with little or no resulting venous dilation. Thus, 24-hour therapy with nitrates is of no value to the patient. A minimum daily 10-hour nitrate-free interval is necessary for the intracellular regeneration of sulfhydryl groups and to maintain the effectiveness of the nitrate preparation.

Indications: Second-choice management of Class 2 and 3 stable angina; angina with concomitant LV dysfunction (shortness of breath and effort tolerance may be improved by nitrate therapy); angina with concomitant mild or moderate hypertension; combination therapy with β-blockers or if β-blockers are contraindicated combined with verapamil or diltiazem; pre- and postoperative management of the cardiac patient undergoing surgery; intraoperative hypertension.

Contraindications: Hypertrophic cardiomyopathy (HCM), constrictive pericarditis, or cardiac tamponade; hypovolemia; right ventricular infarction; severe uncontrolled glaucoma with very high-nitrate dosing, especially intravenous (IV) nitrates.

Adverse effects: Syncope, especially in the elderly, and an increased incidence with added angiotensin-converting enzyme (ACE) inhibitors, diuretics, alcohol, or alpha blockers. Tachycardia, mild palpitations, dizziness, and flushing commonly occur. Headaches are often bothersome; greater than 25% of patients are intolerant and discontinue the drug. Indigestion and halitosis may occur. High-dose nitrates may cause a ↓ in arterial O_2 tension and are relatively contraindicated in severe COPD and hypoxemic situations. Methemoglobinemia has been noted with prolonged high dosage and withdrawal symptoms have been observed with high-dose, long-term use.

Interactions: Heparin resistance with high-nitrate dosage. ACE inhibitors, alpha blockers, and diuretics also ↓ preload tachycardia may be increased when nitrates are used with dihydropyridine Ca antagonists.

Nitroglycerin: *Supplied*: Sublingual tablets 0.15 mg, 0.3 mg, and 0.6 mg (in the UK, glyceryl trinitrate: 300 μg, 500 μg, 600 μg). Spray; nitrolingual spray, 0.4 mg/metered dose, 200 doses/vial. *Dosage*: 0.3 mg is given if the systolic BP is less than 130 mm Hg, 0.6 mg if greater than 130 mm Hg systolic. The patient should be instructed on how and when to use nitroglycerin.

- Sit and put one tablet under the tongue or use the sublingual spray: Avoid taking the drug while standing except when accustomed to such usage. Nitroglycerin is less effective when used with the patient lying,

since less pooling occurs in the limbs and the drug is thus less effective in relieving pain.
- Take a nitroglycerin tablet before activities that are known to precipitate angina.
- Take a second tablet if pain is not relieved in 2 minutes. After taking the second nitroglycerin tablet, chew and swallow a junior aspirin (80 mg) or a regular 325 mg aspirin tablet. Aspirin is used here for its effect in preventing coronary thrombosis.
- Go to the nearest emergency room if pain persists beyond 10 minutes, using a third nitroglycerin during transport if marked weakness or faint like feeling is not present.
- Take nitroglycerin for acute shortness of breath but not if the symptoms are dizziness or palpitations in the absence of pain.
- Keep nitroglycerin tablets in dark, light-protected bottles. If exposed to light, they may only last a few months.
- Use two bottles, one for stock supply with the cotton wool within a well-stoppered bottle, kept in the refrigerator. This will last 1–2 years. The second bottle containing no cotton wool should contain a few months' supply and be refilled when needed.

Dosage: Dosage of other nitrates is given in Table 2.2.

Calcium Antagonists

- *Verapamil* is the most potent antianginal Ca antagonist but is not the safest agent for general use. The pharmacologic and clinical effects of Ca antagonists are given in Table 2.4. Verapamil is more effective than diltiazem because of a more prominent negative inotropic effect; in addition, verapamil causes a greater ↓ in systemic vascular resistance. If β-blockers are contraindicated, verapamil is a reasonable choice, provided that there are no contraindications to the use of this agent [CHF in past, suspect LV dysfunction, or ejection fraction (EF), less than 40% as can precipitate CHF and bradycardia].
- *Dihydropyridines* only amlodipine and low-dose nifedipine are advised because they are well tested; they have no EP and minimal negative inotropic effects. Diltiazem and dihydropyridines have about equal antianginal effects but diltiazem should not be combined with β-blocker as bradycardia occurs.
- *Calcium antagonist–beta-blocker combination*: Verapamil should not be combined with a β-blocker since there is a high incidence of bradyarrhythmias, including life-threatening sinus arrest and asystole; CHF may be precipitated. Diltiazem combined with a β-blocker may cause sinus arrest or asystole. Although the occurrence is rare, caution is necessary and patients should be properly selected prior to prescribing this combination. Sinus bradycardia is not uncommon. Dihydropyridines

can be safely combined with β-blockers since they have no effect on the sinus or A-V nodes.
- Care is needed when dihydropyridines or diltiazem is added to β-blockers in patients with LV dysfunction, since CHF can be precipitated.

Indications: Consider Ca antagonists as second line in the management of stable angina Class 1, 2 and 3, advisable only when β-blockers are contraindicated or produce bothersome effects.

Disadvantages: Sinus node dysfunction, A-V block with verapamil or diltiazem. High incidence of constipation with verapamil. Ca antagonists do not significantly ↓ the incidence of fatal MI. Verapamil and diltiazem ↑ the risk of CHF in patients with LV dysfunction and should be avoided in this subset when the EF is less than 40%. Nifedipine may be given a trial in patients without overt CHF and EF greater than 35% if a β-blocker is contraindicated. Ca antagonists are commonly and inappropriately used in this large group of cardiac patients in whom β-blockers, when used with due caution, are often effective, well tolerated, and likely to have salutary effects on prognosis. The Ca antagonists may, however, have to be used judiciously when β-blocking agents are ineffective or contraindicated.

Contraindications: Aortic stenosis; sick sinus syndrome and A-V block with verapamil and diltiazem; CHF or suspected LV dysfunction; MI with CHF (EF <40% for verapamil and diltiazem; EF <35% for nifedipine).

Table 2.4: Dosages of calcium antagonists for angina.

Preparation	Initial	Dosage maintenance (daily mg)	Maximum (daily mg)
Amlodipine (Norvasc)	5 mg/d	5–10	10
Nifedipine extended Release	30 mg once	60–90	90
Procardia XL; Adalat XL (C) 30, 60, 90 mg tabs	daily		
Adalat Retard 20 mg (UK)	20 mg BID	40–80	80
Diltiazem 60, 120 mg tabs (30, 60, C)	60 mg TID	180–240	360
Cardizem 60, 90,	60 mg TID	180–240	360
Cardizem SR (C) 60, 90, 120 mg capsules	60–90 mg BID	180–240	360
Tildiem (UK) 60 mg			
Adizem SR (UK) 120 mg			
Verapamil 80, 120 mg tablets	80 mg TID	240–360	360

Interventional Therapy

- The COURAGE investigators (2015) did not find a difference in survival between an initial strategy of PCI plus medical therapy and medical therapy alone in patients with stable IHD.
- The trial of patients with stable angina compared an initial strategy of PCI plus optimal medical therapy with optimal medical therapy alone. A follow-up of 4.6 years showed conclusively that patients in the two groups had similar rates of death or MI (Boden et al. 2007).
- They studied 2,287 patients who had objective evidence of myocardial ischemia: 1,149 patients to undergo PCI with optimal medical therapy (PCI group) and 1,138 to receive optimal medical therapy alone (medical therapy group).

At 4.6 years, there were 211 primary events in the PCI group and 202 events in the medical therapy group.

The 4.6-year cumulative primary event rates were 19% in the PCI group and 18.5% in the medical therapy group cause and nonfatal MI during a median follow-up.

- Percutaneous coronary intervention did not reduce the risk of death, MI, or other major cardiovascular events when added to optimal medical therapy (Boden et al. 2007).
- Rapidity of improvement in health status occurred in both groups; the majority of patients who received optimal medical therapy alone had improved symptoms within 3 months. Optimal medical therapy consisted of antiplatelet therapy, anti-ischemic therapy, and aggressive lipid and BP control.
- Optimal medical therapy is a proven option for chronic stable angina.
- The *COURAGE investigators* (Sedlis et al. 2015) did not find a difference in survival at 15 years between an initial strategy of PCI plus medical therapy and medical therapy alone in patients with stable IHD.

Coronary artery bypass grafting (CABG): Strongly advise a left internal mammary artery anastomosis to the LAD. The artery remains attached at its origin from the left subclavian. This is the surgical procedure of choice for all patients, but especially for the relatively young; the 10-year occlusion rate is 5%, as opposed to 15% for internal mammary graft and 50% for vein graft. Even so, internal mammary graft or anastomosis is deferred, if possible, by angioplasty in the younger patient.

Although bypass surgery is superior to drug therapy when severe proximal stenosis of the LAD artery is present, there is no evidence indicating that the procedure is superior to angioplasty in patients with good LV function (EF >50%) where the lesion is suitable for angioplasty. Therefore, young patients in this group with relatively good LV function, EF greater than 40%, should be given a trial of angioplasty/STENT. Bypass is reserved for later use, utilizing left internal mammary artery anastomosis and often in diabetics.

UNSTABLE ANGINA

Pathophysiology

In the majority of cases of unstable angina, atheromatous plaques are eccentric with irregular borders and a narrow neck on angiography. A ruptured or fissured plaque with overlying platelet thrombus is a common finding confirmed by several investigators during angioscopy. In addition, silent ischemia is frequently observed in patients with unstable angina, and prognosis is worse in this subset.

Therapy

Manage as non-STEMI (see Chapter 3).
- Aspirin, 240–325 mg, chewed or swallowed for a rapid effect, interventional therapy for most at 24–48 hours.

BIBLIOGRAPHY

1. Al-Lamee R, Thompson D, Dehbi HM, et al. Percutaneous coronary intervention in stable angina (ORBITA): a double-blind, randomised controlled trial. Lancet. 2018;391(10115):31-40.
2. Bally M, Dendukuri N, Rich B, et al. Risk of acute myocardial infarction with NSAIDs in real world use: Bayesian meta-analysis of individual patient data. BMJ. 2017;357:j1909.
3. Bhattacharyya AK, Connor WE. Beta-sitosterolemia and xanthomatosis. A newly described lipid storage disease in two sisters. J Clin Invest. 1974;53(4):1033-43.
4. Boden WE, O'Rourke RA, Teo KK, et al. Optimal medical therapy with or without PCI for stable coronary disease. N Engl J Med. 2007;356(15):1503-16.
5. Cox D, Maree AO, Dooley M, et al. Effect of enteric coating on antiplatelet activity of low-dose aspirin in healthy volunteers. Stroke. 2006;37:2153-8.
6. Fox KA, Poole-Wilson PA, Henderson RA, et al. Randomized Intervention Trial of unstable Angina (RITA) investigators. J Am Coll Cardiol. 2015;66(5):511-20.
7. Kapoor JR. Enteric coating is a possible cause of aspirin resistance. J Am Coll Cardiol. 2008;52:1276-7.
8. Khan GM. Sitosterol blood levels are elevated in diabetics and may be the cause of coronary artery disease and stroke. J Med Sci. 2017;3:89-94.
9. Khan MG. Angina. In: Khan MG, Bartlett JG, Chopra S, Topol EJ (Eds). Medical Diagnosis and Therapy, 1st edition. Pennsylvania: Lea and Febiger; 1994.
10. Khan MG. Beta blockers are the only drugs that prevent sudden cardiac death. In: Khan MG. Practical Cardiology. New Delhi: Jaypee Brothers Medical Publishers (P) Ltd.; 2018. pp. 312.
11. Mancini GB, Farkouh ME, Brooks MM, et al. Medical treatment and revascularization options in patients with type 2 diabetes and coronary disease. J Am Coll Cardiol. 2016;68(10):985.
12. Olsson G, Rehnqvist N, Sjogren A, et al. Long-Term Treatment With Metoprolol After Myocardial Infarction: Effect on 3 Year Mortality and Morbidity. JACC. 1985,5(6):1428-37.

13. Pagidipati NJ, Hemal K, Mark DB, et al. Sex differences in functional stress test versus CT angiography in symptomatic patients with suspected CAD: insights from PROMISE. J Am Coll Cardiol. 2016;67:2607-16.
14. Peters RW, Muller JE, Goldstein S, et al. Propranolol and the morning increase in the frequency of sudden cardiac deaths (BHAT Study). Am J Cardiol. 1989;63(20):1518-20.
15. Salen G, Horak I, Rothkopf M, et al. Lethal atherosclerosis associated with abnormal plasma and tissue sterol composition in sitosterolemia with xanthomatosis. J Lipid Res. 1985;26:1126-33.
16. Salen G, von Bergmann K, Lutjohann D, et al. Ezetimibe effectively reduces plasma plant sterols in patients with sitosterolemia. Circulation. 2004;109:966-71.
17. Sedlis SP, Hartigan PM, Teo KK, et al. Effect of PCI on long-term survival in patients with stable ischemic heart disease. N Engl J Med. 2015;373(20):1937-46.
18. Williams MC, Hunter A, Newby DE, et al. Use of coronary computed tomographic angiography to guide management of patients with coronary disease. J Am Coll Cardiol. 2016;67(15):1759-68.

CHAPTER 3

Acute Myocardial Infarction

PATHOPHYSIOLOGIC IMPLICATIONS

- An acute myocardial infarction (MI) is nearly always caused by occlusion of a coronary artery by thrombus overlying a fissured or ruptured atheromatous plaque. The ruptured plaque, by direct release of tissue factor and exposure of the subintima, is highly thrombogenic. Exposed collagen provokes platelet aggregation. Coronary angiography performed during the early hours of infarction has confirmed the presence of total occlusion of the infarct-related artery in over 90% of patients. It is not surprising that aspirin, through inhibition of platelet aggregation, reduces the incidence of coronary thrombosis and is especially useful in prevention of the progression of unstable angina to thrombosis and MI.
- Soft chewable aspirin 240 mg is particularly useful when given at the onset of chest pain produced by infarction.
- Aspirin, however, does not block all pathways that relate to platelet aggregation. In addition, aspirin does not ↓ the incidence of sudden death in patients with acute MI but an appropriate β-blocker does.
- Beta-blockers are the only cardioactive agents currently available that are proven to prevent sudden cardiac death (Table 3.1).
- The increased morning incidence of acute MI documented in several studies of the diurnal variation of infarction is related to the early morning catecholamine surges, which induce platelet aggregation, and an ↑ in blood pressure (BP) and hydraulic stress, which may lead to plaque rupture (Flowchart 3.1).
- Beta-adrenergic blockers have been shown to ↓ the early morning peak incidence of acute infarction and sudden death.
- Unfortunately, when an atheromatous plaque ruptures, the thrombogenic effect of plaque contents cannot be completely nullified by the inhibition of all aspects of platelet aggregation, and chemical agents that can arrest the effects of these thrombogenic substances deserve intensive study.
- Use of a β-blocking agent may inhibit plaque rupture perhaps by its ability to ↓ cardiac ejection velocity. This action reduces hydraulic stress on the arterial wall that might be critical at the arterial site where the atheromatous plaque is predisposed to rupture (Flowchart 3.2).

Table 3.1: Total deaths and sudden deaths in beta-blocker randomized control trials of postmyocardial infarction and heart failure patients.

	Control	Drug	% Decrease
Propranolol*			
Total sudden deaths	78	60	64
5 am–11 am	31	11	64
Total deaths	188/1,460	138/1,456	26
Timolol†			
Total sudden deaths^	95	47	50
Instant, within seconds	38	11	71
Total deaths	117/718	67/670	42
Metoprolol#			
Total sudden deaths	21	9	57
Total deaths	31/147	25/154	19##
MERIT-HF^			
Total sudden deaths	132	79	40.2
Total deaths	217/2,001	145/1,990	33.2
Bisoprolol [CIBIS]‡			
Total sudden deaths	83	48	42.2
Total deaths	228/1,320	156/1,327	31.6

*BHAT study, AM sudden death (Peters et al. 1989) follow-up 25 months, 120–240 mg daily.
†Timolol Norwegian MI study; mean duration 17 months.
Follow-up: 10 mg twice daily.
#Metoprolol: A very small study of only approximately 150 patients in each group followed for 3 years.
##"This reduction in cardiac mortality did not reach statistical significance, as was to be expected from our sample size" (Olsson et al. 1985).
^In MERIT-HF, there were fewer sudden deaths in the metoprolol CR/XL group than in the placebo group [79 vs 132, 0.59 (0.45–0.78); p = 0.0002] and deaths from worsening heart failure [30 vs 58, 0.51 (0.33–0.79); p = 0.0023].
‡Bisoprolol in CIBIS; significant decrease in deaths and sudden deaths.
Carvedilol did not prevent sudden death in two large RCTs; total mortality in RCT was not significantly reduced in post-MI patients.

- Occlusion of a coronary artery leads, in about 20 minutes, to death of cells in areas of severely ischemic tissue, which will usually become necrotic over 4–6 hours. Since early and late mortality are directly related to the size of the infarct, limitation of infarct size (or even prevention of necrosis) by means of thrombolytic therapy initiated at the earliest possible moment, is of the utmost importance.
- The ischemic zone surrounding the necrotic tissue provides electrophysiologic (EP) inhomogeneity that predisposes the occurrence of

Flowchart 3.1: Pathophysiology of atheroma formation, erosion, rupture, causing sudden cardiac death and myocardial infarction. Why the coronary arteries?

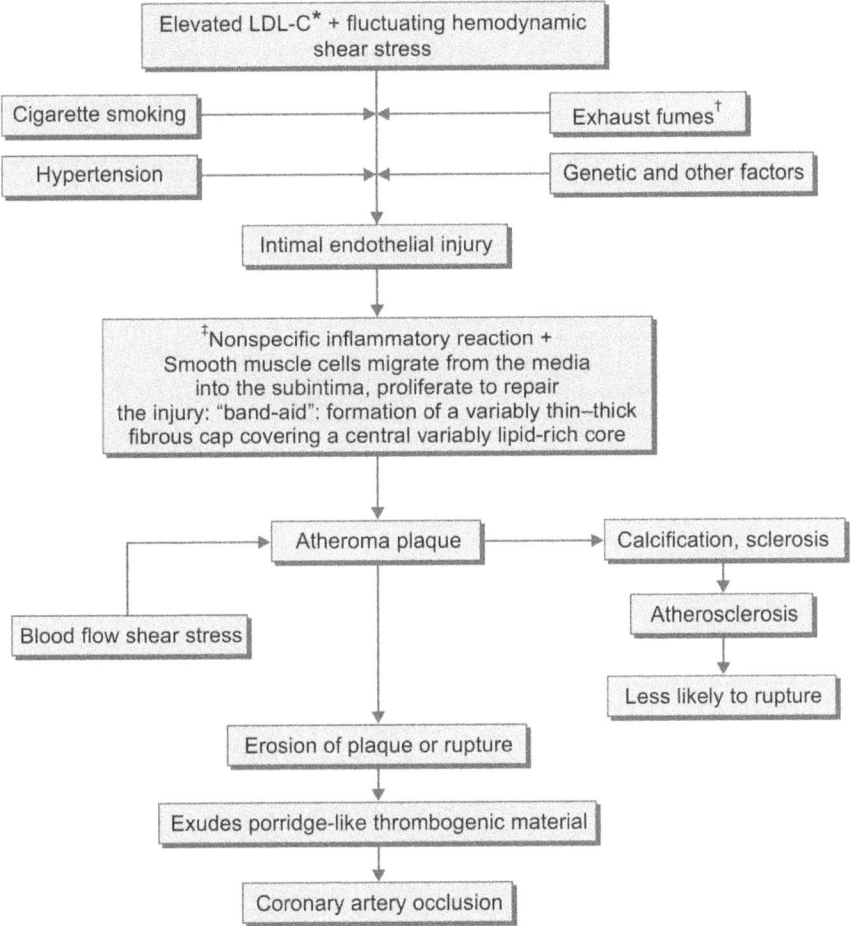

Coronary arteries prone to atheroma: As empty in systole and refilled during diastole, hemodynamically fluctuating shear stress causes injury to the intima; finally erosion or rupture of atheroma plaque occurs particularly in genetically susceptible individuals. Coronary arteries are hydraulically vulnerable unstable channels. During an average lifespan, they empty and fill rapidly at fluctuating shear stress more than 2 billion times with altered arterial hemodynamics at bends, bifurcations and at ostia. Over time the altered shear stress causes erosion and fissuring of plaques. High levels of low-density lipoprotein cholesterol (LDL-C) and in diabetics elevated sitosterol (Khan 2017) cause atheroma and arterial obstruction.

The algorithm suggests that fatal events may be best prevented by:
• Greatly reducing culprit LDL-C levels and sitosterol in diabetics, and administration of an appropriate β-blocker to alter hemodynamic shear stress and prevent erosions. For individuals with diabetes mellitus, blood sitosterol levels must be maintained less than 4.4 mg/L (Khan 2017).
• Fatal or nonfatal MI and sudden deaths were significantly prevented by timolol and propranolol, but by no other cardioactive agents; perhaps β1 and β2 agents are more cardioprotective than β1 agents.

†From motor vehicles, as dangerous as smoking.
‡Aspirin: A double agent; inhibits platelet aggregation and perhaps the inflammatory process.

Flowchart 3.2: Salutary effects of beta-adrenergic blockade. (↑, increase; ↓, decrease).

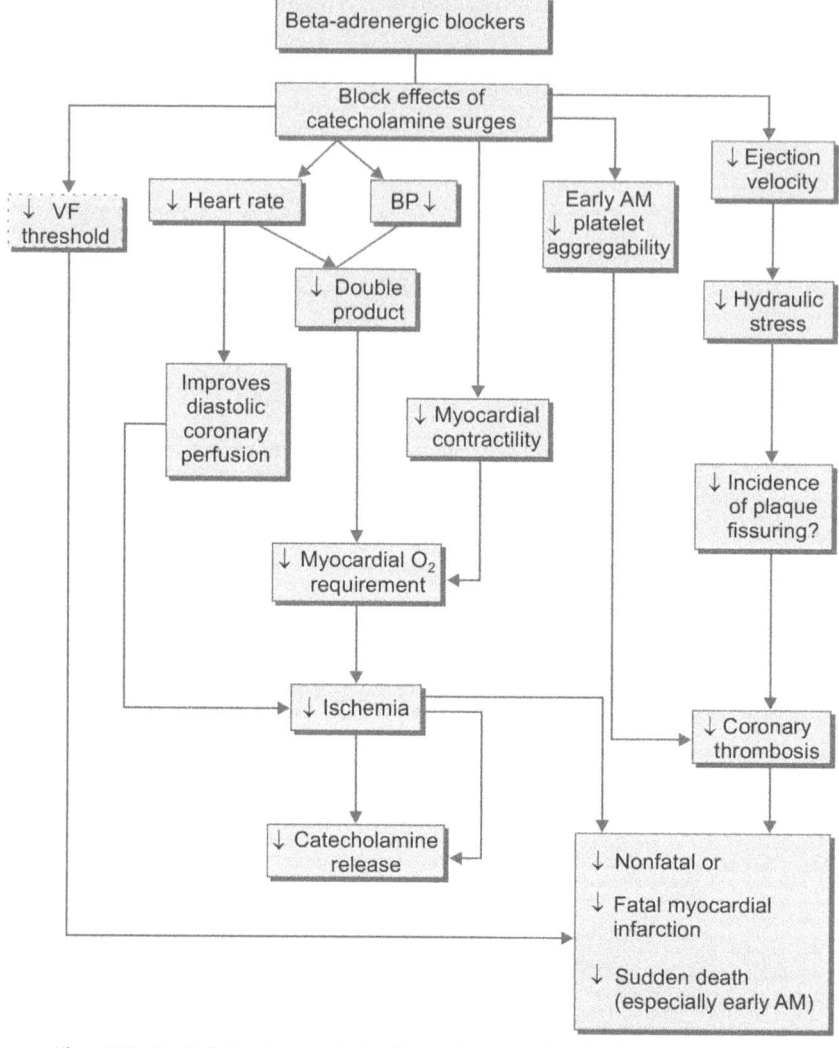

Source: Khan MG. On Call Cardiology, 3rd edition. Philadelphia: WB Saunders, Elsevier Science; 2006.

lethal arrhythmias. These arrhythmias are most common during the early hours after onset and contribute to one of the major mechanisms of sudden death.

Extensive myocardial necrosis is the major determinant of congestive heart failure (CHF); papillary, septal, and free wall rupture; and cardiogenic shock, in which greater than 35% of the myocardium is usually infarcted.

- The most effective means of reducing the extent of myocardial necrosis is timely percutaneous coronary intervention (PCI) (within 60 minutes) or administration of thrombolytic therapy, aspirin, and a β-blocking agent as soon as possible after the onset of symptoms of coronary thrombosis.

Diabetic sitosterolemia: High blood sitosterol causes heart attacks and stroke in diabetics. This important novel discovery is discussed at the end of this chapter.

DIAGNOSIS

Chest Pain

- Usually lasts more than 20 minutes and often persists for several hours. However, the pain of infarction can last for only 15 minutes and, occasionally, fatal infarction is ushered in by only a few minutes of severe pain or even unheralded cardiac arrest. Infarction may be silent, particularly in diabetic patients and in the elderly.
- Typically retrosternal and across the chest.
- Variations of a crushing, vise-like, heavy weight on the chest, pressure, tightness, strangling, aching.
- At times, only a discomfort with an oppression and burning or indigestion-like feeling.
- May radiate to the throat, jaws, neck, shoulders, arms, scapulae, or the epigastrium. At times, pain is centered at any one of these areas, e.g. the left wrist or shoulder, without radiation.
- Usually builds up over minutes or hours, as opposed to aortic dissection, in which pain has an abrupt onset like a gunshot.

  Associated symptoms and factors include:
- Diaphoresis, cold clammy skin, apprehension.
- Shortness of breath, nausea, vomiting, dizziness.
- Presyncope and rarely syncope may occur due to bradyarrhythmias, especially in inferior MI.
- Occasionally, no pain. A marked ↓ in BP with associated symptoms, along with electrocardiogram (ECG) findings, should suffice in making the diagnosis.
- Painless infarcts (in about 10% of patients), especially in diabetics or the elderly. In these patients, associated symptoms are often prominent and serve as clues to diagnosis.
- Over 50% of patients have a history of angina or prior infarction.
- Approximately, 33% of patients with acute infarction have no major risk factors: Death of a parent or sibling less than age 55, hypercholesterolemia, cigarette smoking, hypertension, or diabetes. Absence of these factors should not influence the diagnosis.

Physical Signs

- Patient appears apprehensive, anxious, cold, clammy.
- Area of chest pain may be indicated with a clenched fist.
- Tachycardia 100–120/minute. An ↑ in BP due to increased sympathetic tone is observed in slightly more than half of patients with anterior infarction.

- Bradycardia less than 60 beats/minute and a ↓ in BP in about two-thirds of inferior infarcts; many of these patients become hypotensive, sometimes profoundly.
- S4 gallop is common; S3 and S4 if in CHF or cardiogenic shock.
- Murmur of mitral regurgitation (MR) due to papillary muscle dysfunction.
- Crepitations, more prominent over the lower third of the lung fields, may be present.
- Elevated jugular venous pressure due to left and right CHF or a very high venous pressure in the presence of right ventricular infarction or cardiac tamponade.
- Frequently, there are no abnormal physical signs, and this finding in a patient with suggestive symptoms should not ↓ the level of suspicion that the patient may have an MI.

Although sophisticated tests evolved in the 1980s to improve diagnostic accuracy, they are of limited value in the era of thrombolysis. Thus, a relevant history and correct interpretation of the ECG are of paramount importance in the implementation of early thrombolytic therapy, which will be of greatest benefit if given very early after symptom onset (<60 minutes).

Electrocardiogram

Diagnostic Features of ST-segment Elevation Myocardial Infarction

- ST-segment elevation of greater than 1 mm in more than two-limb leads (Figs. 3.1 to 3.3), or
- At least 2 mm ST elevation in more than two precordial leads (Figs. 3.4 and 3.7).

The above criteria, which have been used in most clinical trials of thrombolytic therapy, have become internationally standard and are considered diagnostic in patients with symptoms suggestive of acute MI. Where symptoms are not typical, the response to nitroglycerin is ascertained. Also, minimal ST-segment elevation in black patients must be reassessed to exclude the occasional normal variant. There is clear recognition that Q waves may evolve early or late and cannot be relied upon for early diagnosis. Thus, the terms "transmural" and "nontransmural" have been abandoned and Q wave or non-Q wave infarction cannot be categorized in the early phase. The best differentiating feature is ST-segment elevation, which is present in 95% of patients with acute coronary thrombotic occlusion.

In addition, later ECG signs of infarction include:
- Diminution of R waves (poor R wave progression)
- Evolving Q waves (Fig. 3.2)
- The simultaneous presence of reciprocal ST-segment depression is important to confirm the electrocardiographic diagnosis (Figs. 3.1 to 3.3).

Acute Myocardial Infarction **71**

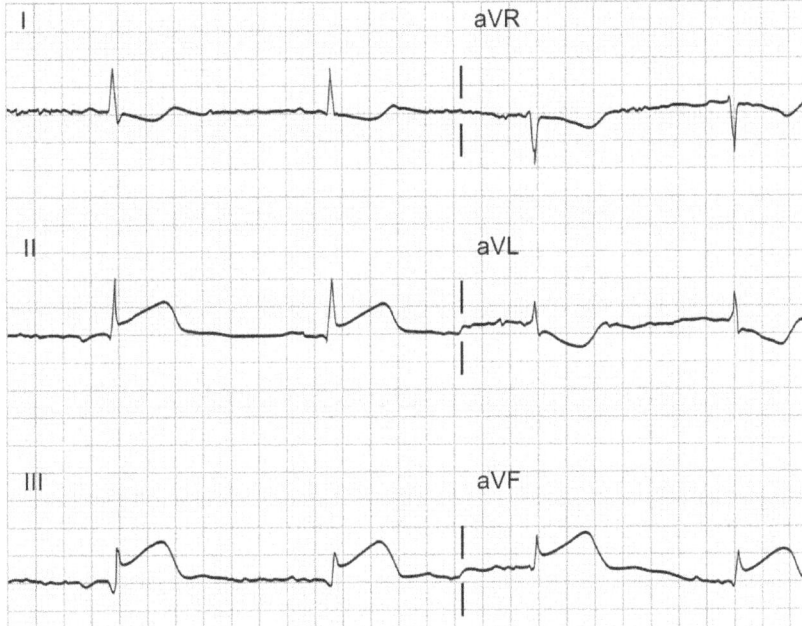

Fig. 3.1: Acute inferior myocardial infarction. ST elevation in three inferior leads; note reciprocal depression in leads I and aVL.
Source: Khan MG. On Call Cardiology, 3rd edition. Philadelphia: WB Saunders, Elsevier Science; 2006. p. 84.

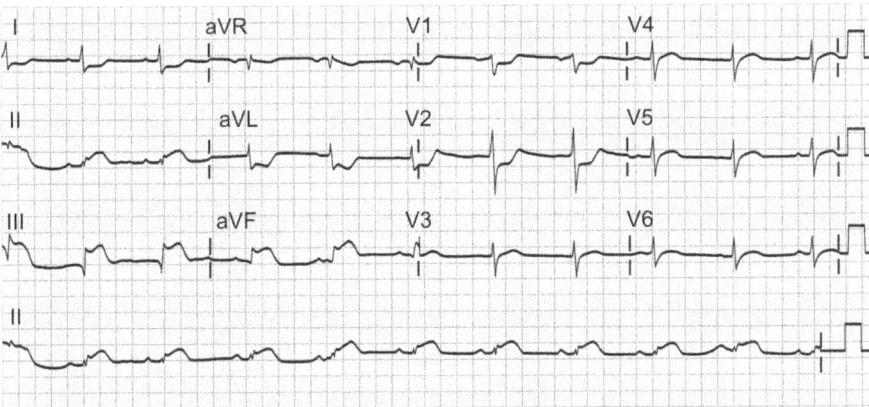

Fig. 3.2: Acute inferior myocardial infarction (STEMI); abnormally shaped high ST segment in inferior leads. Note the reciprocal depression in leads I, aVL, V1 and V2. Reciprocal depression is not diagnostic of infarction but is an important confirmatory sign that strongly supports the diagnosis.

72 *Internal Medicine: Diagnosis and Therapy*

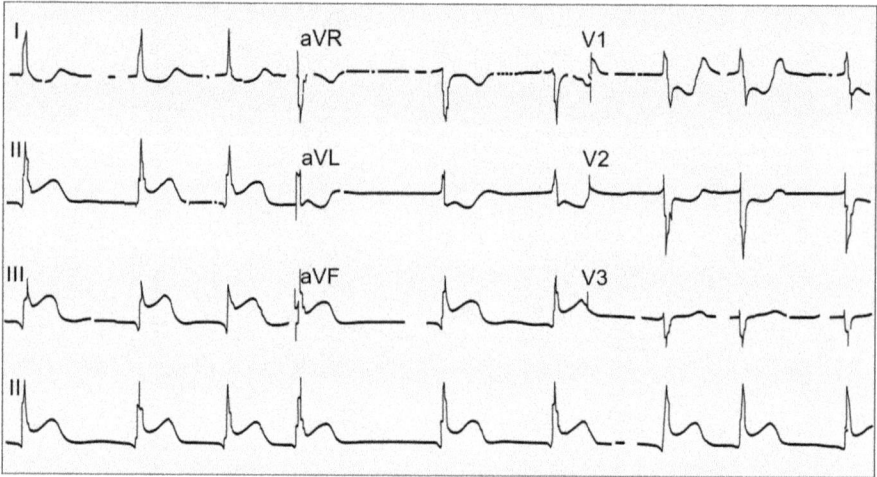

Fig. 3.3: Acute inferior myocardial infarction: ST elevation in leads II, III, and aVF. Note reciprocal depression in leads V1, V2 and aVL.

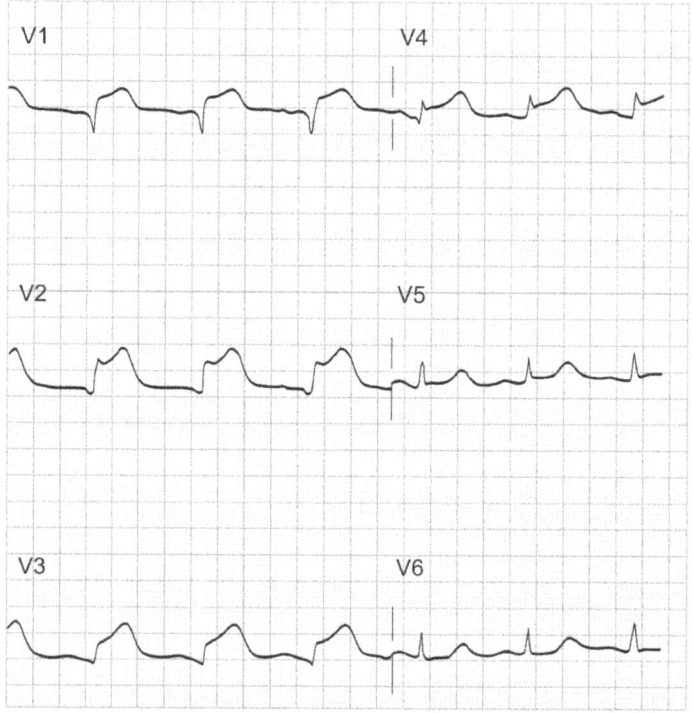

Fig. 3.4: Abnormal ST elevation greater than 2 mm in three precordial leads V1-V3 and V4: anterior STEMI.

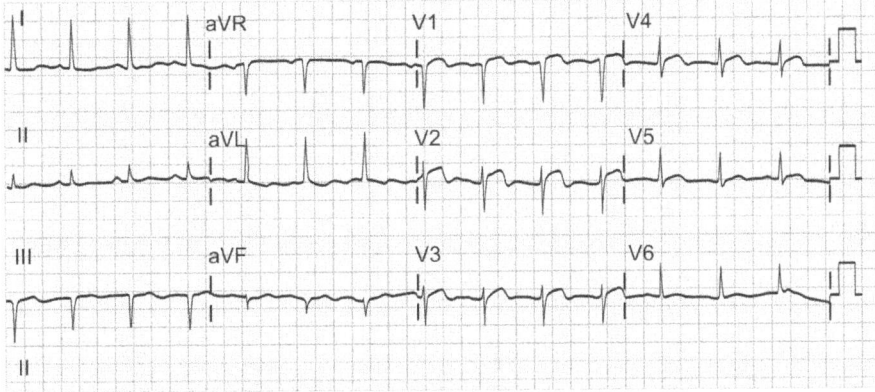

Fig. 3.5: Abnormal ST-segment elevation V1-V6 diagnostic for acute anterior MI.

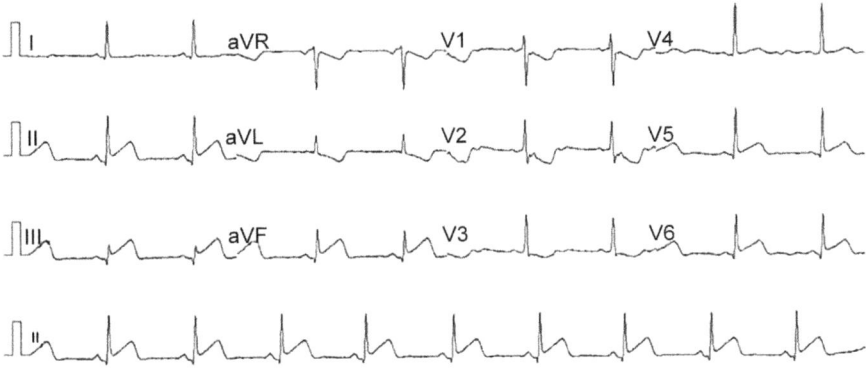

Fig. 3.6: ST-segment elevation leads II, III, aVF and anterolateral leads V5 and V6 acute inferolateral infarction. Note reciprocal ST depression leads aVL, V1-V3 help to confirm the diagnosis of acute MI.
Source: Khan GM. A new electrode placement method for obtaining 12-lead ECGs. Open Heart. 2015;2:e000226.

- Patients who are developing non-Q wave infarction often manifest ST depression, or T wave change.

If the first ECG is not diagnostic of acute injury/infarction, but the patient is strongly suspected of having an acute coronary syndrome, the ECG is repeated q 15 minutes until diagnostic changes are observed or until the creatine kinase (CK) and/or CK-MB results or troponins are reported.

Mimics of Acute MI Pattern on ECGs

An incorrect diagnosis may lead to unneeded coronary angiograms. Mimics include:
- Early repolarization pattern
- In some young individuals, especially African Americans, the ST segment is elevated in V3 to V5 associated with minor T wave inversion

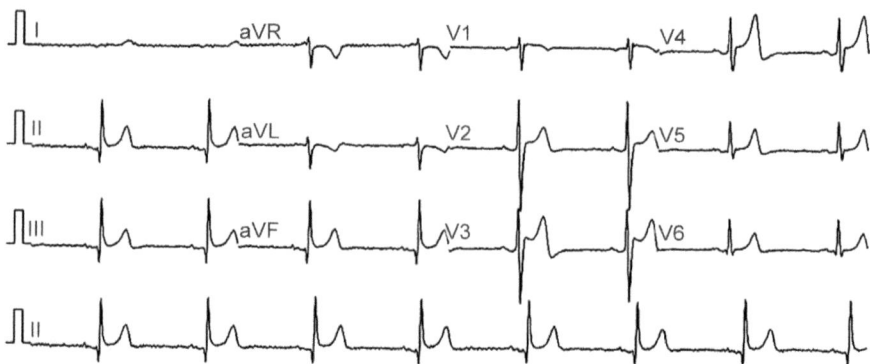

Fig. 3.7: Routine ECG from a 24-year-old male with no heart disease. Sinus bradycardia, ST segment concave (not convex) elevation II, III, aVF, and normal variant in V2, V3, V4; can be misdiagnosed as acute pericarditis or ST-segment elevation myocardial infarction (STEMI). Note the ST segment in V3 has a small notch at its commencement and is concave and not the convex shape of STEMI. There is reciprocal depression in aVR. If the ST elevation in II, III, aVF were due to inferior STEMI, there should be some reciprocal depression in I and aVL.

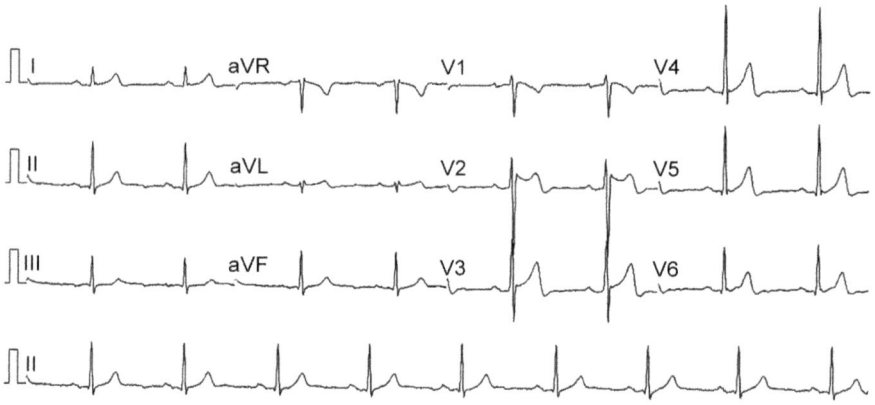

Fig. 3.8: ST-segment elevation V2 and V3; normal variant in a healthy 26-year-old man. Rarely observed in women.

as a normal variant; the ST segment tends to be slightly coved and may mimic acute MI, and caution is required to assess the clinical findings (Fig. 3.8).
- Acute pericarditis: Elevation in lead I is accompanied by elevation in leads II, III, and aVF; the ST elevation is concave, as opposed to convex upward with an injury current of infarction.
  - Reciprocal ST depression and PR-segment elevation in aVR is a typical finding with pericarditis.
  - Characteristic features of acute pericarditis: ST-segment elevation in most leads; I, II, aVL, aVF, V5 and V6, with reciprocal ST depression

and PR-segment elevation in aVR. In addition, note sinus tachycardia and prominent PR-segment depression commonly seen with acute pericarditis.
- *Takotsubo stress cardiomyopathy*: If the ECG is equivocal and there is a strong clinical impression that acute MI is present, valuable confirmatory information may be obtained from an echocardiogram that is diagnostic of Takotsubo stress cardiomyopathy.
- Because the initial abnormality may not be fully diagnostic in up to 40% of cases, it is imperative to correlate the findings with accurate historical details. In patients with chest pain, new or presumably new Q waves in two leads with ST elevation are diagnostic in over 85% of cases.
- Q waves are fully developed in 4–12 hours and may manifest as early as 2 hours from onset of chest discomfort or associated symptoms.
- Evolutionary ST-T changes occur during 12–24 hours but may be delayed up to 30 hours.
- Inferior MI ST elevation in lead II, III and aVF with evolving Q waves and reciprocal depression in V1-V3. The latter depression may be due to reciprocal changes, but there is evidence to suggest that in some patients it is due to left anterior descending (LAD) disease. The evolutionary changes in repolarization that occur with inferior infarction evolve more rapidly than with anterior infarcts.
- Tachycardia may ↑ ischemic injury, causing elevation of the ST segment that must be differentiated from extension of infarction or pericarditis. Importantly, reciprocal depression does not occur in pericarditis.

Nondiagnostic ECG

Acute MI may be present with ECG changes that are nonspecific in 10–20% of cases and may result from:
- Slow evolution of ECG changes. The tracing may remain normal for several hours.
- Old infarction masking the ECG effect of a new infarct.
- Inferior MI associated with left anterior hemiblock in which R waves are expected to be small in leads II, III, aVF.
- Left bundle branch block (LBBB).
- Apical infarction.
- Posterolateral infarction is not usually associated with ST elevation or Q waves.

ST elevation of infarction from the following:
- Acute pericarditis where the ST segment elevation is not confined to leads referable to an anatomic segmental blood supply. Thus, elevation in lead I is accompanied by elevation in leads II, III, aVF; the ST elevation is concave, as opposed to convex, upward with an injury current of infarction; and reciprocal depression is absent.

- Early repolarization changes may mimic infarction but are often observed mainly in leads V5 and V6 with a subtle "fish hook" configuration. This feature is common in blacks.
- Left ventricular (LV) aneurysm, in which there may be permanent ST elevation.

ECG and Location of Infarction Sites

- Anteroseptal: ST elevation V1, V2, V3
- Anterior: ST-segment elevation V2-V4
- Extensive anterior: V1-V6, 1 aVL
- Anterolateral: V4-V6, 1 aVL
- Inferior: 2, 3, aVF
- Posterior infarction: Tall R waves V1, V2, upright T waves occasionally ST depression V1-V2 and often inferior or inferolateral infarct signs
- Right ventricular infarction: ST-segment elevation V2, V4R, often associated with inferior infarction.

ECG and Size of Infarction

The extent of ST-segment elevation gives clues to infarct size, but the correlation is not close. The site of infarction influences mortality but is not as paramount as the size of infarction, which can be reasonably ascertained from the number of leads showing ST elevation, as follows:
- Small MI: 2 or 3 leads
- Moderate: 4 or 5 leads
- Large: 6 or 7 leads
- Extensive: 8 or 9 leads.

Echocardiography in Acute Myocardial Infarction

Echocardiography is not required routinely in an uncomplicated MI, especially where the history and ECG are typical or with non-Q wave infarction.

Indications

- Patients with cardiogenic shock often require assessment to determine the presence of mechanical complications: septal rupture, severe MR, myocardial rupture, and tamponade. Color Doppler can provide quick results and, with the unconscious patient, a transesophageal echocardiogram (TEE) is helpful and accurate.
- To distinguish acute severe MR from papillary muscle rupture.

- In patients with new LBBB with typical chest pain and history suggestive of acute infarction, echocardiography can assist with the diagnosis.
- Patients with an atypical ECG pattern and clinical features of MI.
- Suspected right ventricular infarction with high jugular venous pressure to assess right ventricular involvement and differentiate pericardial tamponade causing a high venous pressure.
- To identify high-risk patients with multivessel disease. The contralateral remote zone should be hyperkinetic, but if it is not, this usually indicates significant noninfarct vessel atherosclerotic disease.
- In patients with moderate CHF not clearing after more than two doses of furosemide, echocardiographic assessment of LV systolic function is useful prior to β-blocker therapy. Although radionuclide ventriculography gives a more accurate assessment of the ejection fraction (EF), the estimate obtained from echocardiography is usually adequate to assist with the evaluation of outcomes and therapy.

PUBLIC EDUCATION AND PHYSICIAN INTERACTION

It is estimated that in areas where thrombolytic therapy is available, 20–30% of patients with acute MI in North America and about 40% in the United Kingdom receive such treatment.

- Thrombolytic therapy has proven valuable and reduces mortality and morbidity. Timing of treatment, however, is of great importance, and until recently it was uncertain as to the outer time boundary of therapy from symptom onset. In the recently completed Late Assessment of Thrombolytic Efficacy (LATE) double-blind placebo-controlled trial of 5,700 patients treated between 6 hours and 24 hours of symptoms, patients receiving tissue plasminogen activator (tPA) within 12 hours had a 27% ↓ of mortality compared with placebo. These data extend the time window of 0–6 hours, established by GISSI-1 and ISSI-2, to 12 hours.
- The first hour of symptoms represents a huge opportunity for benefit for thrombolytic therapy. In the recent MITI trial, patients treated in the first 60 minutes had mortality reduced from 10% to 2%, and 40% of these patients had no infarct on thallium scintigraphy. In the GISSI-1 and ISIS-2 trials, ↓ in mortality was greater than 50% compared with controls treated in the first hours. Unfortunately, less than 3% of patients actually received therapy in this time frame. The average delay in hospital admissions of 80–90 minutes largely accounts for the problem, is inexcusable, and should be reduced to less than 15 minutes.
- Benefit is observed up to 12 hours.
- A major undertaking is the education of patients and the community at large about the importance of minimizing delays between the onset of symptoms of suspected heart attack and attention in the emergency room of the nearest hospital.

- It is not easy to motivate healthy individuals, and efforts to educate the public in this area of their care have not been sufficiently fruitful. Leaflets and health booklets appear to have little impact. A concerted effort must be made by physicians' groups in individual communities in conjunction with audiovisual programs for the public. In addition, hospitals must adopt policies to enforce rapid triage in the emergency room; physicians must be encouraged to institute thrombolytic therapy within a few minutes of the patient's arrival.

Delays to be Avoided

- Reaching the emergency room more than 6 hours after onset of symptoms: Patient and public education should address this issue.
- *Slow emergency room triage*: Patients with chest pain should be allowed quick passage, not exceeding a 1-minute delay at the so-called "triage area", to an area of the emergency room delineated for the rapid assessment of MI.
- Waiting for attending physician.
- *Emergency room physician delay*: The emergency room physician must be well trained to deal with patients who have chest pain. This physician must be allowed to give intravenous (IV) thrombolytic therapy [streptokinase (SK), tPA, or anisoylated plasminogen streptokinase activator complex (APSAC)] to all those who qualify according to an approved, well-outlined hospital emergency room protocol for IV use of thrombolytic agents. The protocol should clearly show the indications and contraindications to IV thrombolysis, but should be simplified. The only well-documented contraindications are active bleeding, stroke, major trauma or surgery in the past 6 months, and uncontrolled hypertension.
- *Waiting for coronary care unit (CCU) beds*: Transfer is advisable after commencement of thrombolysis and initial hemodynamic stability is achieved. Thus, emergency rooms must be equipped to administer all functions that are available in the CCU.
- *Waiting 1–2 hours for CK, CK-MB enzyme results*: The CK is not usually sufficiently elevated within the first 4 hours to establish the diagnosis of infarction and can be used only after the fact. The object is to ↓ or, in some cases, prevent enzyme release by rapid reperfusion of ischemic myocardium.

RISK STRATIFICATION

On admission, risk stratification assists in decision making, especially when relative contraindications to thrombolytic therapy are present. Characteristics of patients with acute MI who, on admission, have a high risk of death or complications, include:

Table 3.2: ISIS-2*: Effects of aspirin and streptokinase given within 4 hours and within 24 hours of onset of myocardial infarction.†

	Placebo (I)	SK	Aspirin	SK + Aspirin	Placebo (I) + Tablets	Neither
35-day vascular mortality; therapy within 4 hours	12.3%	8.2%	8.9%	6.4%	13.1%	
Within 24 hours	12%	9.2%	9.4%	8%	11.8%	13.3%
	1,029/8,595	791/8,592	804/8,587	343/4,292	1,016/8,600	568/4,300

(I, infusion; SK, streptokinase)
*Modified from Randomised trial of intravenous streptokinase, oral aspirin, both, or neither among 17,187 cases of suspected acute myocardial infarction: ISIS-2. ISIS-2 (Second International Study of Infarct Survival) Collaborative Group. Lancet. 1988;2:349-60.Lancet, 2:350, 1988.
†Odds of death, 53% SD 8 Reduction; 2 p <0.00001.

- Large infarcts usually associated with moderate to severe CHF, pulmonary edema, with crackles observed over more than one-third of the lower lung field
- An EF less than 35%
- Cardiogenic shock indicating a large infarct or mechanical complication and high mortality
- Over age 75: The 1-year mortality more than 30% versus less than 10% in patients less than age 70
- New LBBB
- New right bundle branch block (RBBB) with LV failure
- Previous MI and recent infarction with CHF.

Patients with cardiogenic shock and other selected high-risk individuals should be considered for transfer to an interventional cardiac catheterization laboratory for emergency angiography and possible infarct vessel angioplasty.

THERAPY

- Immediate relief of pain is of paramount importance since pain enhances autonomic disturbances that may precipitate sudden death. All patients should take or be given noncoated aspirin, 162–325 mg, immediately and then enteric coated, 160–325 mg qd. This dosage proved very effective in ISIS-2 (Table 3.2) and ISIS-3; a 325-mg dose was used successfully in GISSI-2 (Table 3.3). An initial large dose of 325 mg is strongly recommended because a lower dose may still leave substantial thromboxane activity at this crucial period and may take a few days before achieving greater than 95% of inhibition of platelet activity. Beta-blockers are administered without delay if there are no contraindications, and thrombolytic therapy is commenced in properly

Table 3.3: Timing of thrombolytic therapy and lives saved by GISSI-1 and ISIS-2.

	GISSI-1*		ISSI-2†	
	Control	SK treated	Control	SK and aspirin treated
	5,860	5,852	8,595	8,592
Mortality:	13%	10.7%	11.8%	9.1%
Mortality reduction:	17.7%	Lives saved	22.9%	Lives saved
		130/5,852		233/8,595
		2/100 treated		3/100 treated
	Hours	Lives saved		Lives saved
	<3	3/100		4/100
	3–6	2/100		2.6/100
	6–9	1/123		
	6–24	—		1/100

(SK, streptokinase)
*Modified from Effectiveness of intravenous thrombolytic treatment in acute myocardial infarction. Gruppo Italiano per lo Studio della Streptochinasi nell'Infarto Miocardico (GISSI). Lancet. 1986;1:397-402.
†Modified from Randomised trial of intravenous streptokinase, oral aspirin, both, or neither among 17,187 cases of suspected acute myocardial infarction: ISIS-2. ISIS-2 (Second International Study of Infarct Survival) Collaborative Group. Lancet. 1988;2:349-60.

selected patients. These treatment modalities will be discussed in this chapter.
- In all patients with uncomplicated infarction, treated with thrombolytic agents, a delayed strategy of coronary angiography or "watchful waiting" (with no angiogram unless angina or a positive functional test) is pursued. A conservative strategy has evolved based on the result of the Thrombolysis in Myocardial Infarction (TIMI) 2 trial.
- Patients for whom thrombolytic therapy is contraindicated should be considered for primary (direct) angioplasty of the infarct vessel if they can be transferred quickly (<90 minutes) to a facility with skilled operators and personnel to perform coronary intervention.

Emergency Management

Pain Relief

- Morphine: 4 mg IV over 1 minute, repeated if necessary at a dose of 2-5 mg q 5-30 minutes as needed at the rate of 1 mg/minute.
- A β-blocker, preferably given IV for two doses then orally (Table 3.4), if there is no contraindication. Beta-blockade has been shown to abolish

Table 3.4: Dosage of thrombolytic agents.	
Drug	Dosage
Streptokinase	1.5 million U in 100 mL 0.9% saline IV infusion over 30–60 minutes
Anistreplase (APSAC)	30 U in 5 mL sterile water or saline by slow IV bolus over 2–5 minutes
tPA (alteplase)	6–10 mg IV bolus over 1–2 minutes then 50 mg IV infusion over 1 hour, 20 mg IV infusion over 2nd hour, 20 mg IV infusion over 3rd hour; 100 mg total dose
tPA front-loaded (Author's recommendation)	15 mg bolus 0.75 mg/kg over 30 minutes (not >50 mg) 0.50 mg/kg over 60 minutes (not >35 mg) Total dose ≤100 mg

and may prevent recurrence of chest pain and decrease the need for morphine or nitroglycerin.
- Nitroglycerin is usually given sublingually for two doses. Recurrence of chest discomfort after adequate administration of morphine and a β-blocker should prompt the use of IV nitroglycerin.

Control of Early Life-threatening Arrhythmias

Lives can be saved by:
- Prompt defibrillation or conversion of ventricular tachycardia (VT) by medical teams or paramedics
- *Lidocaine (lignocaine) IV*: Effective for the control of VT, but its prophylactic use is *not* recommended (discussed later in this chapter).
- *Beta-blockers*: It may be required as therapy independent of pain control to abolish ventricular arrhythmias or to prevent their occurrence, especially if these arrhythmias are catecholamine induced. These agents ↓ the incidence of ventricular fibrillation (VF); they should not be given with hypotension, bradycardia, or signs of CHF.

Treatment of Autonomic Disturbances

- Monitoring of the cardiac rhythm is routine practice.
- Autonomic disturbances are triggered by ischemic tissue as well as pain and may result in sinus tachycardia and tachyarrhythmias that are associated with inappropriate catecholamine release, thereby intensifying ischemia, which further increases release of catecholamines. Alternatively, bradycardia may occur and the associated hypotension may enlarge the infarct. This vicious cycle results in an ↑ in infarct size, which can culminate in progressive CHF and shock.
- Autonomic disturbances may be abolished by morphine and β-blockade.

- Symptomatic bradycardias with pulse rates less than 40/minute are controlled with the judicious use of atropine (0.4–0.6 mg) IV given slowly q 5–10 minutes as needed, to a max of 2 mg. *Caution*: Do not ↑ the heart rate (HR) beyond 60/minute. Too rapid administration of atropine may result in sinus tachycardia in some patients and, rarely, VF may be precipitated.

Ancillary Therapy

- Oxygen 2–3 L/minute via nasal prongs is given during the first few hours until assessment is completed, then O_2 is continued if the patient is short of breath, tachypneic, or if there is proven hypoxemia. Pulmonary edema causes hypoxemia, but ventilation–perfusion mismatch plays a role. Cessation of O_2 administration indicates to the patient that some improvement is occurring and helps to allay anxiety.
- *Diet*: Fluids only for 8–12 hours until it is established that the infarction is uncomplicated, then light diet as tolerated with no added salt until the patient is discharged from the CCU.
- A stool softener is routinely prescribed, e.g. docusate (100–200 mg) bid.
- Bedrest and bedside commode for 24 hours, then washroom privileges and ambulation.
- Anticoagulants, for tPA, IV heparin 5,000 U/bolus, with thrombolytic therapy, 1,000 U/h, with careful adjustment of partial thromboplastin time (PTT) between 60 seconds and 85 seconds (or 2.5 × control).
- *Mild sedation*: Oxazepam (15 mg) or a similar agent at bedtime.

Interventional Therapy

Percutaneous coronary intervention versus thrombolytic agent:
- Primary PCI is the preferred mode of reperfusion when performed in a timely fashion by an experienced team. However, significant changes in healthcare delivery in most countries will be required to accomplish the benefits of PCI.
- This accomplishment is probably achieved in less than 50% of patients who have an acute MI in the United States of America and Canada. In cities, approximately 75% reach facilities equipped to deal with cases within 60–90 minutes. Perhaps this can be accomplished in approximately 1% of such patients in Asia, Africa and developing countries. How can we help the unfortunate underprivileged of the world?
- Percutaneous coronary intervention completed within 2–4 hours of onset of chest pain saves lives and reinfarction. This accomplishment is nearly impossible in most countries.
- Percutaneous coronary intervention must be done within 90–120 minutes after arrival to an equipped facility, the procedure is usually

accomplished in approximately 4–6 hours from onset of chest pain, often more than 8 hours. At this time, myocardial necrosis is established.
- In non-facility-equipped areas, doctors and ambulance crews could learn to interpret the ECG of STEMI and administer a thrombolytic agent immediately or within the hour.
- Percutaneous coronary intervention has not been tested against immediate triple noninvasive therapy: aspirin, propranolol, timolol, or metoprolol, and within the hour thrombolytic therapy.
- Among patients, in PCI studies, the better outcome after angioplasty was driven primarily by a reduction in the rate of reinfarction (1.6% in the angioplasty group vs 6.3% in the fibrinolysis group; p <0.001; a 75% reduction).

Thrombolytic Therapy

Reduction in major events and mortality is achieved by thrombolytic therapy instituted within 4 hours of onset of symptoms.
- *It is certainly very effective if given within 2 hours.* Family physicians should commence IV SK, within the hour; ambulance crews should be trained.

The important determinants of outcome are age and administration within 2 hours of onset of symptoms not exceeding a door-to-needle time of 20 minutes. Although the relative survival benefit is greatest for patients aged 65–75 years, the most absolute benefit is in the elderly aged more than 70 years with anterior infarction. Uncomplicated acute inferior MI carries a low risk in the younger and elderly individual.

Caution of intracranial hemorrhage (ICH): Incidence in randomized controlled trials (RCTs) was reported as follows GUSTO III (1997): SK 0.37, tPA 0.72, ASSENT-2: tPA 0.93, TNK/tPA, 0.94.
- Analysis of the Medicare database suggests that thrombolytic therapy is harmful in patients more than 75 years old (Thiemann et al. 2000).
- Reportedly, the incidence of stroke is greater than 4% for tPA and approximately 2.85% for SK in patients older than age 75.
- There appears to be a four- to fivefold greater incidence of ICH in patients older than 75 years who are treated with tPA versus SK.
- Heparin is not required when SK is used; thus, SK is used in many countries outside the United States particularly in patients at low risk and in the elderly over age 75 and particularly in patients seen within 3 hours of onset.
- Assessment of global and regional LV function 3 weeks after a first infarction indicated similar effects for SK and tPA.

Pooled mortality results of recent trials in over 42,000 patients randomized 21,034 to thrombolytic therapy, 20,979 to placebo, were 10% in the treated

Table 3.5: Lidocaine (lignocaine) dosage.		
	Normal dosage, e.g.: 60–90 kg patient	Halve dose: elderly, CHF, shock, hepatic dysfunction, cimetidine, some beta-blockers*, halothane
1st IV bolus Usually	1.5 mg/kg 100 mg	0.75 mg/kg 50 mg
2nd bolus Usually	0.75 mg/kg 50 mg	0.5 mg/kg 25–30 mg
Concomitant Infusion	2–4 mg/min (50 µg/kg/min)	1–2 mg/min (20 µg/kg/min)

Therapeutic level 1.5–5 µg/mL, 1.5–5 µg/L, 6–26 µmol/L.
Seizures: levels >6 mg/L.
*Hepatic-metabolized beta-blockers: propranolol, metoprolol.

group and 11.7% in the control group. These percentages account for 350 lives saved. The treatment of 21,000 patients saved 2 lives in 100 patients less than age 60 treated within 6 hours from onset of symptoms, 7 lives in patients 60–69 years old, and 8 lives in those more than age 70. Thus, the 70- to 75-year-old patients derived the greatest absolute benefits from thrombolytic therapy.

There is currently no ideal thrombolytic agent. From GISSI-2 and ISIS-3, the three approved agents:—(1) SK, (2) tPA, and (3) anistreplase (APSAC)—are equally effective.

Tables 3.1, 3.2 and 3.5 give relevant results of GISSI-1, ISIS- 2, GISSI-2, and ISIS-3.

Thus, until recently no evidence of any real difference in 5-week mortality between SK and tPA or APSAC has been observed despite randomization of over 60,000 patients in ISIS-3 and GISSI-2. Assessment of global and regional LV function 3 weeks after a first infarction indicates similar effects for SK and tPA. It is important to note that tPA must be used in conjunction with IV heparin to achieve excellent late patency rates and avoid reocclusion.

The choice of thrombolytic therapy remains controversial owing to the high cost of tPA and APSAC and the increased incidence of stroke (4/1,000 patients treated) for these two agents (see Fig. 3.3). However, the results of the GUSTO study provided some solution to the controversies and defined the role of IV heparin. The net clinical benefit of the aggressive thrombolytic regimens, of front-loaded tPA which open the infarct vessel faster than previous strategies used along with carefully titrated IV heparin in GUSTO, a 41,021-patient trial in 15 countries and 1,100 hospitals demonstrated a 14% mortality reduction compared with SK or combined tPA and SK published in September 1993. It was shown that a small ↑ in hemorrhagic stroke for these aggressive regimens will be acceptable for the trade-off of a more extensive "net" mortality ↓.

- The choice of tenecteplase, tPA, or SK is of little consequence to public health worldwide, particularly when the real problem is transport to an emergency room (ER) within 2 hours of onset of symptoms and the ER door-to-needle time which is still inexcusably high, in excess of 40 minutes in most hospital facilities.

Indications for Thrombolytic Therapy

- Patients less than or equal to 75 years old, seen within 6 hours of onset of symptoms with clinical and ECG diagnoses consistent with acute MI (with ≥2 mm ST elevation in ≥1 precordial leads or ≥1 mm ST elevation in ≥2 limb leads) are candidates for thrombolytic therapy.

Probable indications include:
- Patients older than age 75 in good general health should *not* be excluded if seen within 6 hours of pain onset where the impending infarction is large or extensive and there is no contraindication to thrombolytic therapy. ISIS-3 indicated that patients older than age 75 showed the greatest benefits. However, thrombolytic therapy should be used with great caution in patients older than age 80 because most studies indicate increased risk of major bleeding in this subset of patients. In one study, SK caused a twofold increased risk of major hemorrhage that resulted in a mortality of 17% in patients older than age 75 and 1% in those younger than age 75. It must be re-emphasized that IV heparin and a thrombolytic agent in patients over age 80 should be used with caution until further large, randomized studies show proven benefit at low risk in these patients. When thrombolytic therapy is considered necessary in healthy patients over age 75 with large infarcts seen within 6 hours, the combination of aspirin and the cautious use of SK is advisable, preferably without heparin use.
- Patients with new LBBB seen within 6 hours of onset of chest pain. This subset represents a high-risk group and was shown to benefit in the ISIS-3 study.
- Patients with new RBBB, proven acute infarction, associated with CHF
- Patients seen within 12 hours from onset of symptoms with evidence of ongoing ischemia: Pain still present or stuttering episodes in the presence of continuing elevation of ST segments and CK and CK-MB elevation (Table 3.6). Caution is required in patients seen after 12 hours because late reperfusion appears to ↑ the risk of myocardial rupture and it is necessary to weigh the risks involved.

Contraindications

Absolute contraindications include:
- Active internal bleeding within the prior weeks
- Suspected aortic dissection

Table 3.6: Effects of allocated treatment on deaths in days 0–35 among (i) all patients and (ii) patients presenting within 0–6 h with ST elevation.

	Fibrinolytic comparisons			Difference %SK–%tPA		Difference %SK–%APSAC	
	SK	tPA	APSAC	%	SD	%	SD
(i) All patients	13,780	13,746	13,773	%	SD	%	SD
Any	1,455 (10.6%)	1,418 (10.3%)	1,448 (10.5%)	0.24	0.37	0.05	0.37
(a) Timing							
Day 0–1	699 (5.1%)	649 (4.7%)	700 (5.1%)	0.35	0.26	-0.01	0.26
Day 2–7	357 (2.6%)	415 (3.0%)	378 (2.7%)	-0.43	0.20*	-0.15	0.19
Day 8–35	399 (2.9%)	3544 (2.6%)	370 (2.7%)	0.32	0.20	0.21	0.20
(b) Antithrombotic allocation							
Aspirin plus sc heparin	726 (10.5%)	684 (10.0%)	722 (10.5%)	0.58	0.52	0.06	0.52
Aspirin alone	729 (10.6%)	734 (10.7%)	726 (10.6%)	-0.09	0.53	0.03	0.52
(ii) 0–6 h, ST elevation	8,643	8,571	8,622	%	SD	%	SD
Any	861 (10.0%)	822 (9.6%)	855 (9.9%)	0.37	0.45	0.05	0.46
(a) Timing							
Day 0–1	421 (4.9%)	389 (4.5%)	408 (4.7%)	0.33	0.32	0.14	0.33
Day 2–7	201 (2.3%)	236 (2.8%)	218 (2.5%)	-0.43	0.24	-0.20	0.23
Day 8–35	239 (2.8%)	197 (2.3%)	229 (2.7%)	0.47	0.24	0.11	0.25
(b) Antithrombotic allocation							
Aspirin plus sc heparin	425 (9.8%)	389 (9.1%)	427 (9.9%)	0.69	0.63	-0.13	0.64
Aspirin alone	436 (10.2%)	433 (10.1%)	428 (9.9%)	0.05	0.65	0.22	0.65

$2p < 0.05$

Source: ISIS-3: A randomized comparison of streptokinase vs. tissue plasminogen activator vs. anistreplase and of aspirin plus heparin vs. aspirin alone among 41,299 cases of suspected acute myocardial infarction. Lancet, 339:759,1992.

- Recent head injury or cerebral neoplasm
- Recent trauma, major surgery within 6 weeks
- Recent prolonged or clearly traumatic cardiopulmonary resuscitation (CPR)
- History of cerebrovascular accident known to be hemorrhagic
- Cerebrovascular accident within 6 months
- Severe hypertension, uncontrolled BP greater than 200/110 mm Hg.

Relative contraindications include:
- Known bleeding diathesis or current use of anticoagulants
- Active peptic ulcer without bleeding; patient on medications
- History of severe hypertension under drug treatment; systolic greater than 180 mm Hg, diastolic greater than 110 mm Hg
- Significant liver dysfunction or esophageal varices
- Underlying malignancy
- Elderly patients who are confused, lethargic, or agitated.

Complications of thrombolytic therapy include:
- Bleeding, especially in patients requiring invasive procedures. Intracranial bleeding reportedly occurs in 0.3-1.4% and is more common in patients older than age 70.
- Rarely myocardial and splenic rupture, cholesterol embolization
- Hypotension and allergic reactions occur in approximately 5-10% with SK or anistreplase.

Streptokinase: *Action*: SK combines with plasminogen to form plasminogen activator complex. The complex converts free plasminogen to plasmin, which causes fibrinogenolysis and independent lysis of fibrin. SK also causes activation of fibrin-bound plasminogen; thus, two independent actions occur. The activator complex has a half-life of about 85 minutes. The extensive coagulation defect begins rapidly after administration, remains intense for about 4-8 hours, and dwindles over the following 36-48 hours.

About 65% of coronary reperfusion rate is observed when 1.5 million U of the drug is given within 3 hours of onset of symptoms of infarction.

Dosage: See Table 3.4. *Adverse effects*: Allergic reactions are seen in about 2% of patients. Edema, bronchospasm, angioneurotic edema, anaphylaxis reported in 0.1-0.5% with apparently no fatalities. Hypotension occurs in 6-8% of patients but usually is responsive to fluid administration.

Anistreplase (Eminase): APSAC is a 1:1 molecular combination of plasminogen and SK with a catalytic center protected by a chemical group.

Anistreplase is activated in the bloodstream; deacylation to the active complex begins immediately and continues at a constant rate with a half-life of about 90 minutes. An advantage over SK is the ease of administration by slow IV bolus. The drug produces about a 60% patency rate in about 40 minutes with persistence of activity for 4-6 hours. This agent is approximately as effective as SK or conventional dosing tPA in achieving vessel patency and this effect is enhanced by routine aspirin use. Concomitant heparin therapy is not advisable. *Dosage*: See Table 3.4.

Tissue plasminogen activator (Activase): Tissue type plasminogen activator is the physiologic activator of plasminogen but has a higher affinity for fibrin-bound plasminogen. However, tPA's specificity for fibrin-bound plasminogen is relative and dose dependent. Activation of free plasminogen occurs with increasing dosage and blood levels of tPA. Thus, bleeding complications are similar to SK.

Because tPA therapy results in a significantly faster-achieved higher vessel patency rate (85% at 90 minutes) than SK, and tPA was used in ISIS-3 without the necessary combination with IV heparin for 6 days, further randomized studies using different heparin regimens are in progress. The net clinical outcome (total death plus stroke) in ISIS-3 was similar (11.1%) in the SK versus the tPA-treated group. As outlined earlier, the GUSTO trial showed accelerated TPA led to a significant 14% mortality reduction compared with SK. The preferred dose of tPA is a 15-mg bolus, 50 mg over 30 minutes, and the remaining 35 mg over the next 30 minutes. Plasma clearance is decreased with hepatic dysfunction and the drug is not advisable in patients who have hepatic disease. *Dosage*: See Table 3.4. *Adverse effects*: These are essentially the same as listed under SK, except that allergic reactions do not occur and hypotension from the drug per se is quite unusual. Hypotension with all thrombolytics can occur as a result of the Bezold–Jarisch reflex.

Reteplase, a recombinant plasminogen activator, is as effective as SK when administered as two IV boluses of 10 million U, 30 minutes apart.

Tenecteplase: TNKase is a genetically engineered triple-combination mutant of native tPA. In ASSENT-2, the drug caused a similar mortality reduction as did tPA in patients administered the drug less than 4 hours from onset, but it was superior in patients treated more than 4 hours. The major advantage is the ease of single bolus injection; TNKase has replaced tPA in many institutions.

The ASSENT-3 trial randomized patients with ST elevation MI to receive one of three treatment strategies: full-dose tenecteplase with unfractionated heparin, full-dose TNKase with enoxaparin, or half-dose TNKase with abciximab and unfractionated heparin.

- Results of the trial indicated that the use of enoxaparin with standard dose fibrinolysis provides a similar reduction in mortality and cardiac events as combination of reduced dose of thrombolytic agent plus abciximab without an increased risk of major hemorrhage.

Dosage for tenecteplase:
- Less than 60 kg   30 mg in 6 mL over 5 seconds
- 60–70 kg   35 mg in 7 mL fluid
- 70–80 kg   40 mg in 8 mL
- 80–90 kg   45 mg in 9 mL
- Greater than 90 kg   50 mg in 10 mL.

Beta-blocker Therapy

Sufficient attention has not been paid by the medical profession and researchers regarding the subtle differences that exist amongst the available β-blocking drugs.
- Of the cardioselective agents only propranolol, timolol and metoprolol have been shown to significantly reduce coronary heart disease mortality and events in RCTs. Bisoprolol has not been tried in trials of patients with MI, but was beneficial in heart failure (HF) trial. A most popular cardioselective agent, atenolol, is used worldwide and is not advisable.
- Brain concentration: Lipophilicity allows high concentration of drug in the brain; appears to block sympathetic discharge in the hypothalamus and elevates central vagal tone to a greater extent than water soluble.

  Hydrophilic agents, such as atenolol, and this may relate to the prevention of sudden cardiac death. It appears that this information has not reached clinicians or researchers.
- Atenolol a widely used β-blocker is poorly effective and is no advisable. The drug should be rendered obsolete and should not be used in clinical trials.

The two agents, timolol and propranolol proven to reduce cardiac deaths particularly sudden death in post-MI patients (= high-risk patients) are rarely used (see Table 3.1).

Acute coronary occlusion producing anteroseptal or anterior MI is often associated with sinus tachycardia. Necrotic tissue is surrounded for a time by a zone of severe myocardial ischemia and injury that causes pain. Both ischemia and pain initiate catecholamine release, and the vicious circle is perpetuated. During the early phase of infarction, the amount of myocardial damage is not fixed and a dynamic process is usually in evolution.

Beta-blockers have a proven beneficial effect when relieving pain, ischemia, and injury current during the early phase of acute MI. Decreased mortality, modest ↓ in infarct size, and ↓ in the reinfarction rates have been documented in patients given IV β-blockers, followed by oral therapy from day 1 and for 30–90 days, as well as up to 2 years postinfarction. The early ↓ in mortality and infarction rates have been modest, but sufficiently significant to warrant early β-blocker therapy for all patients with anterior or anteroseptal infarcts, especially in those with sinus tachycardia, provided that the systolic BP is greater than 100 mm Hg and there is no contraindication to β-blockade. If adverse effects are feared, esmolol IV is advisable since its action dissipates in about 10 minutes. IV use during acute MI. *Dosage*: See Table 3.4.

The merits of β-adrenergic blockade in ischemic syndromes are given in Flowchart 3.2.
- Decrease in HR prolongs the diastolic interval during which coronary perfusion normally occurs. Thus, an ↑ in blood flow may ensue to

ischemic areas of myocardium. Necrotic tissue is not capable of salvage, but the area subject to infarction may remain ischemic for several hours, and increased perfusion to ischemic areas may limit the ultimate size of infarction.
- Sinus tachycardia causes increased O_2 demand and can shift the balance in ischemic tissue toward necrosis; sinus tachycardia decreases VF threshold. Beta-blockers relieve sinus tachycardia and associated hypertension and ↑ VF threshold; some trials showed ↓ in the incidence of VF.
- Beta-blockers ↓ phase 4 depolarization and thus suppress arrhythmias that may arise in ischemic tissue, especially when initiated by catecholamines.
- Decrease in myocardial contractility decreases O_2 requirement.
- Decrease in stress on infarcting tissue by the remaining myocardium appears to be responsible for the modest but important ↓ in the incidence of early myocardial rupture due to acute infarction.
- In patients given thrombolytics, there is currently no confirmation of experimental findings that viability of ischemic myocardium is prolonged. However, β-blockers have been shown to ↓ the incidence of post-thrombolytic ischemic events in patients.
- Where there is some residual patency of the infarct-related artery, β-blockers do exert a strong anti-ischemic effect and will ↓ infarct size; in this group of patients, perhaps equivalent to non-Q wave infarction, β-blockers have been demonstrated to have a major impact on pain and serious events.

Clinical trials have not adequately tested the use of β-blockers during the first 3 hours of onset of symptoms. The metoprolol in acute myocardial infarction (MIAMI) trial is often quoted as showing a lack of effectiveness of early β-blocker use in reducing mortality. However, the mean treatment time was 11 hours. In ISIS-1, 80% of patients were treated up to 8 hours and less than 30% within 4 hours of onset, resulting in a 15% ↓ in cardiovascular mortality with significant prevention of early myocardial rupture. Beta-blockers were given to 720 patients at about 3–4 hours after onset of symptoms in TIMI 2-B and resulted in a 47% ↓ in the incidence of reinfarction in 6 days; also, the incidence of recurrent chest pain was significantly decreased. However, a ↓ in mortality and myocardial rupture was not observed in TIMI 2, probably due to the small number of patients studied, resulting in a type II error. Pooled trial results with the use of β-blockade covering mainly 4–6 hours from onset of symptoms indicate a 23% ↓ in mortality occurring on day 1, then no significant ↓ during the next few weeks.

Early IV followed by oral β-blocker therapy should be strongly considered for all patients presenting with definite or probable acute infarction, in whom contraindications do not exist.

These agents are particularly strongly indicated in the following situations:
- Sinus tachycardia unassociated with hypotension or clinically apparent CHF
- Rapid ventricular response to atrial fibrillation (AF) or flutter
- Administration of thrombolytic agents: To prevent arrhythmias and/or ischemia and improve survival
- Recurrent ischemic pain
- Moderate impairment of LV function with frequent or complex ventricular ectopy after the first week postinfarction.

Nitroglycerin: In patients with anterior infarction, there is an evidence to suggest that IV nitroglycerin causes a slight ↓ in mortality. The American College of Cardiology/American Heart Association (ACC/AHA) Task Force considers the data inadequate to recommend the routine use of IV nitroglycerin in patients with uncomplicated acute MI.

Intravenous nitroglycerin is not recommended in patients with uncomplicated MI. Cutaneous preparations have a role in some patients without hypotension for the relief of chest discomfort.

Indications include:
- Relief of chest pain unresponsive to morphine and β-blockers
- Stuttering pattern of pain indicating continued ischemia
- Moderate to severe CHF or pulmonary edema complicating acute MI and pulmonary capillary wedge pressure (PCWP) greater than 20 mm Hg.

Contraindications include:
- Hypovolemia
- Inferior infarction: Nitroglycerin is used cautiously only when needed to manage postinfarction angina and/or pulmonary edema, since hypotension may be precipitated
- Right ventricular infarction
- Cardiac tamponade
- Significant hypoxemia: IV nitroglycerin may accentuate hypoxemia by increasing ventilation–perfusion mismatch.

Adverse effects: These include worsening of hypoxemia and severe hypotension that may ↑ ischemia. Preload ↓ may cause hypotension. Rarely, nitrates precipitate bradycardia and hypotension responsive to atropine. Oral, cutaneous, and other nitrates, including interaction with heparin, are discussed further in other chapter.

Dosage: See Infusion Pump Chart in Chapter 1. Commence with a 5 mg bolus injection then ↑ the dose by 5–10 µg/minute q 5 or 10 minutes to abolish chest pain and/or to achieve a mean arterial pressure ↓ of 10% and a maximal ↓ of 20% in hypertensive patients. The systolic BP must not be allowed to fall under 95 mm Hg or diastolic less than 60 mm Hg. HR should be maintained less than 110/minute. Nitrate tolerance develops after about

48 hours use of IV nitroglycerin, but in unstable patients, the dose is titrated up as required rather than leaving a nitrate-free interval.

Lidocaine (Lignocaine, UK): In the first 24–48 hours, ventricular premature contractions (VPCs) and short runs of VT bear little relation to the occurrence of VF. R on T is an exception but usually appears less than 2 minutes before VF. Lidocaine is far from completely effective in preventing VF, and inexperienced staff are often tempted quite unnecessarily to push the dose to toxic levels to "control" VPCs, which are, in the main, quite harmless.

Probable indications include:
- Frequent VPCs, causing hemodynamic disturbance in the absence of bradycardia where atropine is advisable
- Sustained VT (see Fig. 6.4)
- Following VT occurring in the first 24 hours of infarction, lidocaine is given for 48 hours
- Post VF or for repetitive VF.

Recent trials and meta-analysis suggest that prophylactic lidocaine may actually ↑ mortality because of its ability to cause asystole.

Contraindications include: Sinoatrial dysfunction, which may precipitate sinus arrest; A-V block, all grades, which can cause asystole; patients recovering from asystole; idioventricular rhythm; severe CHF; porphyria. Relative contraindications include sinus bradycardia.

The prophylactic use of lidocaine in acute MI remains controversial in the United States and its widespread use has been greatly curtailed. The drug is associated with an ↑ in the occurrence of asystole. In the early hours of infarction, VF occurs in approximately 5% of patients and many patients must be treated to prevent some episodes of VF. A meta-analysis of 14 randomized trials indicated that lidocaine reduced the incidence of VF 33% without a ↓ in mortality. In areas where facilities for monitoring cardiac rhythm and/or for defibrillation are lacking or inadequate, the drug has a role. In heavily monitored units, lidocaine is unnecessary, and the cost is not justified. *Dosage*—bolus IV 1.0–1.5 mg/kg, 75–100 mg over 5 minutes, during which time a continuous infusion of 2 mg/minute for a 70- to 80-kg patient younger than age 70 is commenced (Table 3.5). An additional bolus of 50% of the original amount given 10 minutes after the first bolus prevents a dip in plasma level below the therapeutic range, which commonly occurs 20–60 minutes after starting the infusion. In the elderly, bolus 0.75 mg/kg, then if needed, 25–30 mg IV bolus. Do not allow a time lapse of minutes between the bolus and commencement of the infusion, as inadequate blood levels may ensue. Halve the dose in patients with CHF, shock, hepatic dysfunction, or concomitant use of a hepatic-metabolized β-blocker or cimetidine (Box 3.1).

Box 3.1: Warnings to avoid lidocaine (lignocaine) toxicity.
- Reduce bolus dose and infusion rate in the elderly (over age 70).
- Determine the dose utilizing lean body weight.
- Decrease the dose in heart failure, hypotension, cardiogenic shock.
- Decrease dosage with hepatic dysfunction or concomitant use of cimetidine, propranolol, or drugs that decrease hepatic blood flow or metabolism.
- Previous seizure activity or central nervous system disease
- Determine blood levels if infusion rates are high (≥4 mg/mL/min) or neurologic adverse effects

If frequent multiform ventricular ectopy persists, resulting in hemodynamic disturbance, an additional bolus, 0.5–1 mg/kg, is given q 10 minutes for 2 or 3 doses if deemed necessary, and the infusion rate is increased to 3 mg/minute. Re-evaluate the clinical situation, including serum K, magnesium, presence of bradycardia or sinus tachycardia, and contraindications, and factors that ↑ lidocaine toxicity prior to increasing the rate to a maximum 4 mg/minute for a patient less than 200 lbs (90 kg). *Adverse effects*: The incidence of asystole appears to be increased by lidocaine use. Confusion, seizures, drowsiness, dizziness, lip or tongue numbness, slurred speech, muscle twitching, double vision, tremor, altered consciousness, respiratory depression or arrest, complete heart block in patients with impaired A-V conduction, hypotension due to peripheral vasodilation.

Calcium Antagonists

In a very small study of 288 postinfarction patients treated with diltiazem, 11 patients died, as opposed to 9 patients in the placebo group; diltiazem decreased infarction rates at 2 weeks. This small, short-term study has been used to advance the claim that diltiazem is the drug of choice in the management of non-Q wave infarction. Physicians have extended the drug's use to other ischemic syndromes with the hope that the drug will prevent reinfarction, but without bearing in mind that the drug does not significantly ↓ the cardiac death rate.

A second large, well-run study of 2,466 postinfarction patients treated with diltiazem showed an ↑ in total mortality due to diltiazem in patients with LV dysfunction. Thus, diltiazem is not recommended in acute MI, Q wave or non-Q wave, if signs of LV dysfunction are present or if the EF is less than 40% (see Fig. 3.2). There was a trend in favor of a ↓ in total events (death and/or reinfarction) in the small number of patients with non-Q wave infarction treated for 1 year with diltiazem, but the evidence from this overall negative study is not sound enough to recommend diltiazem to all patients with non-Q wave infarction. In the absence of ongoing chest pain, diltiazem has an uncertain role in the management of non-Q wave infarction in patients with good LV function, who are unable to take a β-blocking drug and in whom further interventional therapy in the form of angioplasty or bypass surgery is contraindicated because of underlying ill health or age.

It is clear that Ca antagonists have no role in the routine management of acute MI. Meta-analysis indicates that this group of drugs does not significantly ↓ infarct size, infarction rates, or mortality in patients with acute MI. Nifedipine used without a β-blocking drug in patients with unstable angina may ↑ chest pain and shows no beneficial trend in mortality. Dihydropyridines should be avoided in patients with acute MI since they may ↑ HR and vasodilation may cause a ↓ in BP. Also, Ca antagonists may ↓ BP during the early hours of infarction. A ↓ in BP may contraindicate the use of lifesaving medications: β-blockers, thrombolytic agents, IV nitroglycerin, and/or angiotensin-converting enzyme (ACE) inhibitors.

Verapamil should not be used in patients with acute MI because of its negative inotropic effect and strong propensity to precipitate CHF, sinus arrest, or asystole. The drug is advisable in selected patients with supraventricular tachycardia (SVT) or AF with an uncontrolled ventricular response after a trial of β-blockers or digoxin in the absence of CHF.

Diltiazem is not indicated in acute MI since it increases mortality in patients who manifest LV dysfunction or in those with an EF less than 40%. Ca antagonists are not advisable in patients with acute MI and concomitant, severe chronic obstructive pulmonary disease (COPD) since these agents may increase hypoxemia.

Diabetic Sitosterolemia

Diabetes heart attacks can be prevented by reducing blood sitosterol levels.

Abnormally high blood sitosterol causes atheromatous coronary artery disease (CAD) and fatal MI in young adults with sitosterolemia, in which mutations in either ABCG5 or G8 proteins cause intestinal hyperabsorption of sitosterol.

Diabetics restrict carbohydrates and, of necessity, consume much vegetable plant foods and shellfish containing sitosterol.
- About 1 million diabetics die annually in India. Tight glucose control in RCTs has not shown significantly improved outcomes. Although LDL-C definitely causes atheroma and MI, it cannot account for the epidemic of deaths caused by diabetes (1.5 million in China).
- A novel study conducted by the author is the first to show that 12–14 hours fasting sitosterol blood levels are abnormally high in patients with

type II diabetes mellitus, particularly in those with CAD, with levels reaching 100% more than observed in nondiabetic.
- Dietary restriction of sitosterol-containing foods and treatment with ezetimibe or with more effective agents to be developed would improve outcomes, particularly heart attacks, stroke, nephropathy, amputations caused by atheromatous peripheral vascular disease (PVD) and perhaps blindness in diabetic patients.

BIBLIOGRAPHY

1. A randomised trial of propranolol in patients with acute myocardial infarction. I. Mortality results. JAMA. 1982;247:1707-14.
2. Acute myocardial infarction in women. Lancet. 2016;387(10018):506.
3. Assessment of the Safety and Efficacy of a New Thrombolytic (ASSENT-2) Investigators, Van De Werf F, Adgey J, et al. Single-bolus tenecteplase compared with front-loaded alteplase in acute myocardial infarction: The ASSENT-2 double-blind randomised trial. Lancet. 1999;354:716-22.
4. Chen ZM, Pan HC, Chen YP, et al. Early intravenous then oral metoprolol in 45,852 patients with acute myocardial infarction: randomised placebo-controlled trial. Lancet. 2005;366:1622-32.
5. Collins R, Peto R, Baigent C, et al. Aspirin, heparin and fibrinolytic therapy in suspected acute myocardial infarction. N Engl J Med. 1997;336:847-60.
6. Effectiveness of intravenous thrombolytic treatment in acute myocardial infarction. Gruppo Italiano per lo Studio della Streptochinasi nell'Infarto Miocardico (GISSI). Lancet. 1986;1:397-402.
7. Global Use of Strategies to Open Occluded Coronary Arteries (GUSTO III) Investigators. A comparison of reteplase with alteplase for acute myocardial infarction. N Engl J Med. 1997;337:1118-23.
8. Goyal A, Spertus JA, Gosch K, et al. Serum potassium levels and mortality in acute myocardial infarction. JAMA. 2012;307(2):157-64.
9. Gruppo Italiano per lo Studio della Sopravvivenza Nell 'Infarto Miocardico (1990) GISSI-2: a factorial randomised trial of alteplase versus streptokinase and heparin versus no heparin among 12,490 patients with acute myocardial infarction. Gruppo Italiano per lo Studio della Sopravvivenza nell'Infarto Miocardico. Lancet. 1990;336:65-71.
10. GUSTO Investigators. An international randomized trial comparing four thrombolytic strategies for acute myocardial infarction. N Engl J Med. 1993;329:673-82.
11. Henderson RA, Jarvis C, Clayton T, et al. 10-year mortality outcome of a routine invasive strategy versus a selective invasive strategy in non-ST-segment elevation acute coronary syndrome: the British Heart Foundation RITA-3 Randomized Trial. J Am Coll Cardiol. 2015;66:511-20.
12. ISIS Steering Committee. Intravenous streptokinase given within 0-4 hours of onset of myocardial infarction reduced mortality in ISIS-2. Lancet. 1987;1:502.
13. ISIS-3: a randomized comparison of streptokinase vs tissue plasminogen activator vs. anistreplase and of aspirin plus heparin vs aspirin alone among 41,299 cases of suspected acute myocardial infarction. ISIS-3 (Third International Study of Infarct Survival) Collaborative Group. Lancet. 1992;339:753-70.

14. Khan GM. A new electrode placement method for obtaining 12-lead ECGs. Open Heart. 2015;2:e000226.
15. Khan GM. Sitosterol blood levels are elevated in diabetics and may be the cause of coronary artery disease and stroke. J Med Sci. 2017;3(2):89-94.
16. Khan MG, Topol EJ. Acute myocardial infarction. In: Khan MG, Bartlett JG, Chopra S, Topol EJ (Eds). Medical Diagnosis and Therapy, 1st edition. Pennsylvania: Lea and Febiger; 1994.
17. Norwegian Multicenter Study Group. Timolol-induced reduction in mortality and reinfarction in patients surviving acute myocardial infarction. N Engl J Med. 1981;304:801-7.
18. Randomised trial of intravenous streptokinase, oral aspirin, both, or neither, among 17,187 cases of suspected acute myocardial infarction: ISIS-2 (Second International Study of Infarct Survival) Collaborative Group. Lancet. 1988;2:349-60.
19. Six-month effects of early treatment with lisinopril and transdermal glyceryl trinitrate singly and together withdrawn six weeks after acute myocardial infarction: the GISSI-3 trial. Gruppo Italiano per lo Studio della Sopravvivenza nell'Infarto Miocardico. J Am Coll Cardiol. 1996;27:337-44.
20. Thygesen K, Alpert JS, Jaffe AS, et al. Third universal definition of myocardial infarction. J Am Coll Cardiol. 2012;60:1581-98.
21. Widimsky P, Budesinsky T, Vorac D, et al. Long distance transport for primary angioplasty vs immediate thrombolysis in acute myocardial infarction. Final results of the randomized national multicentre trial: PRAGUE-2. Eur Heart J. 2003;24:94-104.

CHAPTER 4

Sitosterolemia

INTRODUCTION

Sitosterol is elevated in diabetics and causes coronary artery disease (CAD), myocardial infarction (MI), and stroke.

Patients with type 2 diabetes mellitus have an extraordinarily high incidence of MI and stroke. Our medical therapies that effectively control hyperglycemia do not significantly reduce the incidence of MI and stroke caused mainly by atheroma. Thus, the author searched for culprits other than hyperglycemia and low-density lipoprotein cholesterol (LDL-C). A *"Holmes"* deduction dictated the following thinking.

- Meat consumption is harmful for a few individuals; elevation of LDL-C is known to cause atheroma and MI.
- Carbohydrates are harmful for some by causing hyperglycemia and overweight.
- If two of three much consumed foods cause harm, should we exempt the third large group, vegetable plant foods? A culprit may be lurking within.
  - In addition, diabetics consume much vegetable plant foods that contain sitosterol.
  - This plant sterol, sitosterol, is used worldwide as an herbal remedy.
  - Clinicians and researchers are unaware that sitosterol is a harmful substance consumed by most diabetics.
  - Sitosterol is known to cause severe atheromatous CAD, resulting in fatal MI in children and young adults with genetic familial sitosterolemia.[1,2]
  - In this disease, mutations in either ABCG5 or G8 proteins cause intestinal hyperabsorption of sitosterol.[3,4]
  - This genetic intestinal defect is present in diabetics and in a small genetic study of six diabetics. Postprandial levels of sitosterol were significantly higher in than in six nondiabetic subjects.[5] 12-hour fasting sitosterol was not assessed.

AN OVERVIEW

The genetic disease sitosterolemia alerted the attention of the author to two genuine causes of atheroma of vital arteries, LDL-C and sitosterol.
- Elevated blood sitosterol is the culprit, causing heart attacks, stroke, and probably nephropathy, neuropathy and retinopathy in diabetics because glucose or its metabolism cannot cause these pathologic changes.
- Bhattacharyya and Connor (1974) reported on a lipid storage disease in two sisters. Because of markedly elevated plasma and tissue sitosterol levels, premature atherosclerosis develops.
- Salen et al. (1985) described the autopsy findings from an 18-year-old white male who died suddenly of an acute MI. From age 10, he had noted tendon xanthomas that began on the left elbow and back and then subsequently in the Achilles tendons, knees, and wrists. Measurements of plasma sterols 4 years prior to death revealed high concentrations of plant sterols with mild hypercholesterolemia and a diagnosis of sitosterolemia with xanthomatosis was established.
- Plasma concentrations of sitosterol above 10 mg/L are diagnostic of sitosterolemia.
- Sitosterolemia is a recessively inherited disorder that results from mutations in either ABCG5 or G8 proteins, with intestinal hyperabsorption of dietary sterols and decreased hepatic excretion of plant sterols.[3,4]
- Diabetics have a genetic defect in the pancreas and a genetic defect in the intestine that causes increased absorption of sitosterol.
- At present, this intestinal genetic defect that causes increased intestinal absorption of sitosterol and other plant sterols is virtually unknown to the medical profession or public at large.
- There is no doubt that elevated blood sitosterol causes rampant atherosclerosis and is harmful.
- The author conducted a study of 40 patients with type 2 diabetes and controls that showed abnormally high blood levels of sitosterol in diabetic subjects.[6]

Twelve-hour fasting blood sitosterol levels were assessed. 78.3% of diabetic subjects with CAD showed elevated levels 5.1–9.5 mg/L[6] (Tables 4.1 and 4.2). Normal reference ranges 0–5 mg/L.
- 44% of diabetic patients showed levels beyond 5 mg/L.
- 100% control subjects [17] showed levels 0.7–3.5 mg/L.
- Vegetarians 4.0–4.2 mg/L.
  - Importantly, mild diabetics on no medications or one oral drug had high levels.
  - The intensity of hyperglycemia bears no relation to the finding of elevated blood sitosterol. The defect genetic defect in the pancreas and intestine are independent.

Table 4.1 Albumin–creatinine ratio, (ALB/CR), sitosterol and campesterol blood levels, and presence of CVD for each diabetic subject.

Subject	Albumin–creatinine ratio	Microalbumin	Diabetes severity	Sitosterol mg/L	Campesterol	Vascular disease
*1	271	2336	+++	9.0	8.3	CAD, nephropathy
2	1.3	13.7	+	5.3	8.3	CAD
3	0.5	<5	+	9.2	7.2	CAD
4	<2	22	+	5.1	7.8	CAD
5	13.2	179	+++	5.4	6.8	CAD; nephropathy
**6	3.9	42.8	+++	6.6	7.4	CAD; nephropathy
7	<2	<5	+++	6.3	9.2	CAD
**8	185	77	+++	8.3	11.2	CAD, nephropathy
9	<1.0	6.9	+	5.2	6.4	CAD
10	11	3.7	+	3.2	4.1	CAD
11	<1	7.3	++	2.9	4.2	BP
12	<1	7.3	+	2.6	4.1	BP
13	<1	5.6	+	4.1	4.8	CAD
14	<2	<5	+	3.0	4.5	BP
15	<2	<5	+	2.3	5.2	BP
**16	5.7	78.7	+	4.4	6.2	CAD
17	1.9	5.3	+	6.1	8.0	CAD
18	<2	<5	+++	8.7	15.7	CAD
19	<2	<5	+	5.2	8.0	CAD
20	<2	<5	++	1.2	4.2	BP
**21	<1	5.9	+	7.9	12.5	CAD
22	<2	<5	+	1.2	2.0	BP
23	1.2	15.2	+	6.4	10.8	CAD
24	<2	<1	+	0.7	1.7	BP
**25	3.3	36	+	4.2	6.0	BP
26	8.9	96	+	2.8	4.2	Arrhythmia
**27	5.4	87.5	+++	3.3	5.2	CAD
28	4.3	73	+	3.7	6.8	BP
29	5.2	20.2	+	6.9	7.8	CAD
**30	<1.0	7.9	+	3.2	4.2	BP

Contd...

Contd...

Subject	Albumin–creatinine ratio	Microalbumin	Diabetes severity	Sitosterol mg/L	Campesterol	Vascular disease
31	<2.0	<2	+	3.6	6.5	BP
32	<2	<2	+	3.6	6.8	BP
*33	102.3	880.2	+	6.4	7.9	CAD; nephropathy
34	1.2	9.5	+	3.6	2.5	BP
35	2.7	17.3	++	3.7	5.3	arrhythmia
#36	253.9	802.0	++	3.4	5.0	CAD; nephropathy
#37	<1	<5	-	5.4	9.4	CAD
38	<2	<5	++	7.8	6.0	CAD
**39	<2	<5	+	4.2	7.5	BP
40	0.8	3	++	3.5	6.5	BP

CAD: Coronary artery disease; BP: Blood pressure; +Mild diabetes: One oral drug or two at half dosage; ++Moderate intensity: Duration >10 years: On two oral drugs; one at full dose, second at half dosage; #36: Patient disabled, vegetable metal intake night before test, unknown unreliable; #37 proven diabetes mellitus: (-) very mild, on no medications: mother, father and 4 siblings all are diabetics; +++m Moderately severe: Two oral drugs at maximum dose or added insulin; *e-glomerular filtration rate <25 mL/min; **Test done ~16 hours after food.

EZETIMIBE: A NEW DRUG FOR DIABETICS

Ezetimibe reduces both blood cholesterol and sitosterol levels and is used to treat sitosterolemia. Sitosterol concentrations decreased by 21% (P <0.001) in patients treated with ezetimibe compared with a nonsignificant 4% rise in those on placebo (between group P <0.001.[7] A more effective agent that can decrease sitosterol more than 40% is needed.

- In IMPROVE-IT, a RCT of patients with acute MI, the benefit of the simvastatin-ezetimibe combination, was *"particularly pronounced in patients with diabetes mellitus"*.[8-11] This salutary effect was likely due to lowering of LDL-C and importantly, sitosterol.

Recommended New Therapy for Diabetics

- Ezetimibe is indicated as adjunctive therapy to diet for the reduction of elevated sitosterol and campesterol levels in patients with homozygous familial sitosterolemia.
- Our study shows that diabetics have hypersitosterolemia[6] and ezetimibe is therefore indicated as adjunctive therapy to diet for the reduction

Table 4.2. Nondiabetic subjects.			
Control subjects	Sitosterol, mg/L	Campesterol	Vascular disease
1	1.5	2.3	CAD
2	2.4	3.5	CAD
3	2.8	4.5	BP
4	2.9	3.8	CAD
5	2.8	5.9	CAD
6	2.6	3.8	CAD
7	1.2	3	Cardiomyopathy
8	2.4	3.6	CAD
9	2.0	3.3	CAD
10	1.0	1.8	CAD
11	1.4	1.6	CAD
12	1.5	2.2	CAD
13	3.6	6.5	BP
14	2.3	2	CAD
#15	4.2	6.7	Cardiomyopathy
#16	4	6.8	BP
#17	4.2	8.5	BP

CAD: Coronary artery disease; BP: Blood pressure;
#Vegetarian requested to have large vegetable meal with added avocado.

of elevated sitosterol.[6] More effective sitosterol inhibitors should be developed.
- All diabetic patients with elevated sitosterol levels should be treated with a statin and ezetimibe and diet restriction of sitosterol-containing foods.
- All diabetics particularly those with family history of CAD or stroke require treatment with ezetimibe 10 mg/day added to their statin medication, preferably atorvastatin or rosuvastatin.
- Elevated blood sitosterol 4.5–10 mg/L may be the cause of nephropathy and retinopathy and caution is required. Further studies are underway in diabetic patients with retinopathy.
- Until results are available all patients with retinopathy should be treated with ezetimibe and diet.

Ezetimibe Suggested Dosage

About 50% of diabetic patients are expected to have sitosterolemia.
- Ezetimibe reduces blood sitosterol approximately 21%.[7]
- For each category given below consumption of sitosterol-containing foods should be minimized (see later).

Dosage: 12-hour Fasting Sitosterol Level
- 8–10 mg/L   20 mg daily
- 4.5–7.9 mg/L   10 mg daily
- *Sitosterol level not determined because of cost, or unavailable*: advise 10 mg daily, diet and statins.

FOODS WITH HIGH-SITOSTEROL CONTENT

- Avocado
- Pistachio, peanuts and other nuts, olives, chocolate
- Shellfish
- Canola, corn, safflower, coconut oils have a high content of sitosterol and should be minimized.
- *Soyoil and flaxseed has a much lower level.*
- Bran rice, red rice, polished rice are high in sitosterol and used much in China and far East. White rice, fruit and several vegetables are relatively low in sitosterol content.

SITOSTEROL IN NONDIABETIC PATIENTS

Most important, it is not inconceivable that some nondiabetic patients with MI or stroke may have increased sitosterol levels.
- Patients with mild diabetes had high sitosterol levels;[6] thus, the genetic defect may not be confined to diabetics.
- Luister et al. (2015) in a small study of 104 patients evaluated the relationship between phytosterols, oxyphytosterols, and other markers of cholesterol metabolism and concomitant CAD in patients with severe aortic stenosis who were scheduled for elective aortic valve replacement.[12]
- The absolute values for the cholesterol absorption markers, sitosterol and campesterol were increased by 18.18 ± 11.59 ng/mg (38.8%) and 11.40 ± 8.69 ng/mg (30.4%) in aortic valve tissues from patients with documented CAD compared to those without concomitant CAD.
- The study of aortic valve tissues did not assess fasting sitosterol blood levels; diabetics were few.

Miettinen et al. (2005) found that the higher the absorption of cholesterol the higher is the plant sterol content of serum and atherosclerotic plaques, which they studied following carotid endarterectomy.[13]
- In that study, in which they divided the plaques into high, medium and low cholesterol, the low cholesterol plaques had the highest noncholesterol sterols.[13]
- In 4S, no reduction was observed in recurrence of coronary heart disease (CHD) with simvastatin in patients with high baseline plant sterol contents and with marked increase of serum plant sterols during the 5-year treatment period and only assessed desmosterol, lathosterol,

and Campesterol, not sitosterol.[14] Only sitosterol, not tested by these investigators, is known to cause atheroma formation and progression.
- Also, simvastatin does not decrease levels of sitosterol because it does not prevent hyperabsorption of plant sterols.
- PROCAM studied each of 159 men who suffered an acute MI or sudden coronary death within 10 years of follow-up and were matched with two controls (N = 318) by age, smoking status, and date of investigation.[15]
Analysis was performed using conditional logistic regression. Plasma sitosterol concentrations were mildly elevated in cases compared with controls (4.94 ± 3.44 µmol/L vs 4.27 ± 2.38 µmol/L; P = 0.028).
- The upper quartile of sitosterol (>5.25 µmol/L) was associated with a 1.8-fold increase in risk (P <0.05) compared with the lower three quartiles.[15-17]
- Among men with an absolute coronary risk greater than or equal to 20% in 10 years as calculated using the PROCAM algorithm, high sitosterol concentrations were associated with an additional threefold increase in the incidence of coronary events.[18-20]
- Because the intestinal genetic abnormality that exists in patients with diabetes mellitus is variable and may occur in those with mild diabetes regardless of glucose levels, it remains possible that some nondiabetics with CAD may have this genetic disturbance.
- The available data cannot confirm an increased risk in nondiabetics with sitosterol, but cannot rule it out either.
- Studies are needed in nondiabetics, particularly in individuals age 25-35 with a family history of CAD and in patients admitted with acute coronary syndrome.
- Most important sitosterol is not a marker of CAD but is a genuine cause as is LDL-C.

REFERENCES

1. Bhattacharyya AK, Connor WE. Beta-sitosterolemia and xanthomatosis. A newly described lipid storage disease in two sisters. J Clin Invest. 1974;53:1033-43.
2. Salen G, Horak I, Rothkopf M, et al. Lethal atherosclerosis associated with abnormal plasma and tissue sterol composition in sitosterolemia with xanthomatosis. J. Lipid Res. 1985;26:1126-33.
3. Lee M, Lu K, Patel SB. Genetic basis of sitosterolemia. Curr Opin Lipidol. 2001;12(2):141-9.
4. Hazard SE, Patel SB. Sterolins ABCG5 and ABCG8: regulators of whole body dietary sterols. Pflugers Arch. 2007;453:745-52.
5. Lally SE, Owens D, Tomkin GH. Sitosterol and cholesterol in chylomicrons of type 2 diabetic and non-diabetic subjects: the relationship with ATP binding cassette proteins G5 and G8 and Niemann-Pick C1-like 1 mRNA. Diabetologia. 2007;50(1):217-9.
6. Khan GM. Sitosterol blood levels are elevated in diabetics and may be the cause of coronary artery disease and stroke. J Med Sci. 2017;3(3):89-94.

7. Salen G, von Bergmann K, Lutjohann D, et al. Ezetimibe effectively reduces plasma plant sterols in patients with sitosterolemia. Circulation. 2004;109:966-71.
8. Cannon CP, Blazing MA, Giugliano RP, et al. Ezetimibe added to statin therapy after acute coronary syndromes. N Engl J Med. 2015;372:2387-97.
9. Go AS, Mozaffarian D, Roger VL, et al. Executive summary: heart disease and stroke statistics—2013 update: a report from the American Heart Association. Circulation. 2013;127:143-52.
10. Centers for Disease Control and Prevention. National Diabetes Fact Sheet: national estimates and general information on diabetes and prediabetes in the United States, 2011. Atlanta, GA: US Department of Health and Human Services, Centers for Disease Control and Prevention; 2011.
11. Duckworth W, Abraira C, Moritz T, et al. Glucose control and vascular complications in Veterans with type 2 diabetes. N Engl J Med. 2009;360:129-39.
12. Luister A, Schött HF, Husche C, et al. Increased plant sterol deposition in vascular tissue characterizes patients with severe aortic stenosis and concomitant coronary artery disease. Steroids. 2015;99(Pt B):272-80.
13. Miettinen TA, Railo M, Lepäntalo M, et al. Plant sterols in serum and in atherosclerotic plaques of patients undergoing carotid endarterectomy. J Am Coll Cardiol. 2005;45(11):1794-801.
14. Miettinen TA, Gylling H, Strandberg T, et al. Baseline serum cholestanol as predictor of recurrent coronary events in subgroup of Scandinavian simvastatin survival study. Finnish 4S Investigators. BMJ. 1998;316:1127-30.
15. Assmann G, Cullen P, Erbey J, et al. Plasma sitosterol elevations are associated with an increased incidence of coronary events in men: results of a nested case-control analysis of the Prospective Cardiovascular Münster (PROCAM) study. Nutr Metab Cardiovasc Dis. 2006;16:13-21.
16. ADVANCE Collaborative Group, Patel A, MacMahon S, et al. Intensive blood glucose control and vascular outcomes in patients with type 2 diabetes. N Engl J Med. 2008;358:2560-72
17. The Action to Control Cardiovascular Risk in Diabetes Study Group, Gerstein HC, Miller ME, et al. Effects of intensive glucose lowering in type 2 diabetes. N Engl J Med. 2008;358:2545-59.
18. Jaceldo-Siegl K, Lütjohann D, Sirirat R, et al. Plant sterol concentration in plasma and intake in plant-based diets. FASEB J. 2016;30(1):145-8.
19. Nicolas A, Fatima S, Lamri A, et al. ABCG8 polymorphisms and renal disease in type 2 diabetic patients. Metabolism. 2015;64(6):713-9.
20. Ng DP. Prognostic value of the insertion/deletion polymorphism of the *ACE gene* in type 2 diabetic subjects: results from the Non-insulin-dependent Diabetes, Hypertension, Microalbuminuria or Proteinuria, Cardiovascular Events, and Ramipril (DIABHYCAR), Diabete de type 2, Nephropathie et Genetique (DIAB2NEPHROGENE), and Survie, Diabete de type 2 et Genetique (SURDIAGENE) studies: response to Hadjadj et al. Diabetes Care. 2008;31:e78.

CHAPTER 5

Heart Failure

INTRODUCTION

The term "heart failure" (HF) is preferred to "congestive heart failure" (CHF) because manifestations of congestion may be absent at rest in some patients with moderate or severe left ventricular (LV) dysfunction. Indeed, there may be no clinical manifestations of forward or backward failure at rest.

The management of HF requires the application of five basic principles to actuate a salutary effect.
- Ensure a correct diagnosis, excluding *mimics* of HF.
- Determine the underlying heart disease, if possible, and treat.
- Define precipitating factors, because HF can be a result of underlying disease and is often precipitated by conditions that can be prevented or easily corrected.
- Understand the pathophysiology of HF.
- Know the actions of the pharmacologic agents and their appropriate indications.

DIAGNOSTIC HALLMARKS

Symptoms

Dyspnea, orthopnea, paroxysmal nocturnal dyspnea (PND), weakness, fatigue, edema, weight gain of greater than 2 lbs within 2-3 days and an ↑ in abdominal girth are common complaints.

Signs

- Crepitations (crackles) over the lower lung fields.
- Many patients are treated for HF based on the presence of crepitations.
- Heart failure may be present without pulmonary crepitations, and crepitations may be present in the absence of HF.
- Crepitations that fail to clear on coughing may be due to atelectasis, fibrosis and restrictive lung disease, pneumonia, *Pneumocystis* infection, lymphangitic carcinomatosis, and other causes of noncardiogenic pulmonary edema.

- S3 gallop or summation gallop (S3 and S4). An S3 gallop may elude auscultation in patients with coronary heart disease (CHD), although a corresponding movement associated with rapid diastolic filling may be visible on careful inspection of the precordium.
- An S3 or summation gallop is virtually always present in patients with dilated cardiomyopathy (DCM), even in the absence of HF.
- An ↑ in jugular venous pressure (JVP) greater than 2 cm above the sternal angle. The most common cause of right ventricular failure is left HF, and signs of this should be sought.
- A prominent V wave of tricuspid regurgitation or an A wave of atrial hypertrophy.
- A positive hepatojugular reflux usually indicates a right atrial pressure greater than 9 mm Hg and a pulmonary capillary wedge pressure (PCWP) greater than 15 mm Hg where right HF is secondary to left HF.
- Bilateral leg or sacral edema. Edema may be absent with severe HF, and when present, edema is often assumed to be due to HF.
- If a diagnosis of HF is not confirmed by other findings and a basic cause for HF is not present, consider the edema to be due to stasis, venous insufficiency, or deep venous thrombosis (DVT), of lymphangitic origin, or induced by drugs such as nonsteroidal anti-inflammatory drugs (NSAIDs) or calcium (Ca) antagonists.

Chest X-ray

Look for the following:
- Constriction of lower lobe vessels with dilation of those in the upper lobes. This sign is observed with pulmonary venous hypertension in LV failure, mitral stenosis, severe chronic obstructive pulmonary disease (COPD), or X-ray taken in the recumbent position.
- Interstitial pulmonary edema: Pulmonary clouding, perihilar haze, Kerley B or A lines caused by edema and thickening of interlobular septa. Kerley B lines usually are localized to the periphery of the lower zones and appear as horizontal lines 1–3 cm in length and no wider than 0.1–0.2 cm (Fig. 5.1).
- They occur transiently when pulmonary venous pressure exceeds about 22 mm Hg. A lines are less common, reflect thickened intercommunicating lymphatics, and appear as thin nonbranching lines, several inches in length, extending from the hilar region. The transient appearance of A and B lines is caused by LV failure and may persist if the lymphatic channels are obstructed by tumor, choked by dust particles in pneumoconiosis, or thickened by fibrosing alveolitis or hemochromatosis. They may be caused by viral infections or drug hypersensitivity.
- Pleural effusions: Subpleural or free pleural, blunting of the costophrenic angle, the right usually greater than the left.

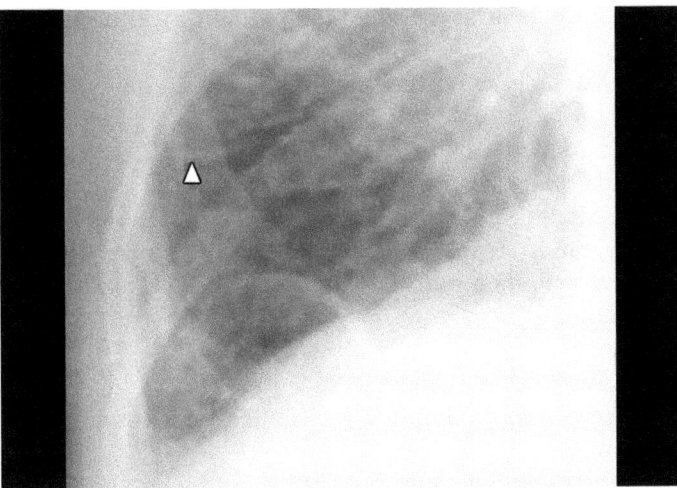

Fig. 5.1: Kerley B lines in interstitial pulmonary edema. These are short opaque lines (arrowhead) seen best along the lateral aspects of the lungs. Thickened interlobular septa from lymphangitic spread of tumor can produce an identical appearance.
Source: Khan MG. On Call Cardiology, 3rd edition. Philadelphia: WB Saunders, Elsevier Science; 2006; p. 172.

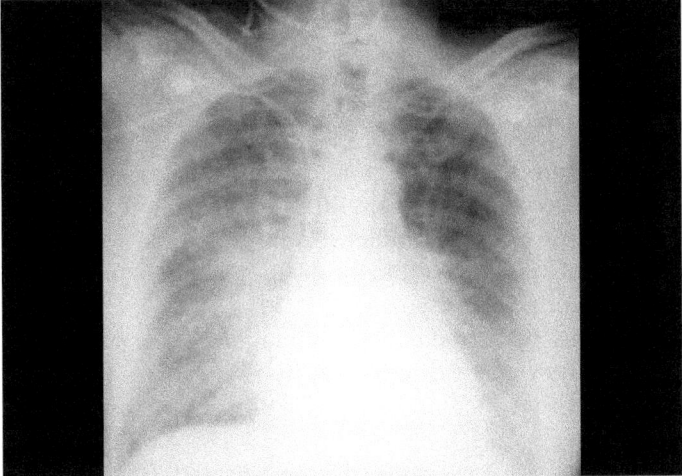

Fig. 5.2: Diffuse alveolar pulmonary edema showing ill-defined opacification in both lungs that is most prominent in the perihilar regions.
Source: Khan MG. On Call Cardiology, 3rd edition. Philadelphia: WB Saunders, Elsevier Science; 2006; p. 173.

- Alveolar pulmonary edema, a butterfly pattern (Fig. 5.2), may be unilateral.
- Interlobar fissure thickening due to accumulation of fluid, seen best on the lateral film.

- Dilatation of the central right and left pulmonary arteries (PAs).
- Cardiomegaly.

The heart size may be normal on chest X-ray, in many instances, with HF present due to:
- Acute myocardial infarction (MI) in patients with CHD. Cardiac dilation may not take place in a transverse direction and patients with more than 1 old infarcts may present with HF and a normal heart size on chest radiograph. Hypokinetic, dyskinetic areas may be observed on inspection or palpitation of the chest wall and are readily observed on echocardiography
- Mitral stenosis
- Aortic stenosis in some patients
- Heart failure due to predominant diastolic dysfunction
- Cor pulmonale.

The following radiologic mimics of HF should be excluded:
- Lung infection, including all causes of acute respiratory distress syndrome (ARDS)
- Allergic pulmonary edema (heroin, nitrofurantoin)
- Lymphangitic carcinomatosis
- Uremia
- Increased cerebrospinal fluid (CSF) pressure
- High altitude pulmonary edema
- Alveolar proteinosis.

Lung Ultrasound

Lung ultrasound can outperform chest X-ray for diagnosing HF.
- Bilateral presence of two or more lung zones with at least three B lines had negative and positive predictive values of 92%.
  The accuracy of lung ultrasound for detecting CHF in patients presenting with acute dyspnea was assessed.
- Ultrasound was performed in the emergency department by trained emergency physicians. Adjudication by two experts who relied on all available data (but were blinded to lung ultrasound results) was the gold standard.
- The final diagnosis was acute decompensated HF in 46%, in 1,005 patients.
- The negative and positive predictive values of clinical assessment plus lung ultrasound were both 97%. Lung ultrasound alone had negative and positive-predictive values of 92%, which were significantly higher than the values of 76% and 77%, respectively, for chest X-ray alone.
- In patients who had measurement of brain-type natriuretic peptide (BNP), lung ultrasound alone had higher negative predictive-value (86% vs 75%) and positive-predictive value (92% vs 75%). Agreement

was excellent between two novice users and an expert in a blind review of a random sample of 200 ultrasound clips (Kappa, 0.92).
- Lung ultrasound may soon replace chest X-ray as the diagnostic modality of choice for pneumonia, and this study suggests the same for CHF.
- Accuracy is operator-dependent, and robust training is required, although this study suggests the technique is easily learned.

Electrocardiography

Scrutinize the electrocardiogram (ECG) for:
- Acute or old infarctions
- Recent ischemia (assess by serial ECGs)
- Left ventricular aneurysm: ST segment elevation in two contiguous leads present greater than 3 months postinfarction
- Bradyarrhythmias or tachyarrhythmias, particularly atrial fibrillation (AF) with a fast ventricular response
- Left or right ventricular hypertrophy
- Left atrial enlargement, which is an early sign of altered LV compliance from LV hypertrophy and a common feature of mitral regurgitation (MR) and/or mitral stenosis.

Echocardiography

Echocardiography provides many diagnostic aids.
- Decreased systolic function: An ejection fraction (EF) 35-40% is often seen in patients with moderate HF. The EF may not be decreased in patients with HF caused by AF, MR or ventricular septal defect (VSD) and in patients with LV diastolic dysfunction (called HF preserved EF).
- The radionuclide evaluation of EF is more accurate than that of echocardiography, but the latter is superior in detecting the presence and significance of valvular lesions and specific chamber enlargement, ventricular wall motion abnormalities, global hypokinesia, and chamber enlargement.
- An approximate assessment of PA pressure is extremely useful.
- Valvular abnormalities: Reasonably accurate assessment of the severity of MR and obstructive lesions can be ascertained by continuous wave Doppler.
- Exclude cardiac tamponade.
- Assess pericardial effusion and pericardial calcification.
- Diastolic dysfunction abnormalities.
- Assess left ventricular hypertrophy (LVH), left atrial enlargement, and right ventricular hypertrophy.
- The diagnosis of hypertrophic, dilated, or restrictive cardiomyopathy (RCM).

N-terminal Probrain Natriuretic Peptide or BNP Assays

- This test is much abused and is not cost effective. Errors are many.
- Clinical use of BNP for the diagnosis of HF is useful but has been criticized in that patients with high concentrations of this peptide typically have classic signs, symptoms, and laboratory values greatly indicative of the disorder, i.e. an accurate diagnosis can be made on clinical grounds and from chest X-ray.
- Asian and Black patients with HF have higher natriuretic peptide levels on admission compared with White and Hispanic patients.
- In obese individuals and in patients who are less symptomatic and are less hemodynamically decompensated, diagnostic thresholds are generally lower and the test may be unreliable.
- In most a quarter of patients with chronic symptomatic HF may have natriuretic peptide levels in the lower ranges (30), and their levels should be explained by other contributing factors (e.g. obesity, ischemia) when clinical presentation is out of proportion to their degree of disease severity by other measures. In contrast, euvolemic patients (particularly older women, likely with lower lean mass) may have higher ranges.
- Meanwhile, natriuretic peptide levels are consistently higher in patients with underlying chronic kidney disease. As patients reach end-stage renal disease, natriuretic peptide levels can be tenfold higher than the operational range common to non-end-stage renal disease patients.

Heart failure is readily diagnosed by the symptoms of severe shortness of breath on minimal effort, shortness of breath in bed, swelling of the ankles caused by accumulation of fluid, edema, and radiologic confirmation. Thus, the value of BNP is exaggerated.

- At a cutoff of 100 pg/mL, the diagnostic accuracy of BNP has been shown to be approximately 83%.
- A level of BNP less than 50 pg/mL indicates the absence of HF. Patients with the diagnoses of HF usually have mean BNP levels greater than or equal to 675 pg/mL.
- Some laboratories report in units ng per liter (ng/L), which is equivalent to pg/mL. For patients with HF, BNP values will, in general, be above 100 pg/mL. Lower levels are often seen in obese patients. Higher levels are seen in those with renal disease, in the absence of HF; renal dysfunction is not uncommon.

CAUSES

A complete cure may be a rare reward if a surgically correctable lesion is uncovered.

- Left atrial myxoma (echo diagnosis)
- Significant MR: It may be missed because of the presence of a poorly audible murmur due to low cardiac output, thick chest wall, or COPD.

- Mitral and aortic stenosis
- Cardiomyopathies
- Atrial septal defect (ASD)
- Arteriovenous (AV) fistula
- Constrictive pericarditis
- Cardiac tamponade: It may simulate HF and must be excluded because usual HF medications, diuretics, angiotensin-converting enzyme (ACE) inhibitors, or nitrates can cause marked hemodynamic deterioration in patients with impending tamponade.
- Pulmonary edema or HF is not a complete diagnosis. The basic cause must be stated as part of the diagnosis and an associated precipitant must be defined, if present.

It is necessary to make a systematic search for the following basic causes of heart disease.

- Myocardial damage: CHD and its complications, myocarditis; cardiomyopathy
- Ventricular overload: *Pressure overload*: Systemic hypertension, coarctation of the aorta, aortic stenosis, pulmonary hypertension. *Volume overload*: MR, aortic regurgitation, VSD, ASD, patent ductus arteriosus.
- Restriction and obstruction of ventricular filling: Right ventricular infarction; constrictive pericarditis; cardiac tamponade (although not truly HF); restrictive cardiomyopathies; specific heart muscle diseases (SHMDs); hypertensive, hypertrophic "cardiomyopathy" of the elderly; mitral stenosis and atrial myxoma.
- Others: Cor pulmonale, thyrotoxicosis, high output failure: AV fistula, peripartum cardiomyopathy, and beriberi.

PRECIPITATING FACTORS

- Reduction or discontinuation of medications, salt binge, increased physical and mental stress.
- Increased cardiac work: Increasing hypertension (systemic or pulmonary), arrhythmias, pulmonary embolism, infections, increased activities, physical and emotional stress.
- Progression or complications of the underlying disease: Acute MI, LV aneurysm, valvular heart disease with progression of stenosis or regurgitation
- Several drugs may precipitate HF: Alcohol, NSAIDs, β-blockers, corticosteroids, disopyramide, procainamide, propafenone, and other antiarrhythmics, Ca antagonists, adriamycin, daunorubicin, mithramycin. Excessive alcohol intake can significantly ↓ LV contractility.

PATHOPHYSIOLOGY

In most patients with HF, cardiac output is reduced due to poor LV systolic function.

However, LV systolic function may be relatively normal in some patients with valvular regurgitant lesions, hypertensive heart disease, and RCM, in which diastolic dysfunction plays a major role in causing HF.

Heart failure is a syndrome identified by well-defined symptoms, signs, and/or hemodynamic findings caused by an abnormality of cardiac function that result in a relative ↓ in cardiac output and compensatory renal and neurohormonal adjustments.

Cardiac output is the product of stroke volume and heart rate (HR). Stroke volume is modulated by:
- Preload
- Myocardial contractility
- Afterload.

Preload: It is the extent of fiber stretch during diastole and is clinically represented by the end-diastolic volume. The LV end-diastolic or filling pressure is closely related, although in a nonlinear fashion, to end-diastolic volume, and is an indication of LV preload. In the absence of obstruction to blood flow through the pulmonary veins and into the ventricle, the LV end-diastolic pressure is in turn reflected by the PCWP or PA end-diastolic pressure.

Decrease preload and diastolic dysfunction: The affected ventricle may contract well if adequately filled but may relax poorly, resulting in a diastolic dysfunction that is more prominent than the commonly occurring systolic dysfunction.

An ↑ in ventricular diastolic stiffness impedes diastolic stretch and causes failure to adequately fill the ventricle. Conditions that alter ventricular compliance, causing diastolic dysfunction, a ↓ in preload, and thus, a ↓ in cardiac output, include: MI (although systolic dysfunction is the main abnormality); cardiac tamponade; constrictive pericarditis; hypertensive heart disease; RCM; DCM; SHMD, e.g. amyloid; the aging heart; and hypertensive, hypertrophic "cardiomyopathy" of the elderly. Approximately 15% of patients with HF have mainly diastolic dysfunction with relatively preserved EF. Over 70% of patients with HF have systolic dysfunction and about 15% have both systolic and diastolic dysfunction.

Diastolic dysfunction: In patients with predominant diastolic dysfunction, the heart size and EF are often normal. The heart fills less and empties less, and the percent ejected may be relatively normal, but the stroke and cardiac index are decreased. Since a ↓ in preload exists in the above conditions, the use of preload-reducing agents is relatively contraindicated. Hemodynamic and clinical deterioration may ensue with the use of diuretics, nitrates, ACE inhibitors, nitroprusside, or prazosin.

Afterload: It is represented by LV wall end-systolic stress, which must be overcome to allow ejection of blood from the ventricle. An ↑ in afterload signifies an ↑ in myocardial O_2 demand.

Afterload is determined by: the radius of the ventricle (A), LV end-systolic pressure (B), and arteriolar resistance or impedance (C). Afterload is highly dependent on A and B. In turn, B is dependent on cardiac index and C. A ↓ in systolic vascular resistance or a ↓ in blood pressure (BP) is not identical with a ↓ in afterload. Also, a ↓ in systemic vascular resistance is not synonymous with a ↓ in arterial BP, as a compensatory ↑ in cardiac output occurs to maintain BP. The peripheral systolic pressure may be maintained because of colliding reflected pressure waves, despite a ↓ in central systolic BP.

Conditions causing an ↑ in afterload include: aortic stenosis, pulmonary stenosis, coarctation, hypertension, and all causes of HF because of activation of the renin angiotensin and sympathoadrenal system.

Left ventricular dysfunction and HF due to systolic dysfunction improve with therapy directed at:
- A ↓ in afterload, which improves ventricular emptying at a lowered demand for O_2
- A judicious ↓ in preload, in order to ↓ symptoms caused by pulmonary congestion but without bringing about an unwanted ↓ in cardiac output or a marked stimulation of the renin angiotensin system.

Myocardial contractility: A ↓ in myocardial contractility or systolic dysfunction is commonly caused by CHD, especially in patients with large areas of infarction. Rarely, DCM and myocarditis are implicated; and with late-stage volume overload due to valvular regurgitant lesions, myocardial damage occurs, culminating in pump failure.

COMPENSATORY ADJUSTMENTS

The body responds to the abnormality of cardiac function and a relative ↓ in cardiac output by bringing several homeostatic mechanisms into action. This situation is similar to the body's reaction to severe bleeding over several hours, but the results are, of course, less than completely appropriate in HF.
- *Activation of the sympathetic system* causes an ↑ in HR, force, and velocity of myocardial contraction in order to ↑ stroke volume and cardiac output. An ↑ in systemic vascular resistance occurs in order to maintain BP. The body's homeostatic response is appropriate but often not sufficient to compensate for the ↓ in cardiac index and increased filling pressures. It is, in fact, counterproductive in some ways. Also, sympathetic stimulation causes sodium (Na) and water retention and an ↑ in venous tone in order to ↑ filling pressure that enhances preload, provided that there is no restriction to ventricular filling.
- *The renin angiotensin system is stimulated.* Patients with mild HF show little or no evidence of stimulation of the renin angiotensin system. Stimulation of the system is observed in response to treatment with

diuretics and is seen in untreated patients with more severe degrees of HF. The secretion of renin causes angiotensin I to be converted by ACE to the vasoconstrictor angiotensin II. This action occurs in the circulation and in the tissues.

Angiotensin II supports systemic BP and cerebral, renal, and coronary perfusion through:
- Arteriolar vasoconstriction and an ↑ in systemic vascular resistance
- Stimulation of central and peripheral effects of the sympathetic system
- Marked resorption of Na and water in the proximal nephron
- Enhanced aldosterone secretion, which brings about Na and water retention in the renal tubules, distal to the macula densa. Since the distal tubules only handle about 2% of the nephron's Na load, this latter contribution is small, compared to proximal Na resorption, but is a final tuning of Na balance.
- Stimulating thirst and vasopressin release, thereby increasing total body water.

Renal blood flow is preserved by selective vasoconstriction of postglomerular efferent arterioles. The adjustments, however, made to maintain BP and cerebral, coronary, and renal perfusion, cause a marked ↑ in afterload, which unnecessarily increases cardiac work and myocardial O_2 demand. Thus, HF increases.

THERAPY: NONSPECIFIC

- Bedrest, 24 hours only, is necessary for patients with the New York Heart Association (NYHA) Class IV or acute HF requiring admission to the hospital. After 36 hours of furosemide intravenous (IV), most patients are able to walk to the bathroom, with assistance, but some may require a bedside commode for the first 24 hours. It is important to quickly ambulate in order to avoid deep vein thrombosis and pulmonary embolism.
- Heparin, subcutaneous (SC), is advisable until the patient is mobilized.
- In patients ill enough to be admitted to the hospital and suspected of having hypoxemia because of a history of orthopnea, PND, and symptoms of pulmonary congestion or when hypoxemia is proven by arterial blood gas (ABG) analysis, O_2 is given to some for 12–24 hours. ABG analysis is not necessary in the majority of patients with HF. Oxygen, 2–3 L/minute, by nasal prongs is usually adequate but most do not require this therapy.
- Overweight patients with HF benefit from weight ↓. The physician must have a basic understanding of salt intake to confidently advise the patient.
- *Salt*: Patients must recognize that salt added to meals at the table is only a minor part of the daily salt consumption and that increased salt in the diet can precipitate HF and an expensive admission to hospital. Table 1.1 lists a few commonly used foods and their Na content (*see* Chapter 1).

DRUG-COMBINATION CHOICE

In clinical practice, an appropriate drug or combination for patients with HF due to ventricular systolic dysfunction requires consideration of the patient's functional class. It is appropriate to utilize the NYHA functional class since several major clinical trials have incorporated this parameter in study design.

NYHA Functional Class

- Class I: Asymptomatic on ordinary physical activity associated with maximal oxygen consumption greater than 20 mL/kg/minute.
- Class II: Symptomatic on ordinary physical activity with maximum VO_2 of 16–20 mL/kg/minute.
- Class III: Symptomatic on less than ordinary physical activity with maximum VO_2 of 10–15 mL/kg/minute.
- Class IV: Symptomatic at rest or on any activity with maximum VO_2 of less than 10 mL/kg/minute.

Drug Therapy, NYHA Class IV Heart Failure

CONSENSUS studied only NYHA Class IV HF patients. In 253 randomized patients, the 6-month mortality was 44% in patients treated with diuretics and a digoxin combination and 26% in patients given enalapril in addition (p <0.002). Forty-two percent of the group treated with added ACE inhibitors showed an improvement in functional class, compared with 22% in the control group (p = 0.001). A significant ↓ in mortality attributable to ACE inhibitor therapy was observed mainly during the first 6 months.
- The current recommendation to treat NYHA Class III–IV HF patients with furosemide, beta-blocker, digoxin, an ACE inhibitor, aldosterone antagonist (amiloride) is appropriate, given the short-life expectancy of Class IV patients, and is, of course, supported by the obvious symptomatic benefit, improved survival, and ↓ in sudden death that results from therapy. Amiloride should replace spironolactone that causes hormonal adverse effects including gynecomastia in men and abnormal symptoms and signs in women.

Drug Therapy, NYHA Class II Heart Failure

- Clinical trials have confirmed that monotherapy with diuretics, digoxin, or ACE inhibitors is not satisfactory for NYHA Class II patients in sinus rhythm who have an EF 35–40% and who have had overt HF.
- Sufficient data strongly indicate that these patients should be managed with triple therapy:
  - Furosemide: Diuretic, beta-blocker, and ACE inhibitor.

- All patients with EF less than 35, or cardiomegaly on chest X-ray, or gallop rhythm, should be administered digoxin to prevent recurrent HF (*see* Class III–IV treatment).
- In the few patients in whom ACE inhibitors are contraindicated or cause adverse effects, and angiotensin receptor blocker (ARB) is advisable but may not be equal to ACE inhibitor efficacy.
- If angioedema-like symptoms occurred with ACE inhibitor do not give ARB.
- *Losartan* and candesartan appear to have poof of some efficacy.
- *Telmisartan* is not recommended because of adverse profile (probable increased cancer risk).
- *Olmesartan* is not advisable; the Food and Drug Administration (FDA) remarked on sprue and cancer.
- African origin—the combination of hydralazine, isosorbide dinitrate and diuretic proved effective in a sound randomized controlled trial (RCT).
- The African-American Heart Failure Trial (A-HeFT) (2004)—the combination significantly reduced mortality and hospitalizations.

Diuretics

The main action of diuretics is to ↓ preload. Although this effect does not improve cardiac output or survival, diuretics are still first-line agents in the management of HF because they ameliorate bothersome, congestive symptoms and prevent costly hospitalization. No need for emergency room for many.

Furosemide

Furosemide can be used alone as first-line therapy in patients with NYHA Class II HF with mild systolic dysfunction, especially when HF is precipitated by a reversible cause such as pneumonia, infection, AF, arrhythmia, NSAIDs or other drugs. These patients are often controlled with furosemide IV 80 mg, 40 mg approximately 12 hours later + oral 40 mg/day. Visit to an ER and expense can be avoided.

In many furosemide 20–40 mg + amiloride 5 mg should suffice and maintained without ACE inhibitor or digoxin therapy.
- If underlying heart disease is present and LV function is abnormal, ACE inhibitor and beta-blocker are indicated.

Action: Furosemide inhibits Na and chloride reabsorption from the ascending limb of the loop of Henle, with weak effects in the proximal tubule, which excretes the drug. Intravenous furosemide has a venodilator effect; thus, preload ↓ occurs within minutes and relief of symptoms may occur before the appearance of increased urinary flow.

- The potency of action allows furosemide and other loop diuretics to retain beneficial effects in renal failure patients with glomerular filtration rates (GFRs) as low as 10 mL/minute.
- In patients with elevated serum creatinine, greater than 2.3 mg/dL (203 μmol/L) estimated GFRs (eGFR) less than 30 mL/minute, furosemide retains activity, whereas thiazides, except metolazone, are not effective.
- Furosemide: *Supplied*: tablets; 20 mg, 40 mg, 80 mg. *Dosage*: IV 40–80 mg given as a slow IV bolus, 20 mg/minute.
- *Caution*: If renal failure is present, do not exceed 4 mg/minute to prevent ototoxicity.
- For acute HF of mild to moderate severity in patients with acute MI, small doses are advisable (20–40 mg IV repeated 1–2 h after careful assessment) in order not to ↓ cardiac output or produce further stimulation of the renin angiotensin system. For acute HF in patients with known NYHA Class III or IV, large doses may be required, depending on the extent of pulmonary congestion and the degree of respiratory distress (80 mg IV followed by 80–120 mg in 2–4 h and repeated q 8 or 12 h as needed; maintenance 40–120 mg once daily).
- Larger dosages may be required if urinary output is poor or if chronic renal failure is present (with serum creatinine >2.3 mg/dL, 203 mmol/L) or if severe pulmonary congestion with respiratory distress persists (with a JVP >5 cm), having excluded cardiac tamponade or mimics of HF. See earlier discussion on this topic.
- Maintenance dose should be given before 9 am on an empty stomach. Split doses are rarely needed at 7 am and 2 pm.
- The afternoon dose should not be given later than 2 pm in order not to disturb the patient's sleep.
- It is preferable to give 160 mg once daily rather than 80 mg bid since the tubules may be resistant to the 80-mg dose in patients with severe HF.
- Doses greater than 160 mg are preferably divided into 120 mg in the morning and 80 mg in the afternoon.
- Patients with Class IV ventricles and graded as NYHA Class IV require greater than or equal to 120 mg in 1 day, alternating with 80 mg the next day to achieve adequate control.
- *Serum potassium (K) caution*: Always maintain the serum K greater than 4 mEq (mmol)/L. Patients who require large doses of furosemide greater than 80 mg qd benefit from added aldosterone antagonists (amiloride 5 mg) which enhances diuretic effectiveness of furosemide and normalizes serum K.
- When the combination is used, K supplements or K-sparing diuretics should not be given, except with carefully monitored serum K levels. Also, salt substitutes contain K and can cause hyperkalemia. Periodic measurements of serum K are advisable for all patients taking daily diuretics.

Adverse effects: Hypokalemia, hypersensitivity in patients allergic to sulfur compounds, very rarely leukopenia, thrombocytopenia, precipitation of gout, hypocalcemia, hypomagnesemia.

Drug interactions: Cephalosporin or aminoglycoside antibiotics may show increased nephrotoxicity in patients with renal dysfunction when given large doses of loop diuretics.
- An increased reabsorption of lithium may occur, resulting in lithium toxicity; with chloral hydrate, hot flushes, sweating, and tachycardia may occur
- NSAIDs antagonize the action of loop diuretics as well as thiazides; the effect of tubocurarine is increased.

Metolazone

Supplied—tablets; 2.5 mg, 5 mg, 10 mg.

Dosage: 2.5–5 mg once daily; maximum 10 mg (rarely indicated).

This thiazide diuretic has a unique property of retaining effectiveness when other thiazides become ineffective with GFR less than 30 mL/minute.
- The combination of metolazone and furosemide is very useful in patients with refractory HF who fail to respond to large doses of furosemide or ethacrynic acid.

Aldosterone Antagonists

- These agents are most useful for patients with class II-IV HF. Requiring 40 mg daily of furosemide to obtain greater than 90% relief of HF symptoms and or signs.
- They enhance the diuretic action of furosemide and also conserve K.
- But caution is required to prevent hyperkalemia. Thus, do not use if renal dysfunction particularly if the eGFR is less than 50 mL/minute
- Spironolactone causes breast tenderness gynecomastia in males and has hormonal adverse effects in females. The drug is no longer (1990) used in the United Kingdom for hypertension

Beta-blockers

Team do blocks for most drugs.

Bisoprolol: *Supplied*—5 mg, 10 mg tablets. *Dosage*—2.5 mg, first test dose, increase over days to 5 mg; maximum 10 mg.

Bisoprolol was proven effective in CIBIS and prevented sudden death (Table 5.1).

CIBIS-II was stopped early, after the second interim analysis, because bisoprolol showed a significant mortality benefit. All-cause mortality was significantly lower with bisoprolol than on placebo [156 (11.8%) vs 228

Table 5.1: Conditions in which there is an increased sensitivity to digoxin and conservative dosing is recommended.

Elderly patients (age >70)	Hypercalcemia
Hypokalemia	Hypocalcemia
Hyperkalemia	Myocarditis
Hypoxemia	Low-skeletal mass
Acidosis	Hypothyroidism
Acute myocardial infarction	Amyloidosis
Hypomagnesemia	

(17.3%) deaths] (42% reduction), with a hazard ratio of 0.66 (95% CI 0.54–0.81, p <0·0001).
- *Sudden death*: There were significantly fewer sudden deaths among patients on bisoprolol than in those on placebo [48 (3.6%) vs 83 (6.3%) deaths], with a hazard ratio of 0.56 (0.39–0.80, p = 0·0011). Treatment effects were independent of the severity or cause of HF.
- Total mortality 228 (17%) versus 156 (12%)—31.5% reduction and 35.7% reduction.
- 96% ACE inhibitor 51% digoxin.
- A 32% lower risk of mortality and admission to hospital.

Metoprolol: *Supplied*—tartrate 12 hours acting 50 mg, 100 mg. *Dosage*—50 mg twice daily, if needed 100 mg twice daily. 24 hours acting preparation may not cover 24 hours.

Metoprolol succinate controlled-release/extended-release (CR/XL) is advisable; the tartrate preparation 24 hours action is not as reliable.

Metoprolol succinate 24 hours acting is advisable (extended-release tablet intended for once daily administration) 25–100 mg daily in a single dose; increase to 200 mg if needed.

Metoprolol CR/XL Randomised Intervention Trial in Congestive Heart Failure (MERIT-HF) trial used metoprolol CR/XL once daily, in addition to standard therapy. The study was stopped early on the recommendation of the independent safety committee. Mean follow-up time was 1 year. All-cause mortality was lower in the metoprolol CR/XL group than in the placebo group [145 (7.2%, per patient-year of follow-up)] vs 217 deaths (11.0%), relative risk 0·66 (95% CI 0.53–0.81); p = 0.00009 or adjusted for interim analyses p = 0.0062]. There were fewer sudden deaths in the metoprolol CR/XL group than in the placebo group (79 vs 132).

Carvedilol was proven effective in the Carvedilol Prospective Randomized Cumulative Survival (COPERNICUS) trial (2001).

But because of alpha activity BP may decrease causing lightheadedness and falls. Also sudden death not prevented significantly.

The COPERNICUS trial studied 2,289 patients with severe HF, a low EF 16–24% but free from overt fluid retention or recent treatment with

IV diuretics or positive inotropic drugs showed: a highly significant 35% reduction in all-cause mortality with carvedilol. There were 190 placebo deaths and 130 with carvedilol, a 35% decrease in the risk of death, p = 0.0014. The dose of carvedilol was 6.25 mg, with slow increase to 25 mg twice daily. ACE inhibitor, digoxin, and spironolactone were used in 97%, 66%, and 20% of patients, respectively.

Atenolol: It is poorly effective and not recommended.

Nebivolol: The effect of beta-blockade with nebivolol in elderly patients with HF in this study was similar in those with preserved and impaired EF (van Veldhuisen et al. 2009). *Nebivolol dosage* is 5 mg once daily.

Digoxin

After more than 200 years of use and controversies in the 1970s regarding its efficacy and role, digoxin has been fully restored as the only oral positive inotropic agent available that significantly improves symptoms, signs, EF, and other hemodynamic parameters in patients with all grades of acute, recurrent, or chronic HF, with salutary effects occurring when combined with a diuretic, beta-blocker and/or ACE inhibitor. Most useful for HF with low BP less than 120 mmHg, and severe or recurrent HF.

- Clinicians who have used this drug for more than 30 years in patients with ventricular systolic dysfunction (NYHA Class III and IV HF) recognize the effectiveness of the drug when combined with diuretics and have documented the recurrence of HF when digoxin is discontinued.
- An S3 or summation gallop present during several days of treatment with diuretics and ACE inhibitors disappears within days of digitalization. Also, objective hemodynamic data are now available that clearly indicate the drug's salutary effects.

Digoxin has been shown to further improve cardiac function in patients with abnormal hemodynamic variables when stabilized on diuretics and ACE inhibitors.

Contraindications: Patients with sick sinus syndrome or AV block of all grades.

Cautions: Many physicians avoid the use of digoxin in the first 24 hours of MI, except in the management of patients with AF with hemodynamic compromise, in whom electrical cardioversion is preferred.

Indications:
- Heart failure associated with AF; patients in sinus rhythm (severe HF due to systolic dysfunction, particularly patients with NYHA Class III or IV, or EF <35% regardless of the presence of an S3 gallop).

- In these patients, the drug is combined with diuretics and ACE inhibitors; as part of triple therapy in patients with NYHA Class II HF and EF less than 35%; as the second-line agent for management of NYHA Class II HF patients with EF greater than 35% in combination with diuretics (salutary effects are equal to those of ACE inhibitors combined with diuretics); where ACE inhibitors or ARBs are contraindicated because of hypotension, renal failure.

Action: Inotropic effect: Digoxin increases the force and velocity of myocardial contraction and improves the EF. It combines with and partially inhibits the Na pump, the enzyme Na, and K-activated adenosine triphosphatase (Na-K-ATPase) located in the sarcolemmal membrane of the myocardial cell and increases the availability of intracellular Ca to contractile elements, resulting in enhanced myocardial contractility. This effect causes the Frank-Starling function curve to move upward and to the left.

Increase of vagal activity and a modest ↓ in sympathetic activity slow conduction velocity in the AV node. This action is important in slowing the ventricular response in AF and the termination of paroxysmal supraventricular tachycardia (PSVT). Mild slowing of the sinus rate occurs due to the mild ↓ in sympathetic activity.

Increase in Phase 4 diastolic depolarization increases the activity of ectopic pacemakers.

Pharmacokinetics: About 66% of the oral tablet dose is absorbed mainly in the stomach and the upper small bowel.
- Following absorption, the drug is widely distributed, but binding to skeletal muscle is particularly important because a low muscle mass in the elderly calls for a smaller loading dose. The mean serum half-life is approximately 36 hours.
- It is advisable to wait until equilibration is reached to obtain a digoxin level that represents myocardial concentration.
- Dosing at bedtime is advisable so that an assay during a morning assignment would be appropriate.
- Bioavailability is reduced as a result of decreased absorption due to: malabsorption syndrome; colestipol, cholestyramine, Metamucil (or similar agents); antacids, metoclopramide, phenytoin, phenobarbital.
- Absorption is enhanced by lomotil and decreased intestinal motility. An increased serum digoxin level may result from antibiotics, especially neomycin, and some broad-spectrum antibiotics that may eliminate *Eubacterium lentum*, which partially metabolizes digoxin to inactive dihydrodigoxin and may thus cause increased digoxin absorption. However, this effect occurs in less than 10% of patients. Digoxin levels are also increased by quinidine, some Ca antagonists, and amiodarone. Excretion is by the kidneys.

- Thus, undetected or unnoticed renal insufficiency is the most common cause of digoxin toxicity.

After 1 mg oral dosing, peak onset of action occurs in 1–6 hours, with serum levels usually greater than 1 mg/mL; maximum inotropic action is observed in 4–6 hours.

Dosage: 0.5–1 mg over 24 hours prescribed as follows:
- Orally: 0.5 mg immediately, 0.25 mg q 12 hours for two doses, followed by an appropriate maintenance dose depending on age, renal function, and presence or absence of conditions that ↑ sensitivity to the drug. If such conditions are present, halve the initial dose (or 0.25 mg bid) for 2 days, followed by maintenance dosage depending on age or renal function.
- Alternative dosage: Recommendation is 0.125 for those age older than 75 mg; 0.25 mg bid for 3 days then once daily, having regard to renal function. However, 0.5 mg qd for 1 week may cause toxicity if an unsuspected ↓ in creatinine clearance is present, especially in the elderly, or if sensitivity exists. Also, in patients younger than age 70 with normal renal function, the initial 0.25 mg daily dose may not achieve adequate levels or salutary effects for several weeks.
- Rapid oral method for AF with a ventricular response: 110–140/minute in patients with HF not receiving digoxin. *Caution*: The patient is reassessed prior to each dose and the order for the drug is then written: 0.5 mg immediately, 0.25 mg q 4 or 6 hours for three doses, followed by maintenance.

Suggested maintenance dosage with normal serum creatinine:
- Age younger than 70 (0.25 mg qd preferably at bedtime)
- Age more than 70 (0.125 mg at bedtime).

In patients with AF requiring further control of ventricular response, a 0.125-mg daily dose in addition to the maintenance dose indicated is often necessary.

Avoid digoxin if known renal failure is present or eGFR less than 45 mL/L.

Caution: Digoxin toxicity may occur in patients with known or unsuspected renal dysfunction, and especially in the elderly, in whom creatinine clearance is frequently reduced in the presence of a normal serum creatinine. In patients less than age 70 with serum creatinine of 1.3–2.3 mg/dL (115–203 mmol/L), give 0.125 mg on alternate days and assess digoxin levels in about 10 days. In patients over age 70 with abnormal serum creatinine greater than 2.3 mg/dL (203 mmol/L), it is advisable to avoid digoxin use because toxicity is a major concern. In this situation, treatment with diuretics and vasodilators is indicated and digoxin is relatively contraindicated.

Box 5.1: Digoxin interactions.

Increase serum levels
  Quinidine displaces digoxin at binding sites, decreases renal elimination
  Verapamil, diltiazem, nicardipine, felodipine, amiodarone, propafenone
  ACE inhibitiors may decrease renal elimination
  NSAIDs decrease renal elimination
  Lomotil, probanthine decrease intestinal motility
  Erythromycin, tetracycline eliminate Eubacterium lentum
  Spironolactone, digoxin assays falsely elevated
  Electrophysiologic interactions may occur with amiodarone, diltiazem, verapamil

Decrease serum levels or bioavailability
  Antacids, metoclopramide, cholestyramine, colestipol
  Metamucil, neomycin, phenytoin, phenobarbital, salicylazosulfapyridine

Digoxin Toxicity

A ↓ in the incidence of definite or serious digitalis intoxication has materialized because of physician awareness of the pharmacokinetics: absorption, binding, distribution, and excretion of the drug. In particular, the hazard in patients with renal dysfunction, including elderly patients with unsuspected impaired renal function with a normal serum creatinine, has sharply curtailed digitalis toxicity.

A *lean skeletal mass*, especially in the elderly, carries two important connotations:
- Digoxin binds to skeletal muscle; thus, in individuals with lean skeletal mass, more digoxin is available in the serum for myocardial binding. Therefore, there is a higher probability of toxicity in patients with lean skeletal mass, especially if renal dysfunction inhibits elimination of the drug.
- Low skeletal muscle mass in the elderly reflects a lowered serum creatinine that leads the physician to believe that renal function is normal, when creatinine clearance may be reduced by greater than or equal to 50%.

Reduction of the maintenance dose in patients with conditions that ↑ sensitivity to digoxin (*see* Table 5.1) and the appropriate use of digoxin serum assay are important precautionary measures. Conditions that ↑ or ↓ the bioavailability of digoxin, particularly drugs that cause interactions, are listed in Box 5.1.

Symptoms and signs of digitalis intoxication include:
- *Gastrointestinal (GI):* Nausea, anorexia, vomiting, diarrhea, abdominal pain, weight loss.

Table 5.2: Major manifestations of digoxin toxicity.

Manifestations	%
Non-life-threatening arrhythmias	
Multifocal VPCs	30
First-degree AV block	15
Supraventricular tachycardia	25
Life-threating arrhythmias	
Third-degree AV block	25
Second-degree AV block	15
Ventricular tachycardia	20
Ventricular fibrillation	10
Asystole	8
Noncardiac	
Nausea and vomiting	50
Hyperkalemia*	25

*Due to renal failure and/or inhibition of the sodium pump.

- *Central nervous system (CNS)*: Visual hallucinations; blue, green, or yellow vision; blurring of vision and scotomas; dizziness, headaches, restlessness, insomnia, and rarely mental confusion and psychosis.
- *Cardiac*: There is a spectrum from occurrence of arrhythmia in digoxin-free state, through latent arrhythmia precipitated by digoxin, to arrhythmia directly secondary to digoxin. First-degree, second-degree or third-degree AV block; sinus pause more than two seconds; paroxysmal atrial tachycardia (PAT) with block (ventricular rate is often 90–120/min; the P waves may be buried in the T waves); accelerated junctional rhythm; ventricular premature beats (VPBs), bigeminal or multifocal; VT; and rarely VF. Table 5.2 shows the incidence of arrhythmias caused by digoxin toxicity. In addition, deterioration in HF may be due to digoxin toxicity.
- No single serum digoxin concentration drawn at the appropriate time interval, greater than 6 hours after oral dosing, can indicate toxicity reliably, but the likelihood increases progressively through the range 1.5–3 ng/mL or mg/L (1.2–3.5 nmol/L).
- Concentrations greater than 2.5 ng/mL must be avoided.
- Levels less than 1.5 ng/mL drawn at the appropriate time are rarely associated with toxicity, except in patients with myocardial sensitivity as listed in Table 5.2.
- Digoxin toxicity in the patient with the absence of the conditions listed and a level less than 1 ng/mL is so rare as to exclude the diagnosis.

- Reviews indicate that digoxin-intoxicated patients have a mean serum digoxin level of 3.3 ng/mL.

Management of Digoxin Toxicity

- Discontinue digoxin.
- Replace K if hypokalemia is present. Hold diuretics until serum K is in the normal range.
- Clarify conditions that ↑ sensitivity to digoxin (Table 5.2). Toxicity is likely to be present if suggestive symptoms are manifest and if there is a precipitating cause for renal impairment or if the serum creatinine is elevated.
- Assess digoxin level.
- Assess ECG signs: Digitalis effect does not mean toxicity. (See bradyarrhythmias and tachyarrhythmias as listed under Adverse Effects).

Drug therapy is indicated for arrhythmias causing a threat to life, hemodynamic deterioration, or worsening of HF.

ACE Inhibitors

When HF occurs, sensors in the heart, the aortic arch, and arterioles of the juxtaglomerular apparatus actuate a host of neurohormonal responses that are necessary for the perfusion of vital tissues, especially of the brain, heart, and kidneys. These responses, initiated by sympathoadrenal activation and enhanced by stimulation of the renin angiotensin system, result in marked vasoconstriction, which increases systemic vascular resistance in order to maintain central BP. Unfortunately, an ↑ in systemic vascular resistance increases afterload and contractile myocyte energy costs.

- ACE inhibitors prevent formation of the vasoconstrictor angiotensin II and, at the appropriate dose, provide sufficient vasodilation to bring about a ↓ in afterload and a ↓ in systolic ventricular workload.
- Thus, ACE inhibitors play a major role in drug therapy of HF (NYHA Class II, III, and IV). Although these agents have greatly improved the management and survival of HF patients, they do not replace loop diuretics and are used in combination with a diuretic, with or without added digoxin therapy; see earlier discussion of drug therapy, NYHA Class II, III, and IV HF.
- Outcomes are not significantly prevented by the use of ACE inhibitors or ARBs. These are useful drugs for HF but they have modest and overrated benefits. They have not significantly halted the epidemic. They do reduce rehospitalization for HF but this is a modest effect.

They have not been shown to prevent sudden cardiac death in any subset of cardiovascular disease (CVD); their mechanism of action does not lend to prevention of sudden cardiac death.

Enalapril

Supplied: tablets; 5 mg, 10 mg, 20 mg. *Dosage*: 2.5 mg orally and observe for 2–6 hours. If there is no hypotension, give 2.5 mg bid for a few days, and ↑ slowly over days or weeks to 5 mg to a maximum of 10 mg bid. If HF is refractory, systolic pressure exceeds 120 mm Hg and active ischemia is not present; a maximum dose of 20 mg in the morning and 10 mg at night may be tried cautiously. In patients with severe HF, the dose can be increased more rapidly when under supervision with careful monitoring of BP to avoid hypotension. As with captopril, the dose is often given once daily in patients with very mild renal dysfunction or in patients more than age 70. It is advisable to ↓ the dose of loop diuretics prior to giving the first dose of enalapril, as with other ACE inhibitors.

An initial effect of hypotension is usually observed within 1–2 hours after administration of captopril and within 2-1/2 to 5 hours with enalapril. Withdrawal of diuretics does not always prevent marked hypotension or syncope, and caution is required at all times with the initiation of ACE inhibitor therapy.

Interaction: Important interaction occurs with NSAIDs. Aspirin has been shown to nullify the salutary hemodynamic effects of enalapril and a similar interaction is expected with other ACE inhibitors.

Angiotensin Receptor Blockers

None have proved to decrease total mortality in large well run RCTs. Significance is only achieved by statistical manipulations; significant results are shown only by addition of recurrent HF + deaths due to HF + total deaths.
- They are not all alike and thus caution is needed in choice.
  In PRoFESS study, it failed to prevent stroke.

Olmesartan: The safety of the ARB olmesartan is questionable after two ongoing trials among patients with type 2 diabetes suggested.
- Increased risk for cardiovascular death with the drug. FDA reported 2013 on sprue-like enteropathy may occur.
- Angiotensin II receptor blockers appear to be associated with a modestly increased risk for cancer, according to a meta-analysis published in the Lancet Oncology (Should we be concerned about all ARBs or a single drug, telmisartan?).

BIBLIOGRAPHY

1. Adams KF, Gheorghiade M, Uretsky BF, et al. Clinical benefits of low serum digoxin concentrations in heart failure. J Am Coll Cardiol. 2002;39:946-53.
2. Buckley LF, Carter DM, Matta L, et al. Intravenous diuretic therapy for the management of heart failure and volume overload in a multidisciplinary outpatient unit. JACC Heart Fail. 2016;4(1):1-8.

3. Cohn JN, Tognoni G; Valsartan Heart Failure Trial Investigators. A randomized trial of the angiotensin-receptor blocker valsartan in chronic heart failure. N Engl J Med. 2001;345:1667-75.
4. Effects of controlled-release metoprolol on total mortality hospitalizations, and well-being in patients with heart failure: the Metoprolol CR/XL Randomized Intervention Trial in congestive heart failure (MERIT-HF). MERIT-HF Study Group. JAMA. 2000;283:1295-302.
5. Francis GS, Felker GM, Tang WH. A test in context: critical evaluation of natriuretic peptide testing in heart failure. J Am Coll Cardiol. 2016;67(3):330-7.
6. Khan MG. Heart failure. In: Khan MG (Ed). Cardiac Drug Therapy, 8th edition. New York: Springer; 2015.
7. Khan MG. Heart failure. In: Khan MG, Bartlett JG, Chopra S, Topol EJ (Eds). Medical Diagnosis and Therapy, 1st edition. Pennsylvania: Lea and Febiger; 1994.
8. Khan MI. Treatment of refractory congestive heart failure and normokalemic hypochloremic alkalosis with acetazolamide and spironolactone. Can Med Assoc J. 1980;123:883-7.
9. McMurray JV, Packer M, Desai AS, et al. Angiotensin-neprilysin inhibition versus enalapril in heart failure. N Engl J Med. 2014;371:993-1004.
10. Meine M, Cramer MJ, van der Wall EE. Current aspects of cardiac resynchronisation therapy. Neth Heart J. 2016;24(1):1-3.
11. Nissen SE. Angiotensin-receptor blockers and cancer: urgent regulatory review needed. Lancet Oncol. 2010;11:605-6.
12. Packer M, Coats JS, Fowler MB, et al. Effect of carvedilol on survival in severe chronic heart failure. New Engl J Med. 2001;344:1651-8.
13. Packer M, Gheorghiade M, Young JB, et al. Withdrawal of digoxin from patients with chronic heart failure treated with angiotensin-converting-enzyme inhibitors: RADIANCE Study. N Engl J Med. 1993;329:1-7.
14. Packer M, O'Connor CM, Ghali JK, et al. Effect of amlodipine on morbidity and mortality in severe chronic heart failure: Prospective Randomized Amlodipine Survival Evaluation Study Group. N Engl J Med. 1996;335:1107-14.
15. Pitt B, Pfeffer MA, Assmann SF, et al. Spironolactone for heart failure with preserved ejection fraction. N Engl J Med. 2014;370:1383-92.
16. Pivetta E, Goffi A, Lupia E, et al. Lung ultrasound-implemented diagnosis of acute decompensated heart failure in the ED: a SIMEU Multicenter Study. Chest. 2015;148(1):202-10.
17. Poole JE, Singh JP, Birgersdotter-Green U. QRS duration or QRS morphology: what really matters in cardiac resynchronization therapy? J Am Coll Cardiol. 2016;67(9):1104-17.
18. Sipahi I, Debanne SM, Rowland DY, et al. Angiotensin-receptor blockade and risk of cancer: meta-analysis of randomised controlled trials. Lancet Oncol. 2010;11:627-36.
19. Taylor AL, Ziesche S, Yancy C, et al. Combination of isosorbide dinitrate and hydralazine in blacks with heart failure. N Engl J Med. 2004;351:2049-57.
20. Telmisartan Randomised AssessmeNt Study in ACE iNtolerant subjects with cardiovascular Disease (TRANSCEND) Investigators, Yusuf S, Teo K, et al. Effects of the angiotensin-receptor blocker telmisartan on cardiovascular events in high-risk patients intolerant to angiotensin-converting enzyme inhibitors: a randomised controlled trial. Lancet. 2008;372:1174-83.
21. The Cardiac Insufficiency Bisoprolol Study II (CIBIS-II): a randomised trial. Lancet. 1999;353:9-13.

22. Van Veldhuisen DJ, Cohen-Solal A, Bohm M, et al. Beta-blockade with nebivolol in elderly heart failure patients with impaired and preserved left ventricular ejection fraction: data from SENIORS (Study of Effects of Nebivolol Intervention on Outcomes and Rehospitalization in Seniors with Heart Failure). J Am Coll Cardiol. 2009;53:2150-8.
23. Yusuf S, Diener HC, Sacco RL, et al. Telmisartan to prevent recurrent stroke and cardiovascular events. N Eng J Med. 2008;359(12):1225-37.
24. Zsilinszka R, Mentz RJ, DeVore AD, et al. Acute heart failure: alternatives to hospitalization. JACC Heart Fail. 2017;5(5):329-36.

CHAPTER 6

Arrhythmias

INTRODUCTION

Accurate diagnosis, in particular, differentiation of ventricular tachycardia (VT) and supraventricular tachycardia (SVT) is essential for appropriate management. The electrocardiogram (ECG) diagnostic points for tachy-arrhythmias are shown in Tables 6.1 and 6.2, and Figures 6.1A and B:
- Determine whether the rhythm is regular or irregular then
- Divide into narrow QRS or wide QRS.

The treatment of underlying conditions may cause amelioration and/or prevention of arrhythmia recurrence. The severity of the underlying diseases, particularly the degree of left ventricular (LV) dysfunction, may dictate the choice of antiarrhythmic agent and the outcome. The prognosis of ventricular arrhythmias is closely linked to the degree of LV dysfunction. Echocardiography ejection fraction (EF) is more cost-effective than radionuclide because structural abnormalities including left atrial enlargement may be detected.
- Ejection fraction greater than 50% carries a good prognosis.
- Ejection fraction 40–50% is commonly associated with benign arrhythmias and a fair prognosis.
- Ejection fraction 25–39% is often associated with potentially lethal arrhythmias.
- Ejection fraction less than 25% indicates a poor prognosis.

Adverse effects of drug therapy are related to the degree of LV dysfunction. Drugs that may be used in patients with an EF less than 30% and other scenarios are given in Table 6.3.

The emergency management of arrhythmias calls for a quick assessment of the followings:
- Hemodynamic status: Is the blood pressure (BP) less than 90 mm Hg and are there signs of peripheral hypoperfusion?
- Symptomatic status: Chest pain, shortness of breath, presyncope, syncope, or clouding of consciousness.
- Cardiac decompensation: Signs of congestive heart failure (CHF).

Table 6.1: Differential diagnosis of narrow QRS tachycardia.

Regular	Irregular
Supraventricular tachycardia (SVT); AVNRT Rate = 140–220 P waves usually buried and not apparent in the QRS or less commonly retrograde P barely visible in terminal QRS of V1, forming an rsr1 or forms a pseudo-Q in the very early ST segment, in II, III, aVF, or P hidden in the QRS • In approximately 50% of cases, P waves are hidden within the QRS complex and are not visible; the QRS complex is similar to that of a tracing when in sinus rhythm • In more than 40% of cases, P waves in leads II, III, and aVF occur at the end of the QRS complex and distort the terminal forces of the QRS complex, resulting in pseudo-S waves in leads II, III and aVF and a pseudo-r1 wave in lead V1 (*see* Fig. 6.1A). • In more than 5% of cases, P waves are discernible at the beginning of the QRS complex and cause pseudo-Q waves in leads II, III and aVF	Atrial fibrillation R-R intervals completely irregular Absent P waves
Wolff–Parkinson–White (WPW) with AV reentry, negative P wave lead I suggest left-sided bypass tract **Marked alternation in QRS amplitude highly suspect WPW**	Atrial flutter: AR >250 Variable AV conduction VR 100–220 Note no flutter waves in lead I and V6 but most marked flutter waves in lead II and other leads is a clue to presence of flutter
Paroxysmal atrial tachycardia (PAT) with block, AR 150–200 VR usually <140 P wave often buried in T isoelectric intervals between P waves	Multifocal atrial tachycardia (MAT) Three different P wave morphologies in any lead, variable P-P, PR, R-R intervals AR = 100–200/minute R-R intervals completely irregular; may progress to AF
Sinoatrial tachycardia Average rate = 140/minute Sinus P waves present: Upright P waves in the ST segment	

Contd...

Contd...

Regular	Irregular
Atrial flutter AR = 250–350 often 300/minute VR often 150–160/minute Conduction ratio often 2:1 Sawtooth pattern leads II, aVF Sharp-pointed "P" waves in V1 Note no flutter waves in lead I and V6 but most marked flutter waves in lead II and other leads is a clue to presence of flutter	
Ectopic atrial tachycardia	

(AVNRT, atrioventricular nodal reentrant tachycardia; AR, atrial rate; VR, ventricular rate; AF, atrial fibrillation)

Table 6.2: Differential diagnosis of wide QRS tachycardia.

Regular	Irregular

Ventricular tachycardia
Hallmarks:
• Absence of an RS complex in all precordial leads
• QRS duration:
• R to S interval >100 msec* in one precordial (chest) lead
• Right bundle branch block (RBBB) QRS >140 msec*
• Left bundle branch block (LBBB) QRS >160 msec*
• AV dissociation† (cannon waves in neck) excludes atrial but not nodal tachycardia
• Suggested features:
  ▪ Positive concordance [except Wolff–Parkinson–White (WPW) type A]
  ▪ Left axis −90 to +180 (−60 to −90 suggest VT)
  ▪ QS or rS in V6 (R to S, ratio <1) or net negative QRS in V6
  ▪ V1 "left rabbit ear" taller than the right: slurred
	Atrial fibrillation (AF) and WPW rate (200–300/min with aberrancy[§])

Supraventricular tachycardia (SVT) with known right or LBBB	AF and prior intraventricular conduction defect on recent electrocardiogram (ECG)
SVT with aberrant conduction: visible on aberrant atrial ectopic: small normal q: qRs in V6	
Atrial flutter: with wide QRS[‡] with WPW[§] (rare)	
WPW anterograde through bypass tract[§] (resembles VT)	

*milliseconds.
†AV block or dissociation excludes bypass tract.
‡AF treated with Class IC or IA agents may induce this arrhythmia.
§RR less than 205 milliseconds suggests WPW, treat as VT.

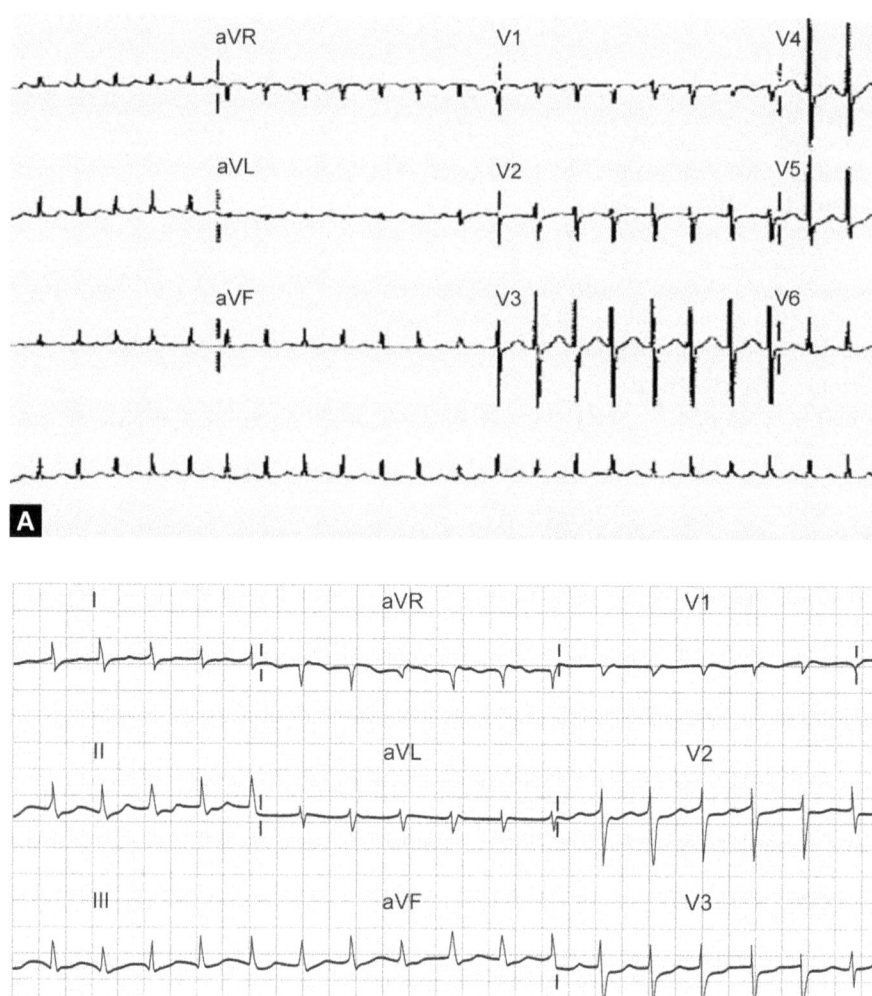

Figs. 6.1A and B: (A) Narrow, regular QRS tachycardia, rate 170 beats/minute: supraventricular tachycardia, common variety of atrioventricular nodal reentrant tachycardia (AVNRT); (B) ECG shows AVNRT: note the distortion of terminal forces, pseudo-S waves, in leads II, III, and aVF, and a pseudo-r' wave in lead V1.
Source: Adapted with permission from Khan MG. On Call Cardiology, 3rd edition. Philadelphia: WB Saunders/Elsevier Science; 2006.

An essential step is to rapidly define the clinical setting and correct a precipitating cause in order to obviate the need for antiarrhythmic therapy or to appraise and prevent deleterious proarrhythmic effects of these agents.

Table 6.3: Ejection fraction (EF) may dictate choice of antiarrhythmic agent.

Group I	Group II	Group III
EF <30%	EF >30%	EF >40%
Only safe agents*	Beta-blockers and agents used for Group I*	Agents given under Group I, II plus Class IA, IB
Amiodarone		Propafenone†
Mexiletine		Flecainide‡
Quinidine		Verapamil
Beta-blockers†		Diltiazem

*All other agents: hazard of precipitating heart failure.
†Used judiciously in properly selected patients, absence of overt heart failure, EF down to 25%.
‡Limited indications (see text).

Precipitating factors and/or clinical setting include:
- Ischemia: As with acute myocardial infarction (MI) or acute myocardial ischemia
- Those characterized by myocardial reperfusion: Post-thrombolytic therapy in acute MI, balloon deflation during coronary angioplasty, release of coronary artery spasm
- Hypotension
- Sick sinus syndrome or atrioventricular (AV) block
- Congestive heart failure
- Hypokalemia, hypomagnesemia, hyperkalemia
- Alkalemia, e.g. may develop rapidly in ventilated patients
- Acidemia
- Hypoxemia
- Pulmonary disease, cor pulmonale, atelectasis, pneumothorax, and carcinoma of lungs. May precipitate atrial flutter or atrial fibrillation (AF)
- Infection
- Fluctuations in autonomic tone
- Acute blood loss
- Thyrotoxicosis
- Digoxin toxicity
- Proarrhythmic effects of antiarrhythmic drugs: Quinidine and other Class IA drugs may cause torsades de pointes, also caused by Class III agents (sotalol and rarely by amiodarone). More typical monomorphic VT and other lethal arrhythmias may be initiated by antiarrhythmic drugs.
- Nonantiarrhythmics: β-agonist, theophylline, terfenadine, and astemizole, especially in combination with erythromycin or ketoconazole
- Ruptured esophagus: May initiate atrial flutter or AF.

SUPRAVENTRICULAR ARRHYTHMIAS

Atrioventricular Nodal Reentrant Tachycardia

Paroxysmal supraventricular tachycardia (PSVT) in patients younger than age 35 usually occurs in an otherwise normal heart and has a good prognosis. However, atrioventricular nodal reentrant tachycardia (AVNRT) is not uncommon with organic heart disease caused by coronary, rheumatic, or other valvular heart disease, and rarely can be life threatening. The onset and termination are abrupt; heart rate (HR) varies from 140/minute to 220/minute, with a regular rhythm (see Table 6.1 and Figs. 6.1A and B).

Treatment

Carotid sinus massage, patient rhythm monitored.
- Response is either reversion to sinus rhythm or no effect at all, in contrast to atrial flutter, where slowing of HR virtually always occurs
- Not recommended in the elderly or in patients with known or highly suspected carotid disease, ischemia, or digitalis toxicity
- With the patient supine (head slightly hyperextended, turned a little toward the opposite side), locate the right carotid sinus at the angle of the jaw. Apply firm pressure in a circular or massage fashion for 2-6 seconds, using the first and second fingers. It is necessary to monitor the cardiac rhythm and gauge exactly when to stop massage because asystole, although rare, can occur. If unsuccessful, after an interval of 2 minutes to allow acetylcholine to be manufactured in the AV node, massage the left carotid sinus. If asystole occurs during the procedure, ask the patient to cough and/or give the patient more than one light chest thumps, which usually reverses transient asystole.
- *Caution:* Never massage for more than 10 seconds.

Verapamil: Caution Verapamil intravenous (IV) is contraindicated in patients with severe hypotension, CHF, LV dysfunction, cardiomegaly, acute MI, sick sinus syndrome (Flowchart 6.1), suspected digitalis toxicity and concurrent use of β-blockers, disopyramide, or amiodarone; do not use in wide QRS tachycardia, antidromic Wolff-Parkinson-White (WPW), or if the refractory period of the accessory pathway is less than 270 milliseconds.

Dosage: Verapamil (5 mg IV) is given slowly over 1-2 minutes. Use 2.5 mg initially if LV function is believed to be slightly impaired. Resistance or recurrence of arrhythmia without a marked ↓ in BP should be treated with an additional 2.5- to 5-mg dose 10 minutes after the first dose. Occasionally, an IV infusion is used, 1 mg/minute to a total of 10 mg or 5-10 mg over 1 hour; 100 mg in 24 hours. Mild hypotension is not a contraindication, and further hypotension can be partially avoided by the administration of calcium chloride (CaCl): 10 mL of a 10% solution over 5-10 minutes;

Flowchart 6.1: Suggested steps in how to treat atrioventricular nodal reentrant tachycardia (AVNRT).

```
                        Is cardiac pathology present?
                        /                           \
                       No                           Yes
                       |                             |
              Systolic blood pressure                |
                   <90 mm Hg?                        |
                   /         \                       |
                  No          Yes          Acute MI, ischemia
                  |            |               present?
             Commence        Either            /        \
                  |            |              No         Yes
                  |         Adenosine          |          |
                  |            |         Other significant*
            Verapamil or       |          heart disease
             adenosine         |            present?
                  |            |             /     \
             Sinus rhythm?     |            No      Yes      Either
              /      \         |             |       |         |
             No      Yes       |             |    Adenosine     |
             |       |         |             |       |          |
        Cardioversion          |         If recurrent       Consider
                               |           AVNRT          cardioversion
                               |          consider
                               |         maintenance
                               |           digoxin
                               |             |
    *    e.g.: Heart failure, cardiomegaly   |
    **   if heart failure is not present   Beta-blocker**
    MI = Myocardial infarction               |
                                          Control? ——— No
                                             |
                                            Yes
```

calcium gluconate is an alternative; for sinus arrest or AV block give CaCl and atropine 0.5 mg IV.

Adenosine (adenocard): This ultrashort-acting agent has decreased the need for IV verapamil (Table 6.4), digoxin, or β-blockers in the acute management of PSVT (*see* Flowchart 6.1).

Dosage using a peripheral vein: 6 mg by rapid IV bolus injection over 2 seconds rapidly flushed into a peripheral vein; if given via an IV line, the

Table 6.4: Adenosine versus verapamil for the management of paroxysmal supraventricular tachycardias.

Parameters	First choice	Second choice
Uncomplicated cases: Ventricular rate <220/min	Verapamil	Adenosine
Hypotension: Mild	Adenosine	Verapamil after pretreatment with calcium chloride or gluconate
Moderate/severe	Adenosine	Verapamil CI
Left ventricular dysfunction: Heart failure cardiomegaly	Adenosine	Verapamil CI
Suspect preexcitation [Atrioventricular reentrant tachycardia (AVRT)]	Adenosine	Verapamil CI
Wide QRS: ? Aberrancy	Adenosine	Verapamil CI
Ectopic or multifocal atrial tachycardia	Verapamil	Adenosine ineffective

drug should be given as proximal as possible and followed by a rapid saline flush. Termination of arrhythmia is expected in less than 1 minute, and the action of the drug lasts for less than 30 seconds after injection. A second bolus injection of 12 mg is repeated 2 minutes after the first if the arrhythmia persists or recurs. The 12-mg dose may be repeated in 2–5 minutes, if required, and may be given via a larger vein than used in prior IV injection. Further recurrence of the arrhythmia calls for alternative therapy. In 10–30% of cases, arrhythmia recurs within minutes of the first injection of adenosine. A smaller dose is required if the drug is given through a central vein. A dose of 6 mg administered through a central vein in the same patient may have a potent effect, whereas a 12-mg dose may be ineffective when administered through a small peripheral vein. The drug should be used cautiously in patients with right to left shunting and must not be administered into the distal port of a balloon-flotation catheter.

Action:
- The drug has a depressant effect on the sinoatrial (SA) node and slows impulse conduction through the AV node. These effects appear to be mediated at the cellular level by an increase in potassium (K) and a decrease in calcium (Ca) conductance. These electrophysiologic (EP) effects are not antagonized by atropine.
- After IV quick bolus injection, adenosine has a rapid onset of action within 5–30 seconds and converts less than 90% of PSVTs to sinus rhythm.

- The drug has a very short half-life (<2 seconds) because it is avidly taken up and metabolized by adenosine deaminase in endothelial and red blood cells.

Indications:
- Termination of AVNRT and AV reentrant reciprocating tachycardia. The drug causes termination of these arrhythmias in greater than 90% of cases. It is the agent of first choice for these arrhythmias in patients with hypotension (*see* Flowchart 6.1) or other situations where rapid conversion to sinus rhythm is needed or as an alternative to electrical cardioversion.
- In patients with PSVT that fails to terminate with a 10-mg dose of verapamil, or when contraindications or relative contraindications to verapamil exist.
- The drug has advantages over verapamil in patients with AVNRT utilizing an accessory pathway in the reentry circuit; adenosine may unmask latent preexcitation when sinus rhythm is restored and can only produce very transient episodes of rapid preexcited arrhythmia, as opposed to verapamil, which is contraindicated in these situations. Thus, adenosine is much safer than verapamil for use in patients with WPW or suspected WPW arrhythmias.
- Adenosine, in decreasing AV conduction, unmasks atrial flutter and assists with diagnosis.
- Adenosine also has a role in patients with suspected SVT or wide complex tachycardia of uncertain type. In patients with misdiagnosed VT, verapamil may precipitate CHF and other life-threatening complications. Adenosine, in this situation, causes reversion if the rhythm is due to AV nodal reentry, and its effect on VT is transient and not detrimental because of its ultrashort half-life.
- Adenosine appears to have an important role and is relatively safe in infants with rapid PSVT with hemodynamic compromise, because repeat electrical cardioversion with 20 J can cause deleterious effects on the myocardium at this age. Adenosine pediatric dosage: 50 mg/kg; increase at 50 mg/kg increments if needed to 150 mg/kg (not included in the drug's product monograph but appears to be relatively safe at this dose range).

Adenosine indications may be limited by cost; adenosine is 60 times more expensive than verapamil. A multicenter study indicated that a 12-mg dose is usually required to achieve about a 90% success in conversion of the arrhythmia to sinus rhythm at a cost of $30 compared with a $0.50 for 10 mg verapamil. Also, there is a high incidence of recurrence of the arrhythmia within minutes of the first successful conversion. The incidence varies from 10% to 33%, a second injection is usually successful. Adenosine is not effective in ectopic atrial tachycardia and multifocal atrial tachycardia (MAT).

Contraindications: Second-degree or third-degree AV block, except in patients with a functioning pacemaker; sinus node disease; known hypersensitivity to adenosine; asthma; chronic pulmonary disease with theophylline usage; unstable angina; acute MI (not given in the product monograph).

Adverse effects: Minor adverse effects occur in 30-60% of patients. It is wise to advise the patient that minor transient adverse effects may occur, lasting 0.5-1 minute. These effects include: facial flushing, dyspnea, chest pain or pressure, mild bronchospasm in patients with chronic obstructive pulmonary disease (COPD), and, less commonly: nausea, vomiting, headache, transient hypotension, and sinus pauses with ventricular standstill of several seconds.

Caution: Safety in patients with myocardial ischemic syndromes is not established. A dose of 12 mg may be ineffective if given through a small peripheral vein, but 6 mg given through a central vein may have a potent effect. Do not administer the 12-mg dose through a central vein or porthole of a balloon-flotation catheter. Avoid the use of adenosine in the presence of a prolonged QT interval because induced bradycardia may promote the precipitation of torsades de pointes.

Interactions
- Dipyridamole markedly enhances the SA and AV nodal effects of adenosine. Dipyridamole decreases cellular uptake of adenosine, thereby inhibiting its metabolism. This interaction may be important in patients being given oral dipyridamole.
- Aminophylline, caffeine, and other methylxanthines completely antagonize adenosine.

Esmolol: It has an ultrashort action that confers major advantages over propranolol, atenolol, and metoprolol. The onset of action is rapid. The drug is quickly metabolized by esterases of red blood cells and has a half-life of 9 minutes that is unaffected by renal failure, CHF, or hepatic dysfunction. The drug is cardioselective and has the same contraindications as other β-blocking agents. Esmolol has a role in the management of uncomplicated cases of SVT not terminated by adenosine and where adenosine or verapamil is contraindicated, especially during acute MI or other ischemic syndromes.

Dosage: Initial loading infusion of 3-40 mg (usually 6 mg), IV infusion over 1 minute (30 mg/kg to maximum 500 mg/kg given over 1 min), and then maintenance infusion 1-5 mg/minute (maximum 50 mg/kg/min).

Adverse effects: Mild transient hypotension occurs in less than 25% of patients, more commonly in those with systolic BP less than 100 mm Hg, and improvement occurs within minutes of discontinuing the IV infusion.

Propranolol: Dosage 1 mg IV given over 2 minutes, repeated q 5 minutes to a maximum of 5 mg.

Metoprolol: Dosage: 5 mg IV bolus over 3 minutes; then, if required after 5 minutes, an additional bolus is given and repeated if needed 5-10 minutes later.

Phenylephrine: It has a role only in young patients with a normal heart when the BP is less than 90 mm Hg, when adenosine is not available, or when cardioversion is felt to be unnecessary. This alpha-agonist increases BP, and vagal activity results in sinus rhythm. *Dosage:* 0.1 mg diluted with 5 mL or 5% dextrose IV bolus over 2 minutes; the BP is measured at 30-second intervals and must not be allowed to exceed 140 mm Hg. Allow 1-3 minutes after each bolus for the BP to return to baseline value before giving an additional bolus. Maximum dose—0.5 mg. If this fails to produce sinus rhythm but stabilization of BP is achieved, verapamil can be given.

Digoxin: It is preferred only if there are signs of CHF, hypotension, or severe cardiomegaly, or signs and symptoms of a sick heart. However, digoxin takes more than 2 hours to have an effect and is not recommended where rapid restoration of sinus rhythm is required. *Dosage:* In the absence of digoxin use during the previous week, 0.5 mg IV by infusion over 10 minutes, followed in 30 minutes with 0.25 mg, then PO 0.25 mg once daily.

Direct current (DC) cardioversion: It may be necessary for patients who are hemodynamically unstable and should be used prior to drug therapy, or if such therapy appears unsuccessful.

Chronic maintenance: Chronic maintenance for bothersome, frequently recurring SVT usually requires digoxin or a β-blocker and occasionally a combination of both drugs. Verapamil 120 mg taken at the onset of SVT has a role in aborting attacks within 1-2 hours and prevents emergency room (ER) visits.

Paroxysmal Atrial Tachycardia with Block

- The arrhythmia is usually due to digoxin toxicity. Atrial rate less than 200 excludes atrial flutter (*see* Table 6.1). If the HR is 90-120/minute with a normal serum K, no treatment is usually required.
- If the serum K is less than 3.5 mEq/L and a high degree of AV block is absent, give KCl IV (60 mEq) in 1 L normal saline over 5 hours.

Multifocal Atrial Tachycardia

- Multifocal atrial tachycardia is usually seen in patients with COPD, hypoxemia, and theophylline toxicity. Treat the underlying cause.
- If tachycardia is symptomatic or causes cardiac embarrassment, give verapamil 2.5-5 mg IV repeated in 30 minutes. Verapamil IV is usually successful, and it should be followed by 80 mg three or four times daily until the underlying problem resolves. Often the arrhythmia causes no

hemodynamic disturbances, especially at rates of 100–130/minute and requires no drug therapy, or the initial dose of verapamil can be given orally.
- Magnesium has a direct effect on K channels, increases intracellular K, and is effective in some patients.
- A β-blocker is more effective than verapamil, but caution is needed in patients with COPD. Metoprolol IV or oral may be given a trial if asthma or severe COPD is not present.

Atrial Flutter

- Atrial flutter is often due to underlying pathology, in particular coronary heart disease (CHD), MI, hypoxemia due to pulmonary embolism, pneumothorax, and COPD; also mitral valve disease and thyrotoxicosis. Removal of the underlying causes may be followed by spontaneous reversion to sinus rhythm.
- The rhythm may be regular or irregular (Figs. 6.2 and 6.3).
- Atrial flutter is easily converted to sinus rhythm by synchronized DC shock 25–50 J. This should be carried out if the patient is hemodynamically compromised, a ventricular response is greater than 200/minute, or the patient is known or suspected to have WPW.
- Patients with ventricular response less than 200/minute: propranolol or other β-blockers may be used to slow the ventricular response.
- Digoxin converts atrial flutter to AF and slows the ventricular response.
- Verapamil reduces the ventricular response and may occasionally cause conversion to sinus rhythm. Verapamil, digoxin, and β-blockers are contraindicated in patients with WPW presenting with atrial flutter or AF. In this setting, verapamil or digoxin may precipitate ventricular fibrillation (VF).

Atrial Fibrillation

- Diagnosis is readily made from the ECG (Figs. 6.4A and B).
- Causes of AF include rheumatic and other valvular heart disease, CHD, hypertension, cardiomyopathies, cor pulmonale, pulmonary embolism, thyrotoxicosis, sick sinus syndrome producing tachy- and bradyarrhythmias, WPW syndrome, alcohol abuse, post-thoracotomy, esophagojejunostomy, ruptured esophagus, carbon monoxide poisoning, and idiopathic.
- Investigations should include echocardiogram to confirm underlying causes and evaluate left atrial size and presence of thrombus.

Digoxin: It is used in the majority of patients to control the ventricular response, except with HR greater than 240/minute, likely due to WPW. Symptomatic patients ventricular rate 150–220/minute; give digoxin IV

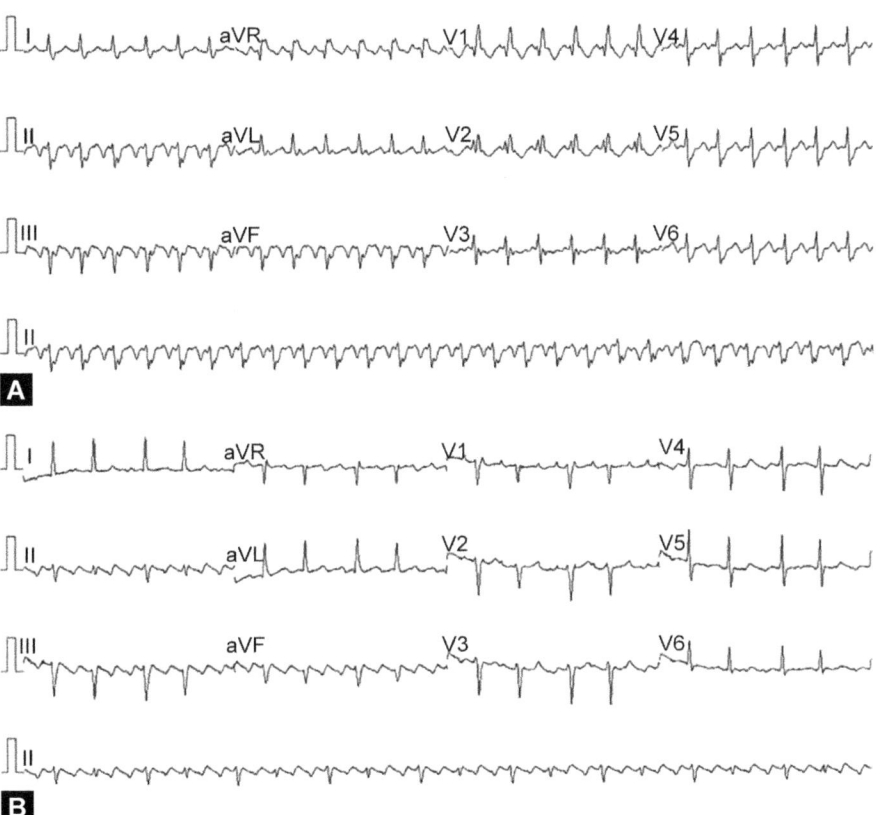

Figs. 6.2A and B: (A) Rapid narrow QRS regular tachycardia; flutter waves lead II, III, aVF. Note no such waves in lead I V6 is a clue to confirming the diagnosis of atrial flutter; (B) Atrial flutter at variable conduction ratio; irregular rhythm, note spiky P waves in V1.
Source: Adapted with permission from Khan MG. On Call Cardiology, 3rd edition. Philadelphia: WB Saunders/Elsevier Science; 2006.

0.5 mg slowly followed by 0.25 mg IV q 2 hours to control the ventricular response. A total dose of 1 mg is usually necessary if the patient has not taken digoxin in the past 2 weeks. For patients who have taken digoxin recently, a dose of 0.125 IV should be tried followed by a further 0.125 mg 2 hours later, if needed, followed by maintenance doses of 0.125–0.25 mg qd. The serum K must be maintained above 4 mEq (mmol)/L.

Diltiazem: Diltiazem IV slows the ventricular response, has less negative inotropic effect than verapamil, and can be given as a continuous infusion up to 24 hours in patients in whom digoxin maintenance is not considered essential. Diltiazem should not be administered in patients with suspected LV dysfunction or known to have EF less than 40%.

Patients with recent onset of AF should be anticoagulated. Conversion to sinus rhythm may be achieved in some patients if it is felt desirable:

142 Internal Medicine: Diagnosis and Therapy

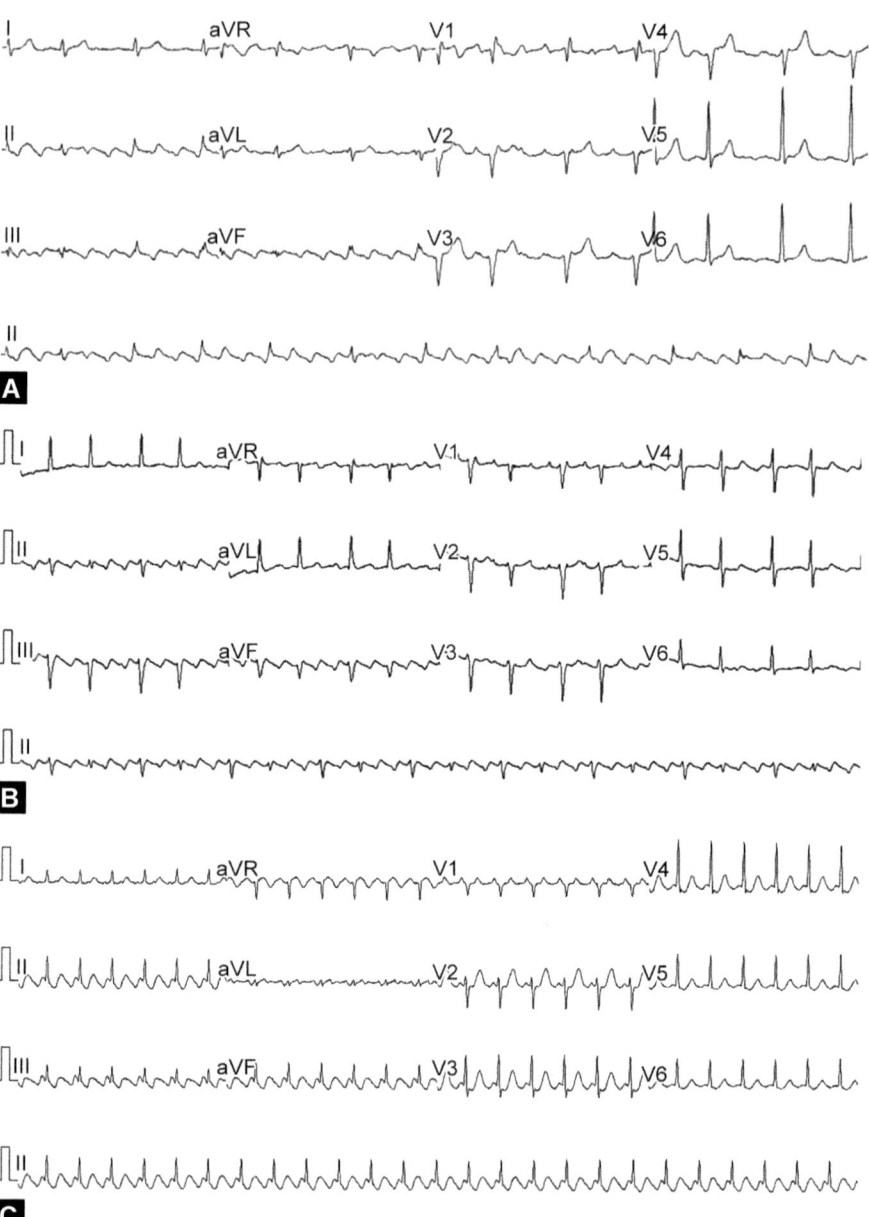

Figs. 6.3A to C: (A) Atrial flutter; irregular rhythm note sawtooth pattern II, III, aVF, spiky waves V1, and no activity in lead I, V6; (B) Atrial flutter; note lead I no flutter waves is a tip off to flutter versus artifact; spiky P waves V1; (C) Atrial flutter rapid regular rhythm.

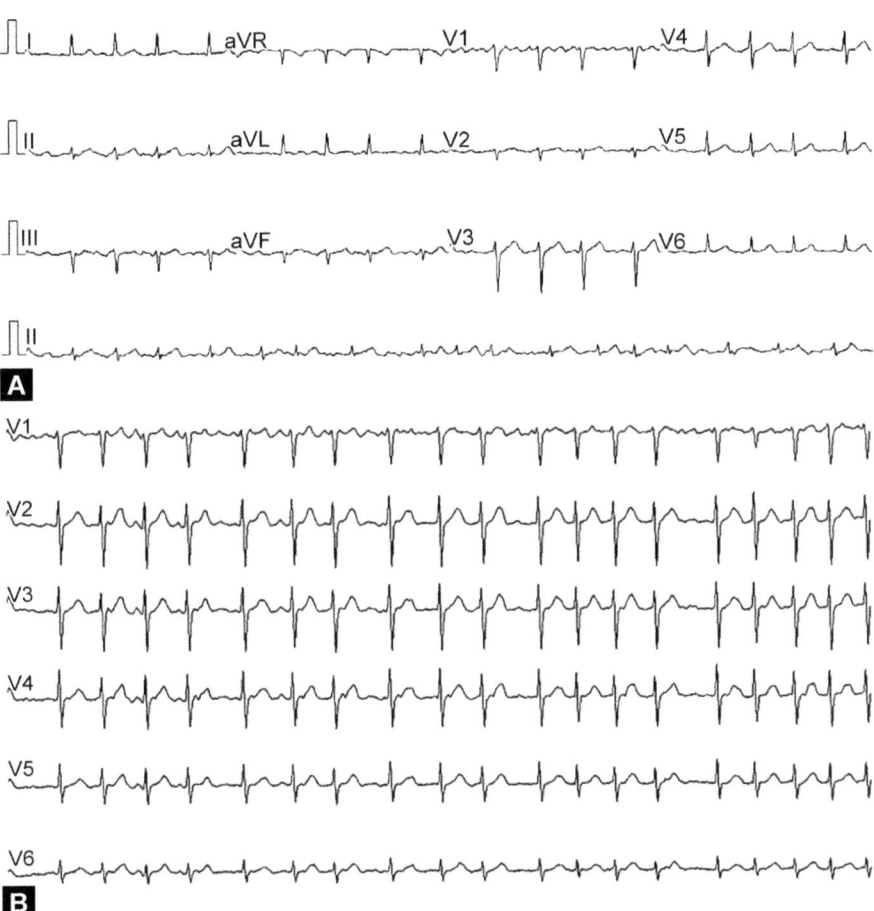

Figs. 6.4A and B: (A) Atrial fibrillation quick ventricular response; (B) Atrial fibrillation rapid ventricular response.

conversion may be achieved after full digitalization and control of ventricular response by adding quinidine 200–300 mg q 6 hours, or, if ventricular function is unimpaired, disopyramide may be used instead of quinidine. Conversion to sinus rhythm is achieved in about 50% of patients. DC conversion should be utilized in individuals with suspected WPW or HR greater than 240, or unstable patients and acute MI with hemodynamic compromise. DC conversion is also deemed necessary in patients with severe aortic stenosis, obstructive cardiomyopathy, and right ventricular infarction in whom atrial transport function is of great importance. Patients with chronic AF benefit from slowing the ventricular response with digitalis, and those who have a fast ventricular response on exercise gain further benefit with the addition of small doses of a β-blocker or oral verapamil.

Synchronized DC cardioversion: It is usually contraindicated in:
- Atrial fibrillation duration more than 1 year because sinus rhythm is usually not maintained.

- Cardioversion is often not considered worthwhile with chronic AF since less than 40% of patients remain in sinus rhythm 1 year postconversion. Other reasons for not electing to convert include the course of anticoagulation 1-2 weeks prior and 3-4 weeks post. Embolization occurs in about 2% of patients as well as transient postconversion arrhythmias.

Wolff-Parkinson-White Syndrome

Electrocardiographic changes are not always typical and depend on the distance between the SA node and the accessory pathway, and the resulting conducting times: intra-atrial, AV node-His, bundle branch, and accessory pathway. Thus, when AV nodal conduction is slowed, ECG features are more prominent and less apparent during exercise or when the accessory pathway is distant from the SA node. ECG hallmarks include:

- A PR interval less than 0.12 second is observed in less than 80% of cases. In approximately 20% of patients, the PR interval is 0.12 second or slightly longer, especially with advancing age (Fig. 6.5).
- A QRS greater than 0.12 second is not necessary for the diagnosis; in about 20% of cases, the QRS duration is less than 0.11 second.
- A delta wave is not always present.
- Occasionally, a pseudoinfarction pattern "Q in leads II, III or AVF" is present
- R wave as the sole or main deflection in V1, V2 referred to as type A WPW suggests localization of the bypass tract in the left ventricle.
- Type A pattern and a negative delta wave in leads II, III and aVF; consider posteroseptal bypass tract.
- Type A and isoelectric or negative delta in one of the following leads: I, aVL, V5, V6; consider a left lateral bypass tract.

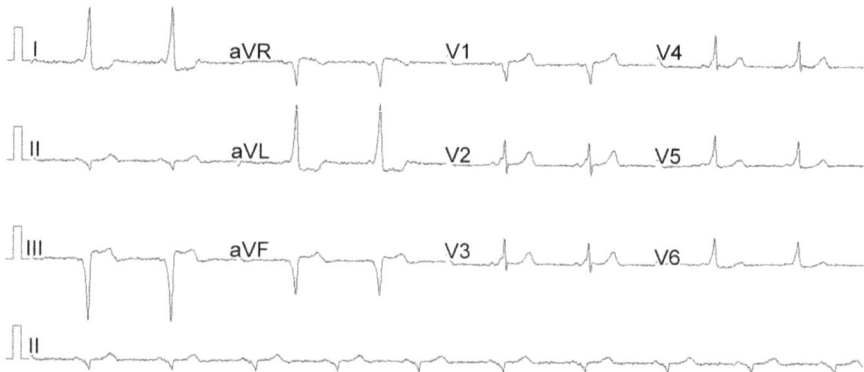

Fig. 6.5: Typical Wolff-Parkinson-White (WPW); short PR slightly widened QRS, delta waves lead I, V2-V6; note pattern in inferior leads mimics old inferior myocardial infarction.

- A negative P wave in lead I during tachycardia suggests a left-sided bypass tract.
- In so-called type B WPW, an S or QS is the dominant deflection in V1, V2, and may be mistaken for incomplete left bundle branch block (LBBB) or voltage criteria for left ventricular hypertrophy (LVH). Type B pattern is more commonly seen with right-sided bypass tracts. The terms type A and type B are no longer considered important hallmarks, but they are ingrained in history and may serve to remind the physician of certain scenarios, e.g. tall R in V1 is not always due to right ventricular hypertrophy or true posterior MI, but may be due to preexcitation; also, type B is present in less than 25% of cases of Ebstein's anomaly (Figs. 6.6 and 6.7).
- Atrial fibrillation occurs in 15–39% of cases; if the refractory period is very short, a very fast ventricular response (240–300) may occur and precipitate VF.

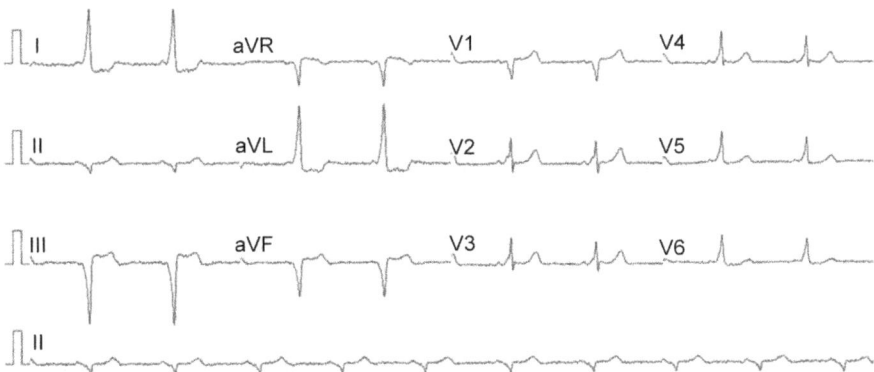

Fig. 6.6: Wolff–Parkinson–White syndrome can mimic old inferior myocardial infarction.

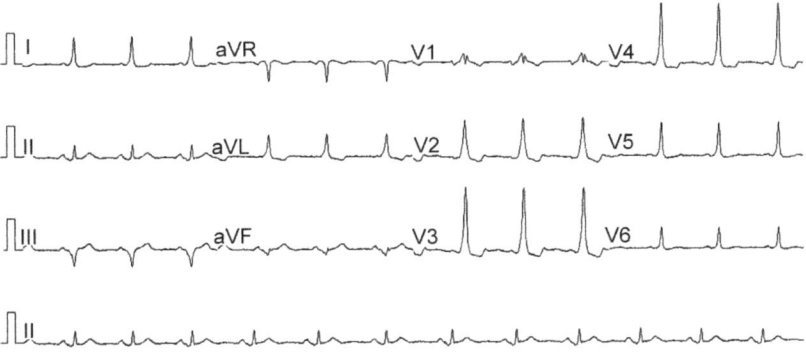

Fig. 6.7: Wolff–Parkinson–White syndrome may cause a RBB pattern or LBBB, incomplete RBBB or may mimic old inferior myocardial infarction.

- Very rarely a wide QRS regular tachycardia may be caused by multiple mechanisms, including the antidromic form of tachycardia.
- A clearly observed retrograde P wave in the ST segment suggests WPW tachyarrhythmia, whereas in AVNRT the P wave is usually lost in the QRS complex and is rarely seen in the ST segment.
- The presence of alternation in QRS amplitude during tachycardia suggests the participation of a bypass tract.
- Rate-related LBBB: Consider WPW.

Also, patients can have more than two pathways with reciprocation, using them and not the AV node, or may have AVNRT with conduction to the ventricles by the bypass tract.

The most common orthodromic arrhythmia in WPW syndrome is a circus movement in which the reentrant circuit uses the AV node in the anterograde direction and the accessory pathway in the retrograde direction and is a reciprocating tachycardia. This situation is present in greater than 85% of WPW arrhythmias. Rarely, a spontaneous change occurs in some patients from orthodromic to the rare antidromic tachycardia.

Antidromic tachycardia is an uncommon but clinically important form of tachyarrhythmia that occurs in 7–15% of patients with WPW; greater than 66% have multiple bypass tracts. In antidromic WPW, the tachycardia uses the accessory pathway in the anterograde direction and the AV node in the retrograde direction, resulting in rapid tachycardia (Fig. 6.8).

Dizziness and syncope occur in greater than 66% of patients with antidromic tachycardia and in less than 10% of patients with orthodromic tachycardia. Antidromic tachycardia may present as AF with rapid ventricular rates, RR less than 205 milliseconds with a wide QRS complex. Table 6.5 gives types of tachyarrhythmias observed with WPW and their approximate incidence.

Associated diseases and mimicry include:
- An increased incidence of WPW in patients with hypertrophic cardiomyopathy; echocardiographic assessment is advisable in all patients with WPW.
- Approximately 25% of Ebstein abnormalities have type B ECG pattern.
- Q waves in two of the three inferior leads II, III and aVF may be incorrectly diagnosed as inferior infarction.
- Absence of R in V1, and initial Q in V2, simulate anteroseptal infarction.
- Tall R waves in V1 may incorrectly suggest right ventricular hypertrophy or true posterior infarction.
- High QRS voltage may incorrectly suggest LVH.
- Type B or type A ECG pattern can be mistaken for incomplete LBBB or right bundle branch block (RBBB), respectively.

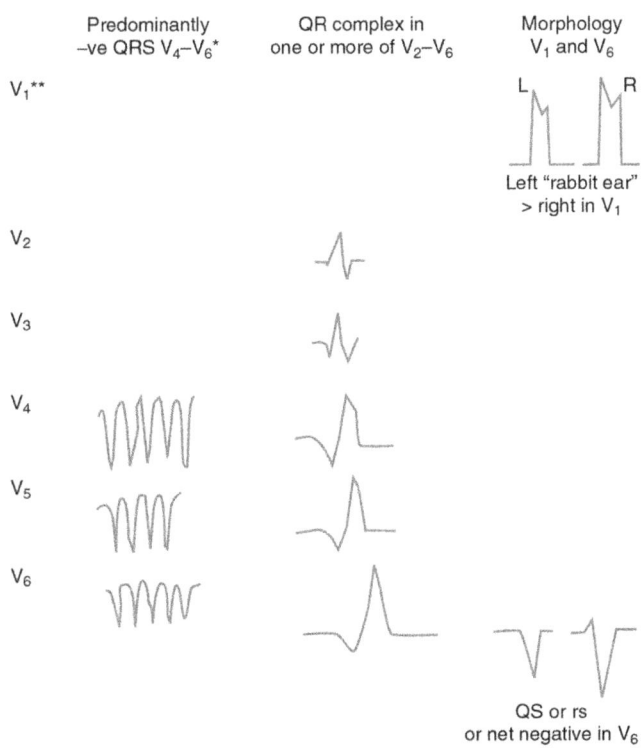

Fig. 6.8: Ventricular tachycardia: negative concordance. Positive concordance in leads V1 to V6 can be caused by ventricular tachycardia or Wolff–Parkinson–White antidromic (preexcited) tachycardia and other tachyarrhythmias. It is necessary to study the entire 12-lead tracing with particular emphasis on leads V1 to V6; lead II may be useful.
*Or concordant negativity in leads V1 to V6; positive concordance in leads V1 to V6 can be caused by ventricular tachycardia or Wolff–Parkinson–White antidromic (pre-excited) tachycardia.
**It is necessary to study the entire 12-lead tracing with particular emphasis on leads V1 to V6; lead II may be useful for assessment of P waves and atrioventricular dissociation.
Source: Adapted with permission from Khan MG. On Call Cardiology, 3rd edition. Philadelphia: WB Saunders/Elsevier Science; 2006.

Table 6.5: Types and approximate incidence of tachyarrhythmias in WPW syndrome.

Tachycardia	Approximate %
• Atrioventricular reentrant tachycardia (AVRT)	60
• Atrial fibrillation	15–39
• Atrial flutter	1
• Regular wide complex QRS indistinguishable from VT (atrial flutter or BBB during AVRT)	1
• Ventricular flutter VF	3

Therapy

- Emergency room management of atrioventricular reentrant tachycardia (AVRT) previously in patients with WPW: Adenosine rapid bolus injection as indicated in the section, Management of AVNRT.
- Patients with rapid ventricular response greater than 240/minute should be managed with IV procainamide. *(Caution:* Avoid in patients with hypertrophic cardiomyopathy.) In tachycardia, which could be pre-excited (e.g. AF or flutter), procainamide less than 10 mg/kg IV over 30 minutes, maximum 1 g in 1 hour, is reasonably safe provided that the patient is not hypotensive and does not become so. Failure to convert the arrhythmia or hemodynamic deterioration is an indication for prompt electrical conversion.
- Amiodarone has a role in the prevention of paroxysmal AF with rapid rates. Failure to respond is an indication for EP studies with a view to ablative therapy.

MANAGEMENT OF VENTRICULAR PREMATURE BEATS AND VENTRICULAR TACHYCARDIA (FIGS. 6.9 AND 6.10)

Ventricular premature beats: Coffee or alcohol consumption is the most common culprits in those with normal or slightly abnormal hearts.

Cessation of coffee, alcohol or other drinks cures the condition in many.

- If the arrhythmia is bothersome; and there is no contraindication (asthma, COPD), give a β-blocker; bisoprolol 2.5–5 mg/day (metoprolol 25 mg BID).
- Sotalol should not be used for the treatment of ventricular premature beats (VPBs) because this is the only β-blocker that may precipitate torsades de pointes.
- Do not use atenolol because it is a poorly effective β-blocker.
- Higher in patients with rheumatic heart disease and congestive cardiomyopathy, thus anticoagulation is strongly recommended. Patients with atrial flutter, however, do not require anticoagulants for conversion or for chronic use because embolization is not a complication.
- Guidelines for the management of benign, potentially lethal, and lethal arrhythmias are given in Table 6.6. An algorithm for the management of sustained VT is given in Flowchart 6.2.
- The selection of an antiarrhythmic agent is often dictated by the efficacy, proarrhythmic effect, and propensity to cause serious adverse effect, especially CHF (Table 6.7)
- *Dosage* of antiarrhythmic drugs is given in Table 6.8.
- Patients with benign arrhythmias require drug therapy only if symptoms are very bothersome. A β-blocker should be given a 3-month trial. Benign

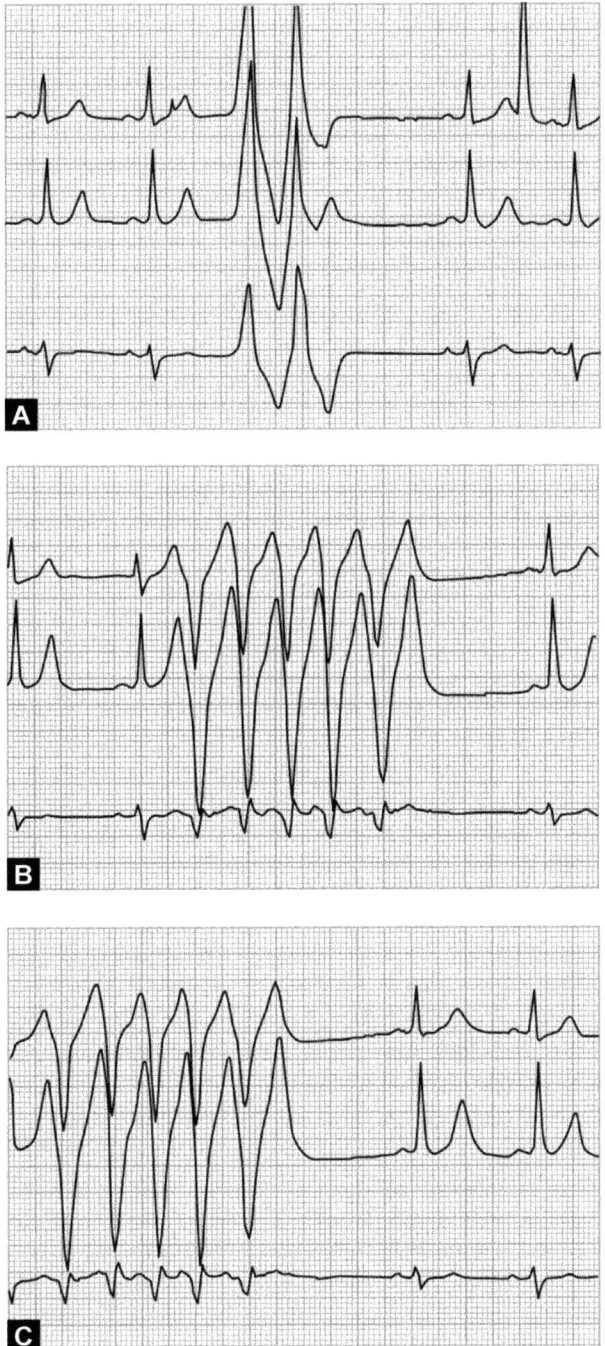

Figs. 6.9A to C: (A) Holter monitor showing multifocal ventricular premature beats, couplets; (B and C) Salvo: nonsustained ventricular tachycardia.
Source: Adapted with permission from Khan MG. On Call Cardiology, 3rd edition. Philadelphia: WB Saunders/Elsevier Science; 2006.

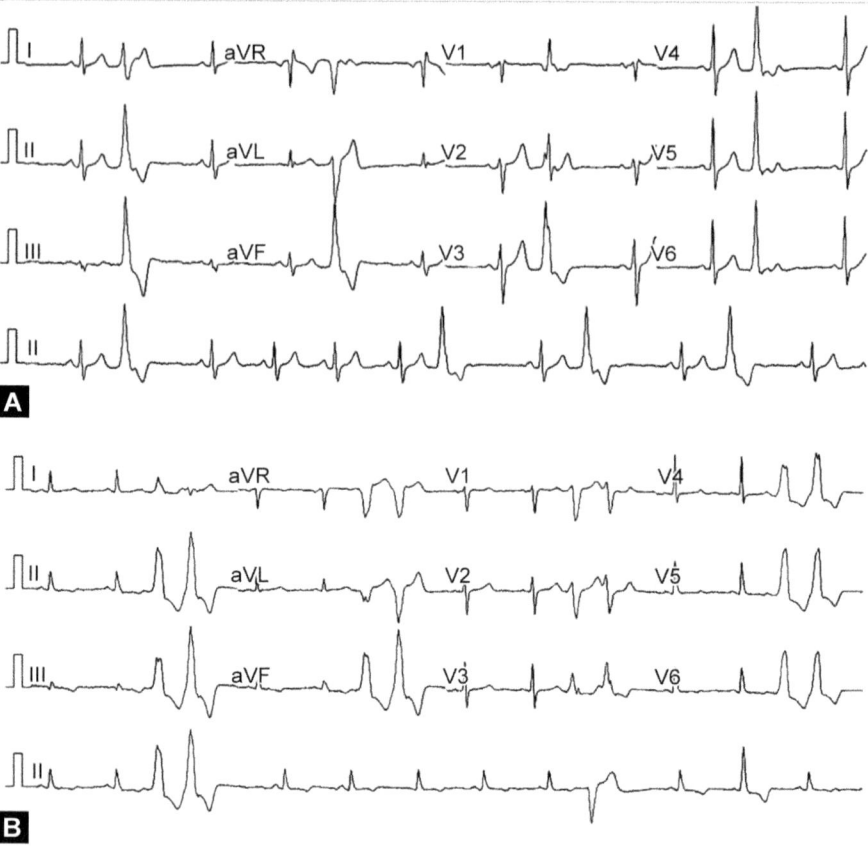

Figs. 6.10A and B: (A) Ventricular premature beats (VPBs)—compensatory pause; (B) VPBs—doublets; pairs of VPBs, multifocal.

arrhythmias may disappear or wax and wane; prolonged therapy may not be justified. Propafenone is of some value but is contraindicated with bundle branch block and significant COPD. Although rare, agranulocytosis has been reported.

- In patients with potentially lethal arrhythmias but with EF 25–30%, only three agents can be considered: (1) amiodarone, (2) mexiletine, and (3) quinidine (*see* Table 6.8). They have only a mild negative inotropic effect. Encainide can precipitate CHF, and the manufacturer's caution must be observed; the drug is also markedly proarrhythmic. The result of the Cardiac Arrhythmia Suppression Trial (CAST) indicates that flecainide, encainide, and moricizine are contraindicated in benign or potentially lethal arrhythmias; *encainide is not approved for general use.*

Table 6.6: Guidelines for the management of ventricular arrhythmias.

Benign arrhythmias	Potentially* lethal	Lethal (malignant arrhythmias)
Normal heart: VPCs, couplets, bigeminy ↓ No treatment reassurance if symptoms very bothersome or VT normal heart ↓ Beta-blocker and reassurance; consider mexiletine 2nd choice	Abnormal heart, e.g. postmyocardial infarction: Frequent VPCs multifocal, nonsustained VT ↓ EF >30%; no overt CHF ↓ Beta-blocker† ↓ Not controlled and symptomatic ↓ Mexiletine (unproven to improve survival) ↓ Not controlled ↓ Consider ↓ Amiodarone‡	a. Cardiovascular collapse b. Postcardiac arrest (VF) ↓ EP studies: In approximately 25% of cases, can initiate and suppress with drug or combination and improve outcome ↓ In majority EF <30% trial sotalol† or amiodarone or amiodarone + beta-blocker§ or Multiprogrammable implantable pacemaker-cardioverter-defibrillator, especially if EF <25% or ablative treatment c. Torsades de pointes (see text)

*Only beta-blockers significantly prolong life; amiodarone appears to do so only in the absence of heart failure.
†Used judiciously, EF down to 25% (see text).
‡Flecainide, moricizine, and propafenone not recommended for benign or potentially lethal arrhythmias.
§Not sotalol.

Classification of Antiarrhythmics

A knowledge of the EP classification of antiarrhythmics is useful in understanding arrhythmia suppression, drug combinations, and proarrhythmic and some adverse effects. Class I drugs inhibit influx of Na into the cardiac myocyte (Fig. 6.11 and Table 6.9). Class IA drugs (quinidine, disopyramide, and procainamide) slow phase zero and prolong the duration of the action potential. Class IB drugs (lidocaine, mexiletine, and tocainide) have relatively no effect on phase zero. Class IC drugs (flecainide, encainide, and propafenone) slow phase zero but have little or no effect on action potential duration. Class II comprises β-blockers. Class III comprises amiodarone and sotalol.

Flowchart 6.2: Management of sustained ventricular tachycardia.

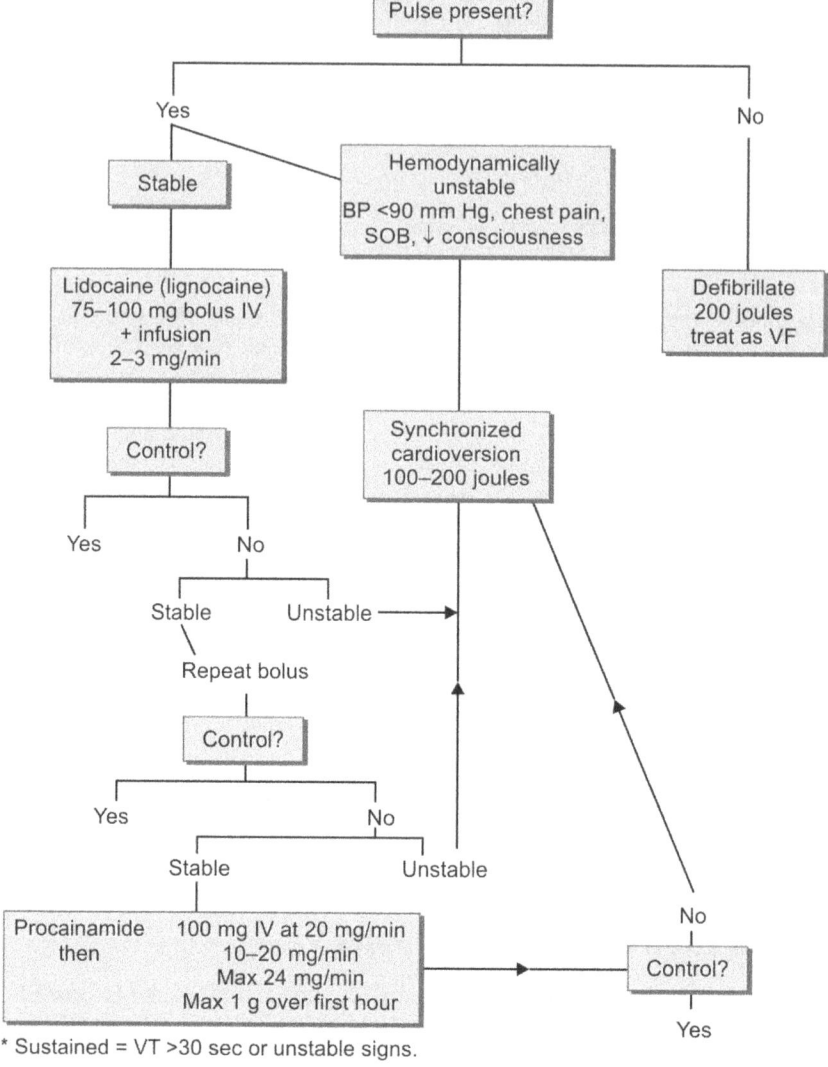

* Sustained = VT >30 sec or unstable signs.

Antiarrhythmic Agents

Caution is needed because these agents except lidocaine β-blockers and procainamide cause serious adverse effects and are successful in occasional cases.

Lidocaine (Lignocaine, UK): It is used in the presence of acute MI to treat frequent ventricular premature contractions (VPCs) more than 6/minute, multifocal or R on T. Lidocaine is the drug of first choice for the management of sustained VT where the patient is hemodynamically stable (Flowchart 6.2) (VT >30 seconds or unstable signs = sustained). *Dosage:* IV

Table 6.7: Drugs for ventricular arrhythmias, adverse effects, and efficacy with lethal arrhythmias.

Drug	Negative inotropic effect	Precipitates heart failure?	Serious side effects	Efficacy with lethal arrhythmias
Quinidine	+	No EF <25 yes +	Yes proarrhythmic ++++ precipitates torsades, VF, platelets ↓	Minimal
Procainamide IV Oral	+++ ++	Yes if EF <40	Yes agranulocytosis + lupus, torsades	Poor
Disopyramide	++++	Yes if EF <40	No; precipitates torsades +	Poor
Mexiletine	+	No EF <25, Yes	No High minor effects Low proarrhythmic +	Minimal
Tocainide	+	EF <25 yes +	Yes agranulocytosis +++ pulmonary alveolitis	Poor
Encainide*	++	Yes if EF <30 +	No, but proarrhythmic ++++	Poor if EF <30
Felcainide*	+++	Yes if EF <35	No, but proarrhythmic ++++	Not recommended if EF <35
Propafenone	+++	Yes if EF <35	Yes; rare agranulocytosis + proarrhythmic ++	Not if EF <35
Amiodarone	+	No EF <25 yes +	Yes; low proarrhythmic +	Yes +++
Beta-blocker	++	Yes if EF <35	No; not proarrhythmic†	Yes +++

*Not recommended for benign or potentially lethal arrhythmias.
†Except sotalol mildly proarrhythmic.
(EF, ejection fraction (%); ++++, maximum effect; +, minimal effect)

rapid bolus 75-100 mg (1-1.5 mg/kg) with immediate infusion of 2-3 mg/minute. A second bolus of 50-75 mg is administered within 5 minutes for VPCs, and earlier if VT persists. A further bolus may be required. In the presence of severe hepatic disease, CHF, or cardiogenic shock, the dose should be halved. A maximum infusion of 4 mg/minute should be given only after careful re-evaluation.

Table 6.8: Antiarrhythmic drug dosage.

Drugs	Dosage
Quinidine	200-mg test dose: If no hypersensitivity, syncope, or ↓ BP, 200–400 mg q 4 h × 4 doses then q 6 h then long-acting forms
Procainamide	375–500 mg q 3 h × 1 week then, q 4 h × 2–4 months. RF*
Disopyramide	300 mg, then 150 mg q 6 h. RF* SR 300 mg bid
Mexiletine	200–400 mg, then 2 h later 200–250 mg q 8 h RF* or MI q 12 h or q 24 h or elderly: 100–150 mg bid
Flecainide[†]	50–200 mg bid maximum 400 mg daily RF* caution
Sotalol[‡]	160–240 mg daily × 1–7 days, then 160–240 mg once or twice daily (investigational 320–720 mg daily for lethal arrhythmias, *see* text) RF*
Amiodarone	200 mg tid or qid × 1–2 weeks, then 200 bid × 4–6 weeks reduce weekly dose[§] by about 400 mg every 4 weeks until patient is taking 200 mg on 5–7 days/week (final maintenance according to Holter)

*Renal failure: increase dosage interval.
[†]See restrictions within text.
[‡]Other beta-blocker dosages (*see* Table 1.3).
[§]Higher doses previously used in the United States of America cause increased pulmonary toxicity.
(bid, twice daily; tid, three times daily; qid, four times daily; h, hours; q, every)

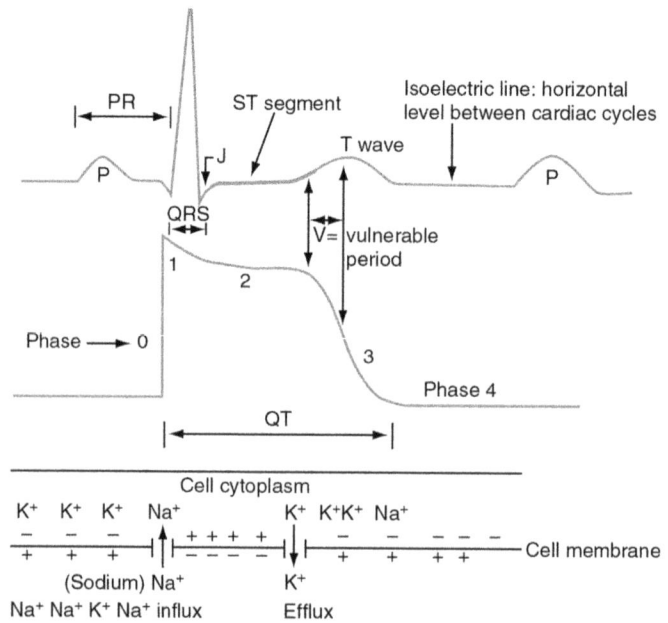

Fig. 6.11: Antiarrhythmic drug action.
Source: Adapted with permission from Khan MG. Cardiovascular system, pharmacology. In: Dulbecco R (Ed). Encyclopedia of Human Biology, Vol. 2. San Diego: Academic Press; 1991. pp. 167-77.

Table 6.9: Electrophysiologic classification or antiarrhythmic drugs.*

Class	Effect on the action potential (AP)†

Sodium channel blockers
• Sodium channel (+ +); blocks potassium efflux (+)
  ▪ Disopyramide
  ▪ Quinidine
  ▪ Procainamide
	Slows phase zero (+ +)
	Moderately prolongs the AP:
	↑ repolarization time, ↑ QT

• Sodium channel (+)
• Other effects
  ▪ Lidocaine (lignocaine)
  ▪ Mexiletine
  ▪ Moricizine (also IA IC actions)
  ▪ Tocainide
	Minimal slowing phase zero (+)
	Minimal narrowing of the AP
	↓ repolarization time

• Sodium channel (+ + + +)
  ▪ Encainide
  ▪ Flecainide
  ▪ Lorcainide
  ▪ Propafenone
	Marked slowing phase zero:
	Marked depression of upstroke
	Marked inhibitory effect on His–Purkinje conduction: ↑ QRS duration
	Shortens AP but only of Purkinje fibers: marked depression on conduction‡
	Repolarization time unchanged‡

Inhibition of the effects of sympathetic stimulation beta-adrenergic blockers	No effect on AP or repolarization§ ↓ phase 4 spontaneous depolarization: Decrease automaticity
Potassium channel efflux blockade Amiodarone + + + +, also sodium block. Sotalol (+ +) (no sodium block and usual Class II effects) Bretylium partly Class III	Slows phase zero (Class I effect) Markedly prolongs the AP: Markedly prolongs repolarization time. ↑ QT; amiodarone brings about a more uniform AP throughout the myocardium: Enhances electrophysiologic (EP) homogeneity
Calcium channel blockers	No effect
Alinidine	Investigational

*Modified from Vaughan Williams.
†See Figure 6.11.
‡May explain proarrhythmic effect.
§Except sotalol, Class III effect.
(+, minimal effect; + + + +, maximal effect; K, potassium)

Procainamide: *Dosage*: See Table 6.8. Indications include management of VT that fails to terminate with a second bolus of lidocaine (lignocaine).

Chronic oral therapy is not advisable since the drug does not improve survival in this category of patients with ventricular arrhythmias. If the drug is prescribed, it should generally not be given for greater than 6 months because of the incidence of drug-induced lupus and the occurrence of agranulocytosis, albeit rare. *Adverse effects:* The IV preparation has moderate negative inotropic effects, and the oral preparation has a mild risk of precipitating CHF. Torsades de pointes is not uncommon. Lupus occurs in greater than 33% of patients treated greater than 6 months; agranulocytosis appears to occur more commonly with the sustained-release preparation. *Interactions:* ACE inhibitors may enhance immune effects; cimetidine increases procainamide levels.

Mexiletine (Mexitil): It is a very weak antiarrhythmic agent and rarely shows salutary effects in the treatment of lethal arrhythmias. However, because of its weak negative inotropic effect, it can be combined in selected cases with sotalol, amiodarone, or quinidine if sinus node disease, hypotension, bradycardia, and AV block are absent. The drug can precipitate CHF in patients with EF less than 24%.

Beta-blockers: Beta-adrenergic blocking agents are effective antiarrhythmic agents that have no proarrhythmic effects, with the exception of sotalol which, because of its unique Class III effects, is the most effective β-blocking antiarrhythmic agent.

Beta-blockers are:
- Effective in all grades of ventricular arrhythmias
- May not completely suppress VPCs, nevertheless, may prevent the occurrence of VF in the same individual
- Particularly useful for ventricular arrhythmias initiated by ischemia or catecholamine release
- Effective for supraventricular arrhythmias. (This aspect was discussed earlier in this chapter.)

Dosage: See Table 1.3 for oral dosage.

Atenolol is not recommended (*see* Chapter 3).

In one study, sotalol and propranolol caused less than 65% and 44% ↓ in VPCs, but sotalol caused less than 99% ↓ of ventricular couplets versus less than 50% ↓ obtained with propranolol.
- In general, β-blockers are avoided in patients with EF less than 30% because CHF may be precipitated. However, recent trials indicate benefit and relative safety of β-blockers in the management of patients with EF as low as 22% who are at high risk for sudden death following episodes of monomorphic VT. Often a combination of acebutolol 200–400 mg

or nadolol 40–80 mg with amiodarone proves effective and safer than amiodarone combined with a Class I agent.
- Several clinical trials have shown sotalol to be a well-tolerated, effective antiarrhythmic agent in patients at high risk for sudden death. The drug may be effective in patients who did not benefit from multiple drug treatment. A dose of sotalol ranging from 160 mg to 720 mg with a mean dose of 240 mg is usually required for suppression that is more frequent in patients with VF, 58% versus 24% in patients with VT. When sotalol is used, it is necessary to maintain a normal serum K. Thiazide diuretics should not be used in combination. If a diuretic is necessary, it is advisable to give amiloride, a K-retaining diuretic.
- Beta-blockers and amiodarone are the only two antiarrhythmics that have been shown to cause prolongation of life in patients with potentially lethal or lethal arrhythmias.

Amiodarone (Cordarone): Amiodarone blocks the efflux of K from myocytes and markedly prolongs the action potential, thus increasing repolarization time and the effective refractory period. Although the QT interval is prolonged, torsades de pointes is, in fact, a rare complication of amiodarone, mainly because the drug enhances homogeneity of the action potential throughout the myocardium. Fortunately, the drug has a very mild negative inotropic action that allows its use in patients with lethal arrhythmias, which often have underlying severe LV dysfunction with EF less than 30%. *Dosage*: IV for life-threatening arrhythmias: Infusion less than 5 mg/kg; usually 300 mg over 2 hours with ECG monitoring; often given over 0.5 hours if life is threatened; maximum dose 1.2 g in 24 hours. Central venous cannulation is required for prolonged infusion. Additional 150-mg boluses can be given if required during the infusion. *Caution*: Hypotension may occur. Oral dosage: See Table 6.8.

Pharmacokinetics:
- About 50% of the oral dose is absorbed; bioavailability is 20–80% and plasma levels occur in 6–12 hours. The lipophilic compound is extensively metabolized to desethylamiodarone, which has pharmacologic activity. The drug is highly bound (95%) to protein, and widespread distribution occurs in most tissues, especially the liver, lungs, and adipose tissue. The concentration in the myocardium is about 20–40 times that in plasma. The volume of distribution is high; an adequate loading dose is necessary; half-life is about 30–110 days.
- With dosages of 200 mg tid, a therapeutic effect is observed in 1–4 days, but increases less than 6 months; the action of the drug may persist for greater than 50 days after cessation of therapy, although most side effects show a decrease after 4–7 days, depending on the oral loading dose. When given IV, a therapeutic effect is observed within a few minutes. A loading dose of 10–12 g in the first 2 weeks and maintenance of 400 mg qd 5 days weekly achieves steady-state plasma amiodarone

and desethylamiodarone concentrations of 1.7 ± 1.3 mg/mL and 1.1 ± 0.5 mg/mL, respectively, only after about 1 month of therapy. Patients usually experience therapeutic benefits to amiodarone at plasma concentrations less than 1.0 mg/mL, and toxicity is not often manifest with concentrations less than 2.0 mg/mL. The action of the drug appears to relate to tissue stores, and myocardial concentration is important.

Indications:
- Lethal ventricular arrhythmias: Sustained VT, recovery from VF, or cardiac arrest. Patients with a first occurrence of lethal arrhythmias in the absence of precipitating factors have about a 50% mortality. Survivors have a high mortality; some have a mortality of greater than 90% in 1 year. The overall mortality in survivors of cardiac arrest is about 66% over 5 years. In these high-risk patients, amiodarone has a role. Alternatively, an antiarrhythmic device may be implanted. The BASIS trial indicated that in patients at high risk for sudden death (i.e. potentially lethal arrhythmias), amiodarone at low dose 200 mg qd caused a decrease in mortality in the first year in post-MI patients.
- For conversion of acute AF to sinus rhythm, especially in patients *with* hypertrophic cardiomyopathy.
- Paroxysmal AF that is *highly symptomatic*, with rapid ventricular rates refractory to other therapy and deemed bothersome and incapacitating.
- Wolff-Parkinson-White: Management of AF or atrial flutter with rapid ventricular rates due to anterograde conduction over the accessory pathway.

Contraindications: Sinus bradycardia, sinus node disease, or AV *block* (requires pacing to allow amiodarone therapy); hypokalemia; severe *hepatic* dysfunction; iodine sensitivity; pregnancy and breastfeeding; porphyria.

Interactions:
- Class IA antiarrhythmic agents prolong the QT interval and may induce torsades de pointes; also erythromycin increases the QT interval and must not be given concomitantly.
- Oral anticoagulant activity is increased.
- Verapamil and diltiazem may produce a sinus arrest or AV block, and quinidine and digoxin levels increase.
- Sotalol should not be used in combination, but any of the available β-blocking drugs can be combined with amiodarone.
- Tricyclics and phenothiazines, including moricizine, may induce torsades de pointes.
- Diuretics may produce hypokalemia and increase the risk of torsades.

Adverse effects:
- Cardiac side effects: Severe bradyarrhythmias, asystole, and rarely torsades de pointes, especially in patients *with* a low serum K. The incidence of serious proarrhythmic effects in patients administered amiodarone is less than 1%.

- Hypothyroidism or, less often, hyperthyroidism occurs in about 5% of patients. Asymptomatic corneal microdeposits develop in most patients after about 3 months of therapy.
- Hepatitis with grossly elevated transaminase levels occurs very rarely but may progress to cirrhosis, which may be fatal; immediate discontinuation of amiodarone is necessary if hepatic transaminases rise to more than three times normal.
- Photosensitivity, metallic taste, nausea, and vomiting; slate-gray skin, rarely seen, is related to high loading and maintenance doses.
- Nervous system effects are common, especially sleep disturbance, twitching, and paresthesia, but they usually respond to decreases in dosage.
- Pulmonary infiltrates and alveolitis should occur in less than 1% of patients with modern conservative dosing schedules.

Necessary monitoring: Because of the high potential for adverse effects, amiodarone should be administered in the hospital or outpatient setting under close supervision. Monitor at 2-4 weeks for 2-4 months, assessing the following:
- Serum K and magnesium levels: If a diuretic is necessary, ensure that a K-sparing diuretic is used, or administer supplemental K
- ECG for bradyarrhythmias and QT prolongation
- Liver function tests
- Free T_4, thyroid-stimulating hormone (TSH), and T_3
- Digoxin serum assay and the dose of digoxin should be halved. If oral anticoagulants are used concomitantly, the dosage should be halved.
- Amiodarone and desethylamiodarone plasma levels
- Request chest X-rays at 3 and 6 months, then 6-monthly or annually thereafter, or earlier if dyspnea occurs
- Holter monitoring early in the course of therapy confirms arrhythmia suppression and is useful in screening for intermittent bradycardia.

Torsades de Pointes

Torsades de pointes is a life-threatening arrhythmia often associated with a prolonged QT interval. The rate is usually 200-250/minute. It is rarely precipitated by drugs that prolong the QT interval (quinidine, disopyramide, procainamide, sotalol, rarely amiodarone, tricyclics, astemizole, pentamidine), severe hypokalemia hypomagnesemia and the congenital QT prolongation syndrome.

Therapy

- Immediately identify and withdraw the offending agent (antiarrhythmics and other drugs known to increase the QT interval).
- Rapidly correct K and magnesium deficiency.

- Magnesium sulfate 1–2 g is usually highly successful, even in the absence of magnesium deficiency; 2 g (10 mL of a 20% solution) is given IV over 10 minutes and is followed by 4 g over 4–8 hours as an infusion of 30 mg/minute. Also, a low K is corrected by KCl infusion. Magnesium is a cofactor of membrane Na, K, adenosine, triphosphatase, or Na pump known to keep the intracellular K-level constant. Magnesium sulfate given IV at higher doses occasionally causes marked hypotension. The substance also has a mild negative inotropic action. Patients with moderate to severe renal failure generally have high magnesium levels, and great caution is required in this situation.
- Accelerating the HR is the simplest and quickest method to shortening the QT interval.
- Temporary transvenous pacing is the safest and most effective method of management since the HR can be quickly and easily controlled for long periods. If available, atrial or atrial ventricular sequential pacing is preferable, but ventricular pacing is a simple procedure and the catheter obtains a more stable position with reliable capture. As an immediate measure, transthoracic pacing may be used while preparations are being made for electrode placement. If there is chronic bradycardia, the patient progresses to permanent atrial sequential pacing.
- An infusion of isoproterenol 2–8 mg/minute is sometimes used if pacing is not readily available. This agent is carefully infused to increase the HR to about 120/minute. Isoproterenol is contraindicated in acute MI, angina, or severe hypertension. However, isoproterenol infusion needs to be carefully monitored to maintain a HR of 100–120. Myocardial ischemia may be precipitated, and the drug may precipitate VT or VF.
- Amiodarone has been successfully used to manage torsades de pointes precipitated by sotalol or Class IA agents. This approach requires further confirmation; however, patients with congenital QT or prolongation syndrome are best managed with β-adrenergic blockers because these agents reduce mortality. Phenytoin has a role if β-blockers are contraindicated. Resistant cases are managed with permanent pacing plus β-blockers or left stellate ganglionectomy. Isoproterenol is contraindicated in the congenital QT prolongation syndrome.

Prevention of torsades depends on the removal of the cause and maintenance of normal K. Amiloride has Class III antiarrhythmic activity; the drug retains K and is the diuretic of choice in patients treated with agents that have the propensity to prolong QT interval.

Although β-blockers do not usually shorten the QT interval, they are the agents of choice in this syndrome and have been shown, in symptomatic patients, to reduce patients' mortality. In patients with congenital long QT syndrome, with or without deafness, torsades de pointes represents the predominant form of VT. Agents that shorten the QT (e.g. Ca, K, lidocaine, digitalis) are not effective. Because syncope or sudden death occurs in these patients, consideration must be given for intervention with cervicothoracic

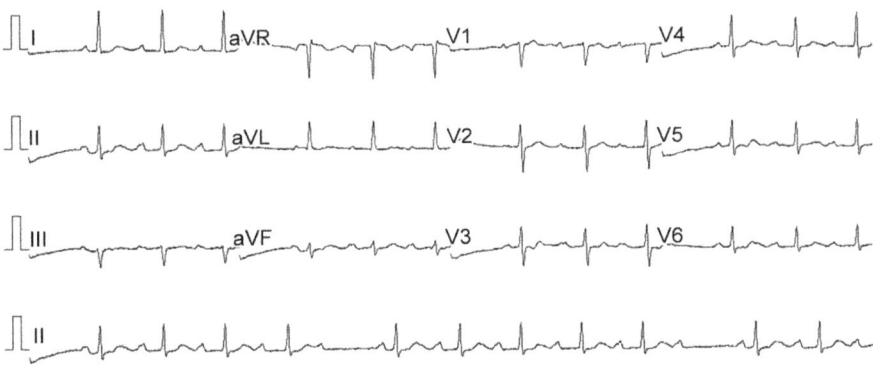

Fig. 6.12: Type 1 AV block. Typical Wenckebach phenomenon: Note beat 3, PR prolongation a QRS complex then followed by a dropped beat (the P wave is on the T wave of the third beat); then a long pause as failure to conduct this P wave. After a pause, the PR following is the shortest. The PR interval is shortest after the pause. Other clues to presence of Wenckebach: (1) the QRS are grouped in pairs or trios; (2) the longest cycle is longer the twice the shortest. Note not all type 1 blocks reveal a Wenckebach pattern. Wenckebach in 1999 without an ECG concluded from the venous pulse waves the phenomenon. Mobitz in 1924 with the ECG defined type 1 and type 2 AV blocks. No treatment is required but reassurance for type 1 block. The typical Wenckebach phenomenon may not be present in all type 1 blocks; the minor electrical disturbance is above the AV node.

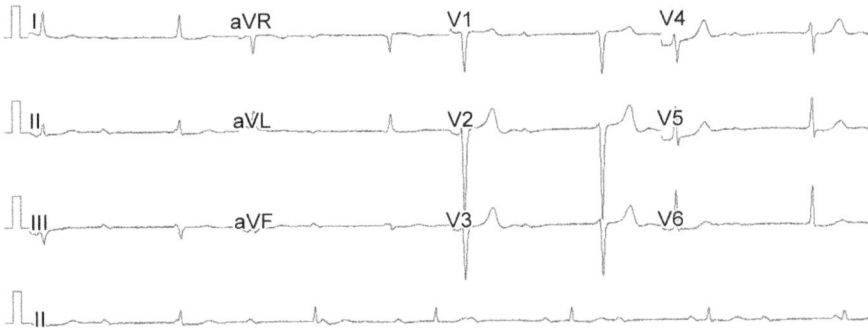

Fig. 6.13: Complete AV block; slow rate 37/minute; AV junctional escape rhythm, idiojunctional: the junction has a private (idio-) pacemaker beating independent of the sinus beat.

sympathectomy or implantation of an automatic implantable cardioverter-defibrillator (AICD).

Bradyarrhythmias

Severe bradycardia-producing symptoms are usually treated with atropine 0.5–0.6 mg q 2 minutes to a maximum of 2–2.4 mg. However, when atropine is used to treat asystole prior to pacing, a dose of 1 mg is given immediately followed by a further 1 mg 2 minutes later.

Figure 6.12 shows Mobitz type 1 and type 2 blocks, and Figure 6.13 shows complete heart block.

Mobitz type 2 block and complete heart block must be managed with ventricular pacing.

BIBLIOGRAPHY

1. Khan MG. A new electrode placement method for obtaining 12-lead ECGs. Open Heart. 2015;2(1):e000226.
2. Khan MG. Arrhythmias. In: Khan MG (Ed). Practical Cardiology. New Delhi: Jaypee Brothers Medical Publishers (P) Ltd.; 2018.
3. Page RL, Joglar JA, Caldwell MA, et al. 2015 ACC/AHA/HRS Guideline for the management of adult patients with supraventricular tachycardia: a report of the American College of Cardiology/American Heart Association Task Force on Clinical Practice Guidelines and the Heart Rhythm Society. J Am Coll Cardiol. 2016;67(13):e27-e115.

CHAPTER 7

Pericarditis/Cardiac Tamponade

PERICARDITIS

The common causes of pericarditis are listed in Flowchart 7.1. The division into obvious causes based on the presence of an easily recognizable underlying disease, and causes that are not obvious, but easily excluded by history and physical and finally nonspecific pericarditis probably caused by viral infections, provides for easy recall. Chest pain
- Is typically retrosternal or left precordial.
- Occasionally radiates to the trapezius ridge (a radiation that does not occur with angina).
- May radiate to the neck or left arm and may simulate angina or myocardial infarction (MI).
- At times, it is localized to the epigastrium or left upper quadrant
- Is sharp, pleuritic, but may be described as an oppressive, dull, vague ache.
- Is increased by deep inspiration, coughing, swallowing, recumbency.
- Is relieved by sitting and leaning forward.

Genuine shortness of breath or forced, shallow breathing due to pain, as well as palpitations, are common features. Underlying infection may cause fever and myalgia. A pericardial friction rub is characteristically:
- Heard between the lower left sternal edge and apex
- Localized to any area or over most of the precordium
- Heard with the diaphragm pressed firmly against the chest wall, with the patient leaning forward with the breath held
- Absent if effusion develops.

The four stages of electrocardiogram (ECG) abnormalities are given in Table 7.1 and Figure 7.1 shows ECG findings.
- Sinus tachycardia is common and may be the only ECG finding if ST elevation has resolved and the T waves remain normal.
- ST-segment elevation, when present, is concave upward with no T wave inversion. With MI, the ST segment is convex, often with Q waves present, and the T waves begin to invert before the ST segment normalizes.

Echocardiography is necessary to detect and quantitate associated pericardial effusion and to assess tamponade.

Flowchart 7.1: Causes of pericarditis.

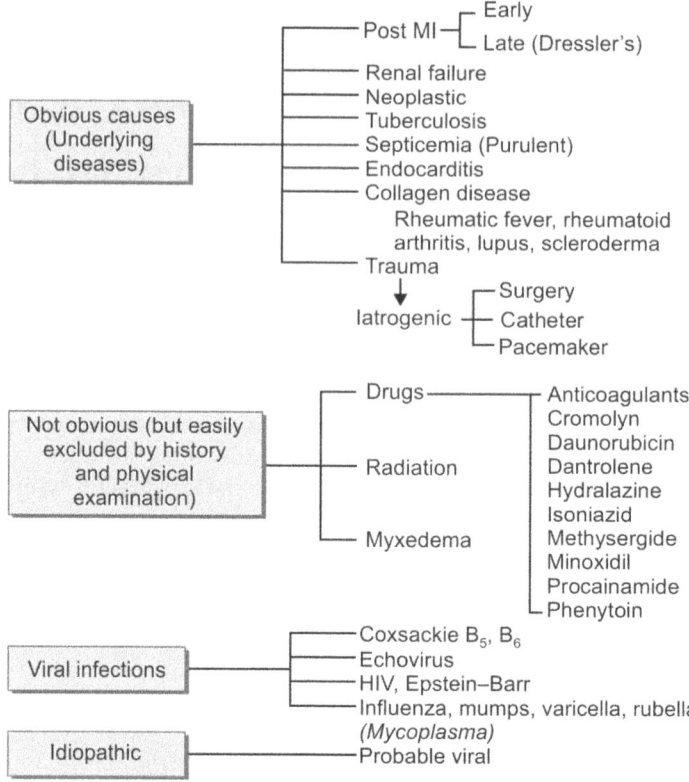

Table 7.1: Electrocardiographic clues to pericarditis.	
Stage I (hours to days)	Widespread ST-segment elevation 2–5 mm concave upward LI, II, III, V2–V5; reciprocal depression aVR V1
Stage II (few days later)	ST and PR segments isoelectric, upright or flattened T
Stage III	After normalization of ST segment, diffuse T wave inversion occurs
Stage IV (days to weeks)	T waves normalize, rarely remain inverted

Idiopathic and Viral Pericarditis

Most cases of idiopathic pericarditis are caused by viral infections (Flowchart 7.1). The patient should be hospitalized and observed for tamponade.

The occurrence of tamponade is manifested by: hemodynamic compromise; elevation of the jugular venous pressure (JVP); pulsus paradoxus; and usually hypotension, which may mask pulsus paradoxus.

Echocardiography helps confirm the pericarditis or tamponade. Pericardiocentesis is not done routinely, even with moderate-sized effusions, if

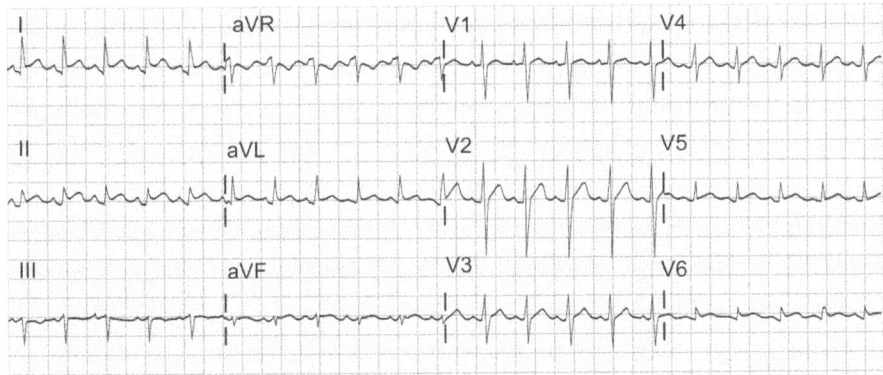

Fig. 7.1: Characteristic features of acute pericarditis: ST-segment elevation in most leads: I, II, aVL, aVF, V5, and V6, with reciprocal ST depression and PR-segment elevation in aVR. In addition, note sinus tachycardia commonly seen with acute pericarditis.

tamponade is not present. If pain is bothersome, the patient should rest in bed and chair for a few days, followed by slow ambulation over 1–2 weeks.

Management of Pain

Pain is relieved by aspirin or other nonsteroidal anti-inflammatory drugs (NSAIDs): ibuprofen, 400 mg q 6 or 8 hours, indomethacin, 25–50 mg q 8 hours, or naproxen, 250 mg tid for 4–10 days. Modified bedrest and increasing dosage of NSAIDs with adequate gastric cytoprotection usually brings relief of pain without major adverse effects.

It is not advisable to commence corticosteroids solely for the relief of pain, because these agents may increase viral replication. Corticosteroids are indicated when there is total failure of high-dose NSAIDs used over several weeks and with relapsing pericarditis not controlled by NSAIDs.

Dexamethasone: Dosage: IV 4 mg may relieve pain in a few hours.

Prednisone: Dosage: 60 mg qd for a few days, decreased by 10 mg q 3–5 days until a dose of 15 mg is reached. If symptoms are controlled, it is advisable to give 15 mg on alternate days for 5 days, and then 10 mg on alternate days for 5 days, 5 mg on alternate days for 5 days, and discontinue. The course of prednisone should be tapered as quickly as feasible. NSAIDs are added at adequate dosage when the corticosteroid dose has reached 15 mg qd, and gastric cryoprotective agents are used if there is a history of previous peptic ulceration or if gastric symptoms are present.

Approximately 25% of patients experience recurrence; if effusion develops, the risk of tamponade is high. In the absence of congestive heart failure (CHF) or tamponade, patients with severe recurrent chest pain unrelieved by adequate doses of NSAIDs may require corticosteroids for control of pain, fever, and shortness of breath. Alternate-day therapy carries less risk of adverse effects.

Pericarditis due to Specific Causes

Postinfarction Pericarditis

Acute pericarditis occurs in approximately 10% of patients within 12 hours to 10 days after infarction. The pain may be confused with postinfarction angina, extension of infarction, or pulmonary embolism. Most cases occur on the third or fourth day postinfarction. Chest pain is best treated with aspirin. NSAIDs such as indomethacin, ibuprofen, and naproxen should be avoided because they appear to interfere with the healing of infarcted tissue and have been shown to cause infarct expansion and to accelerate remodeling.

Dressler's syndrome occurs in less than 0.1% of patients, usually weeks or months after MI, and may be an immune reaction. Pleuritic chest pain, fever, friction rub, leukocytosis, and increased sedimentation rate simulate nonspecific pericarditis. Enteric-coated aspirin, 650 mg bid or tid for 1-2 weeks, should suffice. If pain remains bothersome or is recurrent, NSAIDs should be tried. Occasionally, corticosteroids are necessary and should be given as prescribed under idiopathic and viral pericarditis.

Purulent Pericarditis

Purulent pericarditis usually occurs during septicemia caused by pneumococcus, meningococcus, *Haemophilus*, gonococcus, and other organisms. Pericardiocentesis is indicated in patients suspected of purulent pericarditis in order to isolate microorganisms and determine sensitivities and the appropriate choice of antibiotics. Cardiothoracic surgical assistance often is required for open pericardial drainage or creation of a pericardiopleural window.

Tuberculous Pericarditis

In Asia, Africa, the Middle East, Latin America, and some nonindustrialized countries, tuberculosis is the most common cause of pericarditis. In North America and Europe, tuberculosis is responsible for about 4%, 7%, and 6% of acute pericarditis, tamponade, and constrictive pericarditis, respectively. Diagnosis requires isolation of *Mycobacterium tuberculosis* in pericardial fluid or a histologic examination of pericardial tissue or proven active tuberculosis in other organs. Tuberculous pericarditis is more common in blacks, is commonly seen in patients with acquired immunodeficiency syndrome (AIDS), and has a peak incidence in patients 30-60 years of age.

Symptoms and signs include:
- Cough
- Weight loss
- Dyspnea, occasionally orthopnea

- Fever, chills, and night sweats sometimes for several months before signs of pericarditis occur
- Cardiomegaly
- Possibly a pericardial friction rub plus signs of tamponade
- Hepatomegaly (>90% of patients)
- Ascites (fairly common)
- Cardiac arrhythmias, especially atrial fibrillation (AF) or flutter.

Echocardiographic and computed tomography (CT) examination may reveal pericardial effusion and pericardial thickening.

The patient should be hospitalized, observed for tamponade, and given therapy with isoniazid (300 mg), pyridoxine (50 mg), rifampin (600 mg), and ethambutol (15 mg/kg) qd for at least 9 months, allowing a minimum of 6 months of drug treatment following culture conversion. The combination of isoniazid (300 mg) and rifampin (600 mg) qd for 9 months has been shown to produce a satisfactory response in 95% of patients with extrapulmonary tuberculosis.

Corticosteroid therapy is indicated for recurrent or persistent pericardial effusion in patients receiving adequate courses of antituberculous therapy. This therapy may cause the avoidance of pericardial resection, which appears to be required in 7-40% of patients adequately treated with antituberculous drugs. Although some series show a high incidence of pericardial constriction, pericardiectomy is not routinely recommended.

Uremic Pericarditis

Pericardiocentesis is required only if there is suspicion of purulent infection or tamponade. The condition usually subsides with more frequent dialysis. Recurrent effusions uncontrolled by dialysis may respond to instillation of triamcinolone into the pericardial sac.

The instillation of sclerosing agents is of benefit in some patients with neoplastic pericarditis.

CARDIAC TAMPONADE

Tamponade may occur acutely secondary to:
- *Chest trauma*: An individual who has sustained recent chest trauma and appears in shock with increased venous pressure should be suspected of having cardiac tamponade.
- Acute MI with free wall rupture
- Dissecting aneurysm.

Acute or subacute presentations occasionally occur with:
- Neoplastic involvement
- Nonspecific pericarditis
- Uremia or purulent infections.

Sudden progressive severe shortness of breath, chest tightness, or dysphagia may herald the shock-like state. The JVP is usually elevated; hypotension and tachycardia are usually present.

Diagnostic Hallmarks

Significant pulsus paradoxus is usually detectable, except when severe hypotension or elevation of the diastolic pressure of either ventricle is present; for example, with uremic pericarditis and hypertension. Thus, the physician should not be lulled into a sense of false security by the absence of paradoxus. Pulsus paradoxus is an exaggeration of the normal inspiratory decline of systemic arterial pressure. To determine the presence of significant pulsus paradoxus, the patient's respirations are observed while slowly deflating the blood pressure (BP) cuff. Initially, the Korotkoff sound is heard only on expiration, but as the cuff pressure is lowered, Korotkoff sounds are heard during inspiration; the difference in systolic BP recorded at the commencement of the Korotkoff sounds in inspiration and expiration is an estimate of pulsus paradoxus. Normally, this difference is less than 10 mm Hg. Pulsus paradoxus greater than 12 mm Hg is significant. Muffled heart sounds represent another hallmark. Pulsus paradoxus may be observed in several conditions, including:
- Severe chronic obstructive pulmonary disease (COPD)
- Status asthmaticus
- Pneumothorax
- Massive pulmonary embolism.

However, in COPD and asthma, the JVP falls normally on inspiration. With right ventricular infarction, the venous pressure is high but increases on inspiration (Kussmaul's sign), and pulsus paradoxus is absent. Massive pulmonary embolism may produce a shock-like state with markedly elevated JVP and represents a diagnostic challenge, but the clinical setting usually assists in differentiating the two conditions.

Cardiac tamponade and cardiogenic shock secondary to acute MI may be difficult to differentiate, and both may occur during the course of massive infarction, but tamponade is uncommon. Heart sounds may be faint in both conditions.

Severe CHF causing marked elevation of JVP can be confused with cardiac tamponade. It is important to differentiate the two conditions, since the use of diuretics is contraindicated in the presence of tamponade. Because the most common cause of right heart failure (HF) is left HF, pulmonary congestion is usually detectable with the presence of crackles, third heart sound, radiologic evidence of pulmonary congestion, and left ventricular (LV) failure. Pulsus paradoxus is not a feature of severe CHF, and the presence of a prominent V wave in the venous pulse indicates tricuspid regurgitation and CHF.

Cardiac regional tamponade causing hemodynamic deterioration may occur within the first 2 weeks of cardiac surgery or in conditions causing adhesions and loculation. In these situations, pulsus paradoxus may be absent and the echocardiogram may fail to show effusion all around the heart. In patients with suspected cardiac tamponade, urgent echocardiography is mandatory. Echocardiographic features include:
- An early finding of right atrial collapse, which occurs in most cases except regional tamponade, in which right or left atrial collapse may be observed.
- Right ventricular collapse.

Therapy

- Maintenance of an adequate preload so as to generate stroke volume. Thus, diuretics and preload-reducing agents such as nitrates and angiotensin-converting enzyme (ACE) inhibitors must be avoided. Volume expansion with saline and even transfusion with packed red cells may provide hemodynamic stability until pericardiocentesis is accomplished. It is important to maintain volume expansion so that right atrial pressure may be maintained above intrapericardial pressure in order to prevent right atrial or ventricular collapse.
- Pericardiocentesis carried out by an experienced cardiologist under echocardiographic control or by a cardiac thoracic surgeon. An indwelling pericardial catheter with multiple side holes may be used for drainage and for installation of antibiotics, triamcinolone, or chemotherapeutic agents. Failure of pericardiocentesis is usually due to a posteriorly located effusion. Reaccumulation of fluid and recurrent tamponade are indications for subxiphoid pericardial window drainage carried out by a cardiothoracic surgeon.

CONSTRICTIVE PERICARDITIS

The proper management of constrictive pericarditis begins with correct diagnosis. Common causes include:
- Neoplastic disease, especially carcinoma of lung, or breast asbestosis and lymphoma
- Mediastinal irradiation
- Nonviral pericardial infections
- Viral pericarditis
- Tuberculosis
- Postcardiac surgery
- Chest trauma
- Connective tissue diseases
- Chronic renal failure and dialysis.

Table 7.2: Constrictive pericarditis versus restrictive cardiomyopathy.

	Constrictive pericarditis	Restrictive cardiomyopathy
Clinical features		
Heart size	Usually normal	Usually large
Heart impulse	Quiet	LV and/or right ventricular dilatation
Jugular venous pressure	M pattern*	M pattern
Kussmaul's sign	Present	Present
Systolic (v) waves	Absent	Present (tricuspid regurgitation)
Systolic murmurs	Rare	Common
S3 gallop†	Present	Present (except in amyloid)
Chest X-ray	Clear lung fields	Similar
	Normal heart size	Similar or moderately enlarged
	Pericardial calcification (50%)	Rare
		Myocardial calcification not uncommon
Electrocardiogram	P mitrale	Uncommon
	Atrial fibrillation 33%	Common
	Conduction defects uncommon	Common
	Flat or inverted T waves common	Widespread T wave inversion common
	May show low voltage	Low voltage common
	Q waves *very* rare	QS precordial leads, pseudoinfarction pattern common
Echocardiogram	Thickened pericardium	
	Calcified pericardium	No pericardial calcification, myocardial calcification
	Normal septal motion	
Systemic disease (associated)	Tuberculosis	Amyloid; sarcoid; tuberculosis (see text)
CT or MRI scan	Thickened pericardium	**Normal pericardium**

*Due to exaggerated x- and y-descents.
†Pericardial knock.

Diagnostic Hallmarks

- If the JVP is both markedly and chronically elevated and the history and physical examination fail to suggest an apparent cardiac cause in the presence of a small quiet heart, then a restrictive syndrome must be considered, the most common cause being constrictive pericarditis. Neck vein examination should reveal Kussmaul's sign, which may be difficult to elicit when the venous pressure is severely elevated. The venous pulse usually has a prominent y-descent, coincident with the early rapid diastolic filling of the ventricle. A prominent x-descent, coincident with

filling of the atrium, is often observed in patients with sinus rhythm. The exaggerated x- and y-descents give the venous pressure a characteristic M- or W-shaped pattern (Table 7.2).
- Auscultation should reveal the presence of an early high-frequency third heart sound (S3) caused by abrupt cessation of early diastolic filling. This sound, referred to as a pericardial knock, occurs earlier than the conventional third heart sound of CHF and has a sharp, high-pitched quality that is easily heard with the diaphragm and may mimic an opening snap or early filling sound heard in endomyocardial fibrosis.
- Atrial fibrillation occurs in approximately 33% of cases of constrictive pericarditis.
- The presence of marked ascites, occurring days to weeks before the presence of significant edema, points strongly to constrictive pericarditis and serves to distinguish the condition from CHF, in which prominent edema occurs, followed weeks later by mild ascites. In a few patients with long-standing constriction and congestion, protein-losing gastroenteropathy may ensue.
- Patients who present with noncalcific constrictive pericarditis pose a diagnostic problem. Table 7.2 gives diagnostic points for constrictive pericarditis versus restrictive cardiomyopathy (RCM).

Investigations

A few or all of the following investigations may be required to ascertain the diagnosis.
- Chest X-ray may show pericardial calcification, especially of the apex and posteriorly, which is best seen on lateral views. The heart size is usually normal.
- Electrocardiogram is virtually always abnormal but nonspecific and shows diffuse flat or inverted T wave in greater than 75% of patients; the depth of inversion of the T waves is usually proportional to the degree of pericardial adherence to the myocardium, which may make stripping difficult. Low voltage is present in approximately 50% of cases, along with P-mitral. AF is present in approximately 33% of patients.
- Echocardiography is of limited value in identifying thickened pericardium, unless calcification is present. Doppler echocardiography shows typical Doppler features in both mitral and hepatic vein flow in approximately 85% of patients with constriction amenable to surgery.
- Ultrafast cine-CT and/or magnetic resonance imaging (MRI) fairly accurately assess pericardial thickness, pericardial impingement on the right ventricle, and the degree of dilation of the vena cavae and hepatic veins.
- Cardiac catheterization findings are listed in Table 7.3. Elevation and equalization of all diastolic pressures and the dip and plateau or square

Table 7.3: Catheterization data.

Parameters	Constrictive pericarditis	Restrictive cardiomyopathy
Diastolic pressure	Equalization of early and late diastolic pressures	Equalization of early and late diastolic pressures
LVEDP-RVEDP >6 mm Hg (predictive value 87%)*	Usual finding (few exceptions)	Usually >6, but significant overlap
LA pressure	Equal right	Higher than right; may equalize with severe tricuspid regurgitation
RV pressure square root sign	Always present: early dip and plateau during diastole	Present, but may disappear with therapy
Pulmonary hypertension	Mild	Moderate or severe
RV systolic pressure ≥52 mm Hg (predictive value 71%)	Usual finding	Wide range (30–85 mm Hg)
RVEDP/RV systolic ≥0.38 (predictive value 83%)	Usual finding	Variable, significant overlap

*Both measured simultaneously.
(LVEDP, left ventricular end-diastolic pressure; RVEDP, right ventricular end-diastolic pressure; LA, left atrial; RV, right ventricular)

root sign are typical findings, but these may be observed in some patients with RCM. As outlined above, CT and MRI are useful in differentiating these two categories of patients (Table 7.2).
- It is important to avoid diuretics prior to catheter studies, because sodium (Na) and water loss may cause equalization of left and right ventricular filling pressures in patients with RCM.

Therapy

Surgical pericardiectomy is needed with medical therapy with the judicious use of diuretics and digoxin for control of the ventricular response.

BIBLIOGRAPHY

1. Adler Y, Charron P, Imazio M, et al. 2015 ESC Guidelines for the diagnosis and management of pericardial diseases: the Task Force for the Diagnosis and Management of Pericardial Diseases of the European Society of Cardiology (ESC). Endorsed by: the European Association for Cardio-Thoracic Surgery (EACTS). Eur Heart J. 2015;36(42):2921-64.
2. Fuster V. Stethoscope's prognosis: very much alive and very necessary. J Am Coll Cardiol. 2016;67(9):1118-9.
3. Imazio M, Demichelis B, Parrini I, et al. Day-hospital treatment of acute pericarditis: a management program for outpatient therapy. J Am Coll Cardiol. 2004;43:1042-6.

4. Imazio M, Gaita F. Diagnosis and treatment of pericarditis. Heart. 2015;101:1159-68.
5. Imazio M, Lazaros G, Brucato A, et al. Recurrent pericarditis: new and emerging therapeutic options. Nat Rev Cardiol. 2016;13(2):99-105.
6. Khan MG. Practical Cardiology. New Delhi, India: Jaypee Brothers Medical Publishers (P) Ltd.; 2018.
7. Sagar S, Liu PP, Cooper LT Jr. Myocarditis. Lancet. 2012;379:738-47.

CHAPTER 8

Valvular Heart Disease and Rheumatic Fever

AORTIC STENOSIS

Diagnosis

- The causes of aortic stenosis and the average survival of patients are given in Tables 8.1 and 8.2.
- Diagnosis younger than age 30 is typical of congenital aortic stenosis. In patients older than age 70, calcific aortic sclerosis due to degenerative calcification is common, and significant stenosis develops in less than 5% of these individuals. A bicuspid valve occurs in 2–3% of the population, with a male-to-female ratio of 4:1 and is predisposed to degenerative calcification. Between ages 30 years and 70 years, calcification of a bicuspid valve is the most common cause of aortic stenosis, and, much less frequently, cases of rheumatic valvular disease are encountered.

Physical Signs

Physical signs of significant aortic stenosis include:
- A systolic crescendo-decrescendo murmur best heard at the lower left sternal border, the second right interspace, or occasionally at the apex, with radiation to the neck.
- The longer the murmur and the later the peak of the crescendo-decrescendo, the greater the gradient.
- The intensity of the murmur, in the absence of significant aortic regurgitation, is usually Grade 3 or greater, except if cardiac output is low, as with congestive heart failure (CHF); then, even a Grade 2 murmur may be in keeping with severe stenosis. Aortic regurgitation

Table 8.1: Causes of aortic valvular stenosis.

Clinical parameters	Incidence
Biscuspid calcific	60%*
Degenerative calcific	15%
Rheumatic	20%*
Other	5%

*Reverse in Asia, Africa, Middle East, Latin America.

Table 8.2: Average survival in patients with moderate or severe aortic stenosis.

Clinical parameters	Survival years
Left ventricular failure	1.5–2
Severe shortness of breath	2
Mild shortness of breath	3–4
Syncope	3
Angina	4–5

increases flow across the aortic valve and may produce a loud systolic murmur without stenosis.
- An absent or very soft aortic component of the second sound (A2).
- An S4 gallop is usually present and is highly significant in patients younger than age 50.
- A thrill is commonly present over the base of the heart or the carotid arteries; this indicates a murmur of Grade 4 or louder and may relate to the severity of aortic stenosis if aortic regurgitation is absent.
- A thrusting, forceful apex beat of left ventricular hypertrophy (LVH); the apex beat is usually not displaced, except in patients with concomitant aortic regurgitation or with terminal left ventricular (LV) dilation.
- The carotid or brachial pulse in patients younger than age 65 shows a typical delayed upstroke. In the elderly, loss of elasticity in arteries often masks this important sign.
- A bicuspid valve occurs in 2–3% of the population, with a male-to-female ratio of 4:1, and is predisposed to degenerative calcification.
  - Between the ages of 40 years and 70 years, calcification of a bicuspid valve is the most common cause of aortic stenosis in the United States of America and Canada but rheumatic disease remains prominent in Asia, Africa and South America.

Electrocardiographic and Chest X-ray Hallmarks

The electrocardiogram (ECG) in patients with moderate to severe stenosis often shows features of LVH. Chest X-ray usually shows a normal heart size, with some rounding of the left lower cardiac border and apex; occasionally, some posterior protrusion in the lateral view may suggest LVH. The heart size may be increased if cardiac failure supervenes or with concomitant aortic regurgitation. A common hallmark of valvular aortic stenosis is poststenotic dilation of the ascending aorta.

Echocardiographic Features

Echocardiographic features of moderate to severe aortic stenosis are indicated by the following:
- Doppler peak systolic pressure gradient greater than 60 mm Hg in the presence of a normal cardiac output

Table 8.3: Hemodynamic parameters for severe aortic stenosis.

	Aortic valve area* (cm²)	Aortic valve area index (cm²/m²)	Peak systolic gradient (mm Hg)	Mean gradient (mm Hg)
Severe stenosis	<0.75	<0.4	≥80	≥70
Probable severe	0.75–0.9	0.4–0.6	50–79	40–69
Uncertain	>0.9–1.2	>0.6	<50	<40

*In an average-sized adult.

- Maximal instantaneous Doppler gradient greater than 60 mm Hg (range = 64–165 mm Hg)
- Peak systolic flow velocity greater than 4 m/s (range often observed = 4–7 m/s)
- Valve mean gradient greater than 40 mm Hg (range in several clinical studies = 40–120 mm Hg)
- Valve area less than about 0.75 cm² in an average-sized adult, 0.4 cm²/m² of body surface area, severe or critical stenosis (Table 8.3).

Valve area greater than 1.5 cm² indicates mild aortic stenosis, 0.75–1.4 cm² indicates moderate stenosis.

Severe aortic stenosis: The echocardiographic findings usually indicate a valve area less than 0.7 cm² in an average-sized adult and Doppler peak systolic pressure gradient greater than 60 mm Hg, with a maximal instantaneous gradient in the range of 64–145 mm Hg. If the cardiac output is low or the valve gradient appears inadequate to account for symptomatology, the valve area index should be calculated (*see* Table 8.3).

Patients with LV failure or LV dysfunction require emergency surgery. Others require prompt surgery. During the waiting period, dental work under antibiotic coverage should be completed. The patient should be instructed concerning the risk and strictness of long-term anticoagulant regimen.

Diuretics are indicated if CHF is present and digoxin is used if systolic dysfunction is documented. CHF is not a contraindication to surgery.

Coronary angiography is necessary in patients older than age 35 or in those with chest pain.

Moderate aortic stenosis: Patients who have a valve area of 0.75–1.4 cm² are usually categorized as having moderate aortic stenosis.

However, the situation in patients with valve area of 0.75–1 cm² is regarded by some as a "fool's paradise" (*see* Table 8.3). Some determine severe stenosis by valve area of less than or equal to 0.9 cm² and/or valve area index less than or equal to 0.6 cm²/m². Patients who have moderate aortic stenosis, if minimally symptomatic, should be regarded as being at high risk for development of complications during the following 1–2 years, especially if the ejection fraction (EF) is less than 50% or if there is hemodynamic evidence of LV decompensation. In a study of 66 patients who had moderate aortic stenosis, 31% with minimal symptoms experienced serious complications within 4 years. Also, patients who have EF less than 50% at catheterization appear to have less than or equal to 64% chance of complications due to aortic stenosis over a 4-year period. The absence of severe symptoms does not ensure a favorable outcome. The elderly, mildly symptomatic patient with degenerative calcific aortic stenosis of a moderate degree is at high risk. Thus, if underlying diseases such as respiratory failure, stroke, renal failure, anemia, or cancer are not present, surgery is recommended.

Truly asymptomatic patients with moderate or severe aortic stenosis are not offered surgery but should be followed closely for a change in effort tolerance and breathlessness or other cardiac complications.

The patient should be advised to carry on with activities that are normal and to report any changes immediately.

Patients with a moderate degree of aortic stenosis should be considered at high risk if they are mildly symptomatic, especially if the EF is ↓ or there is hemodynamic evidence of LV decompensation.

Surgical Therapy

Mechanical obstruction to the LV outflow due to significant aortic stenosis is a pressure overload situation that leads to progressive LVH, LV strain, and finally CHF or sudden death. Symptoms due to obstruction of outflow are usually the main indications for valve replacement in patients with moderate or severe aortic stenosis (Table 8.4). In most of these patients, the valve area is less than 1.0 cm^2 and the peak systolic gradient is greater than 60 mm Hg. Fortunately, the hypertrophied myocardium often retains mechanical efficiency, and once the valve is replaced, significant improvement in ventricular systolic performance occurs in most patients. Thus, CHF is not a contraindication to valve replacement. Patients with LV failure due to severe aortic stenosis and followed for greater than 1 year because of intercurrent illness contraindicating surgery usually regain adequate LV function with later valve replacement. Since mortality is greater than 50% in 1 year in patients with CHF, surgery should be done promptly.

Indications for valve replacement include:
- LV failure
- Shortness of breath
- Angina
- Presyncope or syncope not due to preload-reducing agents or other causes of syncope (*see* Chapter 13).

Patients with chest pain or those older than age 35 require coronary angiography to assess the degree of atheromatous coronary stenosis and

Table 8.4: Indications for aortic prosthetic valve surgery.

Parameters	Intervention
Severe aortic stenosis	
Aortic valve area <0.75 cm^2	
Valve area index <0.4 cm^2/m^2	
Symptomatic patients:	
Heart failure or dyspnea	Emergency surgery
LV dysfunction or EF <50%	Urgent surgery
Angina	Urgent surgery
Syncope	Urgent surgery (within a few weeks)
Asymptomatic patients:	
Valve area as above	
Hemodynamic deterioration	No surgery
Left ventricular dysfunction	
Ejection fraction <50%	Fairly urgent (within a few months)
Cardiomegaly or LVH on: ECG or echocardiography	
Moderate aortic stenosis	
Valve area 0.75–1.3 cm^2	
Symptomatic:	
Heart failure	
Other symptoms or LV dysfunction or EF <50% (follow-up monthly)	Urgent surgery Fairly urgent (within a few months)
Truly asymptomatic: (Follow-up at least every 2 months)	Surgery (1–5 years) (if becomes symptomatic)

suitability for coronary artery bypass surgery (CABS). Young patients with left anterior descending artery (LAD) disease should be offered left internal mammary artery to LAD anastomosis or graft; in patients older than age 65, vein graft is appropriately recommended by the American College of Cardiology (ACC) and the American Heart Association (AHA) Task Force.

Contraindications to surgery include:
- Serious underlying disease, especially respiratory failure, cancer, severe renal failure, cerebrovascular accident with residual stroke, and contraindication to anticoagulant therapy
- Age more than 80 is a relative contraindication, except in patients with robust health and excellent cerebral status. Severe intercurrent illness should weigh heavily against surgery, except in patients with CHF due only to severe aortic stenosis with a valve area less than 0.75 cm^2. Because angina may require a combination of valve replacement and bypass surgery if there is coronary artery obstruction, care must be taken to individualize the selection. The patient and family must understand the risks.

Table 8.5: Choice of valve prosthesis.		
Clinical parameters	Mechanical valve	Bioprosthesis
Age <30	First choice	Not recommended
Anticoagulant necessary as in atrial fibrillation	Natural choice	Not recommended
Anticoagulant contraindicated	Not recommended	First choice
Aortic valve replacement		
Age 30–70	First choice	Second choice
Over age 70*, sinus rhythm	Second choice	First choice
Mitral (all ages)	First choice	May be considered in patients over age 70 in sinus rhythm

*Higher risk of bleeding with anticoagulants, and average life span 10 years.

Prosthetic Valve Choice

Problems exist with all types of valve prostheses; none is ideal. Scientific studies have indicated a superiority of mechanical valves over bioprosthetic valves, especially in patients younger than age 30 or at all ages in the mitral position, and mechanical valves are the obvious choice in patients with atrial fibrillation (AF) in whom anticoagulation is already necessary (Table 8.5). Importantly, Collins points out that of 1,117 isolated mitral valve replacements done at Brigham and Women's Hospital since 1971, 620 (54%) had AF and a need for anticoagulation. Bloomfield reiterates that 60% of mitral valves currently implanted in patients in the United States are mechanical; in 1988, the UK Registry reported that 68% of mitral valves implanted were mechanical. The surgeon's background and personal preferences, however, often dictate the choice of valve, taking into consideration the patient's age and the possible presence of contraindications to anticoagulant therapy. In underdeveloped countries, a mechanical valve is still considered first choice because it is preferable to monitor anticoagulation than to run the risk of two operations in 20 years (reoperation carries a >10% mortality and is costly). In the aortic position, it is expected that the durability of the mechanical valve is superior over a 10- to 20-year period because of a high reoperation rate with the use of bioprosthetic valves. The major disadvantage of mechanical valves is the small risk of bleeding due to anticoagulant therapy, and this must be weighed against possible reoperation over 7–15 years with a bioprosthetic valve.

It is well established that reoperation is required much more frequently with bioprosthetic valves, but the complications of thromboembolism, endocarditis, and valve obstruction are similar. A bioprosthetic valve may be considered a reasonable choice in patients older than age 70 whose life expectancy may be shorter than that of the bioprosthesis. In patients in whom anticoagulants are contraindicated or compliance is expected to be poor, a prosthetic valve is appropriate. In women who intend to become pregnant, a bioprosthetic valve is advisable but a mechanical valve with the use of heparin subcutaneously (SQ) for the first 4 months and during the last few weeks of pregnancy is an alternative.

Accelerated calcification of glutaraldehyde-treated bioprosthetic valves in patients younger than age 30 is of concern. However, cryopreserved tissue valves are being tested and appear to maintain tissue flexibility with considerably less tendency to calcify.

Two studies compared the mechanical valve with the bioprosthesis. The Veterans Administration (VA) study reported 10-year follow-up in 575 patients randomized between mechanical valve and bioprosthesis: reoperation for primary valve failure was necessary in 35 patients fitted with bioprostheses, compared to 19 patients with mechanical valves; repeat surgery was performed for perivalvular regurgitation in only 6 bioprosthetic versus 13 mechanical valves. There was a significantly higher incidence of bleeding due to anticoagulant therapy in patients with mechanical valves.

A 12-year comparison in Scotland of the Bjork–Shiley spherical disk valve with bioprosthesis in 261 mitral, 211 aortic, and 61 in both positions indicated no difference in reoperation or survival at 5 years. However, at 12 years, reoperation was necessary in 68 (37%) patients with bioprosthetic valve and 17 (8.5%) with mechanical valve. Porcine valve failure was usually due to rupture of one or more cusps, causing severe regurgitation, with a much greater risk in the mitral position. Importantly, 16 patients died as a result of reoperation for porcine valve replacement. Also, valve failure may cause death before further surgical intervention. Using death and reoperation as endpoints for an actuarial assessment of survival with the original prosthesis intact, the survival rate in patients with Bjork–Shiley prostheses was 48%, versus a 30% survival rate in patients 12 years after porcine valve replacement. This effect was significant for mitral valves but inconclusive for the aortic position.

As a result of the study, the Scottish group advises that a bioprosthesis appears to be contraindicated in the mitral position; replacement in young patients should be with a mechanical valve, but an aortic bioprosthesis has a role in patients older than age 70 who are in sinus rhythm.

The results of balloon aortic valvuloplasty have been disappointing and valve replacement is preferred even in the very elderly.

Complications of Valve Replacement

The major differences in complication rates in mechanical and bioprosthetic valves relate to the incidence of primary valve failure and major bleeding; primary valve failure is very high with bioprosthesis after 5 years, and major bleeding is a drawback of the mechanical valve (Table 8.6).

Table 8.6: Prosthetic valve complications.

Clinical parameters	Mechanical valve (%)	Bioprosthetic valve (%)
Reoperation		
Veterans administration* (10 year)	6.6	12
Scottish study† (12 year)	8.5	37
Major bleeding (12 year)	19	7
Perivalvular leak	4.5	2
Major embolism	8.8	9
Endocarditis	3.7	4.6
Survival rate (12 year)	51.5	44.4

*Bialy D, Lehmann MH, Schumacher DN, et al. Hospitalization for Arrhythmias in the United States: Importance of Atrial Fibrillation. J Am Coll Cardiol. 1992;19:41A.
†Modified from Bloomfield P, Wheatley DJ, Prescott RJ, et al. Twelve-year comparison of a Bjork-Shiley mechanical heart valve with porcine biorostheses. N Engl J Med. 1991;324:573-9.

Transcatheter Aortic Valve Replacement

- In patients with severe aortic stenosis who are at increased surgical risk, transcatheter aortic valve replacement (TAVR) with a self-expanding transcatheter aortic valve bioprosthesis is currently as good as aortic valve replacement.
- It appears to have a better 1-year survival. This intervention is proving most useful in selective patients.
- Patients have to have an adequate size to their aortic valve, not too big and not too small. Their other heart valves have to work reasonably well. Their aorta has to be of reasonable size.
- Increasing experience has not been associated with a decrease in the rate of periprocedural stroke or major vascular complications.
- This suggests that additional measures (i.e. embolic protection devices, improved antithrombotic regimens) may be required to systematically further lower periprocedural stroke rates during TAVR.

AORTIC REGURGITATION

Over the past 25 years, there has been a major change in the pattern of underlying conditions associated with diseases causing aortic regurgitation. Whereas rheumatic fever and syphilis comprised 70% and 20% of cases, respectively, they now account for less than 30% and 1%. With the fall in prevalence of these diseases, bicuspid valve, endocarditis, and diseases causing aortic root dilation have emerged as the common causes (Table 8.7).

Table 8.7: Causes of aortic regurgitation.	
Acute	Chronic
Bacterial endocarditis Aortic dissection Prosthetic valve surgery Aortic balloon valvuloplasty Trauma Rheumatic fever	Rheumatic Endocarditis Congenital: bicuspid valve, ventricular septal defect, sinus of Valsalva aneurysm Aortic root dilatation: connective tissue disorder: Marfan's, ankylosing spondylitis, Reiter's syndrome, rheumatoid arthritis, lupus erythematosus Takayasu arteritis, cystic medionecrosis, myxomatous degeneration, psoriatic arthritis, Behçet's syndrome, relapsing polychondritis, giant cell arteritis, osteogenesis imperfecta, ulcerative colitis Whipple's disease Hypertension Arteriosclerosis Syphilis

Diagnostic Hallmarks

With chronic aortic regurgitation, the left ventricle tolerates regurgitant volume overload and compensates adequately; an asymptomatic period of 10-30 years is not uncommon. Many patients with a moderate degree of aortic regurgitation deny shortness of breath on walking 3-5 miles and/or 3 flights of stairs. Complaints of shortness of breath on exertion, fatigue, palpitations, or dizziness are generally associated with moderate or severe regurgitation over a prolonged period or severe regurgitation of recent onset. Rarely, angina with diaphoresis occurs as the diastolic blood pressure (BP) falls, frequently at night, causing a ↓ in coronary perfusion. Symptoms and signs of CHF at rest are late manifestations.

Hallmarks on physical examination include:
- Typical collapsing pulse: Water-hammer or Corrigan's pulse or a bounding pulse. The underlying mechanism is a rapid ↑ in upstroke followed by an abrupt collapse due to a quick diastolic runoff from the arterial tree. Indeed, all conditions that cause a brisk runoff produce a collapsing or bounding pulse (Table 8.8). The collapsing quality is detected by the examiner placing his or her fingers or palm closed firmly over the radial pulse with the entire limb extended to the ceiling. Pulsus bisferiens, a double peak to the pulse, may be observed with the combination of aortic regurgitation and significant aortic stenosis.
- The patient's head often bobs with each cardiac pulsation
- The BP reveals a wide pulse pressure due to an an increase (↑) in systolic BP and a diastolic that is often less than 50 mm Hg. Occasionally, Korotkoff sounds persist to zero with diastolic arterial pressure still greater than 60 mm Hg

Table 8.8: Causes of a collapsing bounding pulse.	
Cardiac causes	Noncardiac causes
Aortic regurgitation Patent ductus arteriosus	Arteriovenous fistula Paget's disease Pregnancy Fevers Thyrotoxicosis Vasodilator drugs

- Arterial, neck pulsations are usually prominent
- Quincke's sign: Exerting mild pressure on the nail beds brings out intermittent flushing
- Finger pulsations: Collapsing pulsations in the finger pulps or tips
- Traube's sign: Pistol-shot sounds over the femorals
- Duroziez's sign: Compression of the femoral artery proximal to the stethoscope produces a systolic murmur and a diastolic murmur with distal compression.

The apex beat is virtually always displaced downward and outward to the left, indicating LV enlargement in patients with moderate or severe aortic regurgitation. A diastolic thrill may be palpated in the second right interspace or third interspace at the left sternal border, where the murmur of aortic regurgitation is most prominent.

Hallmarks on auscultation include:
- Typical high-pitched blowing, early decrescendo murmur begins immediately after the aortic second sound (A2). The early decrescendo murmur beginning immediately after A2 is unmistakable to the trained ear and is best heard with the diaphragm pressed firmly against the chest, with the patient leaning forward and the breath held in deep expiration. The listener should then listen to the murmur with the patient breathing normally and in the recumbent position in order to train the ear for detection of the softest diastolic murmur.
- The degree of aortic regurgitation correlates best with the duration of the murmur and may be pandiastolic with severe regurgitation
- Perforation of an aortic cusp may change the quality of the murmur to one that resembles the cooing of a dove
- A mid or late diastolic rumble at the apex, the Austin Flint murmur, may be heard as the regurgitant jet hits the anterior mitral leaflet, as it opens and closes during diastole. The leaflet's shuddering can be heard with the stethoscope or observed with the help of Doppler echocardiography
- The A2 may be increased, decreased, or normal, and the accompanying aortic systolic murmur and thrill may represent flow rather than stenosis.

The ECG commonly shows nonspecific ST-T wave changes, and with LVH, the pattern of LVH with volume overload is often present.

Chest X-ray: In patients with moderate or severe aortic regurgitation, dilation of the left ventricle with elongation of the apex inferoposteriorly is almost invariably visible. Progressive further enlargement occurs over years in patients with severe aortic regurgitation. Dilation of the ascending aorta is common in Marfan's syndrome and other causes of aortic root dilation (*see* Table 8.7). The typical appearance of linear eggshell calcification of the ascending aorta is a hallmark of syphilitic aortitis, which is now rare.

Echocardiographic findings include:
- Detection of the type of aortic valve abnormality and underlying disease, e.g. aortic regurgitation due to bicuspid valve or vegetations caused by endocarditis
- Left ventricular chamber dimensions: estimates of LV volume and ventricular function measurements (LV end-systolic dimensions, LV end-diastolic dimensions, fractional shortening or EF)
- Dilation of the aortic root
- Aortic dissection
- Other valve disease
- Other associated states, e.g. perivalvular abscesses in infective endocarditis.

Management of Chronic Aortic Regurgitation

Medical therapy plays an important role, since the timing of valve surgery presents an ongoing challenge for both physician and patient. A review of the natural history of the condition indicates that:
- Greater than 75% of patients with moderate aortic regurgitation survive for more than 5 years
- Greater than 50% are alive 10 years after diagnosis
- Greater than 90% of patients with relatively mild aortic regurgitation survive more than 20 years
- As with aortic stenosis, the occurrence of CHF carries about a 2-year survival, while for angina survival is about 5 years.

A VA study, completed in 1991, comparing the survival of 102 medically treated and 147 surgically treated patients with severe aortic regurgitation, and followed for 7.5 years, indicated that valve replacement may not prolong survival in these patients.

Valve replacement should be considered prior to irreversible myocardial deterioration. However, because timing is often difficult, close follow-up of the patient with minimal or absent symptoms is essential.

Timing of Valve Replacement

- There is general agreement that symptomatic patients with severe chronic aortic regurgitation should have valve surgery in the absence of contraindications.

- Valve surgery is not indicated in asymptomatic patients with severe chronic aortic regurgitation who have good effort tolerance and normal LV function.

Between these two extremes, there is a large group of patients for whom firm data comparing the effect of prognosis of medical with surgical management are lacking, as are widely accepted criteria or a task force consensus that may guide the physician.

Patients with moderate or severe aortic regurgitation should be followed at least every 3 months. A careful history is necessary, including questioning of a spouse or relative who may be able to describe symptoms that are denied by the patient. A cardiovascular examination and ECG are done at each visit. Echocardiography is advisable every 6 months if LV end-systolic dimension is greater than 50 mm or if fractional shortening is less than 30%. A biannual exercise test is useful to assess functional capacity.

If symptoms manifest (dyspnea on mild or moderate exertion, orthopnea, or chest discomfort), cardiac catheterization is necessary for verification of echocardiographic dimensions with a view to surgery.

Patients with prolonged severe LV dysfunction and marked LV dilation are not expected to benefit from surgery. Although there are no fixed rules giving clear contraindications, surgery generally is not advisable in patients who have:

- Ejection fraction less than 30%
- Prolonged severe LV dysfunction (≥18 months).

In these patients, symptoms, signs, and hemodynamic parameters of LV dysfunction may persist or worsen after successful valve replacement. Patients with EF less than 45% and less than 1 year of LV dysfunction usually have a successful postoperative outcome, but those with EF less than 45% and prolonged LV dysfunction (>18 months) have a poor postoperative survival. Repeated radionuclide or echocardiographic assessment of EF and end-systolic volume, especially at rest, is necessary for decision making. It must be emphasized that radionuclide EF is not accurate in patients with AF.

The role of the cardiologist is to consider interventional therapy prior to the occurrence of significant LV dysfunction. At this stage of careful follow-up, surgery is offered if LV function is impaired, if exercise capacity is reduced, or if LV dimensions are "highly abnormal" or show significant deterioration. Management of the asymptomatic patient with severe aortic regurgitation, depressed LV function, and abnormal dimensions, as indicated, should be individualized.

The following echocardiographic or catheter dimensions may be used to help serve in decision making regarding timing for valve surgery. No single estimation should be accepted for making decisions. Marked changes or rate of change at 3- or 6-month visits should guide the physician.

- LV end-systolic dimension of 50–55 mm Hg. A dimension greater than 55 mm usually indicates LV dysfunction and, as outlined earlier, one does not wait for such ominous signals
- LV end-diastolic dimension greater than 70 mm
- LV end-systolic volume index greater than 60 mL/m^2; greater than 90 mL/m^2 indicates severe LV dysfunction
- LV end-diastolic volume index 140–150 mL/m^2; greater than 180 mL/m^2 indicates severe LV dysfunction
- EF less than 50% or fractional shortening less than 30%; fractional shortening less than 25% indicates severe LV dysfunction, LV EF less than 45% represents moderately severe LV dysfunction, and less than 35% indicates very severe dysfunction.

The asymptomatic patient with severe aortic regurgitation should meet more than or equal to one of the abovementioned criteria and should show a marked change from the evaluation done 4–6 months previously in order to be considered a candidate for surgery.

It must be re-emphasized that no single measurement is ideal and that most of them must be obtained to enable the cardiologist to apply the best clinical judgment, taking into account other variables such as age, occupation, and intercurrent illness.

Preparations for surgery include attention to dental work under antibiotic cover. Coronary angiography is necessary in patients older than age 35 or in those with angina.

The choice of prosthetic heart valve is discussed in this chapter under aortic stenosis. Elective valve surgery has a 3–6% operative mortality and emergency surgery greater than 10%. The 5-year survival for valve implant is 60–85%.

- Current clinical indications are unsuitability for surgical aortic valve replacement (SAVR) (Class I) and high surgical risk (Class IIa) (Bonow et al. 2016)

There is little doubt that TAVR with a balloon-expandable device improves survival, as compared with medical therapy, in patients with severe aortic stenosis who cannot undergo surgery.

- Transcatheter aortic valve replacement and SAVR are associated with similar survival rates at 1 year among patients considered to be at high surgical risk, although the frequency of neurologic events is higher among patients treated with balloon-expandable TAVR than among those treated surgically (Adams et al. 2014).
- The results reported by Leon et al. (2016) seem to confirm that TAVR is the treatment of choice in most patients with aortic stenosis who are at high risk for early death and major complications from conventional surgery, particularly if the patient has clinical and vascular features such that he or she can be treated by a TAVR although it can accomplish excellent results with moderately severe disease in patients at moderate risk the following caveats apply:

- The valve replacement may not be possible in approximately 25% of patients because of anatomical problems.
- Calcification close to the valve or aorta aortic regurgitation may coexist; bicuspid valve importantly because tissue valves are used, patients under age 69 are not candidates because reoperation is likely within 15 years.

MITRAL STENOSIS

Mitral stenosis is almost always due to previous rheumatic fever. It takes greater than or equal to 2 years following the rheumatic episode for sufficient fibrosis and thickening of the valve to produce the typical murmur. Most patients remain asymptomatic for 15–20 years following an episode of rheumatic fever, which is subclinical in greater than 50%.

Over the past 30 years, the problem of rheumatic valve disease has shown a marked decline in North America, the United Kingdom, and Europe. However, the disease is still endemic in much of Asia, Africa, the Middle East, Latin America, and the West Indies. Indeed, in these countries, significant mitral stenosis may emerge within a few years of the initial acute rheumatic fever and result in symptomatic disease in juveniles and young adults.

Diagnosis

- The patient with mild mitral stenosis, valve area 1.6–2.0 cm^2, may develop mild dyspnea on moderate to severe exertion but is usually able to do all normal chores; lifestyle is not altered. Symptoms progress slowly, if at all, over the next 5–10 years. However, infection, pregnancy, or tachycardias, including AF, may precipitate severe dyspnea.
- Patients with moderately severe mitral stenosis, valve area 1–1.5 cm^2, usually have symptoms that affect or interfere with daily living. Dyspnea due to progressive pulmonary venous hypertension becomes bothersome. Breathlessness is precipitated by moderate activity such as walking 100 yards briskly, walking up an incline, or even running slowly for 20 yards. Some patients with mild mitral stenosis may reduce activities and tolerate symptoms for several years. Pulmonary infection or AF often precipitates pulmonary congestion, emergency room visits, or hospitalization. Cough, shortness of breath, wheeze, and hemoptysis may mimic bronchitis for several months because the subtle signs of mitral stenosis can be missed by the untrained auscultator. Palpitations are usually due to AF, and some patients may present with a very rapid tachycardia or systemic embolization.
- Severe mitral stenosis, valve area less than 1 cm^2 and valve area index less than 1 cm^2/m^2, usually causes symptoms on mild exertion. The patient presents with more than or equal to one of the following symptoms:

progressive dyspnea, palpitations, marked fatigue, and occasionally cough, hemoptysis, hoarseness, or chest pain. Progression may be rapid, with increasing edema, orthopnea, paroxysmal nocturnal dyspnea (PND), and marked breathlessness. However, some patients tolerate dyspnea and are able to continue work that is not strenuous, at their own pace, for 3-12 months prior to interventional therapy. Fortunately, with mitral stenosis, patients with the most bothersome symptoms benefit the most from mitral valvotomy.

Physical Signs

- On inspection, a malar flush is common in the presence of long-standing, moderately severe mitral stenosis.
- A lower left parasternal lift of heave due to right ventricular hypertrophy may be present.
- The apex beat is tapping in quality, usually not displaced.
- A diastolic thrill localized to the apex beat may be palpated.
- Auscultation reveals a loud slapping first heart sound and is so typical that it warns the examiner to search for other signs of mitral stenosis. Immobility of the cusps reduces this valuable sign.
- The pulmonary second sound is intensified and this vibration associated with pulmonary valve closure is often palpable with significant pulmonary arterial hypertension.
- An opening snap, a sharp high-pitched sound, is a hallmark of mitral stenosis. The opening snap is best heard with the diaphragm pressed firmly just internal to the apex beat and occurs from 0.04-0.14 seconds after the second heart sound. The opening snap may be heard over a wide area and, with severe mitral stenosis, usually occurs less than 0.08 seconds following the second heart sound, audible immediately rather than after a definite gap. The opening snap disappears if the valve becomes heavily calcified and nonpliable.
- The loud slapping first heart sound and opening snap produce a particular cadence that alerts the examiner.
- The opening snap is followed by a low-pitched, mid-diastolic rumbling murmur that is associated, if there is sinus rhythm, with presystolic accentuation, best heard with the bell lightly applied over the apex beat. The murmur often is localized to an area the size of a coin and can easily be missed; it is brought out by exercising the patient and listening with the patient lying on the left side. Occasionally, critical mitral stenosis may cause a marked ↓ in transmitral flow, and the murmur may be hardly audible. There is evidence that in these cases, the disease and contracted chordae ↑ the impedance to ventricular filling so that the reduced mitral valve area is no longer the limiting factor.

- The severity of mitral stenosis correlates best with the length of the murmur rather than the intensity.

Chest X-ray Hallmarks

- Straightening of the left heart border due to left atrial enlargement.
- Larger than normal double density, seen through the right half of the cardiac silhouette, indicating left atrial enlargement
- Elevation of the left main stem bronchus caused by distension of the left atrium with widening of the angle between the two main bronchi.
- Redistribution: restriction of lower lobe vessels and dilation of the upper lobe vessels.
- If CHF is present, signs of interstitial edema are present: Kerley B lines due to lymphatic engorgement and fibrosis, perihilar haze, and eventually frank pulmonary edema are observed.
- Fluoroscopy is no longer commonly done, but shows posterior displacement of the barium-filled esophagus.
- The heart size on posteroanterior X-ray is generally normal or near normal, and the lateral film should be assessed for right ventricular enlargement: "creeping up the sternum".

Electrocardiographic Hallmarks

- Signs of left atrial enlargement are common with moderate and severe mitral stenosis: broad bifid P waves in lead II and, more specifically, an ↑ in the P terminal force (PTFV1) greater than or equal to 40 msec/mm, measured in V1 (area subtended by the terminal negative portion of a biphasic P wave). Hazen et al. have shown that when PTFV1 is greater than 40 msec/mm, 95% of individuals had left atrial size greater than 4 cm; when PTFV1 is greater than or equal to 60 msec/mm, 75% had left atrial size greater than 6 cm.
- Right axis deviation of 90–150° reflects severe mitral stenosis.
- Right ventricular hypertrophy may be present with severe stenosis but does not correlate well with the degree of pulmonary hypertension.
- Atrial fibrillation is common with moderate long-standing rheumatic disease, with the left atrial size greater than 4.5 cm, and is characteristically coarse in appearance.

Echocardiographic Assessment (Figs. 8.1 to 8.3)

- Signs of left atrial enlargement are common with moderate and severe mitral stenosis: broad bifid P waves in lead II and, more specifically, an increase in the P terminal force (PTF1) greater than or equal to 40 msec/mm, measured in lead V1 (area subtended by the terminal negative portion of a biphasic P wave). When the PTF1 is greater than 40 msec/mm, 95% of individuals have left atrial size greater than 4 cm; when the PTF1 is greater than or equal to 60 msec/mm, 75% have left atrial size greater than 6 cm.

- The mitral diastolic gradient can be defined.
- Excellent quantification of mitral valve orifice area.
- Left atrial enlargement is uniformly present, and the size can be accurately determined.
- The degree of calcification of the mitral valve leaflets can be verified.
- Decreased posterior leaflet movement is often observed (Figs. 8.2A and B).
- The degree of right ventricular enlargement can be documented.
- Left ventricular size is expected to be small.
- Right ventricular systolic pressures reflect the degree of pulmonary hypertension.
- The degree of concomitant mitral regurgitation (MR) can be assessed.

A flat E to F slope or EF slope less than 10 mm/sec may indicate severe mitral stenosis, but this measurement is no longer used for quantitating the degree of obstruction. Marked alteration of the E to F slope may be observed in patients with aortic stenosis and regurgitation with no evidence of mitral stenosis and in patients with impaired LV filling caused by reduced LV compliance.

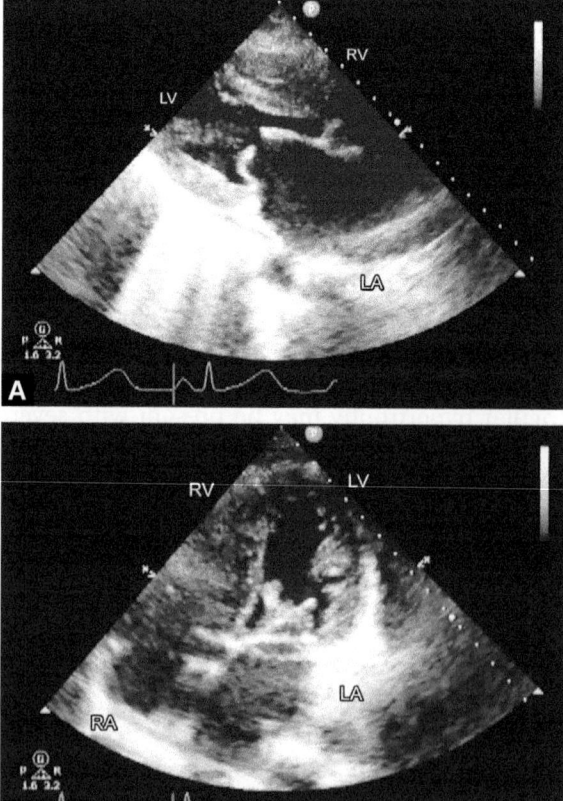

Figs. 8.1A and B

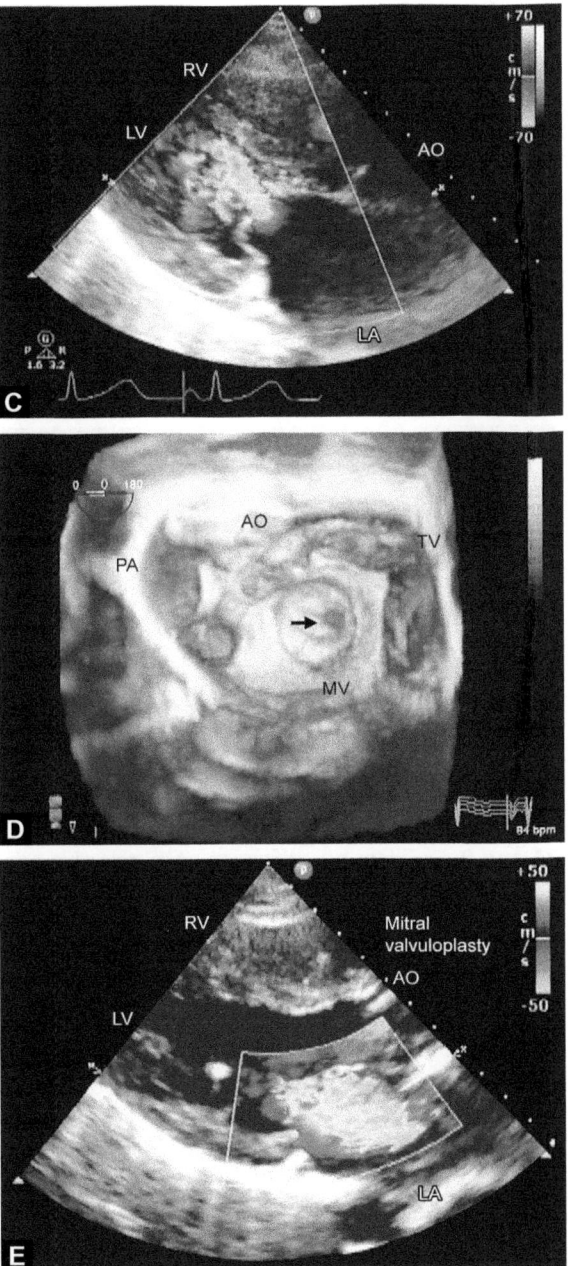

Figs. 8.1A to E: Echocardiographic assessment for mitral stenosis.

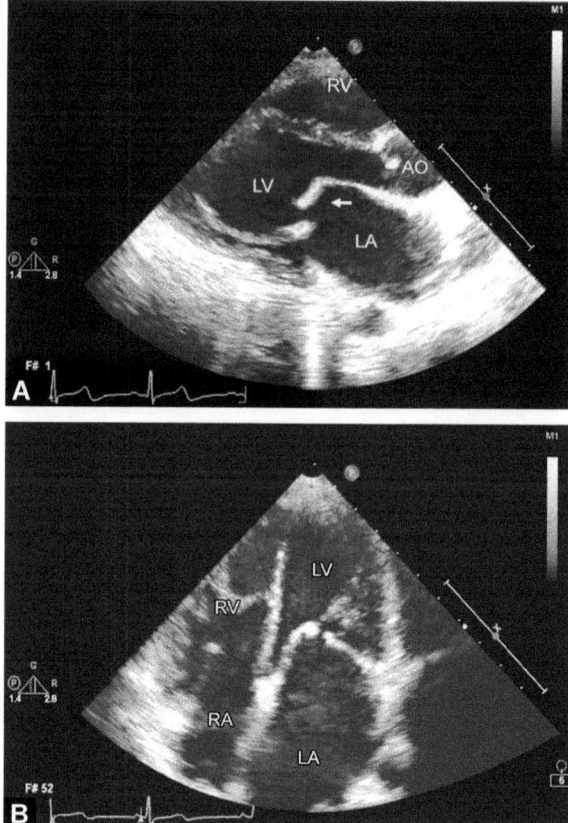

Figs. 8.2A and B: Excellent quantification of mitral valve orifice area.

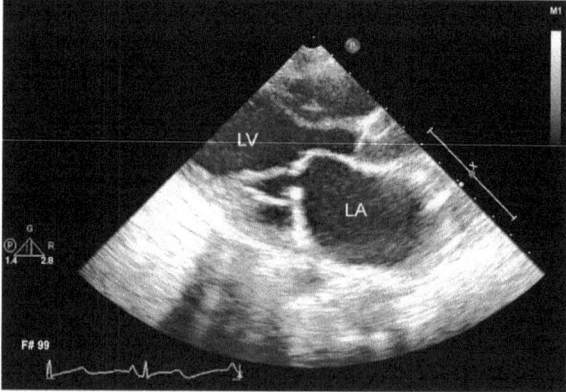

Fig. 8.3: Left ventricular size is expected to be small.

Medical Therapy

All patients should receive prophylaxis for the prevention of rheumatic fever for greater than or equal to 25 years from the acute episode and up to age 45, whichever is the longest. Although pure mitral stenosis is rarely the site of endocarditis, trivial MR is often present, and endocarditis prophylaxis should be strongly enforced.

Mild Mitral Stenosis

- Patients are usually asymptomatic and should be followed annually. A chest X-ray and echocardiogram are done initially, or if needed because of worsening symptomatology. Then, about every 5 years should suffice.
- No treatment is indicated, except for advice on mild dietary salt restriction and avoidance of excessive weight gain and physically strenuous occupations.

Moderate Mitral Stenosis

- Moderate mitral stenosis, valve orifice area 1–1.5 cm^2, is usually mildly symptomatic. Salt restriction is advisable. K-sparing diuretics, such as Moduretic (Moduret) ameliorate shortness of breath and prevent K and magnesium loss. If palpitations are bothersome or short runs of supraventricular tachycardia (SVT) are documented, a small dose of a β-blocking drug is useful: metoprolol 25–50 mg bid, atenolol 25 mg qd, or an equivalent dose of another β-blocker should suffice. Digoxin is not indicated for patients with sinus rhythm or CHF with pulmonary congestion, except as prophylaxis against fast ventricular rates and pulmonary edema if AF develops.
- Chest infections must be vigorously treated because hypoxemia increases pulmonary hypertension and may precipitate right CHF. Also, tachycardia may precipitate pulmonary edema.
- If the patient is managing daily chores and enjoying a near-normal lifestyle, the interventional approach can await some progression of the disease or symptoms but is not delayed in very active patients who need to engage in strenuous work or sport. Marked limitation of lifestyle in such individuals may require early corrective measures. A patient with moderate mitral stenosis should be followed at least twice yearly, but annual echocardiography should suffice.

Severe Mitral Stenosis

- Severe mitral stenosis, valve area corrected for body surface area (valve area index) less than 1 cm^2/m^2, usually requires interventional therapy within 3–6 months to abolish symptoms or ↓ complications and/or progressive ↑ in pulmonary vascular resistance.

- Atrial fibrillation with a fast ventricular response decreases LV filling and may precipitate pulmonary congestion. Digoxin is indicated to control the ventricular response. Digoxin is discussed in detail in Chapter 5. If palpitations remain bothersome and the HR cannot be controlled with digoxin, as often occurs in very active individuals, the addition of a small dose of β-blocking drug is useful. The latter agents can also be used to ↓ sinus tachycardia that is easily provoked in some patients without AF. Many physicians regard the development of AF as an indication for intervention when stenosis is of moderate severity, because the prospects for permanent restoration of sinus rhythm ↓ rapidly with time from onset of arrhythmia.
- The patient with AF must be anticoagulated, if no contraindication exists, because systemic embolization is common. Warfarin is given to maintain the prothrombin time, 1.25-1.5 times the control or international normalized ratio (INR) to 2-3 (see Chapter 11 for advice on anticoagulant control). These tests are done at least every 2 weeks until stabilized, then monthly should suffice. If contraindications to anticoagulant therapy exist, enteric-coated aspirin (325 mg qd) is advisable.

Interventional Management

Balloon valvuloplasty or surgery to relieve valvular obstruction is indicated for most symptomatic patients who have moderate to severe mitral stenosis, valve orifice less than 1 cm^2, as determined by Doppler echocardiography. The results of this technique correlate sufficiently well with catheterization data. Cardiac catheterization is not required in patients less than age 40, in whom ischemic heart disease (IHD) is not present or suspected, and who have typical, clinical features of mitral stenosis that are confirmed by Doppler echocardiography.

Mild mitral stenosis, valve area 1.6-2.0 cm^2, often remains minimally symptomatic greater than or equal to 5-10 years. However, as explained earlier, in countries where rheumatic valve disease is endemic, tight mitral stenosis may emerge at a faster rate in the adolescent or young adult.

Moderately severe mitral stenosis, valve area 1-1.5 cm^2, usually does not require intervention, but decisions must be individualized. In these patients, intervention may be required in the following cases:
- For symptomatic young patients engaged in strenuous activity
- If AF supervenes
- To allow a further pregnancy in a patient who manifested pulmonary edema in a previous pregnancy.

Elective procedures are sometimes performed in women who anticipate pregnancy, but relief of obstruction may be required during the second and third trimester of pregnancy, because the valve orifice is no longer large enough to permit the necessary ↑ in cardiac output to occur without an unacceptable ↑ in left atrial and pulmonary venous pressures. Interventional therapy may take the form of: surgical closed commissurotomy, surgical open commissurotomy, balloon valvuloplasty, or valve replacement.

Closed mitral commissurotomy was the technique of choice until the early 1970s for patients with severe mitral stenosis with noncalcified pliable valves. Open commissurotomy has largely replaced the closed technique, except in much of Asia, Africa, Latin America, and the West Indies, where closed valvotomy has remained the treatment of choice.

Mitral Balloon Valvuloplasty

Percutaneous mitral balloon valvuloplasty appears to give hemodynamic results comparable with surgical closed commissurotomy, as shown by an 8-month follow-up study. The valve area is increased 100% from 1 cm^2 to 2 cm^2 in less than or equal to 77% of cases. A mortality of less than or equal to 2.7% has been reported by the Valvuloplasty Registry. The National Heart, Lung and Blood Institute 30-day follow-up report on 738 patients indicates an 83% overall clinical improvement and mortality of 3%; 4% of patients require valve surgery. An iatrogenic atrial septal defect (ASD) has been reported to occur in 20–87% of patients, depending on criteria used for defining the ASD, which takes less than 6 months to close. However, the defect is usually small, the magnitude of the shunt being less than 2:1, and only few of these ASDs are clinically significant. Currently, complication rates are still high (Table 8.9). The procedure should be done only by highly trained and experienced operators. In such hands, the procedure is first choice in appropriately selected patients for relief of severe mitral stenosis.

Mitral balloon valvuloplasty must have a mortality of less than 1% to be considered an acceptable alternative to surgical commissurotomy. The proper selection of patients and technical aspects are changing such that morbidity and mortality from the procedure are expected to fall.

The patient selection for mitral balloon valvuloplasty is crucial to obtaining a salutary effect with a minimum number of complications. The patients are

Table 8.9: Complications of mitral balloon valvuloplasty.	
Clinical parameters	Complications, incidence (%)
Mortality	2.7
Emergency surgery	6.7
Cardiac tamponade	6.7
Embolism	2.7
Significant mitral regurgitation	13
Emergency valve replacement	4
Restenosis	16
Iatrogenic atrial septal defect	20–87

usually selected based on two-dimensional (2D) echocardiographic results. Ideally, the patients should have:
- Very symptomatic severe mitral stenosis, mitral valve area less than 1 cm^2
- Noncalcified, mobile valve with no subvalvular fibrosis (echo score <8). Valve rigidity, valve calcification, thickening, and subvalvular fibrosis are graded from 0 to 4, and the points are added together. The best candidates are patients who have an echo score less than 8.

Contraindications include:
- Bleeding disorder: Abnormal prothrombin time, prolonged partial thromboplastin time (PTT), increased bleeding time (the patient must discontinue aspirin compounds for greater than or equal to 1 week prior to the procedure)
- Left atrial or appendage thrombus
- Recent embolization
- Severe mitral valve calcification of subvalvular fibrosis
- Moderate or severe MR
- Cardiothoracic deformity.

Transesophageal echocardiography (TEE) has a role in obtaining information needed for the selection of patients for balloon valvuloplasty such as calcification, thickening, mobility, and subvalvular fibrosis. Atrial or appendage thrombus is best visualized with TEE. The technique is also of value in assessing the magnitude of the ASD following the procedure.

Mitral Valve Replacement

A prosthetic valve implant may be required because of the presence of moderate to severe MR coexisting with mitral stenosis. Replacement may also be selected for management of heavily calcified and immobile valves, which are often conical in shape, when they are considered to be beyond repair at the time of surgery. In general, a mechanical valve is preferred in the mitral area. See earlier discussion of prosthetic valve choice and Table 8.5. In less than or equal to 50% of patients, AF is present; a mechanical valve is a natural choice because anticoagulants are necessary. In the young female who may wish to become pregnant, a bioprosthesis is sometimes recommended. However, a mechanical valve can be used in this situation with discontinuation of oral anticoagulants; heparin can be used SQ for the first 4 months of pregnancy and again for the last 3 weeks. Importantly, in the young patient, accelerated calcification of a bioprosthesis may occur. Calcification, as well as pannus formation, may require a second operation.

MITRAL REGURGITATION

While mitral stenosis is nearly always due to rheumatic disease, MR is a common valvular lesion caused by a number of conditions that alter the mitral valve apparatus: valve leaflets, annulus, chordae, and papillary muscles. Common causes of acute and chronic MR are given in Flowchart 8.1.

Flowchart 8.1: Causes of mitral regurgitation.

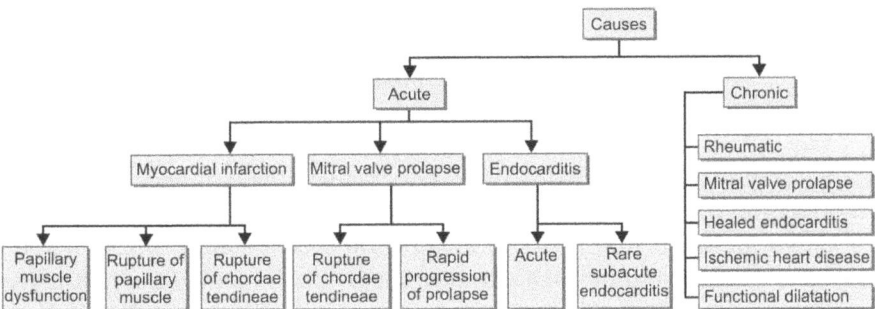

Acute mitral regurgitation: Commonly occurs during acute myocardial infarction (MI), which causes papillary muscle dysfunction, and less commonly, chordal or papillary muscle rupture. Other causes of acute MR are listed in Flowchart 8.1.

Chronic mitral regurgitation: Patients may tolerate a mild to moderate degree of MR for 10 or more years without the appearance of CHF. Chronic volume overload, however, causes slow progressive dilation and mild hypertrophy of the left ventricle. Characteristically, a loud holosystolic murmur is heard maximal at the apex with radiation to the axilla, accompanied by a third heart sound gallop if regurgitation is moderate to severe. In patients with posterior papillary muscle dysfunction causing MR, however, the murmur radiates anteriorly and is best heard at the left sternal border without radiation to the axilla.

Mild to moderate shortness of breath indicates pulmonary congestion or LV dysfunction and should be managed with afterload-reducing agents, particularly angiotensin-converting enzyme (ACE) inhibitors, to encourage forward flow at the expense of regurgitation. Small doses are advisable: captopril, 6.25 mg bid for several days, increasing slowly to avoid hypotension to maintenance of 37.5 mg bid (maximum 75 mg in two or three divided doses or equivalent doses of enalapril).

If concomitant IHD with angina is present and LV dysfunction is not severe, nifedipine is preferred to ACE inhibitors, which may ↑ angina. Also, digoxin and the judicious use of diuretics in combination with nifedipine may be beneficial before considering early valve repair or valve replacement.

Atrial fibrillation with a rapid ventricular response is managed with digoxin and anticoagulants to prevent embolization.

Progressive dyspnea is a late stage and CHF should be anticipated and prevented by timely surgical intervention.

Surgical Treatment

- The timing of valve surgery, whether for repair or replacement due to chronic MR, remains a trial in decision making, as with aortic

regurgitation. Patients with mitral valve prolapse and acute complications are often suitable for valve repair.
- There is an increasing tendency to attempt valve reconstruction. It is advisable to repair as many and as often as feasible, but success depends on the skill of the surgeon. For mitral stenosis and regurgitation, many valves are beyond repair and require replacement.
- Surgery should be considered in patients who have moderately severe MR prior to the development of severe pulmonary arterial hypertension and prior to a ↓ in EF to less than 50%. The interpretation of EF has to be adjusted downward to take into account the low impedance to retrograde flow resulting from MR. A patient with severe MR and an EF less than 40% will have a prohibitively high surgical mortality and will fare better with afterload ↓ and digoxin. Because of the problems of assessing EF in the presence of MR, other parameters of LV function have been used, including end-systolic volume index greater than 50 mL/m^2.
- If surgery is done prior to the manifestations of the aforementioned parameters, survival, functional class, and LV systolic function should show significant improvement. If MR is moderately severe and LV dysfunction is present, it is hazardous to procrastinate. Early surgery is preferable.
- In patients with predominant posterior leaflet prolapse, repair of the posterior leaflet followed by insertion of a nonflexible ring, as recommended by Carpentier, appears to be successful in preventing postoperative systolic anterior motion of the mitral valve.
- In some patients with heavily calcified valves, the mitral valve annulus can be decalcified, and valve repair, decalcification, and annuloplasty should be considered based on Doppler echocardiographic data. TEE gives a more accurate visualization of the mitral valve, however, and is advisable in potential candidates; the latter is justifiable and cost-effective, especially in view of the difficult decision as to timing of surgery.
- The tricuspid valve is also often severely incompetent; tricuspid annuloplasty is advisable in such cases.
- Intraoperative TEE is of considerable value in assessing valve repair. The surgeon ensures excellent coapting edges and lines of closure; if the geometry is ideal, saline is pumped into the ventricle.

MITRAL VALVE PROLAPSE

- Mitral valve prolapse is said to be a common condition affecting an estimated 5% of the US population. The incidence of mitral valve prolapse has been exaggerated because of the inclusion of a large number of patients with a normal variant of mitral valve closure but with correct coaptation; leaflets may only billow slightly into the left atrium with normal coaptation. Also, the appearance may result from the normal saddle shape of the normal mitral ring.

- The minor variant with a click, without a murmur and nondiagnostic echocardiographic features commonly labeled mitral valve prolapse, is subject to interpretation, and this "normal variant" disappears after age 40. Probably because of the inclusion of normal variants with billowing leaflets without true prolapse, the incidence of mitral valve prolapse is reported to be as high as 30% at age 10-20, 15% at age 30, 10% at age 50, 3% at age 70, and less than 1% at age 80. Under age 30, the female-to-male ratio is 3:1, but at age 70, both men and women are about equal. The incidence of significant mitral valve prolapse is about 6% in adult women and 3% in men.
- Genuine mitral valve prolapse has a familial incidence of about 33%, as noted in first-degree relatives.

Causes

These include:
- In developed countries, the common underlying process is a degenerative nonrheumatic condition of unknown etiology described as a dyscollagenosis or myxomatous degeneration of the mitral valve. An ↑ in the spongiosa, myxomatous tissue, in the middle layer of the mitral valve leaflet, encroaches upon the fibrosa. The anterior and posterior leaflets become elongated, thickened, voluminous, and grossly redundant. The chordae become thin and elongated and have a propensity to rupture. Herniation of the posterior leaflet above the anterior leaflet may occur. A mural endocardial fibrous plaque is often observed beneath the posterior leaflet in patients who die suddenly from mitral valve prolapse. The mitral valve annulus is often dilated in patients with significant regurgitation, and in those patients who die suddenly, calcification and fibrosis of the annulus appears to be a common finding.
- Myxomatous changes and mitral valve prolapse are associated with Marfan's syndrome, Ehlers–Danlos syndrome, and osteogenesis imperfecta.
- Rheumatic heart disease, where this disease is still endemic. A dilated annulus allows elongation of chordae with, sometimes, prolapse of the anterior leaflet, but marked billowing or redundancy of leaflets are unusual.
- Papillary muscle dysfunction due to IHD.

Symptoms

Most patients are asymptomatic. Dyspnea is rather vague, often occurs at rest, and is commonly out of proportion with the degree of MR that is usually asymptomatic in greater than 80% of patients. Extreme fatigue, dizziness, anxiety, panic disorders, palpitations, presyncope, syncope, and chest pain may occur without a satisfactory explanation. Psychogenic factors play a role in the varied symptomatology.

Some symptoms relate to the presence of autonomic dysfunction with increased levels of circulating catecholamine, and a hyperadrenergic state; in some patients, increased vagal activity is present. In this condition, there is a tendency for the sinus rate to ↑ steeply in the early part of exercise, and the high frequency of palpitations has been attributed to this pattern of response in these patients. It is not surprising, therefore, that Holter monitoring commonly shows sinus tachycardia, when palpitations are a complaint.

Signs

One or multiple mid or late systolic clicks of nonejection type may be constant or intermittent, changing with posture or maneuvers, but do not prove the existence of mitral valve prolapse. The timing of clicks may be misinterpreted as gallop sounds, but apart from their timing, clicks can be differentiated from a third heart sound by the high-pitched quality and by being most audible with a diaphragm. In some patients, the click is followed by a murmur; in others, only a murmur is present. The murmur has typical features.

- A typical late systolic murmur is unmistakable and confirms the diagnosis.
- The murmur is usually crescendo-decrescendo, the auscultator gets the impression that the murmur is occurring synchronously with the second heart sound, and the murmur often extends through the aortic second sound.
- A whoop, a short honking sound, or a sound of other musical quality may highlight the murmur, which changes in intensity depending on LV volume and BP.
- The late systolic murmur or click is heard earlier and made louder by the following maneuvers that reduce LV volume: standing, tilting upright, Valsalva, and tachycardia. Amyl nitrite decreases ventricular volume and BP; therefore, the murmur is heard earlier but is made softer.
- The murmur or clicks are heard later and are softer with maneuvers that ↑ LV volume or ↓ BP: squatting, bradycardia, β-blocking agents. Thus, the physician should listen to the patient lying, standing, and squatting because the murmur may be heard only on standing. With more severe MR, the duration of the murmur is longer and may become pansystolic.
- When chordal rupture occurs, the murmur changes in quality and radiation.

- The posterior mitral leaflet often has three scallops; rupture of the chorda to the middle scallop of the posterior leaflet is the most common chordal rupture. The resulting murmur radiates anteriorly, is maximal at the lower left sternal border, and radiates toward the upper right sternal edge. The crescendo-decrescendo quality may simulate an aortic systolic murmur. However, the late timing of the murmur of mitral valve prolapse is a distinguishing feature that differentiates the murmur from the early timing of aortic valvular murmurs.
- Chordal rupture of the anterior leaflet causes the murmur to radiate to the posterior axilla.
- The flail mitral valve produces a loud murmur, the intensity of which is characteristically accentuated over the spine and may be heard from the occiput to the sacral spine.
- The MR jet can be identified by TEE; it moves in a counterclockwise direction with flail anterior leaflet, and clockwise with posterior leaflet involvement.

Approximately 15% of patients with mitral valve prolapse have skeletal abnormalities: "straight back," pectus excavatum or carinatum, scoliosis, or some features of Marfan's syndrome.

Complications

These include:
- Severe MR occurs in approximately 10% of patients with true mitral valve prolapse and is five times more common in men older than age 45 than in women. Although mitral valve prolapse occurs most commonly in women, severe MR requiring surgery occurs in about 5% of men and less than 1.5% of women. Chordal rupture is a common occurrence in patients with severe MR.
- Arrhythmias commonly occur and include ventricular premature complexes (VPCs), atrial ectopics, paroxysmal supraventricular tachycardia (PSVT), and occasionally AF. Lethal arrhythmias have been reported (see Chapter 6).
- Sudden death, although rare, occurs in healthy young active individuals and is unexplained. Table 8.10 lists clinical and morphologic features in 15 patients who died suddenly secondary to mitral valve prolapse. These data and a review of previously reported studies on 63 patients indicate that patients with mitral valve prolapse who die suddenly have the following clinical and morphologic hallmarks.
  - Women aged 21–51, without significant MR (70%)
  - Dilated mitral valve annulus (80%)
  - Elongated anterior mitral valve leaflet (>80%)
  - Abnormal elongated posterior mitral leaflet, often with herniation of the posterior leaflet above the anterior leaflet (approximately 80%)

Table 8.10: Clinical and morphologic features in 15 patients dying suddenly secondary to mitral valve prolapse.

Clinical features

Pt. no.	Age (years)	Race	Gender	MVP diagnosed clinically	Marfan's syndrome	Location of death	Last activity	Auscultatory findings		
								SC	SM	SH
1	16	W	M	+	+	Basketball court	Sitting after playing	–	+	0
2	18	W	F	+	0	Home	Arguing	–	0	0
3	21	W	F	+	0	Work	Talking on phone	–	–	0
4	23	W	F	+	0	Work	Drinking water	+	+	0
5	26	W	F	+	0	Work	Talking	+	+	0
6	30	B	M	0	0	Work	Sitting alone	–	–	–
7	30	W	M	0	0	Golf course	Playing golf	–	–	0
8	40	W	F	0	+	Home	Playing with children	–	–	0
9	47	W	F	0	0	Home	Gardening	–	–	0
10	51	W	M	+	0	Restaurant	Sitting after fast dancing	+	+	0
11	53	W	F	+	0	Church	Sitting	–	–	0
12	53	W	F	0	0	Restaurant	Getting up to dance	–	–	–
13	55	W	F	+	0	Home	Standing	+	+	0
14	55	W	M	+	0	Home	Sleeping	–	–	0
15	69	W	F	0	0	Home	–	–	–	–

Contd...

Contd...

Morphologic features

Pt. no.	CHF	VPCs on ECG	HW (g)	MV annulus (cm)	TV annulus (cm)	AML length (cm)	PML length (cm)	Chords missing	Grade of MVP (1-3+)	Plaque under PML	MAC (0-4+)	VC PFO	Redundant of membrane
1	0	+	325	12.5	12	3	2.5	+	2	0	0	–	–
2	0	+*	220	9.6	11.5	2	1.5	0	1	+	0	0	0
3	0	–	360	14	–	3	1.5	+	2	0	1	–	–
4	0	–	280	10	9	2.5	2	0	3	+	0	+	+
5	0	0†	265	12	11	3	3	0	3	+	0	+	+
6	0	–	570	15.5	13	3	2.5	0	3	+	0	0	0
7	0	–	475	10	11	3	2	0	1	+	0	0	0
8	0	–	355	13	12	–	–	+	2	0	2	–	+
9	0	+	445	12.5	12.5	2.5	2	0	3	+	0	0	0
10	0	0	500	10.5	12	2	1.5	0	1	0	0	0	0
11	0	+	325	12.6	10.5	2.5	3	0	2	+	3	0	0
12	0	–	390	13.6	11	3.5	3	0	3	+	1	+	+
13	0	+	390	13	13	3	2.5	+	3	+	0	0	0
14	+	+	670	>12	14	3.5	2	0	3	+	0	+	0
15	0	–	400	15.4	14.5	2.5	3	+	3	+	0	0	0

*This patient had survived a cardiac arrest 2 years earlier.
†This patient had a history of paroxysmal atrial tachycardia.

(AML, anterior mitral leaflet; B, black; CHF, congestive heart failure; F, female; FO, fossa ovale; HW, heart weight; M, male; MVP, mitral valve prolapse; MAC, mitral annular calcification; PFO, patent foramen ovale; PML, posterior mitral leaflet; Pt., patient; SC, systolic click; SH, systemic hypertension; SM, systolic murmur; TV, tricuspid valve; VC, valvular competent; VPC, ventricular premature complex; W, white; +, present; 0, absent; –, no information available)

Source: Adapted with permission from Dollar AL, Roberts WC. Morphologic comparison of patients with mitral valve prolapse who died suddenly with patients who died from severe valvular dysfunction or other conditions. J Am Coll Cardiol. 1991;17:921-31.

- Fibrous endocardial plaque under the posterior mitral valve leaflet (≤75%)
- Significant, moderate to severe prolapse of the mitral valve (53%)
- Raptured chordae (33%)
- Significant, moderate or greater MR (10%)
- MR murmur (50%)
- A click is present (only 25-37%)
- Arrhythmia (>50%); VPCs (about 33%).
• The incidence of endocarditis in patients with true mitral valve prolapse is unknown but estimated to be about 1 in 6,000 in all patients with mitral valve prolapse and about 1 in 2,000 of patients with MR.
• Transient ischemic attacks (TIAs), stroke, retinal arteriolar occlusions, and amaurosis fugax are rare complications of mitral valve prolapse due to embolization of bland emboli. The exact incidence has not been accurately assessed.

Therapy

• The physician must be careful in reassuring patients with mitral valve prolapse syndrome. Patients with billowing leaflets without genuine prolapse rarely get severe MR. Palpitations due to VPCs or occasionally runs of SVT usually require no drug therapy. Following reassurance, if episodes of VPCs or SVT are bothersome, and Holter monitoring demonstrates multiform VPCs, couplets or runs, nonsustained VT, or short bouts of SVT, a very small dose of a β-blocking drug is appropriate and the safest remedy. Metoprolol (25-50 mg bid) or atenolol (25-50 mg once daily) is advisable since both cause less fatigue than propranolol. Sotalol (80-160 mg once daily) is useful, but fatigue and the propensity to precipitate torsades de pointes, albeit rare, do not justify its use in this benign condition. Potentially lethal arrhythmias are rare with mitral valve prolapse and require higher doses of β-blockers. Chest pain requires reassurance or the use of enteric-coated aspirin (325 mg qd). If pain is bothersome or "angina like", a β-blocking drug should be administered with avoidance of nitrates, which reduce ventricular volume and thus ↑ the prolapse.
• Small, bland emboli consisting of platelet and fibrin, which form in relation to the slightly abnormal valve apparatus, may cause TIAs or stroke. Management is with enteric-coated aspirin (160-325 mg qd) or one-fourth of a regular 325-mg aspirin qd. If TIAs continue, it is advisable to add dipyridamole (75 mg tid). This drug is more effective when given on an empty stomach or 30 minutes before meals. However, it is expensive and of unproven value except when combined with aspirin. (The drug is ineffective when used without aspirin).
• Severe MR due to mitral valve prolapse is managed with surgical reconstruction where possible, but in some cases, valve replacement is necessary. The same considerations apply as in other varieties of MR as discussed earlier in this chapter.

RHEUMATIC FEVER

Rheumatic fever is now rare in North America and the Western world but is still prevalent in Asia, the Middle East, Africa, and Latin America, and is the most commonly acquired heart disease in childhood.

Clinical Features

The peak incidence is from age 5 to 15; rheumatic fever is uncommon less than age 5 and virtually unknown less than age 2. Symptoms are manifest 2-3 weeks after Group A streptococcal pharyngitis, which causes a hyperimmune reaction in susceptible individuals.

Symptoms and signs include the following:
- Fever for 2-3 weeks
- Anorexia
- Weight loss
- Arthritis in greater than 80% of patients, especially in older patients. It takes the form of flitting or migratory polyarthritis. Pain, redness, and swelling usually occur in large joints, knees, elbows, wrists, and shoulders; notably, the last joint is rarely involved in other arthritides. A single joint is inflamed for about 1 day to 1 week; the pain resolves completely and then moves on to the second joint. There is typically no deformity of joints.
- Sinus tachycardia
- Subcutaneous nodules in less than or equal to 12% of cases
- Erythema marginatum in less than or equal to 10% of individuals. This is an effervescent, nonpruritic rash with pink circumscribed circles with a pale center mainly involving the trunk
- Sydenham's chorea (St. Vitus dance), which may last for weeks to months, rarely for a few years
- Pancarditis, which is more common in the young, who have minimal or no arthritis. When rheumatic fever "licks" the joints, the disease often spares the heart
- New murmurs, friction rub, cardiomegaly, and CHF, which indicate pancarditis
- An apical pansystolic murmur Grade I-II, which is common with valvular involvement and is usually accompanied by the Carey Coombs murmur. A short, low-pitched rumbling, mid-diastolic apical murmur. Its presence serves to distinguish the systolic murmur of carditis from common innocent systolic murmurs that are typically early or midsystolic vibratory murmurs or a scratchy short ejection systolic murmur located between the pulmonary area and the lower left sternal edge.
- First-degree atrioventricular (AV) block or, rarely, bundle branch block.

Therapy

- Prophylaxis of rheumatic fever requires aggressive treatment of the initial attack of pharyngitis with oral penicillin G, 500 mg immediately then 250 mg qid for 10 days, or intramuscular (IM) benzathine penicillin G, 1.2 million U in patients greater than 60 lbs. and 600,000 U for patients less than 60 lbs. Erythromycin (250 mg qid) or clindamycin (150 mg q 8 hours) is administered to patients allergic to penicillin.
- Arthritis is controlled with enteric-coated aspirin (100 mg/kg qd) in four divided doses to achieve a blood level of 20-25 mg/dL. Corticosteroids should be avoided because they produce no better results than aspirin.
- Pancarditis requires modified bed rest for several weeks until signs of carditis are improved or unchanging. The sedimentation rate should revert to normal, and the C-reactive protein should become negative. Enteric-coated aspirin should be given if fever and carditis are present, as well as for arthritis. Corticosteroids are not usually indicated and are used only if carditis is progressive with manifestation of cardiomegaly and CHF. When required, prednisone (60-80 mg/day; 1.0-1.5 mg/kg/day) is administered in four doses for a period of 4-6 weeks. The dose is then reduced slowly with maintenance of aspirin. The possibility of steroid rebound may be reduced by employing aspirin as overlapping therapy with steroids for 2-3 weeks, during which time the steroids are weaned off. Pericarditis should be managed with aspirin.
- Secondary rheumatic fever prevention is important to prevent recurrence since valvular damage is more intense with each recurrence of rheumatic fever. Management is with benzathine penicillin G (1.2 million U IM q 4 weeks), commonly used in North America and Europe; in endemic areas, 3 weekly injections are advisable. Penicillin is continued for at least 20 years after the initial attack of rheumatic fever or to age 45, whichever occurs first. Patients allergic to penicillin are treated with sulfonamides: 1 g of oral sulfadiazine daily for patients greater than 60 lbs and 0.5 g once daily for patients less than 60 lbs, with liberal fluid intake.

BIBLIOGRAPHY

1. Honda S, Kawasaki T, Shiraishi H, et al. Mitral valve prolapse revisited. Circulation. 2016;133(6):e380-2.
2. Lazar HL. Robotic mitral valve repair for degenerative mitral valve regurgitation: is it for everyone? Circulation. 2015;132(21):1941-2.
3. Moat NE. Will TAVR become the predominant method for treating severe aortic stenosis? N Engl J Med. 2016;374(17):1682-3.
4. Puri R, Rodés-Cabau J. Transcatheter aortic valve replacement: a revolution in evolution. J Am Coll Cardiol Intv. 2016;9(4):364-6.
5. Remenyi B, ElGuindy A, Smith SC Jr, et al. Valvular aspects of rheumatic heart disease. Lancet. 2016;387(10025):1335-46.
6. Weintraub WS. TAVR in nonagenarians: pushing the boundaries. J Am Coll Cardiol. 2016;67(12):1396-8.

CHAPTER 9

Dyslipidemia and Sitosterolemia

INTRODUCTION

This chapter gives in-depth discussion of the value and adverse effects of statins. What evidence there is for causation of diabetes, cancer, myositis, cataracts, and intolerance. The American College of Cardiology (ACC)/American Heart Association (AHA) guidelines are criticized put in perspective and low-density lipoprotein cholesterol (LDL-C) target goals are given depending on risk. Dyslipidemias are clarified and advise on newer add-on drugs are detailed. Relevant clinical trials are criticized.

- The acclaimed Heart Outcomes Prevention Evaluation-3 (HOPE-3) randomized controlled trial (RCT) is criticized. Similar to the first HOPE trial, optimal therapy was not given to subjects. Aspirin a drug that may prevent outcomes in intermediate-risk patients older than age 65 was used by less than 12% of subjects in HOPE-3.
- Ezetimibe as add-on is put in perspective; it must be emphasized that ezetimibe causes a significant decrease in sitosterol levels. A substance that increases atheroma formation and blood levels are increased in diabetics because of hyperabsorption of sitosterol similar to that observed in genetic sitosterolemia (Khan, 2017).

ATHEROMA

Further research in this area is warranted to produce antiatheroma drugs. Cardiovascular diseases (CVDs) cause 18 million deaths per year globally and a similar number of nonfatal cardiovascular events.

- Atheroma rupture, erosions, fissuring with thrombotic overlay is the basic cause for fatal and nonfatal myocardial infarction (MI) which, within this decade, would be responsible for a staggering greater than 15 million deaths each year. It is estimated that in the year 2025 more than 25 million people will die of this disease, and approximately 12 million will be from acute MI in a world population of nearly 8 billion.
- This epidemic may be halted somewhat when we fully recognize that we must prevent atheroma formation at the earliest stage. In many, this

is before age 35 and rarely but unfortunately in children with genetic disease.
- In patient at high risk, a 40–50% lowering of LDL-C is our main concern.
- Most fatal and nonfatal MI occur in individuals with total cholesterol in the range of 190–250 mg/dL. More than 100 million US adults greater than or equal to 20 years of age have total cholesterol levels greater than or equal to 200 mg/dL; almost 31 million have levels greater than or equal to 240 mg/dL. (2016 AHA Statistical Update: 2009–2012 data). Sound the alarm!
- In order to prevent menacing atheroma, we must learn from the effects of genetic disease in which total cholesterol is greater than 2,000 mg/dL. LDL-C greater than 20 mmol/L and plaques of atheroma abound in coronary and vital arteries from about age 12.

Low-density Lipoprotein Cholesterol: Lower is Better

A case of familial hypercholesterolemia type IIb gives a clear vision of our problems.

A boy, born in 1949, had, at birth, cutaneous xanthomas along the extensor surfaces of his arms and legs, gluteal folds, and Achilles tendons. His cholesterol was 951 mg/dL (24 mmol/L). At age 7, he was hospitalized and died.

- A review of the autopsy in 2003 showed the aortic valve contained atherosclerotic lesions, microscopic examination showed plaques rich in lipid-laden foam cells, with focal areas of collagen. The circumflex coronary artery was involved by chronic atherosclerosis and acute thrombosis, and the acute thrombosis was considered the cause of death. Atherosclerotic plaques were also present throughout the thoracic aorta (Rajamannan, 2003).
- Advances have been made for genetic disease. Alirocumab reduced the frequency of apheresis by 75% compared with placebo and eliminated the need for apheresis for 63%, according to top-line results from the 62-patient phase III ODYSSEY ESCAPE trial in heterozygous familial hypercholesterolemia getting the treatments (Kersten, 2016).
- A once-daily oral drug, gemcabene, cut low-density lipoprotein (LDL) by 23–28% over 8 weeks atop high-intensity statin therapy in two homozygous familial hypercholesterolemic patients according to interim results from the small phase IIb COBALT-1 trial.

We are now certain that LDL-C is the major culprit for atheroma formation; other particles are important but are of lower order. More studies as done in ASTEROID (A Study to Evaluate the Effect of Rosuvastatin on Intravascular Ultrasound-derived Coronary Atheroma Burden, 2006) are needed.

ASTEROID trial: Rosuvastatin administration of 40 mg/day achieved an average LDL-C of 60.8 mg/dL (1.56 mmol/L) and increased high-density lipoprotein cholesterol (HDL-C) by 14.7%. This marked amelioration of lipid levels (approximately 30% reduction) caused significant regression of atheroma for all three prespecified intravascular ultrasound (IVUS) measures of disease burden (Nissen et al. 2006). This is the first clear evidence that coronary atheromatous obstructive plaques can regress significantly when LDL-C is markedly lowered.

Tsujita et al. (2015) reported that patients randomized to atorvastatin plus ezetimibe therapy experienced a greater reduction in the percentage of atheroma volume than those randomized to atorvastatin, and it may be due to the lower mean LDL-C achieved. Perhaps cholesterol lowering itself does not explain the greater reduction in the percentage of atheroma volume with convincing and intriguing pleiotropic effects of ezetimibe (Crea and Niccoli, 2015). I do not give credit to the so-called pleiotropic effects, and the effects of add-on ezetimibe are small.

- Statins should be prescribed and dose increased to attain the goal set. If the goal for the patient is less than 1.4 mmol/L and this is not attained, the dose of statin should be increased to the highest tolerated dose using the more effective statin: rosuvastatin 40 mg or atorvastatin 80 mg before adding ezetimibe.
- Genetic factors appear to be important as individuals in the general population vary in their cholesterol response to a high saturated fat diet. Total serum cholesterol and LDL-C increase in response to a high saturated fat intake. Polygenic hypercholesterolemia is the most common cause of increased total cholesterol and LDL-C observed in the general population. It is not a defined inherited genetic defect and is believed to be a hepatic overproduction of very low-density lipoprotein (VLDL) that is converted rapidly to LDL that VLDL triglyceride concentrations remain within the normal range. The estimate prevalence among adults of European descent is 20–80%.
- A 2015 meta-analysis by Berger et al. found that when study participants increased their dietary cholesterol by up to 650 mg/day, their total cholesterol increased an average of 12.1 mg/dL and LDL-C increased an average of 16.7 mg/dL compared with those who consumed less.

Low-density Lipoprotein Cholesterol Testing Centers

It is vital for governmental and other agencies to set up blood collecting centers to screen all individuals, men from age of 30 years and females from age of 40 years.
- The LDL-C in these individuals must be less than 3 mmol/L for many and for those with family history of MI less than 2.5 mmol/L (96 mg/dL).

Blood cholesterol in the range of 5.0–6.5 mmol/L (190–250 mg/dL) is associated with most heart attacks. Dietary advice can be given by flyers and a physician visit encouraged for those who exceed the target goal. In the general population, the main causes for elevated blood cholesterol are high intake of saturated fats and trans-fatty acids, diabetes, and a relative decrease in LDL receptors that mop up cholesterol from the blood.

- Importantly for acute coronary syndrome (ACS), an on-admission LDL-C greater than 3.5 is a danger zone.
- The ACC/AHA guidelines shift away from targets and endorse 30–40% reduction from baseline for those at risk. This advice is not logical as it is too late in the game. It relates only to those at risk; usually age 45–70 when atheroma is prominent and in most symptomatic. I agree, in this population of patients age 30–40, a 50% reduction is necessary, but setting a goal, less than 1.2, 1.4 or 1.8 mmol/L, 2 mmol/L depending on risks is essential. This goal LDL-C would assist patient compliance and clinician interaction. ACC/AHA guideline 2016, claims to reinstate LDL-C goal levels, but their advice remains unclear and is mixed with voluminous pages of redundant information, not suited for busy clinicians in the field. Determine the risk and set an LDL-C goal; this goal motivates the patients and is simpler for physicians.
- It is cumbersome to work out 40%–50%–75% reductions.

PRIMARY DYSLIPIDEMIA

Fewer than 0.1% of the population appears to have a genetic abnormality characterized by cellular LDL receptor deficiency.

- Individuals with a marked increase in serum levels of cholesterol greater than 350 mg/dL (9 mmol/L), or severe hypertriglyceridemia represent a small group of patients seen in clinical practice. These individuals often show evidence of xanthomas and diffuse vascular disease and are at very high risk for developing premature atheromatous coronary artery disease (CAD). If the situation is suspected, screen first-degree relatives, parents, siblings, and children. Alirocumab reduced the frequency of apheresis by 75% compared with placebo and eliminated the need for apheresis for 63%, according to top-line results from the 62-patient phase III ODYSSEY ESCAPE trial in heterozygous familial hypercholesterolemia getting the treatments (Kersten, 2016).
- The gene for the LDL receptor is located on chromosome 19 and its diminished expression in familial hypercholesterolemia was discovered by Goldstein and Brown in 1974. These workers indicated that mutations of this receptor prevent it from efficient cellular uptake of LDL from tissue fluid because it cannot be transported to the cell surface, cannot bind properly to LDL, cannot be internalized, or is not released from the endosome.

Causes of primary dyslipidemia include the genetic hyperlipoproteinemias. Observation of the standing plasma after storage overnight at 4°C reveals characteristic findings that most often obviate the need for expensive electrophoretic analysis.

These have been classified by Fredrickson as:

- Type I: Elevated chylomicrons normal to mildly elevated total cholesterol; markedly elevated plasma triglycerides; creamy supernatant, clear infranant; fortunately type I is very rare (<1%).
- Type IIa: Elevated LDL lipoproteins; plasma total cholesterol and LDL are elevated but with normal triglycerides and with a clear plasma on standing overnight (frequency approximately 10%).
- Type IIb: Elevated LDL and VLDL lipoproteins; the total cholesterol is elevated, as well as triglycerides: this is the most common hyperlipoproteinemia (approximately 40%).
- Type III: Elevated intermediate-density lipoprotein with a mildly elevated serum cholesterol, markedly elevated triglyceride; the overnight standing plasma is turbid and usually has a separate creamy chylomicron supernatant (<1%).
- Type IV: Elevated VLDL and chylomicrons; serum cholesterol is normal; triglycerides are markedly elevated and the overnight plasma is turbid (approximately 45%).
- Type V: Elevated VLDL and chylomicrons; plasma cholesterol is mildly elevated with markedly elevated triglycerides: a turbid plasma and usually a separate creamy chylomicron supernatant (5%).

Classification describes only rare genetic dyslipidemias; electrophoretic determination is costly and genetic hypolipoproteinemias are observed in less than 0.1% of patients with dyslipidemias. Selected causes of hyperlipoproteinemia are given here.

Familial Hypercholesterolemia

- *Heterozygous familial*: The genetic mutations reduce the number of high-affinity LDL receptors by about 50%. Frequency is reportedly 1 in 500 patients in the Western world. There is a two- to fourfold increase in LDL-C. Tendon xanthomas are commonly present; corneal arcus before age 25; atherosclerotic vascular disease, particularly premature obstructive coronary heart disease (CHD), causes early demise if not aggressively treated. In these patients, a thorough physical examination should record the presence or absence of xanthoma tendinosum, tuberosum, and planum. These lesions are mainly observed in patients with familial genetic severe hyperlipidemias; xanthelasma of the eyelids is not closely associated and is a variable finding.

The higher the LDL-C value, the more likely it is that a person has familial hypercholesterolemia if adults (≥20 years) have LDL-C levels greater than or equal to 190 mg/dL, or children (<20 years) have LDL-C levels greater than or equal to 160 g/dL (Onorato and Sturm, 2016).

Primary Combined Hyperlipidemia; Familial Combined Hyperlipidemia

The frequency is reportedly 1 in every 300 patients (this is an exaggeration and may relate to findings in referrals seen in lipid clinics). There is overproduction of LDL and VLDL or both. This disorder is associated with increased risk for CAD but about 10 years later than in heterozygous familial hypercholesterolemia.

Primary Hypertriglyceridemia

Familial hypertriglyceridemia type IV; triglycerides usually in the range 200–500 mg/dL; and the very rare type V in which triglyceride levels of more than 1,000 mg/dL are observed and demand immediate treatment because of the risk for pancreatitis. Early CAD occurs in some families.

SECONDARY DYSLIPIDEMIA

Secondary causes should always be excluded:
- Diabetes mellitus
- Hypothyroidism
- Nephrotic syndrome
- Chronic liver disease
- Obesity
- Dysgammaglobulinemia (monoclonal gammopathy)
- Obstructive jaundice
- Biliary cirrhosis
- Pancreatitis
- Excess alcohol consumption
- Estrogens/progesterone
- Glycogen storage disorders
- Lipodystrophy
- Medications: Corticosteroids, immunosuppressive agents, retinoids, and antiretroviral therapy cause an increase in triglycerides, total cholesterol, and a decrease in HDL-C levels. Diuretics (thiazides) may cause a mild elevation in total cholesterol (1–4%) and a slight lowering of high-density lipoprotein (HDL) (approximately 1–10%). This effect is minimal, however, and occurs in fewer than 10% of individuals. Chronic treatment for more than 2 years usually produces no significant elevation in total cholesterol or decrease in HDL, and modest changes have been exaggerated. The long-term effects of β-blockers on HDL-C have been poorly studied and an increase of 0–7% has been reported in small studies.

It is clear that LDL-C is not increased by β-blockers. Metoprolol has shown no effect on HDL in one well-run study, and a decrease of 6% in another.

Low-density Lipoprotein Cholesterol

- Presence of CAD or risk equivalent and diabetes mellitus.
- Low-density lipoprotein cholesterol greater than 80 mg/dL (2.0 mmol/L).
- Advise drug therapy preferably with a powerful statin, such as 10 mg of rosuvastatin, 20 mg of atorvastatin, or 40 mg of simvastatin to achieve the goal levels less than 80 mg/dL (2 mmol/L).

If several risk factors are present in the absence of coronary, carotid, or peripheral vascular disease, drug therapy is considered if the LDL-C is greater than 130 mg/dL (3.5 mmol/L), with a goal of less than 100. In patients considered to have average risk for atheromatous disease, drug therapy is considered if the LDL-C is greater than 160 mg/dL (>4 mmol/L) with a goal of less than 120 mg/dL (3 mmol/L) (Table 9.1).

- *Guidelines advise LDL-C reduction- 30–40%.*
- According to 2009–2012 data, greater than 100 million US adults more than or equal to 20 years of age have total cholesterol levels greater than or equal to 200 mg/dL. Almost 31 million have levels greater than or equal to 240 mg/dL.
- Most heart attacks occur in individuals with total cholesterol levels between 210 mg/dL and 240 mg/dL (5.5 mmol/L and 6.2 mmol/L), and approximately 50% of adult Americans have cholesterol levels in this range. The average cholesterol level for North Americans is about 212 mg/dL (5.5 mmol/L). In these individuals with borderline high blood cholesterol, a low level of HDL-C further increases the risk for CHD. The emphasis, therefore, must be placed on the general population, in which mild-to-moderate elevation of total cholesterol LDL-C 3–3.5 mmol/L is a common health problem. Indeed, mild hypertension is a parallel marker and the conditions often coexist, thus increasing CHD risk, which is compounded by cigarette smoking and others.

Table 9.1: Formulate low-density lipoprotein cholesterol (LDL-C) goal based on risk and treat to goal.	
Risk	LDL-C goal assessment*
Very high risk	<1.5 mmol/L (60 mg/dL†)
High risk	<2.5 mmol/L (96 mg/dL)
Average risk	<3 mmol/L (115 mg/dL†)

*Items below apply:
†Stop smoking

- Although total cholesterol and HDL-C can be measured in the nonfasting state, the measurement of LDL-C requires a 12-hour fasting specimen for accurate determination of the triglyceride level, which is required for the estimation of the LDL-C.
- Triglyceride estimation must be performed in the fasting state.
- LDL-C is derived as follows: LDL (mg/dL) = total cholesterol−HDL−(triglyceride ÷ 5); or LDL (mmol/L) = total cholesterol (mmol/L)−HDL−(triglyceride ÷ 2.2). If the triglyceride value is above 200 mg/dL (2.2 mmol/L), the estimation is invalid (conversion for triglyceride: mmol/L × 88 = mg/dL; for cholesterol: mmol/L × 39 = mg/dL). LDL-C mmol/L to mg/dL × 39; 4 mmol/L = 156 mg/dL.
- When a patient has documented high-risk LDL-C levels or premature CHD and familial genetic disease is confirmed, all available first-degree relatives should be tested.

High-density Lipoprotein Cholesterol

Data from the Framingham Study indicate that the mortality risk from CHD increases as HDL-C levels decrease. The average risk of mortality from CHD is at a level of 39 mg/dL (1 mmol/L). Every 1% increase in HDL-C decreases CHD risk by about 2%, and each 1% reduction in total cholesterol should produce a 2% reduction in CHD risk. The HDL-C shows a strong inverse association with incidence of CHD at all levels of total cholesterol, including levels under 200 mg/dL (5.2 mmol/L). A 12-year follow-up indicates that the relationship does not diminish appreciably with time. The study confirms that nonfasting HDL-C and total cholesterol are related to development of CHD in both men and women over age 49.

- High-density lipoprotein cholesterol above 60 mg/dL (1.6 mmol/L) appears to be a protective negative risk factor. HDL acts hypothetically to export nonoxidized LDL from foam cells; LDL-C that is not oxidized can potentially be re-exported.

High-density lipoprotein cholesterol, as well as total cholesterol, is not affected by food eaten within prior hours; thus, a nonfasting specimen is not required. A nonfasting specimen allows the sample to be taken immediately after the physician consultation and saves the time and cost of a return visit to a laboratory.

SITOSTEROL

Sitosterolemia is a genetic defect that has been recently uncovered. This very rare, inherited disorder causes increased absorption and decreased excretion of plant sterols, which increase and appear to cause premature growth of atheroma.

Sitosterol may play a role in atheroma development.

Case report: An 18-year-old white male died suddenly of an acute MI. From age 10, he had noted tendon xanthomas that began on the left elbow and back and then subsequently in the Achilles tendons, knees, and wrists. Measurements of plasma sterols by gas-liquid chromatography 4 years prior to death revealed high concentrations of plant sterols with mild hypercholesterolemia, and a diagnosis of sitosterolemia with xanthomatosis was established (Salen et al. 1985).

Blood levels essential: This most important constituent of many so-called healthy foods may be a culprit. *Sitosterol, the blood levels* must be assessed in all patients at moderate or high risk and in all diabetics (Khan, 2017).

- *The author conducted a study that shows a major increase in sitosterol blood levels in diabetics. This increase in sitosterol is a likely cause of atheromatous CAD and MI in diabetics (Khan, 2017).*
- *In RCT, 10 mg of ezetimibe for 8 weeks caused a 21% decrease in sitosterol levels versus a 4% increase in placebo patients (Salen et al. 1985).*
- Investigators were able to determine that ezetimibe was not associated with an increased risk for cancer by analyzing data from two other clinical trials with a total of more than 18,000 patient-years of follow-up (HOPE-3 Trial).

Apolipoprotein A-I (Apo A-I) Milano: A mutated gene *ApoA-I* Milano passed down from an 18th century ancestor of a patient who was found to have excessively high serum cholesterol but with normal coronary arteries, has led to development of a drug, a gene that is cardioprotective. A variant of apolipoprotein, ApoA-I Milano has been identified in inhabitants of rural Italy who exhibit very low levels of HDL but are atheroma free. Nissen et al. have shown that the intravenous (IV) administration of a synthetic version of the agent into a small group of patients caused significant regression of atheroma in coronary arteries. Patients with coronary atheroma were given 5 weekly IV infusions of a recombinant ApoA-I Milano phospholipid complexes and were compared with controls. Intravascular ultrasonography indicated a 4.2% decrease in volume of atheroma; the degree of regression in this short period was unexpected and long-term trials are required.

It appears that individuals with another cardioprotective isoform, ApoA-I Paris, also show an HDL pattern that consists primarily of HDL-3 particles. An epidemiological study observed that HDL-3, but not HDL-2, was associated with a reduced risk of progression of CHD. The prevention and/or release oxidative damage to LDL by HDL-3 offers a potentially important mechanism of cardioprotection; HDL-2 particles, however, show little cardioprotective activity.

C-reactive protein: Investigators of JUPITER study indicate that C-reactive protein (CRP) monitoring should be used to assess risk, regardless of LDL goal achieved by statin therapy. High-risk patients with ACS who have low CRP levels after statin therapy appear to have better clinical outcomes than those with higher CRP levels. But the test is invalid in many who have arthritides or inflammatory disorders. This was a blunderbuss study and

cannot be taken seriously. Optimal treatment: two cardioprotective drugs aspirin and β-blockers were given to few.
- C-reactive protein testing is low on the list and not worth the expense.

TRIGLYCERIDES

Triglyceride-rich VLDLs are secreted by the liver. The VLDL surface coat contains apolipoprotein B and other lipoproteins. VLDL triglycerides undergo hydrolysis by lipoprotein lipase.

Very low-density lipoprotein remnants have one or two fates. Direct removal by the liver or degradation into LDL by lipolytic removal of remaining triglycerides.

Triglyceride levels of 200–400 mg/dL (2–4 mmol/L) are considered borderline and 400–1,000 mg/dL (4–10 mmol/L) are high. Level more than 500 mg/dL carries a high risk for acute pancreatitis and requires immediate dietary and drug therapy. A positive role for high triglyceride levels in CHD still remains controversial as shown in large clinical studies. Because increased triglyceride and low levels of HDL-C are closely associated, the independent contribution of triglyceride may disappear, particularly in men, once the risk of HDL has been taken into account. In a meta-analysis of 17 studies, triglyceride was shown to be an independent risk factor, particularly in women, after controlling for HDL-C, but the association is modest and unproven. Fortunately, elevations of triglycerides are most often controlled by restriction of carbohydrates and alcohol, weight reduction, and exercise an appropriate management of diabetes.

DIETARY MANAGEMENT (TABLES 9.2A AND B)

Dietary modification is expected to decrease an elevated blood cholesterol by 7–15%, depending on the degree of adherence to a low-saturated fat, low-cholesterol diet, and the previous intake of these substances. Some individuals have a marked increase in total cholesterol in response to dietary cholesterol, whereas in others, an increase in saturated fat or cholesterol intake has little or no effect. Dietary change brings about a salutary effect in only some individuals, but a consistent effort must be made to enforce the change, especially because drug therapy entails costs and risks of adverse effects, and because compliance is poor. Several clinical trials have documented the effect of the dietary approach in significantly reducing total cholesterol. Approximately 28% of Americans with elevated total cholesterol appear to respond to dietary cholesterol and saturated fat restrictions with a 10–15% decrease in cholesterol.

Table 9.2A: Saturated fat and cholesterol content of foods.*

Item*	Cholesterol (mg)	Total fat (g)	Saturated fat recommended (g)	Not recommended	Recommended[†]	Use sparingly
Meats						
Beef liver	395	10	3	X		
Kidney	725	11	4	X		
Sweetbread	420	21	—	X		
Lean beef	82	5	2		∶	
Roast beef:						
Rib	85	33	14	X		•
Rump	85	21	9	X		
Stewing	82	27	11	X		•
Lean cut	82	9	4		∶	•
Ground	85	18	8	X		
Steak:						
Sirloin	85	25	10	X		•
Lean cut	85	5	2		∶	•
Veal	90	12	5		∶	•
Lamb, lean	90	7	4			•
Chop and fat	110	33	18	X		
Ham:						
Fat roasted	80	28	7	X		
Boiled						
Sliced	80	18	5			•
Pork chop	80	30	12	X		

Contd...

Contd...

Item*	Cholesterol (mg)	Total fat (g)	Saturated fat recommended (g)	Not recommended	Recommended†	Use sparingly
Chicken:						
Breast and skin	72	6	1		⁞	
Drumstick (fried)	80	9	2		⁞	
Turkey	80	5	2		⁞	
Fish						
Sole	45	1	Trace		⁞	
Trout	50	13	3		⁞	
Tuna	60	7	2		⁞	
Salmon:						
Fresh	42	7	1		⁞	
Canned	32	11	2		⁞	
Mackerel	85	10	2		⁞	
Halibut	54	6	Trace		⁞	
Crabmeat	91	1	Trace			•
Shrimp	130	1	Trace			•
Lobster (450 g)	80	1	Trace			•
Dairy products						
30 mL butter	460	25	16	X		
Egg (50 g)	275	6	2		⁞	
Substitute	0	0	0		⁞	
Buttermilk††	10	2	1			
Yogurt (250 mL)	16	3	2		⁞	

Table 9.2B: Saturated and unsaturated fat and cholesterol content of foods.

Item*	Cholesterol (mg)	Total fat (g)	Saturated fat recommended (g)	Polyunsaturated fat	Not recommended	Recommended†	Use sparingly
Whole milk 250 mL	35	9	5				•
2%	20	5	3			••	
Skim milk	Trace	Trace	Trace			••	
Ice cream:							
Vanilla reg (125 mL)	32	8	5				•
Rich (125mL)	46	12	8		X		
Butter	30	11	1	Trace			•
Lard	12	13	5	1	X		
Cheese (1 oz):							
Brick	27	8	6	Trace			•
Blue	24			Trace		••	
Cheddar	30	10	6	Trace			•
Cottage††	2	0.6	0.5	Trace		••	
Skim milk, processed, 1 oz (30 g)	0	Trace	Trace	Trace		••	
Oils							
Corn oil	0	14	1	7		••	
Rapeseed	0	14	1	3	X		
Safflower	0	13	1	10		••	

Contd...

Contd...

Item*	Cholesterol (mg)	Total fat (g)	Saturated fat recommended (g)	Polyunsaturated fat	Not recommended	Recommended[†]	Use sparingly
Sunflower	0	14	1	9		••	
Soybean	0	14	2	7		••	
Coconut	0	14	12	0.2	X		
Palm	0		7	0.2	X		
Olive	0	14	2	1		••	
Peanut		14	2	4	X		
Nuts							
Almonds	0	16	1	3		••	
Brazil nuts	0	22	5	8	X		
Cashews	0	13	3	2	X		
Coconut	0	13	11	Trace	X		
Peanuts	0	17	3	4	X		
Peanut butter	0	7.5	1.5	2	X		
Pecans	0	21	2	5			•
Walnuts	0	19	2	11		••	

*Quantity is 3 oz (90 g) unless specified; 15 mL = 1 tablespoonful.
[†]Foods recommended contain less than 5 g saturated fat per 3 oz.
[††]Low-fat milk, 2%.
Note: Coconut oil is a dangerous product used in some countries for frying, stewing and making of rotis and chapatis (breads).

Mediterranean Linolenic Acid-rich Diet

A prospective, randomized, single-blind, secondary prevention trial using a Mediterranean linolenic acid-rich diet has proven that linolenic acid is useful in preventing cardiac deaths and nonfatal infarctions. In a study of 605 patients randomized within 6 months of MI, a total of 302 patients were given a diet containing an increased amount of α-linolenic and oleic acids. This diet was modeled on the Cretan Mediterranean diet that includes a high intake of α-linolenic acid, which has a beneficial effect on platelet reactivity. Oleic acid is derived mainly from olive oil. A canola oil-based margarine with a high content of α-linolenic acid was used daily, and the study was based on the hypothesis that the Cretans and Japanese have the lowest CAD mortality in the world and have a high intake of α-linolenic acid. The Japanese have a high consumption of canola and soybean oils; the Cretans derive their consumption of linolenic acid mainly from walnuts and purslane. At a mean follow-up of 27 months, there were 16 cardiac deaths and 17 nonfatal infarctions in the control versus 3 deaths and 5 nonfatal infarctions in the experimental groups ($p = 0.001$).

Trans-fatty acids are at high levels in several frequently used foods that include: hard margarines, cookies, commercially baked products, and fast foods. Most important, trans-fatty acids are now reduced in some products but are being replaced by saturated fatty acids that maintain the increased coronary risk caused by trans-fatty acids.

DRUG THERAPY

Except in patients with atheromatous disease and patients at high risk for CHD, drugs are used after an adequate trial of dietary therapy, a concerted effort by the patient and physician, and/or the assistance of a dietitian or lipid clinic fail to adequately lower total or LDL-C to the desired level usually less than 3 mmol/L in so-called healthy adults with good family history.

When drugs are prescribed, dietary restrictions must be continued. Dietary therapy can achieve only about a 10% lowering of total cholesterol but can reduce triglyceride levels in most individuals from 25% to 50%.

Low-density Lipoprotein Cholesterol Blood Testing Centers

It is crucial for governmental and other agencies to set up centers to screen all individuals, men age of approximately 30 years and females of approximately 40 years.

Lower is better: The LDL-C in these individuals must be less than 2.5 mmol/L (96 mg/dL). Total cholesterol less than 4.4 mmol/L.
- All patients determined to be at high risk (see Table 9.1) are advised to aim for an *LDL-C less than 1.8 mmol/L (<70 mg/dL)*.

- Moderate risk to be less than 2 mmol/L.
- Average risk less than 2.5 mmol/L
- Most individuals at low risk less than 3.2 mmol/L.

Very high risk—men age 40–70, women 45–75 (any of one to three):
1. Based on parent +ve for MI at age less than 70. LDL-C greater than 3.5 mmol/L, approximately 135 mg/dL.
2. Prior MI and LDL greater than 3.5 mmol/L.
3. Diabetes plus any family member: father, uncles, and aunts, +ve for MI.

High risk:
- Diabetic with –ve familial hypercholesterolemia (FH) but LDL greater than 3.5 mmol/L, approximately 135 mg/dL.
- Prior MI –ve FH, but LDL-C greater than 3.5 mmol/L.
- Blood pressure greater than 160, plus LDL greater than 3.5 mmol/L (135 mg/dL).
- Family history –ve but LDL-C greater than 4 mmol/L.

Formulate LDL-C Goal

Start LDL assessment of males age 35–75, females age 40–75 (see Table 9.1).

Statins (3-hydroxy-methylglutaryl-coenzyme A Reductase Inhibitors)

The statins constitute a major advance in the management of patients with dyslipidemia. Their proven value in reducing mortality from CAD and their ability to cause modest regression and significantly prevent progression of atheroma give a ray of hope that the epidemic of atheromatous disease can be halted. The statins are competitive inhibitors of 3-hydroxy-3-methylglutaryl-coenzyme A (HMG-CoA) reductase, the enzyme catalyzing the early rate-limiting step in the biosynthesis of cholesterol, conversion of HMG-CoA to mevalonate.

A modest reduction in intracellular cholesterol occurs, resulting in an increase in the number of hepatic LDL receptors that bring about clearance of circulating LDL-C.

Randomized Controlled Trials

The Scandinavian Simvastatin Survival Study (4S) reported a remarkable reduction in total mortality of 30%, and revascularization rates fell by 37%.

The study enrolled 4,444 patients with angina or previous MI (79%) and a high total cholesterol 5.5–8 mmol/L. The subjects were randomized to double-blind treatment with simvastatin or placebo with follow-up 5.4 years. Simvastatin caused a 25% decrease in cholesterol and 35% reduction in LDL-C. Two hundred fifty-six patients (12%) in the placebo group died, compared with 182 (8%) in the simvastatin group [relative risk (RR) of death 0.70; p = 0.0003). Coronary deaths 189 in the placebo and 111 in the simvastatin group, while noncardiovascular causes accounted for 49 and 46 deaths, 622 patients (28%) in the placebo group and 431 (19%) in the simvastatin group had one or more major coronary events. Other benefits of treatment included a 37% reduction (p <0.00001) in the risk of undergoing myocardial revascularization procedures (4S, 1994).

In the Scotland Prevention Study, pravastatin administered to men 45–64 years of age with average cholesterol 272 mg/dL (7 mmol/L), significantly reduced the incidence of heart attack. Total mortality was not significantly decreased. Only nonfatal MIs were increased significantly. On probabilities, these MIs could have been prevented by the use of daily aspirin. Thus, it is not justifiable to apply the results of the West of Scotland trial to healthy men with cholesterol concentration in the range of approximately 200–240 mg/dL (5–6.2 mmol/L).

The Cholesterol and Recurrent Events (CARE) 1996—Pravastatin: The CARE study involved post-MI patients with cholesterol concentration in the low range (209 ± 17 mg/dL; 5.4–5.8 mmol/L) that is commonly seen in patients with ACS.

There was no decrease in total mortality rate. The number of fatal MIs was 38 versus 24 (p = 0.07).

- Breast cancer occurred in 12 pravastatin-treated patients versus 1 in the control group (p = 0.002). It is important in women to evaluate the use of statins, particularly in patients who have a positive family history of breast cancer. There was no decrease in total mortality rate. The number of fatal MIs was 38 versus 24 nonsignificant (p = 0.07).

Hague et al. (2016) assessed the long-term effects of treatment with statin therapy on all-cause mortality, cause-specific mortality, and cancer incidence from extended follow-up of the long-term intervention with pravastatin in ischemic disease (LIPID) trial.

Methods and results: LIPID initially compared pravastatin and placebo over 6 years in 9,014 patients with previous CHD. After the double-blind period, all patients were offered open-label statin therapy. Data were obtained over a further 10 years from 7,721 patients, by direct contact for 2 years, by questionnaires thereafter, and from mortality and cancer registries. During extended follow-up, 85% assigned pravastatin and 84% assigned placebo took statin therapy. Patients assigned pravastatin maintained a significantly lower risk of death from CHD (RR 0.89; 95%; p = 0.009), and from any cause (RR 0.91; absolute risk reduction, 2.6%; p = 0.003). Cancer incidence was similar by original treatment group during the double-blind period. There were no significant differences in cancer mortality, or in the incidence of organ-specific cancers. Cancer findings were confirmed in a meta-analysis with other large statin trials with extended follow-up (Hague et al. 2016).

Conclusions: In LIPID, the absolute survival benefit from 6 years of pravastatin treatment appeared to be maintained for the next 10 years, with a similar risk of death among survivors in both groups after the initial period. Treatment with statins does not influence cancer or death from noncardiovascular causes during long-term follow-up (Hague et al. 2016).

LIPID study: In 9,014 patients, aged 31–75 years, the events from 40 mg pravastatin daily were compared with those of a placebo and a long follow-up period of 6.1 years. The patients had a history of MI or hospitalization for unstable angina and initial plasma total cholesterol levels of 155–271 mg/dL (4.0–7.0 mmol/L). Baseline cholesterol was much higher than in the CARE study. Mortality was 633 (14.1%) in placebo group, 498 (11.0%) in the pravastatin group (relative reduction in risk, 22%; p <0.001). Deaths from CHD, the primary end point: 373 versus 287; pravastatin reduced the risk for CHD mortality 24% (p <0.001).

MRC/BHF heart protection study (2002): The study indicated that in vascular high-risk patients, 40 mg simvastatin safely reduced the risk of heart attack, of stroke, and of revascularization by at least one-third. Among the 4,000 patients with a total cholesterol less than 5 mmol/L (192 mg/dL), a clear reduction in major events was observed. All-cause mortality was significantly reduced [1,328 (12.9%) deaths among 10,269 allocated simvastatin vs 1,507 (14.7%) among 10,267 allocated placebo; p = 0.0003], owing to a highly significant 18% proportional reduction in the coronary death rate [587 (5.7%) vs 707 (6.9%); p = 0.0005]. There were highly significant reductions of about one-fourth in the first-event rate for fatal and nonfatal MI [898 (8.7%) vs 1,212 (11.8%); p <0.0001], for nonfatal or fatal stroke [444 (4.3%) vs 585 (5.7%); p <0.0001], and for coronary or noncoronary revascularization [939 (9.1%) vs 1,205 (11.7%); p <0.0001].

PROSPER: Pravastatin in the Elderly (2002), pravastatin 40 mg was administered to 5,804 randomized elderly patients aged 70–82. At the short, 3.5-year follow-up, there was no difference in the number of strokes, but CHD death was reduced by 24%. There were 245 new cases of cancer in the pravastatin group versus 199 in the placebo group. Breast and gastrointestinal cancers showed the largest increases.

- New cancer diagnoses were more frequent on pravastatin than on placebo (HR 1.25; 95% CI 1.04–1.51; p = 0.020).

Older adults with hypertension and hyperlipidemia might not benefit from taking pravastatin for primary prevention of cardiovascular events, according to an open-label study in JAMA Internal Medicine.

The study, a secondary analysis of a large lipid-lowering trial (ALLHAT-LLT), looked at adults aged 65 years and older who were clear of atherosclerotic CVD at baseline and had moderate hyperlipidemia and hypertension.

No benefit was found when pravastatin was given for primary prevention to older adults with moderate hyperlipidemia and hypertension, and a nonsignificant direction toward increased all-cause mortality with pravastatin was observed among adults 75 years and older.

Hyperlipidemia and hypertension: Roughly 2,900 patients were randomized to pravastatin (40 mg/day) or usual care (Han et al. 2017).

Over 6 years, all-cause mortality was higher with pravastatin than with usual care (19% vs 16%), although the difference was not statistically significant. The mortality gap was wider for patients aged 75 and older (31% vs 23%), but still did not reach statistical significance. There were also no significant differences in secondary outcomes, including CHD events.

An editor's note concludes that statins' musculoskeletal risks and the current findings "should be considered before prescribing or continuing statins for patients in this age category".

The Pravastatin or Atorvastatin Evaluation and Infection Therapy-Thrombolysis in Myocardial Infarction 22 (PROVE IT-TIMI 22): 4,162 patients with ACS, ST segment elevation myocardial infarction (STEMI), NSTEMI or high-risk unstable angina—in the preceding 10 days and with a total cholesterol level of 240 mg/dL (6.21 mmol/L) or less, were randomized to receive atorvastatin 80 mg (intensive statin therapy) or pravastatin 40 mg. The primary end point was a composite of death from any cause, MI, documented unstable angina requiring rehospitalization, revascularization (performed at least 30 days after randomization), and stroke (Cannon et al. 2004). The median LDL-C level achieved during treatment was 95 mg/dL (2.46 mmol/L) in the pravastatin group and 62 mg/dL (1.60 mmol/L) in the atorvastatin group (p <0.001). The triple end point of death, MI, or rehospitalization for recurrent ACS at 30 days occurred in 3% of patients receiving atorvastatin 80 mg versus 4.2% of patients receiving pravastatin 40 mg (p = 0.046).

- *There were nonsignificant reductions in the rates of death from any cause* (p = 0.07) *and of death or MI* (p = 0.06). The risk of the secondary end point of death due to CHD, MI, or revascularization was reduced by 14% in the atorvastatin group (p = 0.029), a poor result with a 2-year event rate of 19.7%, as compared with 22.3% in the pravastatin group.
- *The additions: Risk of death, MI, or urgent revascularization was reduced* by 25% in the atorvastatin group (p <0.001).
- Benefit appeared to be greater among patients with a baseline LDL-C of at least 125 mg/dL (3.5 mmol/L) a prespecified subgroup, with a 34% reduction in the hazard ratio, as compared with only a 7% reduction among patients with a baseline LDL-C below 125 mg/dL (3.5 mmol/L) (Cannon et al. 2004). Clearly LDL-C must be lowered to less than 3 mmol/L in all individuals with intermediate (some) risk.
- Importantly admission LDL-C greater than 3.5 is danger zone.

HOPE-3 evaluated cholesterol lowering with rosuvastatin 10 mg daily, blood pressure lowering with candesartan at a dose of 16 mg plus hydrochlorothiazide at 12.5 mg, and the combination of both interventions for the prevention of cardiovascular events among persons who did not have CVD and were at intermediate risk (defined as an annual risk of major cardiovascular events of approximately 1%) men 55, and women 60 years of age or older and women 65 years of age or older who had at least one of the following cardiovascular risk factors: elevated waist-to-hip ratio, history of a low level of HDL-C, current or recent tobacco use, dysglycemia, family history of premature coronary disease, and mild renal dysfunction.

Estimates indicate a low-risk category for subjects studied; I would not consider the subjects as intermediate risk. These subjects are average type individuals with no family history of MI; diabetics were rare. Risks were:
1. Total cholesterol in subjects: 201 mg/dL (5.2 mmol/L)
2. LDL-C: 127 mg/dL (3.3 mmol/L).

- *Only 10% and 11% received aspirin. A complete failure of expert trialist to see the gaps in their logic and knowledge of internal medicine.*

A total of 20% of the participants were white, 49.1% were Asian, 27.5% were Hispanic, and 3.3% were black or belonged to another ethnic group. The median follow-up was 5.6 years; cumulative nonadherence rates of as high as 23% in the groups receiving active treatment.

Cataracts: HOPE-3 trial, in which patients randomly allocated to rosuvastatin:
- More participants in the rosuvastatin group than in the placebo group underwent cataract surgery [241 (3.8%) vs 194 (3.1%), p = 0.02]
- Higher doses 30–40 mg for a longer period greater than 10 years are needed to assess for cataracts.
- Higher statin doses than used in HOPE-3 may cause more cataracts.
- Other minor decreases in outcomes are not solidly proven in this blunderbuss trial.

In Table 9.3, 12,705 randomized; yet only small numbers had an outcome and no reduction in total mortality, or CVD deaths.

Conclusion: In low and so-called intermediate risk patients, statin use is not proven to be of benefit. Perhaps a more defined group of intermediate risk may be helped.

In HOPE-3, risk was unfortunately determined by vague unproven risk factors.
- Elevated waist-to-hip ratio
- History of a low level of HDL; a presumptive nonproven factor

Table 9.3: Outcome of rosuvastatin group and the placebo group.

	Rosuvastatin	Placebo
Total mortality	334	357
Acute MI	45	69
Cardiovascular deaths	154	171

- Cholesterol 5.2 mmol/L (a non-high level) LDL-C 3.2 mmol/L very slightly high
- Current or recent tobacco use (over 6 years how much of a risk?)
- Family history of premature coronary disease 27%
- Mild renal dysfunction; unproven risk
- Diabetes only 5.5%.

In essence: An average low-risk population studied, and without cardioprotection by aspirin.

Valentin Fuster emphasized, at ACC 2016, the need to avoid hype when reporting the HOPE-3 findings. The results "fulfill the concept of people who think lower LDL is better", he said, adding "we need to be clear about the absolute event rate... we need to be very careful when talking to people about a RR reduction when the absolute event rate was 1.2%. *RR is a way to confuse people. Fuster (2015) has called attention to the delicacy of presenting statistics.*

Which Statin to Choose?

- Hydrophilic agents excreted by the kidney include the pravastatin and rosuvastatin; thus, interactions with hepatic metabolized agents are minimized.
- Lipophilic agents include atorvastatin, lovastatin, and simvastatin; these are hepatic metabolized. Interactions may occur with cimetidine and other agents that use the cytochrome P450 pathway. It appears that atorvastatin increases fibrinogen levels.
- Rosuvastatin must not be used in conjunction with cyclosporine; cyclosporine levels are increased. Caution in individuals allergic to sulfur.

Statin contraindications include porphyria; concomitant use of cyclosporine, nicotinic acid or fibrates, cyclosporine, other cytotoxic drugs; erythromycin and similar antibiotics; also contraindicated in women of childbearing age and during lactation. Hepatic metabolized agents must be avoided in individuals with hepatic dysfunction. Caution in elderly over age 75 and in patients with hypothyroidism.

Atorvastatin: This statin is more effective than pravastatin, fluvastatin, and simvastatin.

Dosage: 10–40 mg daily for patient at intermediate and high risk; 60–80 mg for STEMI for a few months; reduce dose when LDL-C goal is reached; lower is better if no adverse effects.

If the LDL-C goal is not achieved, the addition of ezetimibe is advised.

The REVERSAL investigators randomized 2,163 patients to moderate lipid-lowering (40 mg of pravastatin) or intensive treatment (80 mg of atorvastatin) for 18 months. IVUS was performed during baseline coronary arteriography and repeated at study completion.

Low-density lipoprotein cholesterol (mean: 150.2 mg/dL) was reduced to 110 mg/dL in the pravastatin arm versus 79 mg/dL in the atorvastatin group (p <0.0001). The primary end point (percent change in atheroma volume) showed progression in the pravastatin cohort; +2.7%, p = 0.001, and showed no progression in the atorvastatin arm (−0.4%, p = 0.98). The progression rate was significantly lower in the atorvastatin arm (p = 0.02). In addition, pravastatin caused a 5.2% decrease in CRP versus 36.4% for atorvastatin (p <0.0001). In this subset of patients, LDL-C levels should be maintained less than 80 mg/dL (2 mmol/L).

Simvastatin: Dosage of 5–10 mg is given with the evening meal; increase if needed in 8–12 weeks to maximum 20 mg daily if rosuvastatin or atorvastatin is not available.

- The author does not recommend simvastatin use because of interactions.

Pravastatin; 10 mg with the evening meal; increase over 2–4 months to a maximum of 40 mg once daily. Hyperuricemia and thrombocytopenia have been observed, albeit rarely. The drug should not be administered to patients over age 75 as it is ineffective (Han et al. 2017).

Rosuvastatin: A dosage of 10–20 mg daily should achieve goal if LDL-C at baseline is 3–4 mmol/L. If goal is not achieved at 40 mg, add 10 mg of ezetimibe. The 30 mg with ezetimibe may be required in genetic familial hyperlipidemia.

Rosuvastatin is a potent agent that causes a 40–50% reduction in LDL-C.

Adverse Effects of Statins

Headaches occur in about 10%, stomach pain, flatulence, diarrhea, constipation, nausea, hepatic dysfunction with increased hepatic transaminases occur in 2%, chest pain owing to stomach disturbance or muscular aches may occur. A flu-like illness with myalgia, elevation of creatine kinase (CK), myopathy occurred in 0.5%, and rhabdomyolysis has been observed in patients receiving concomitant niacin, gemfibrozil, cyclosporine, and other immunosuppressive drugs. MedWatch Reporting System listed 3,339 cases of statin-associated rhabdomyolysis over a 12-year period. Myopathy and deaths occurred most commonly with cerivastatin (Baycol), which was withdrawn in 2000.

The risk of rhabdomyolysis is increased in the elderly over age 75 and in patients with hepatic and renal dysfunction, hypothyroidism, and diabetes.

Rhabdomyolysis occurs rarely and is usually the result of the following:
- Too high a dose of statin: Atorvastatin 80 mg or greater, simvastatin greater than 60 mg or greater, rosuvastatin greater than 40 mg.
- Combination with interacting drug, particularly: Cyclosporine, fibrates, niacin, antifungal agents, antibiotics such as erythromycin, azithromycin and clarithromycin.

- *Caution*: With rosuvastatin and pravastatin if the creatinine clearance is less than 55 mL/minute, serum creatinine greater than 1.5 mg/dL (133 μmol/L). Do not use rosuvastatin if the eGFR is less than 30 mL/minute.
- Patients with hypothyroidism.

The mechanism for statin-induced myopathy is unclear; statins appear to reduce the production of small regulatory proteins that are important for myocyte maintenance. Minor muscle pain and weakness was reported in 1–5% of patients.

Intolerance

This is definite in approximately 5% and not greater than 20% as some indicate.

Cataracts: Lens opacity observed in animals given high doses has not been a clinical problem; although minor lens opacification occurs. Recently cataracts have been documented in RCTs (HOPE-3), caution is needed with highest doses rosuvastatin 40 mg or atorvastatin 80 mg greater than 6 months.

Rash is uncommon. Baseline transaminase and CK are advisable. If more than a threefold increase in baseline transaminases or CK occurs, the drug should be discontinued. Pancreatitis occurs rarely. Caution: avoid in renal transplant patients on cyclosporine or immunosuppressives.

- In patients receiving oral anticoagulants, reduction in the dose of warfarin is usually required with atorvastatin.
- Severe myositis may cause hyperkalemia in patients with renal insufficiency, particularly including long-standing diabetics who are also on angiotensin-converting enzyme (ACE) inhibitors.
- Do not combine with fibrates or niacin. Although it is rare for the combination to cause rhabdomyolysis and kidney damage, *the combination of statins with a fibrate or nicotinic acid is not recommended.*

The Controlled Rosuvastatin Multinational Trial in Heart Failure (CORONA) trial assessed the debate regarding the potential role of statin therapy in chronic HF. CORONA was a multicenter, randomized-controlled, placebo-controlled trial of 5,011 older patients (age 60 years, mean age 73 years) with ischemic cardiomyopathy [left ventricular ejection fraction (LVEF) 40% for the New York Heart Association (NYHA) functional class III and IV or LVEF 35% for NYHA functional class II]. Patients were randomized to either rosuvastatin at 10 mg daily or a placebo and received a median of 2.7 years' follow-up (Kjekshus et al. 2007). The study did not reach the primary combined end point of cardiovascular death, nonfatal MI, or nonfatal stroke (p = 0.12) or any coronary event end point.

In the GISSI-HF (Gruppo Italiano per lo Studio della Sopravvivenza nell'Insufficienza Cardiaca-Heart Failure) trial, rosuvastatin also did not demonstrate a reduction in mortality (GISSI-HF 2008).

Thus, statins are not generally advised for the management of heart failure.

NEW DRUG CLASS AND NEW THERAPIES

Ezetimibe

Supplied as 10-mg tablets, with a recommended dosage of 10 mg once daily, with or without food. Ezetimibe localizes and appears to act at the brush border of the small intestine and inhibits cholesterol absorption. The drug is a potent and selective inhibitor of cholesterol absorption and decreases delivery of cholesterol to the liver, thus promoting the synthesis of LDL receptors, with a subsequent 20% reduction in LDL-C. Importantly, this location of action appears to be largely unaffected by the pathophysiology of genetic familial hyperlipidemia, for which treatment is still most unsatisfactory. Ezetimibe's half-life is approximately 22 hours and is not altered by renal or hepatic function. The drug does not use the cytochrome P450 or N-acetyltransferase and there is no significant interaction.

Ezetimibe decreases sitosterol blood levels.
- Ezetimibe is a valuable addition to our therapeutic armamentarium as it is effective and allows for the use of moderate doses of statins in resistant cases of hypercholesterolemia; this will avoid adverse effects of high-dose statin therapy (>60 mg of atorvastatin, 40 mg of rosuvastatin).
- It is advisable to add ezetimibe to all patients with diabetes and most with ischemic heart disease as combination with statin should not await failure to reach a goal.

IMPROVE-IT trial: This double-blind, randomized trial involved 18,144 patients hospitalized for an ACS within the past 10 days and had LDL-C levels of 50–100 mg/dL (1.3–2.6 mmol/L) if they were receiving lipid-lowering therapy or 50–125 mg/dL (1.3–3.2 mmol/L) if they were not receiving lipid-lowering therapy. The combination of simvastatin (40 mg) and ezetimibe (10 mg) (simvastatin–ezetimibe) was compared with simvastatin (40 mg) and placebo (simvastatin monotherapy). The primary end point was a composite of cardiovascular death, nonfatal MI, unstable angina requiring rehospitalization, coronary revascularization (≥30 days after randomization), or nonfatal stroke. The median follow-up was 6 years. Results are shown in Table 9.4.

A greater proportion of patients in the simvastatin–ezetimibe group than in the simvastatin monotherapy group achieved the dual goal of an LDL-C level of less than 70 mg/dL (1.8 mmol/L) and a high-sensitivity CRP level of less than 2.0 at 1 month.
- The beneficial effects of ezetimibe were found mainly in patients with diabetes, with a recent coronary event (Cannon et al. 2015).

Table 9.4: IMPROVE-IT trial results.

	Simvastatin	Simvastatin + Ezetimibe
Total mortality	1,231	1,215
Cardiovascular disease (CVD)	538	537
Coronary heart disease	461	440
Any myocardial infarction (MI)	1,083 (14.4%)	1,414 (13.1%)
Fatal MI	49	41
CVD + MI + Stroke	1,704	1,544 (p = 0.003)

- The benefit of simvastatin–ezetimibe was consistent across nearly all prespecified subgroups. The greatest absolute benefit was seen in high-risk patients. *The benefit appeared to be particularly pronounced in patients with diabetes mellitus* and in patients 75 years of age or older. [This beneficial effect is likely due to lowering of sitosterol blood levels by ezetimibe along with LDL-C (Khan, 2017].
- Approximately 27% of subjects had diabetes mellitus, and 70% had undergone percutaneous coronary intervention (PCI) during the index hospitalization. The PCI in probabilities decreased the number of deaths observed and diluted the immense value of ezetimibe added to simvastatin that caused reduction in outcomes.
  Average LDL-C level was 69.5 mg/dL (1.8 mmol/L) in the simvastatin monotherapy group and 53.7 mg/dL (1.4 mmol/L) in the simvastatin-ezetimibe group. The lowering of LDL-C to 1.4–1.2 mmol/L is a necessary goal in patients admitted with ACS, particularly those at higher risk: anterior MI, ejection fraction (EF) less than 40%, evidence of heart failure during the first few days of infarction.
- For most higher risk patients, the new guidelines recommend considering ezetimibe (10 mg) as the first add on to statin therapy.
- Recommendations on incorporating the proprotein convertase subtilisin-kexin type 9 (PCSK9) inhibitors evolocumab and alirocumab, approved in 2015, are also offered for selective patients. The guidelines were presented at the ACC's annual meeting in Chicago (April 2016).

PRECISE-IVUS (Plaque REgression with Cholesterol absorption Inhibitor or Synthesis inhibitor Evaluated by IVUS) trial: The aim of this study was to evaluate the effects of ezetimibe plus atorvastatin versus atorvastatin monotherapy on the lipid profile and coronary atherosclerosis in Japanese patients who underwent PCI, a prospective, RCT. Eligible patients who underwent PCI were randomly assigned to atorvastatin alone or atorvastatin plus ezetimibe (10 mg) daily. Atorvastatin was uptitrated with a treatment goal of LDL-C less than 70 mg/dL. Serial volumetric IVUS was performed at baseline and again at 9–12 months to quantify the coronary plaque response in 202 patients.

The combination therapy (atorvastatin + ezetimibe) resulted in lower levels of LDL-C than atorvastatin monotherapy (63.2 ± 16.3 mg/dL vs 73.3 ± 20.3 mg/dL; p <0.001). For the absolute change in percent atheroma volume (PAV), the mean difference between the two groups (−1.538%; 95% CI: −3.079% to 0.003%) did not exceed the predefined noninferiority margin of 3%, *but the absolute change in PAV did show superiority for the dual lipid-lowering strategy compared with atorvastatin alone.*

- For a PAV, a significantly greater percentage of patients who received atorvastatin/ezetimibe showed coronary plaque regression (78% vs 58%; p > 0.004).
- It is surprising that a small difference of LDL-C, 10–20 mg/dL can achieve a recognizable difference in atheroma regression.

Fibrates

These agents are activators of the enzyme plasma lipoprotein lipase. Fibrates cause a modest decrease in total or LDL-C. A 10–20% reduction in serum cholesterol, a 30–50% reduction in triglycerides, and a 10–15% increase in HDL-C have been observed in most studies.

In patients with high triglyceride levels (>500 mg/dL) resistant to concerted weight reduction and control of diabetes, fibrate therapy is required. In the majority of this subset of patients, LDL-C levels are increased to greater than 130 mg/dL, and some endocrinologists and lipid clinics advocate addition of statins; now, the use of ezetimibe added to fibrate is preferable to prevent the rare but disastrous problem of myopathy, alcoholism, gallstones, and pregnancy.

Fenofibrate

The recommended dosage is 160–200 mg daily with the main meal. The drug decreases LDL-C levels 10–15% increases in HDL-C approximately 20%, and triglycerides decrease more than 30%. Fenofibrate has been shown to decrease small dense LDL, lipoprotein (Lp) (a) and fibrinogen levels. High levels of Lp(a) small dense LDL and fibrinogen are risk factors for CAD.

Gastrointestinal disturbances occur in fewer than 7% of patients. If cholelithiasis is suspected during treatment therapy, ultrasound of the gallbladder is indicated. If gallstones are present, fenofibrate should be discontinued. Thus, it is wise to perform this procedure before commencing therapy. Abnormal liver function tests with an elevation of transaminases and an increase in alkaline phosphatase have been observed but normalized upon discontinuation of the drug. Test liver function monthly and then annually or if there are symptoms that suggest hepatic dysfunction. Rash, pruritus, urticaria or erythema, weight loss, impotence, alopecia, pancreatitis, hepatitis, and CK elevations may occur but subside on discontinuation of the drug.

Contraindications include the following:
- Severe renal or hepatic impairment. Fibrates are excreted by the kidney and should be used with caution in patients with renal dysfunction.
- Gallbladder disease
- Pregnancy, women of childbearing potential, and during lactation
- Primary biliary cirrhosis.

Fibrates may potentiate the effects of oral anticoagulants. Myositis has been reported with the combination of other fibrates and statins, thus careful monitoring is essential.

Bezafibrate

A dosage of 200 mg twice daily with or after food is used. The drug can be taken once daily. Contraindications include severe renal or hepatic impairment, hypoalbuminemia, primary biliary cirrhosis, gallbladder disease, nephrotic syndrome, and pregnancy.

Adverse effects include nausea, abdominal pain, myositis, urticaria, headache, and impotence. Bezafibrate causes a fall in glucose levels; also, an increase in serum creatinine occurs and monitoring is necessary. Long-term trials are necessary to document efficacy in reducing mortality and to assess adverse effects. The drug may cause alopecia.

Interactions:
- Oral anticoagulants: The dosage of anticoagulants should be reduced with careful management of prothrombin time or international normalized ratio.
- HMG-CoA reductase inhibitors: severe myositis and rhabdomyolysis have been observed with the combination of fibrates and lovastatin, with marked elevation of serum potassium, which may be life-threatening.

Niacin

Use of niacin is not recommended; the drug should be rendered obsolete.
- The AIM-HIGH study confirmed that use is nonjustified. The trial was stopped after a mean follow-up period of 3 years owing to a lack of efficacy. There was a small excess of ischemic strokes in the niacin group.

MANAGEMENT OF ELEVATED SERUM TRIGLYCERIDES

A triglyceride level up to 200 mg/dL (2.0 mmol/L) is considered to be within normal limits. About 200–400 mg/dL (2–4 mmol/L) is borderline high. 400–600 mg/dL (4–6 mmol/L) is high and more than 500 mg/dL carries a risk for pancreatitis.

Treatment of hypertriglyceridemia becomes urgent if triglyceride levels are above 500 mg/dL (5 mmol/L) because of the risk of pancreatitis and avascular necrosis of the femoral head. Fortunately, control is nearly always achieved with a low-carbohydrate diet. Weight loss almost always reduces triglyceride levels. Alcohol abuse is one of the most common causes of high triglyceride levels, and cessation of alcohol consumption is necessary for control. Failure to reduce levels to less than 500 mg/dL (mmol/L) is an indication for a fibrate with weight reduction diet, increase in exercise, and cessation of alcohol.

The evidence linking triglycerides directly with an increased risk of CHD remains controversial.

- Kersten (2016) reported in an editorial on two studies that identify ANGPTL4 as a link between triglycerides and CHD.
- Elevated triglyceride levels virtually always decrease when significant weight loss is achieved, alcohol consumption is curtailed, and diabetes is brought under strict control; fibrates are overused in this setting. It is most important to do no harm.

If the LDL-C is also elevated, the author advises the addition of ezetimibe rather than the addition of a statin; this strategy should obviate the rare but life-threatening occurrence of rhabdomyolysis.

BIBLIOGRAPHY

1. Ascherio A, Rimm EB, Stampfer MJ, et al. Dietary intake of marine n-3 fatty acids, fish intake, and the risk of coronary disease among men. N Engl J Med. 1995;332:977-82.
2. Bellosta S, Paoletti R, Corsini A. Safety of statins: focus on clinical pharmacokinetics and drug interactions. Circulation. 2004;109:III50-7.
3. Blankenhorn DH, Azen SP, Kramsch DM, et al. Coronary angiographic changes with lovastatin therapy. The Monitored Atherosclerosis Regression Study (MARS). Ann Intern Med. 1993;119:969-76.
4. Bohula EA, Morrow DA, Cannon C, et al. Atherothrombotic risk stratification and ezetimibe use in IMPROVE-IT. J Am Coll Cardiol. 2016;67(13 Suppl):2129.
5. Brown MS, Goldstein JL. A receptor-mediated pathway for cholesterol homeostasis. Science. 1986;232(4746):34-47.
6. Brown WV, Bays HE, Hassman DR, et al. Efficacy and safety of rosuvastatin compared with pravastatin and simvastatin in patients with hypercholesterolemia: a randomized, double-blind, 52-week trial. Am Heart J. 2002;144:1036-43.
7. Cannon CP, Blazing MA, Giugliano RP, et al. Ezetimibe added to statin therapy after acute coronary syndromes. N Engl J Med. 2015;372:2387-97.
8. Cannon CP, Braunwald E, McCabe CH, et al. Intensive versus moderate lipid lowering with statins after acute coronary syndromes. N Engl J Med. 2004;350:1495-504.
9. Crea F, Niccoli G. Ezetimibe and plaque regression: cholesterol lowering or pleiotropic effects? J Am Coll Cardiol. 2015;66:508-10.
10. de Lorgeril M, Renaud S, Mamelle N, et al. Mediterranean alpha-linolenic acid-rich diet in secondary prevention of coronary heart disease. Lancet. 1994;343:1454-9.
11. Everett BM, Smith RJ, Hiatt WR. Reducing LDL with PCSK9 inhibitors—the clinical benefit of lipid drugs. N Engl J Med. 2015;373:1588-91.

12. Everett BM. Low-density lipoprotein cholesterol and the on-target effects of therapy: how low is too low? J Am Coll Cardiol. 2017;69(5):483-5.
13. Fuster V. Unraveling the complexities of statistical presentation. Why it is important. J Am Coll Cardiol. 2015;66(25):2909-10.
14. Gagne C, Caudet D, Bruckert E. Efficacy and safety of ezetimibe coadministered with atorvastatin or simvastatin in patients with homozygous familial hypercholesterolemia. Circulation. 2002;105:2469-75.
15. GBD 2013 Risk Factors Collaborators. Forouzanfar MH, Alexander L, et al. Global, regional, and national comparative risk assessment of 79 behavioural, environmental and occupational, and metabolic risks or clusters of risks in 188 countries, 1990-2013: a systematic analysis for the Global Burden of Disease Study 2013. Lancet. 2015;386:2287-323.
16. Gharavi AG, Diamond JA, Smith DA, et al. Niacin-induced myopathy. Am J Cardiol. 1994;74:841-2.
17. Goldberg AC, Hopkins PN, Toth PP, et al. Familial hypercholesterolemia: screening, diagnosis and management of pediatric and adult patients: clinical guidance from the National Lipid Association Expert Panel on Familial Hypercholesterolemia. J Clin Lipidol. 2011;5(3 Suppl):S1-8.
18. Graham DJ, Staffa JA, Shatin D, et al. Incidence of hospitalized rhabdomyolysis in patients treated with lipid-lowering drugs. JAMA. 2004;292:2585-90.
19. Hague WE, Simes J, Kirby A, et al. Long-term effectiveness and safety of pravastatin in patients with coronary heart disease: sixteen years of follow-up of the LIPID study. Circulation. 2016;133:1851-60.
20. Han BH, Sutin D, Williamson JD, et al. Effect of statin treatment vs usual care on primary cardiovascular prevention among older adults: the ALLHAT-LLT randomized clinical trial. JAMA Intern Med. 2017;177(7):955-65.
21. Heart Protection Study Collaborative Group. MRC/BHF Heart Protection Study of cholesterol lowering with simvastatin in 20,536 high-risk individuals: a randomised placebo-controlled trial. Lancet. 2002;360:7-22.
22. Hjalmarson A, Goldstein S, Fagerberg B, et al. Effects of controlled-release metoprolol on total mortality, hospitalizations, and well-being in patients with heart failure: the Metoprolol CR/XL Randomized Intervention Trial in congestive heart failure (MERIT-HF). MERIT-HF Study Group. JAMA. 2000;283:1295-302.
23. HOPE-3.Salim Yusuf, Jackie Bosch, Gilles Dagenais,et al for the HOPE-3 Investigators† Cholesterol Lowering in Intermediate-Risk Persons without Cardiovascular Disease. N Engl J Med; April 2, 2016DOI: 10.1056/NEJMoa1600176
24. Hu FB. The Mediterranean diet and mortality—olive oil and beyond. N Engl J Med. 2003;348:2595-6.
25. Jacotot B, Benghozi R, Pfister P, et al. Comparison of fluvastatin versus pravastatin treatment of primary hypercholesterolemia. French Fluvastatin Study Group. Am J Cardiol. 1995;76:54A-6A.
26. Jarcho JA, Keaney JF Jr. Proof that lower is better—LDL cholesterol and IMPROVE-IT. N Engl J Med. 2015;372:2448-50.
27. Jones PH, Davidson MH, Stein EA. et al. for the STELLAR Study Group. Comparison of the efficacy and safety of rosuvastatin versus atorvastatin, simvastatin, and pravastatin across doses (STELLAR trial). Am J Cardiol. 2003;92:152-60.
28. Keech A, Simes RJ, Barter P, et al. Effects of long-term fenofibrate therapy on cardiovascular events in 9,795 people with type 2 diabetes mellitus (the FIELD study): randomised controlled trial. Lancet. 2005;366:1849-61.

29. Kersten S. The genetics of dyslipidemia—when less is more. N Engl J Med. 2016;374:1192-3.
30. Knoops KT, de Groot LC, Kromhout D, et al. Mediterranean diet, lifestyle factors, and 10-year mortality in elderly European mean and women: the HALE project. JAMA. 2004;292:1433-9.
31. Long-term Intervention with Pravastatin in Ischemic Disease (LIPID) Study Group. Prevention of cardiovascular events and death with pravastatin in patients with coronary heart disease and a broad range of initial cholesterol levels. N Engl J Med. 1998;339:1349-57.
32. MAAS Investigators. Effect of simvastatin on coronary atheroma: the Multicentre Anti-atheroma Study (MAAS). Lancet. 1994;344:633-8.
33. Mullin GE, Greenson JK, Mitchell MC. Fulminant hepatic failure after ingestion of sustained-release nicotinic acid. Ann Intern Med. 1989;111:253-5.
34. Nayor M, Vasan RS. Recent update to the US cholesterol treatment guidelines: a comparison with international guidelines. Circulation. 2016;133:1795-806.
35. Onorato A, Sturm AC. Heterozygous familial hypercholesterolemia. Circulation. 2016;133:e587-9.
36. Park SJ, Kang SJ, Ahn JM, et al. Effect of statin treatment on modifying plaque composition: a double-blind, randomized study. J Am Coll Cardiol. 2016;67(15):1772-83.
37. Randomised trial of cholesterol lowering in 4,444 patients with coronary heart disease: the Scandinavian Simvastatin Survival Study (4S). Lancet. 1994;344:1383-9.
38. Ray KK, Cannon CP, McCabe CH, et al. Early and late benefits of high-dose atorvastatin in patients with acute coronary syndromes: results from the PROVE IT-TIMI 22 trial. J Am Coll Cardiol. 2005;46:1405-10.
39. Ridker PM, Pradhan A, MacFadyen JG, et al. Cardiovascular benefits and diabetes risks of statin therapy in primary prevention. Lancet. 2012;380(9841):565-71.
40. Sacks FM, Pfeffer MA, Moye LA, et al. The effect of pravastatin on coronary events after myocardial infarction in patients with average cholesterol levels. Cholesterol and Recurrent Events Trial investigators. N Engl J Med. 1996;335:1001-9.
41. Salen G, Horak I, Rothkopf M, et al. Lethal atherosclerosis associated with abnormal plasma and tissue sterol composition in sitosterolemia with xanthomatosis. J Lipid Res. 1985;26:1126-33.
42. Schwartz GG, Olsson AG, Ezekowitz MD, et al. Effects of artovastatin on early recurrent ischemic events in acute coronary syndromes: the MIRACL study: a randomized controlled trial. JAMA. 2001;285:1711-8.
43. Shepherd J, Cobbe SM, Ford I, et al. Prevention of coronary heart disease with pravastatin in men with hypercholesterolemia. West of Scotland Coronary Prevention Study Group. N Engl J Med. 1995;333:1301-7.
44. Shor R, Wainstein J, Oz D, et al. Low serum LDL cholesterol levels and the risk of fever, sepsis, and malignancy. Ann Clin Lab Sci. 2007;37(4):343-8.
45. Tsujita K, Sugiyama S, Sumida H, et al. Impact of dual lipid-lowering strategy with ezetimibe and atorvastatin on coronary plaque regression in patients with percutaneous coronary intervention: the multicenter randomized controlled PRECISE-IVUS trial. J Am Coll Cardiol. 2015;66:495-507.
46. Yusuf S, Bosch J, Dagenais G, et al. Cholesterol lowering in intermediate-risk persons without cardiovascular disease. N Engl J Med. 2016;374:2021-31.

CHAPTER 10

Infective Endocarditis

DIAGNOSIS

The diagnosis of infective endocarditis must be considered and excluded in all individuals with a heart murmur and fever of unknown origin. Infection of the heart valves may be caused by bacteria and, less commonly, fungi, *Coxiella*, or *Chlamydia*.

A few hours or days of fever, chills and rigors are common with acute bacterial endocarditis (ABE). An insidious onset over weeks with fever, malaise, chills, and weight loss indicates subacute bacterial endocarditis (SBE). The division of infective endocarditis into ABE and SBE remains helpful to clinicians.

In a patient with a murmur and a fever of undetermined origin, one of the following precipitating or predisposing factors, if present, should produce a high index of suspicion of infective endocarditis:

- Known valvular heart disease, especially rheumatic, bicuspid aortic valve, or mitral valve prolapse, with significant regurgitation; Marfan's and floppy valve
- Prosthetic valve
- Recent dental or oropharyngeal surgical procedure
- Genitourinary instrumentation or surgery of the respiratory tract
- Intravenous (IV) addiction
- *Congenital heart disease:* Patent ductus, ventricular septal defect (VSD), Fallot's tetralogy, and coarctation
- Prolonged use of IV catheters and hyperalimentation
- Burns
- Inflammatory and other bowel disease, suspect *Streptococcus bovis*. If this organism is isolated, exclude polyposis and carcinoma of the colon
- Hemodialysis.

Infective endocarditis is a severe disease, with an in-hospital mortality rate of about 20% (Selton-Suty et al., 2012). Infective endocarditis can also present with a complication, particularly stroke, or systemic embolism.

Infective endocarditis may occur, however, in the absence of previously known valvular disease or other precipitating factors, especially in elderly patients.

Physical Signs

- A heart murmur is usually present with SBE, absent in 1–5%.
- A murmur may be absent in less than 15% of patients with ABE and not heard in about 33% of individuals with right-sided endocarditis, especially if care is not taken to listen for the murmur of tricuspid regurgitation.
- A change in the quality or grade of the murmur is an unreliable indicator.
- Intermittent medium-to-high-grade fever is usually prominent, but in elderly or immunocompromised patients, fever may be mild or absent. Normal body temperature is lower in the elderly, 97°F (36°C) as opposed to 98°F (37°C) in individuals less than age 70.
- Finger clubbing takes about 6 weeks to appear, is seen only with SBE, and disappears a few weeks after successful treatment.
- Osler's nodes, although uncommon, are pathognomonic, manifest as exquisitely painful, SQ papules, pea- to almond-sized on the palms and soles. Lesions disappear in 1–5 days and may be seen during adequate therapy.
- Petechiae with pale centers may be observed on everting the upper eyelids. They may be seen in the oropharynx as retinal cotton wool exudates, canoe-shaped hemorrhages with white spots in their center (Roth's spots).
- Splinter hemorrhages may be due to trauma, but a increase in their numbers is relevant.
- Splenomegaly is observed in about 50% of patients with SBE and in about 15% of those with ABE. The enlarged spleen may be painful and tender and can rupture. An ultrasound of the spleen is advisable in all cases of suspected infective endocarditis.
- *Pigmentation:* Pasty, cafe-au-lait complexion reverts to normal after treatment.
- *Janeway lesions are rare:* 1–4 mm painless flat erythematous macules, nontender on the palms and soles, blanch on pressure.

INVESTIGATIONS

When acute endocarditis is suspected, three separate sets of blood cultures are taken at separate venous sites over 24 hours. It is advisable to put 10 mL of blood in an aerobic culture bottle and 10 mL in an anaerobic bottle. The two subsequent cultures can be done at 20 minutes apart with 10 mL each in aerobic bottle, unless an anaerobic infection is strongly suspected. The increased volume of blood improves the bacteriological yield.

- Three or four separate sets of blood cultures taken from a separate vein puncture site with the first and last samples drawn at least 1-hour apart.
- Urinalysis often shows mild hematuria or increased red blood cells (RBCs) and few RBC casts.

- Increased creatinine, urea, or blood urea nitrogen (BUN) is nonspecific.
- The erythrocyte sedimentation rate (ESR) is virtually always elevated and can be 75–110 mm/h (Westergren) with SBE (note the Wintrobe test gives different normals so care is needed).
- The rheumatoid factor is positive in approximately 50% of patients.
- Anemia is seen in more than 30% of patients with SBE.
- The white blood count may be slightly increased or remain normal. There is almost always a shift to the left, however, with an increase in band forms.
- It is advisable to check the Gram stain of the blood and buffy coat for organisms.
- 4–6 blood cultures are taken over a 1–2-hour period and carry a 90% chance of recovering organisms.
- Urinalysis often shows mild hematuria or increased RBCs and few RBC casts.
- Increase in creatinine, urea or BUN is nonspecific.
- The ESR is virtually always elevated and can be 75–110 mm/h (Westergren) with SBE.
- The rheumatoid factor is positive more than 50% of patients.
- Anemia is seen in more than 30% of patients with SBE.
- The white blood cell (WBC) may slightly increase or remain normal. There is almost always a shift to the left, however, with an increase in band forms.
- Check Gram's stain of the blood, buffy coat for organisms.

A sterile blood culture is observed in less than or equal to 25% of cases due to—prior antibiotic therapy; fastidious organisms (as with slow-growing streptococci); fungal infection (request fungal precipitins); Q fever (serology should be requested); and chlamydia infection.

A sterile blood culture is observed in up to 25% of cases owing to the following:
- Prior antibiotic therapy
- Fastidious organisms as with slow-growing streptococci
- Fungal infection; request fungal precipitins
- Q fever; serology should be requested
- Chlamydia infection.

Bacteria Causing Endocarditis

- *Staphylococcus aureus* is responsible for more than 85% of cases of acute endocarditis
- *Streptococcus pneumoniae* causing acute fulminant endocarditis is now rare. *Gonococcus, Pseudomonas,* and *Serratia marcescens* may cause right-sided acute endocarditis.
- Streptococci are implicated in 60–80% of subacute endocarditis.

Table 10.1: Detection of vegetations by transesophageal versus transthoracic 2D echocardiography.

	Overall	>10 mm	6–10 mm	<5 mm
TTE	100%	100%	100%	100%
Transthoracic 2D color Doppler	63%	70%	65%	25%

(TTE: transesophageal echocardiography)

- Fecal streptococci, commonly termed "enterococci," cause less than or equal to 10% of infective endocarditis, but with a higher incidence in the geriatric population.
- Nutritionally, variant streptococci—*Streptococcus anginosus, Streptococcus mitis*, and similar organisms require special media for their growth. *Staphylococcus aureus* approximately 40% with Enterococcal species approximately require special media for their gr. *S. mitis, S. bovis, S. anginosus, Haemophilus influenzae, Pseudomonas aeruginosa, P. cepacia*, and *S. marcescens*.
- Infective endocarditis is a severe disease, with an in-hospital mortality rate of about 20% (Selton-Suty et al. 2012). Infective endocarditis can also present with a complication, particularly stroke or systemic embolism.
- Infective additional episodes of endocarditis (Alagna et al. 2014).

Echocardiography

Echocardiography is of major benefit. Transthoracic echocardiography (TTE) detects approximately 63% of vegetations (see Table 10.1). *S. aureus* and some streptococci may produce small lesions of less than 5 mm, which are poorly detectable by transthoracic echocardiography.

Transthoracic echocardiography is superior and can be crucial to the management of endocarditis (Table 10.1). Transthoracic 2-dimensional Doppler echocardiography gives poor detection of prosthetic heart valves, especially in the mitral position and of calcific sclerotic native valves.

Transthoracic echocardiography plays a vital role in the following:
- Failure of TTE to show vegetations in patients strongly suspected of having endocarditis
- All prosthetic heart valves
- Calcific sclerotic native valves
- Valvular destruction secondary to infective endocarditis, especially perivalvular abscesses.

THERAPY

It is imperative that therapy be started immediately after 4–6 blood cultures are taken and relevant clinical information is forwarded to the microbiology laboratory.

Vegetations that are less than 1 cm are usually cured by 4–6 weeks of antibiotic therapy. Vegetations more than 1 cm that do not respond to 3 weeks of antibiotic therapy often necessitate surgery.

See Box 10.1 for a description of antimicrobial agents and therapy for various microorganisms.

Box 10.1: Prevention of bacterial endocarditis-cardiac conditions.*
Endocarditis prophylaxis recommended:
- Prosthetic cardiac valves, including bioprosthetic and homograft valves
- Previous bacterial endocarditis, even in the absence of heart disease
- Surgically constructed systemic–pulmonary shunts or conduits
- Most congenital cardiac malformations
- Rheumatic and other acquired valvular dysfunction, even after valvular surgery
- Hypertrophic cardiomyopathy
- Mitral valve prolapse with valvular regurgitation.

Endocarditis prophylaxis not recommended:
- Isolated secundum atrial septal defect
- Surgical repair without residua beyond 6 months of secundum atrial septal defect, ventricular septal defect, or patent ductus arteriosus
- Previous coronary artery bypass graft surgery
- Mitral valve prolapse without valvular regurgitation†
- Physiologic, functional, or innocent heart murmurs
- Previous Kawasaki disease without valvular dysfunction
- Previous rheumatic fever without valvular dysfunction
- Cardiac pacemakers and implanted defibrillators.

*This table lists selected conditions but is not meant to be all-inclusive.
†Individuals who have a mitral valve prolapse associated with thickening and/or redundancy of the valve leaflets may be at increased risk for bacterial endocarditis, particularly men who are 45 years of age or older.
Source: Dajani AS, Taubert KA, Wilson W, et al. Prevention of bacterial endocarditis. Recommendations by the American Heart Association. JAMA. 1990;264(22):2920.

Empiric therapy can be tailored based on the following:
- *Native valve endocarditis*: In patients with native valve endocarditis, SBE presentation in patients less than age 65 requires obvious coverage of *S. viridans*, which is the causative organism in less than or equal to 70% of cases, and fecal streptococci in less than or equal to 15%—penicillin (2 million U q 4 hours IV) plus gentamicin (1.3–2 mg/kg q 8 hours IV) until the organism has been defined and sensitivities and the minimum inhibitory concentration (MIC) of the drug against the isolated organism are known.

- Highly penicillin-susceptible bacteriological cure rates more than or equal to 98% may be anticipated in patients who complete 4 weeks of therapy with parenteral penicillin or ceftriaxone for infective endocarditis caused by highly penicillin-susceptible viridans group streptococci (VGS) or *S. gallolyticus (bovis)*. Ampicillin is a reasonable alternative to penicillin and has been used when penicillin is not available because of supply deficiencies [American Heart Association (AHA) 2015].

  The addition of gentamicin sulfate to penicillin exerts a synergistic killing effect in vitro on VGS and *S. gallolyticus (bovis)*.

  Both aqueous crystalline penicillin G and ceftriaxone are reasonable options for a 4-week treatment duration. A 2-week treatment regimen that includes gentamicin is reasonable in patients with uncomplicated infective endocarditis, rapid response to therapy, and no underlying renal disease.

- *Geriatric endocarditis*: As above, but in elderly patients, fecal streptococci are more common and occur in less than or equal to 25% of patients; it is advisable to use—ampicillin or sulbactam (2 g q 4 hours) plus gentamicin (1.3-2 µg/kg q 8 hours). Penicillin is the second choice and an alternative to ampicillin or sulbactam, provided the SBE is present for less than 3 months. The dose interval of aminoglycosides must be increased in patients more than age 65 or in individuals with renal impairment, and titrated to blood levels to avoid renal and ototoxicity. A predose level (trough) more than 2 µg/mL (2 mg/L) reflects decreased excretion rate and accumulation of the drug—extend the dosing interval. Keep predose level 1-2 µg/mL. Peak level 30 min postinfusion 6-10 µg/mL, depending on sensitivities and type of organism.

- *Acute endocarditis:* Acute presentation requires coverage for *S. aureus*, which causes more than 85% of ABE and less than or equal to 50% occurring on valves not known to be abnormal, especially bicuspid aortic valves—cloxacillin (2 g IV q 4 hours for 4-6 weeks) or nafcillin (2 g IV q 4 hours for 4-6 weeks) or flucloxacillin (2 g IV q 4 hours).

  Antibiotics should be commenced immediately after collection of blood cultures in patients with rapidly progressive acute endocarditis or in those presenting with hemodynamic decompensation. Urgent IV antibiotic therapy may halt tissue damage and is necessary to prepare patients for surgical intervention.

- *Prosthetic valve endocarditis*: Infective endocarditis occurs in approximately 3% of patients within the 1st year of surgery and thereafter in about 1%/year. The incidence is highest in the first 2 months, and the most common organisms at that stage are *S. epidermidis* (in 25-30%) and *S. aureus* (in 20-25% of cases). *S. epidermidis* continues to be an important organism during the ensuing years but with a decreasing incidence. Within the first 2 months, gram-negative organisms, fungi, diphtheroids, and enterococci are infecting organisms. *S. epidermidis*

is nearly always methicillin resistant, and the use of vancomycin is necessary.
- *Dosage:* Vancomycin 15 mg/kg IV q 12 hours in combination with gentamicin 1-1.2 mg/kg IV q 8 hours; the addition of rifampin 300 mg po q 8 hours may cause a modest improvement in the cure rate but increases the incidence of toxicity.

Late prosthetic valve endocarditis should be treated in a similar method, as outlined, pending results of culture and sensitivities since the offending organism is usually *S. viridans*, fecal streptococci, *S. aureus*, and *S. epidermidis*.
- *Right-sided endocarditis:* It is most common in IV drug addicts and may present with a pneumonic illness. Infecting organisms include *S. aureus* (60%), *S. epidermidis* (10%), and *Pseudomonas* and *Serratia* (10%).

Organism Isolated and Sensitivities Determined

Once the microorganism has been isolated and antibiotic sensitivities are available, an appropriate antibiotic combination is selected. Organisms that commonly cause endocarditis and appropriate antibiotic combinations include the following:
- *Streptococcus viridans or S. bovis*: If the MIC-to-penicillin is less than 0.1 mg/L, give—penicillin (IV 2 million U q 4 hours for 2 weeks), then amoxicillin (po 500 mg q 6 hours for 2 weeks), or ampicillin or sulbactam (2 g q 6 hours for 2 weeks IV), then amoxicillin (po 500 mg q 6 hours for 2 weeks).
- Partially sensitive *S. viridans* or *S. bovis*, MIC penicillin more than 0.1 mg/L—penicillin (3 million U q 4 hours IV) plus gentamicin (1.3-2 mg/kg q 8 hours IV for 2-4 weeks) or from the 3rd week, amoxicillin (500 mg po q 6 hours for 2 weeks).
- *Streptococcus faecalis, S. faecium, S. durans*, or similar fecal streptococci are difficult to eradicate—if the length of illness is less than 3 months, give ampicillin or sulbactam (IV 2-3 g q 6 hours for 4 weeks) plus gentamicin (1.3-2 mg/ kg q 8 hours) and monitor levels and adjustment for renal function. Gentamicin is given for 4 weeks. The combinations of ampicillin or penicillin and the β-lactamase inhibitor sulbactam have been shown to be the most active antimicrobials tested against gentamicin-resistant β-lactamase producing *S. faecalis*.
- *Staphylococcus aureus*: Methicillin-sensitive strains constitute most cases of *S. aureus* endocarditis and are treated with nafcillin or cloxacillin (at doses given above) or flucloxacillin (IV 2 g q 4 hours) plus gentamicin (1.3-2 mg/kg q 8 hours IV), the dose to be monitored by levels. The dose is reduced in elderly patients and those with renal dysfunction, while the dosing interval is increased. Gentamicin is discontinued after 1 week, and nafcillin or flucloxacillin IV is continued for 3-4 weeks. The length of treatment is usually 4-6 weeks.
- *Streptococcus pneumoniae* is highly sensitive to penicillin and is managed with penicillin G (2 million U q 4 hours) for 2 or more weeks.

For patients allergic to penicillin or methicillin-resistant *S. aureus* give vancomycin (15 mg/kg IV q 12 hours given slowly over 6 hours) for 4-6 weeks. Monitor serum levels, peak 20-40 µg/mL 2 hours postcompletion of infusion, trough levels 5-10 µg/mL reduce dose and ↑ the dosing interval in renal failure.

Bacterial Endocarditis Prophylaxis

Recommendations are given in Box 10.2 and in Tables 10.2 to 10.4.

Box 10.2: Prevention of bacterial endocarditis—dental or surgical procedures.*
Endocarditis prophylaxis recommended:
- Dental procedures known to induce gingival or mucosal bleeding, including professional cleaning
- Tonsillectomy and/or adenoidectomy
- Surgical operations that involve intestinal or respiratory mucosa
- Bronchoscopy with a rigid bronchoscope
- Sclerotherapy for esophageal varices
- Esophageal dilatation
- Gallbladder surgery
- Cystoscopy
- Urethral dilatation
- Urethral catheterization, if urinary tract infection is present†
- Urinary tract surgery, if urinary tract infection is present†
- Prostatic surgery
- Incision and drainage of infected tissue†
- Vaginal hysterectomy
- Vaginal delivery in the presence of infection†.

Endocarditis prophylaxis not recommended:‡
- Dental procedures not likely to induce gingival bleeding, such as simple adjustment of orthodontic appliances or fillings above the gumline
- Injection of local intraoral anesthetic (except intraligamentary injections)
- Shedding of primary teeth
- Tympanostomy tube insertion
- Endotracheal intubation
- Bronchoscopy with a flexible bronchoscope, with or without biopsy
- Cardiac catheterization
- Endoscopy with or without gastrointestinal biopsy
- Cesarean section
- In the absence of infection for urethral catheterization, dilatation and curettage, uncomplicated vaginal delivery, therapeutic abortion, sterilization procedures, or insertion or removal of intrauterine devices.

*This box lists selected procedures but is not meant to be all-inclusive.
†In addition to prophylactic regimen for genitourinary procedures, antibiotic therapy should be directed against the most likely bacterial pathogen.
‡In patients who have prosthetic heart valves, a previous history of endocarditis, or surgically constructed systemic-pulmonary shunts or conduits, physicians may choose to administer prophylactic antibiotics even for low-risk procedures that involve the lower respiratory, genitourinary, or gastrointestinal tracts.
Source: Dajani AS, Taubert KA, Wilson W, et al. Prevention of bacterial endocarditis. Recommendations by the American Heart Association. JAMA. 1990;264(22):2920.

Infective Endocarditis

Table 10.2: Recommended standard prophylactic regimen for dental, oral, or upper respiratory tract procedures in patients who are at risk.*

Drug	Dosing regimen†
Standard regimen	
Amoxicillin	3.0 g orally 1 hour before procedure; then 1.5 g 6 hours after initial dose
Amoxicillin or penicillin-allergic patients	
• Erythromycin or • Clindamycin	• Erythromycin ethylsuccinate, 800 mg, or erythromycin stearate, 1.0 g orally 2 hours before procedure; then half the dose 6 hours after initial dose • 300 mg orally 1 hour before procedure and 150 mg 6 hours after initial dose

*Includes those with prosthetic heart valves and other high-risk patients.
†Initial pediatric doses are as follows—amoxicillin, 50 mg/kg; erythromycin ethylsuccinate or erythromycin stearate, 20 mg/kg; and clindamycin, 10 mg/kg. Follow-up dose should be one half the initial dose. Total pediatric dose should not exceed total adult dose. The following weight ranges may also be used for the initial pediatric dose of amoxicillin—less than 15 kg, 750 mg; 15–30 kg, 1,500 mg; and >30 kg, 3,000 mg (full adult dose).
Source: Dajani AS, Taubert KA, Wilson W, et al. Prevention of bacterial endocarditis. Recommendations by the American Heart Association. JAMA. 1990;264(22):2920.

Table 10.3: Alternate prophylactic regimens for dental, oral, or upper respiratory tract procedures in patients who are at risk.

Drug	Dosing regimen*
Patients unable to take oral medications	
Ampicillin	Intravenous or intramuscular administration of ampicillin, 2.0 g, 30 minutes before procedure; then intravenous or intramuscular administration of ampicillin, 1.0 g, or oral administration of amoxicillin, 1.5 g, 6 hours after initial dose
Ampicillin- or amoxicillin- or penicillin-allergic patients unable to take oral medications	
Clindamycin	Intravenous administration of clindamycin, 300 mg, 30 minutes before procedure and intravenous or oral administration of 150 mg 6 hours after initial dose
Patients considered high risk and not candidates for standard regimen	
Ampicillin, gentamicin, and amoxicillin	Intravenous or intramuscular administration of ampicillin, 2.0 g, plus gentamicin, 1.5 mg/kg (not to exceed 80 mg), 30 minutes before procedure; followed by amoxicillin, 1.5 g orally 6 hours after initial dose; alternatively, the parenteral regimen may be repeated 8 hours after initial dose
Ampicillin- or amoxicillin- or penicillin-allergic patients considered high risk	
Vancomycin	Intravenous administration of 1.0 g over 1 hour, starting 1 hour before procedure; no repeated dose necessary

*Initial pediatric doses are as follows—ampicillin, 50 mg/kg; clindamycin, 10 mg/kg; gentamicin, 2.0 mg/kg; and vancomycin, 20 mg/kg. Follow-up dose should be one-half the initial dose. Total pediatric dose should not exceed total adult dose. No initial dose is recommended in this table for amoxicillin (25 mg/kg is the follow-up dose).
Source: Dajani AS, Taubert KA, Wilson W, et al. Prevention of bacterial endocarditis. Recommendations by the American Heart Association. JAMA. 1990;264(22):2921.

Table 10.4: Prevention of bacterial endocarditis—regimens for genitourinary or gastrointestinal procedures.

Drug	Dosing regimen*
Standard regimen	
Ampicillin, gentamicin, and amoxicillin	Intravenous or intramuscular administration of ampicillin, 2.0 g, plus gentamicin, 1.5 mg/kg (not to exceed 80 mg), 30 minutes before procedure; followed by amoxicillin, 1.5 g orally 6 hours after initial dose; alternatively, the parenteral regiment may be repeated once 8 hours after initial dose
Ampicillin- or amoxicillin- or penicillin-allergic patient regimen	
Vancomycin and gentamicin	Intravenous administration of vancomycin, 1.0 g, over 1 hour plus intravenous or intramuscular administration of gentamicin, 1.5 mg/kg (not to exceed 80 mg), 1 hour before procedure; may be repeated once 8 hours after initial dose
Alternate low-risk patient regimen	
Amoxicillin	3.0 g orally 1 hour before procedure; then 1.5 g 6 hours after initial dose

*Initial pediatric doses are as follows—ampicillin, 50 mg/kg; amoxicillin, 50 mg/kg; gentamicin, 2.0 mg/kg; and vancomycin, 20 mg/kg. Follow-up dose should be one half the initial dose. Total pediatric dose should not exceed total adult dose.
Source: Dajani AS, Taubert KA, Wilson W, et al. Prevention of bacterial endocarditis. Recommendations by the American Heart Association. JAMA, 1990;264(22);2921.

- Replace penicillin with amoxicillin for dental procedures—amoxicillin 2 g po is given 1 hour prior to dental procedures, including professional cleaning, then 1.5 g 6 hours later.
- Patients allergic to penicillin who can take oral medications are given the choice of erythromycin or clindamycin, 300 mg 1 hour prior and 150 mg 6 hours postprocedure. This is a major improvement in prophylaxis, since erythromycin (at 800 mg as advised by the AHA or 1,500 mg by the British group) causes severe nausea and/or abdominal discomfort. Also, the drug is not extremely effective for fecal streptococci.
- Prophylaxis for mitral valve prolapse has caused confusion over the past 10 years. The AHA advises pro-phylaxis only for individuals with mitral regurgitation (MR), i.e. presence of a mid to late or holosystolic murmur (Box 10.3).

Box 10.3: Recommendations for endocarditis prophylaxis in the UK.
1. *Dental extractions, scaling, or periodontal surgery under local or no anesthesia:*
   a. For patients not allergic to penicillin and not prescribed penicillin more than once in the previous month:
      Amoxicillin
      - *Adults:* 2 g single oral dose taken under supervision 1 hour before dental procedure
      - Children under 10—half adult dose
      - Children under 5—quarter adult dose
   b. For patients allergic to penicillin:
      - *Erythromycin stearate:*
        - *Adults:* 1.5 g orally taken under supervision 1–2 hours before dental procedure plus 0.5 g 6 hours later
        - Children under 10—half adult dose
        - Children under 5—quarter adult dose, or
      - Clindamycin
        - *Adults:* 600 mg single oral dose taken under supervision 1 hour before dental procedure
        - *Children under 10:* 6 mg/kg body weight single oral dose taken under supervision 1 hour before dental procedure
      Under general anesthesia
   c. For patients not allergic to penicillin and not given penicillin more than once in the previous month:
      - Amoxicillin *intramuscularly*:
        - *Adults:* 1 g in 2.5 mL 1% lignocaine hydrochloride just before induction plus 0.5 mg by mouth 6 hours later
        - *Children under 10:* Half adult dose, or
      - Amoxicillin orally
        - Adults 3 g oral dose 4 hours before anesthesia followed by a further 3 g by mouth as soon as possible after operation
        - Children under 10—half adult dose
        - Children under 5—quarter adult dose, or
      - Amoxicillin and probenecid orally
        - *Adults:* Amoxicillin 3 g together with probenecid 1 g orally 4 hours before operation. Special risk patients who should be referred to hospital:
          - Patients with prosthetic valves who are to have a general anesthetic
          - Patients who are to have a general anesthetic and who are allergic to penicillin or have had penicillin more than once in the previous month
      - Patients who have had a previous attack of endocarditis

Recommendations for these patients are:
   d. For patients not allergic to penicillin and who have not had penicillin more than once in the previous month:
      - *Adults:* 1 g amoxicillin intramuscularly in 2.5 mL 1% lignocaine hydrochloride plus 120 mg gentamicin intramuscularly just before induction: then 0.5 g amoxicillin orally 6 hours later
      - Children under 10—amoxicillin, half adult dose; gentamicin 2 mg/kg body weight

Contd...

Contd...

    e. For patients allergic to penicillin or who have had penicillin more than once in the previous month:
- *Adults:* Vancomycin 1 g by slow intravenous infusion over 60 min followed by gentamicin 120 mg intravenously just before induction or 15 min before the surgical procedure
- Children under 10—vancomycin 20 mg/kg intravenously, gentamicin 2 mg/kg intravenously.

2. *Surgery or instrumentation of upper respiratory tract:* Recommended cover is as for 1 (a) or 1(e), but any postoperative antibiotic may have to be given intramuscularly or intravenously if swallowing is painful.
3. *Genitourinary surgery or instrumentation:* For patients with sterile urine the suggested cover is directed against fecal streptococci and is as for 1 (d) or 1 (e) above. If the urine is infected, prophylaxis should also cover the pathogens involved.
4. *Obstetric and gynecological procedures:* Cover is suggested only for patients with prosthetic valves, and is as for 1 (d) or 1(e) because of the risk from fecal streptococci
5. *Gastrointestinal procedures:* Cover is suggested only for patients with prosthetic valves and is as for 1 (d) or 1 (e).

Source: Simmons NA. Antibiotic prophylaxis of infective endocarditis. Recommendations from the Endocarditis Working Party of the British Society for Antimicrobial Chemotherapy. Lancet. 1990;335:89.

BIBLIOGRAPHY

1. Alagna L, Park LP, Nicholson BP, et al. Repeat endocarditis: analysis of risk factors based on the International Collaboration on Endocarditis Society for Antimicrobial Chemotherapy. Lancet. 1990;335:89.
2. Cahill TJ, Prendergast BD. Infective endocarditis. Lancet. 2016;387(10021):882-93.
3. Dayer MJ, Jones S, Prendergast B, et al. Incidence of infective endocarditis in England, 2000-13: a secular trend, interrupted time-series analysis. Lancet. 2015;385(9974):1219-28.
4. Khan GM. Encyclopedia of Heart Diseases, 2nd edition. New York: Springer; 2011.
5. Selton-Suty C, Célard M, Le Moing V, et al. Preeminence of *Staphylococcus aureus* in infective endocarditis: a 1-year population-based survey. Clin Infect Dis. 2012;54(9):1230-9.
6. Thornhill MH, Dayer MJ, Prendergast B, et al. Incidence and nature of adverse reactions to antibiotics used as endocarditis prophylaxis. J Antimicrob Chemother. 2015;70(8):2382-8.

CHAPTER 11

Cardiac Arrest

INTRODUCTION

- Most of cardiac arrests occur at home, mostly unwitnessed. Thus, automatic external defibrillators (AEDs) that improve resuscitation rates for witnessed arrests have limited effectiveness on reducing overall mortality. In addition, the rate of survival to hospital discharge in the United States, with the best CPR and use of AEDs is approximately 9% and it is difficult to avoid neurologic disasters.
- The late JF Pantridge emphasized that every home should have an AED and a fire extinguisher (Personal communication 1970).
- Annually worldwide there are approximately 7 million deaths due to an MI and more than 3 million die suddenly within 1 hour of onset of symptoms.
- 1 million die within 72 hours from cardiogenic shock and this number will increase dramatically, if the new ACC and AHA BP guidelines are followed (normal BP is now <130 systolic, diastolic <80; a serious error has been made by notable experts who should guide the medical profession and physicians in the field) (*see* Chapters 3 and 8).
- Each day in the United States, approximately 1,000 sudden deaths occur.
- Prevention of cardiac arrest requires cure or amelioration of atheroma the basic cause of most arrest by producing obstruction of coronary blood flow that leads to ventricular fibrillation (VF) or cardiogenic shock.
- For the millions of individuals at cardiac risk, it is advisable to maintain a systolic BP greater than 130 mm Hg to curb or ameliorate cardiogenic shock. This statement should engender rethinking amongst the ACC and AHA hypertension experts who formulated the obscure recent guidelines.
- See Chapter 1 and later discussion for probable solutions to prevent sudden deaths because when it occurs the outcome is dismal.
- There is some data indicating that a significant number of cardiac arrest victims do have a small warning that unfortunately is often ignored. Warnings that include, shortness of breath, or chest discomfort that may occur hours–to–days of the arrest.

- About approximately 90% of people who have cardiac arrest die from it, most within minutes. Sudden cardiac death accounts for approximately 50% of all coronary artery disease (CAD) deaths and 15–20% of all deaths (Gillum1990; Myerburg et al. 2004).
- A number of cardiac disorders cause lethal tachyarrhythmias or failure of formation or transmission of the cardiac impulse that results in cardiac arrest, but the mechanisms that initiate these fatal arrhythmias are mostly unknown and are diverse.

Only S propranolol and timolol in post-MI, bisoprolol and metoprolol in heart failure have proven effective in randomized clinical trials (RCTs) to significantly prevent sudden cardiac deaths (Table 11.1).

CAUSES

The basic cardiac causes of cardiac arrest include:
- Ventricular fibrillation or pulseless ventricular tachycardia (VT)—in at least 80%; VF is defined as a pulseless, chaotic, and disorganized rhythm with an undulating irregular pattern that varies in size and shape and a ventricular waveform greater than 150 minutes.

Table 11.1: Beta blockers are the only drugs that prevent sudden cardiac death.			
	Control	Drug	% Decrease
Propranolol:			
*Total sudden death	78	60	23
5–11am	31	11	64
Total deaths	188/1,460	138/1,456	26
**Timolol:*			
^Total sudden death	95	47	50
Instant, within seconds	38	11	71
Total deaths	117/718	67/670	42
#Metoprolol:*			
Total sudden death	21	9	57
Total deaths	31/147	25/154	19##
MERIT-HF metoprolol:			
Total sudden death	132	79	40.2
Total deaths	217/2,001	145/1,990	33.2

Contd...

Contd...

	Control	Drug	% Decrease
CIBIS bisoprolol:			
Total sudden death	83	48	42.2
Total deaths	228/1,320	156/1,327	31.6

(Only four beta-blockers of the ten available definitely prevent sudden cardiac death; they all gain high brain concentration; and atenolol does not and use should become obsolete)
*BHAT study, AM sudden death (Peters et al.) follow-up 25 months, 120–240 mg daily.
**Timolol Norwegian MI study; mean duration 17 months. Follow-up—10 mg twice daily
#Metoprolol—a very small study of only approximately 150 patients in each group followed for 3 years.
##"This reduction in cardiac mortality did not reach statistical significance, as was to be expected from our sample size" (Olsson et al. 1985).
#In (MERIT-HF), there were fewer sudden deaths in the metoprolol CR/XL group than in the placebo group [79 vs 132, 0.59 (0.45–0.78); p = 0.0002] and deaths from worsening heart failure [30 vs 58, 0.51 (0.33–0.79); p = 0.0023].
Bisoprolol in CIBIS; significant decrease in deaths and sudden death.
Carvedilol did not prevent sudden death in two large RCTs; total mortality in RCT was not significantly reduced in post-MI patients
(BHAT, Beta-Blocker Heart Attack Trial; CIBIS, cardiac insufficiency bisoprolol study; MI, Myocardial infarction; MERIT-HF, Metoprolol CR/XL Randomized Intervention Trial in congestive heart failure; RCT, randomized clinical trial)
Source: Gabriel KM. Practical Cardiology. New Delhi, India: Jaypee Brothers Medical Publishers (P) Ltd; 2018.

- Asystole—10%
- Electromechanical dissociation (EMD)—5%
- Myocardial rupture, cardiac tamponade, acute disruption of a major blood vessel, and acute mechanical obstruction to blood flow that includes the pulmonary embolism.
- Severe aortic stenosis
- Hypertrophic cardiomyopathy—cardiac deaths in young athletes are usually caused by hypertrophic cardiomyopathy (Maron, 1997) (35%) and anomalous origin of the left main coronary artery from the right sinus of valsalva (20%).
- Dilated cardiomyopathy
- Complete heart block or sinoatrial disease
- Wolff-Parkinson-White syndrome in patients with very short refractory period of the bypass tract
- Torsades de pointes in patients taking antiarrhythmic drugs, some antibiotics that prolong the QT interval.
- Prolonged QT syndromes (congenital or acquired)
- Structural abnormalities, such as pulmonary embolism or aortic dissection

- Brugada syndrome, younger Asian males night deaths, and arrhythmogenic right ventricular dysplasia
- Always assume VF or pulseless VT because patients who can be saved from cardiac arrest usually have these cardiac arrest rhythms. The single most effective intervention that can save victims of sudden cardiac arrest is the earliest delivery of defibrillation and widespread distribution of AED has saved many lives.

Approximately, 75% of all cases of cardiac arrest involve an unstable atheromatous plaque with overlying thrombus, causing occlusion, or distal embolization of a major coronary artery. Cardiac arrest in coronary disease may occur with little or no warning (plaque emboli), during the acute phase of MI (occlusion) or later, caused by an arrhythmia circuit that may respond to trigger factors (catecholamines, ischemia, hypokalemia, and critically timed ventricular premature beats) to precipitate VF.

- A history of ischemic heart disease (IHD) is present in up to 50% of patients; in a significant number of these patients, atheromatous coronary disease is silent until the time of the event. Most sudden cardiac deaths are the result of coronary atheroma. In these individuals, VF usually occurs either because of a new acute ischemic event or because of myocardial scarring and/or hypertrophy, which probably predisposes the myocardium to reentrant tachycardia that triggers VF.
- In a study by Davies, of 168 consecutive cases of sudden coronary death within 6 hours of symptoms, the proportion of deaths owing to IHD at time intervals of less than 1 hour and less than 6 hours did not differ. In this study, 73.3% showed thrombosis on an unstable plaque. No acute change in the coronary artery was observed in 19%. Overall, it is determined that cardiac sudden death is associated with no acute coronary lesion in approximately 15% of individuals who succumb to unexpected cardiac arrest.

CARDIOPULMONARY RESUSCITATION STUDIES

- A prospective statewide observational study in Arizona had shown that training the population in continuous chest compressions (CCCs) until the arrival of emergency medical services (EMS) increased the rate of bystander-initiated CPR and increased the rate of survival to discharge from the hospital (Svensson et al. 2010).
- The results of a RCT from the Resuscitation Outcomes Consortium (ROC) have greatly improved our approach to the ideal methods for CPR and disqualify CCC.
- Patients received either CCCs or the standard approach of chest compressions that were interrupted for positive-pressure ventilation in a ratio of 30 compressions to two ventilations (termed "interrupted

chest compressions"). A total of 12,653 patients were included in the group that received CCCs (intervention group) and 11,058 in the group that received interrupted chest compressions (control group).
- The overall rate of survival to hospital discharge was 9.0% in the intervention group and 9.7% in the control group—a nonsignificant difference. Survival with favorable neurologic function at discharge did not differ significantly between the two groups.
- A prespecified per protocol analysis that was based on strict adherence to the treatment algorithm showed significantly lower rates of survival among patients in the intervention group than among those in the control group (7.6% vs 9.6%).

If the results of the current ROC study had been available, the guidelines committee might have decided to retain the previous recommendation to give chest compressions interrupted for ventilations and perhaps even to upgrade that recommendation to a class IIa recommendation for EMS providers. Should the AHA reconsider their recommendation? (Koster, 2015).
- This RCT finding should supersede the guidelines derived from the Arizona observational study. Most important 100 compressions at more than 100 (up to 120)/min at proper depth and speed is difficult for many bystanders to accomplish. Intentional rapidity often destroys the depth of compression.

The Arizona strategy makes one logical move—compression first because within the first 3-4 minutes of a witnessed arrest there is sufficient oxygenated blood available.
- Thus, I advise push it to the brain immediately and rapidly for 30 compressions. But after this, the system of all compression is flawed.

Rarely, a sudden cardiac death resulting from electrical dysfunction occurs without discernible cardiac pathology (primary electrical disease). Current information strongly indicates that coronary artery spasm, latent preexcitation, and prolonged QT syndromes do not play a role in patients with idiopathic VF.

Pathogenesis of the syndrome of sudden death during sleep in young apparently healthy Southeast Asian males is undetermined and appears to be unrelated to idiopathic VF in "normal" hearts; see Brugada syndrome in Chapter 27.

MANAGEMENT OF VENTRICULAR FIBRILLATION

Immediate defibrillation within 2-4 minutes of witnessed cardiac arrest is the most important single therapy that may rescue patients in cardiac arrest, without producing tragic iatrogenic brain damage from attempting full CPR and the unavoidable hesitations that occur in many settings of cardiac arrest.

The operation of AEDs does not demand complex learning skills in rhythm analysis and operation of the device can be mastered within hours. A single control activates the defibrillator to quickly analyze the cardiac rhythm, indicates that a shock is required, and, on command, charges and delivers the shock.

DRUG THERAPY

Epinephrine

Salutary effects of epinephrine are:
- Increased myocardial contractility
- Elevated perfusion pressure
- Possible conversion of EMD to electromechanical coupling
- Improved chances for defibrillation
- Improved blood flow to the heart and brain when sinus rhythm is restored.

Epinephrine is an alpha- and beta-adrenergic agonist and is the drug of first choice, administered as an initial 1-mg intravenous (IV) bolus after the third shock fails to defibrillate. Intracardiac epinephrine is not recommended, except when IV or intratracheal routes are not possible.

A high dose of epinephrine is necessary to maintain adequate diastolic BP to produce adequate coronary and cerebral perfusion (Table 11.2).

Indications

- Fine VF is made coarse and more susceptible to removal by electrical countershock
- The VF that fails to respond to countershock may respond after epinephrine
- Asystole and pulseless idioventricular rhythms
- Electromechanical dissociation.

A study indicated—analysis included some 3,000 patients with in-hospital cardiac arrest and a shockable rhythm after the first defibrillation. Roughly half received epinephrine within 2 minutes of the first defibrillation—contrary to AHA guidelines, which recommends deferred epinephrine.
- Patients who received early epinephrine, compared with those who did not, had about 30% lower odds of survival, of return to spontaneous circulation, or of good functional outcome. The data suggest that if adrenaline is given, it should be deferred until at least after the second shock has been delivered.

A second analysis, among hospitalized patients with persistent VT or fibrillation, showed that the rate of deferred second defibrillation (1–3 minutes after the first shock) roses from 26 to 57% from 2004 to 2012—consistent with a 2005 AHA guideline update supporting this strategy.
- Deferred defibrillation was not associated with improved survival.

Table 11.2: Cardiac arrest drugs.

Drug	Dosage	Supplied	Comment
Epinephrine	1 mg IV bolus repeated q 3–5 min 10 mL tracheobronchial (1:10,000)	10 mL (1 mg in 1:10,000 dilution)	Do not give with $NaHCO_3$ in same IV
Sodium bicarbonate	1 mEq IV bolus (mmol)/ kg, usually 50 mEq (mmol) initially; 1 amp = 44 mEq then 0.5 initial dose q 10–15 min	50 mL of 8.4% = 50.0 mEq (mmol)	Used for hyperkalemic arrest Recommended for trial after 7th shock, pH <7.1, or 10 min in asystole
Atropine	1 mg In asystole q 2–5 min (max of 3 mg) 0.5 mg bradycardia q 5 min–2 mg	10 mL = 1 mg 5 mL = 0.5 mg (UK, 1 mL amp = 0.6 mg or 1 mg)	
Lidocaine (lignocaine)	75–100 mg IV bolus simultaneous infusion 2–3 mg/min 100 mg in 5 mL (2%)	50 mg in 5 mL (I%) 100 mg in 10 mL (1%)	Useful in recurrent VF if lidocaine fails; also for VF following electrocution
Propranolol for VF	1 mg over 2–5 min (q 2–5 min to max 5 mg)		
	UK—1 mg over 2 min (q 2 min to max 5 mg)		
Metoprolol	5 mg IV over 5 min		
Calcium chloride	2.5–5 mL 10%, (5–7 mg/ kg 250–500 mg) IV bolus	10 mL 10% $CaCl_2$	Not recommended in cardiac arrest, except with hyperkalemia or postverapamil Do not give with $NaHCO_3$

($CaCl_2$, calcium chloride; IV, intravenous; $NaHCO_3$, sodium bicarbonate; VF, ventricular fibrillation)

Vasopressin

Vasopressin appears to be modestly effective for both VF and asystole. Dosage—a single 40-U IV dose, one time only. There is no evidence to support the value of repeat vasopressin doses. If there is no response 5-10 minutes after a single dose of vasopressin, it is advisable to resume epinephrine.

There is no evidence to support its use in asystole or pulseless electrical activity (PEA).

- Wenzel et al. (2004) showed the success of vasopressin alone and vasopressin followed by epinephrine in refractory asystolic cardiac arrest. In this randomized study, out-of-hospital cardiac arrest patients were assigned to receive two injections of either vasopressin 40 IU or 1 mg of epinephrine followed by additional treatment epinephrine, if needed. 589 patients received vasopressin; 597 received epinephrine. The effects of vasopressin were like those of epinephrine in the management of VF and PEA.
- Vasopressin was superior to epinephrine in patients with asystole. The authors concluded that vasopressin followed by epinephrine may be more effective than epinephrine alone in the treatment of refractory cardiac arrest.

Lidocaine (Lignocaine)

Lidocaine is given after a fourth shock fails to defibrillate as a 100-mg IV bolus, followed after about 1 minute of CPR, by a 360-J shock. If defibrillation is successful, give a 50-mg bolus of lidocaine and an infusion at 2–3 mg/min immediately. The lower dose is used for the elderly or those with heart failure. An additional bolus is given 10 minutes later to maintain therapeutic lidocaine levels.

Lidocaine is not harmful. At ACC 2016, it was emphasized that a RCT showed that in patients with witnessed arrest the drug may provide salutary effects. This is mostly in those in whom there is hope for recovery based on the rapidity of CPR and defibrillation.

Sodium Bicarbonate

This agent is no longer recommended for routine use during cardiac arrest of brief duration except in patients with preexisting hyperkalemia. However, after about 10 minutes of CPR and if a seventh shock fails to result in defibrillation, an IV bolus of sodium bicarbonate (50 mEq) is advisable. The drug should not be used simultaneously with calcium chloride or epinephrine.

Calcium Chloride

Calcium chloride is no longer recommended. The drug may be useful, if asystole is caused by verapamil or in the management of hyperkalemia causing arrest. The drug is, however, of no value in EMD.

Dosage

Give 2.5–5 mL 10% calcium chloride or (UK), calcium gluconate IV bolus; 10 mL of a 10% solution.

Amiodarone

At the ACC 2016, it was emphasized that a RCT showed that in patients with witnessed arrest amiodarone may provide salutary effects. This is mostly in those in whom there is hope for recovery based on the rapidity of CPR and defibrillation.

Amiodarone is useful in the management of witnessed cardiac arrest. A resuscitation trial indicated no benefit from amiodarone or lidocaine but in witnessed arrest, both agents provided salutary effects and are advisable [The Resuscitation Outcomes Consortium Amiodarone, Lidocaine or Placebo Study (Kudenchuk 2016)]

Overall, neither amiodarone nor lidocaine resulted in a significantly higher rate of survival or favorable neurologic outcome than the rate with placebo among patients with out-of-hospital cardiac arrest due to initial shock-refractory VF or pulseless VT (Kudenchuk et al. 2016).

For VF or pulseless VT, give 300 mg IV push and for recurrence 150-500 mg bolus over 5-10 minutes, followed by 10 mg/kg/24 hours (0.5 mg/mL) continuous infusion; maximum 2.2 g over 24 hours.

Magnesium Sulfate

A 1-2 g IV in polymorphic VT (TdP) may expedite ventricular defibrillation and is advisable for suspected hypomagnesemia.

BRADYARRHYTHMIAS: ASYSTOLE OR ELECTROMECHANICAL DISSOCIATION

Severe symptomatic bradycardia is usually treated with 0.5-0.6 mg atropine repeated every 2 minutes to a maximum of 2.4 mg. When atropine is used to treat asystole before pacing, a dose of 1 mg is given immediately, followed by an additional 1 mg after 2 minutes. In severe bradycardia or atrioventricular block without a QRS complex, atropine is worth a trial. No harm can ensue, as if VF is precipitated by atropine; defibrillation may produce a stable rhythm to allow coronary perfusion before pacing. Be aware that VF may masquerade as asystole. Thus, rotate the monitoring electrodes and check the monitor to ensure that VF is not present. Give epinephrine with the hope that fibrillation may ensue and then countershock.

Asystole in a heart that was beating forcefully minutes before the occurrence of asystole may complicate anterior infarction, and pacing may be lifesaving. Asystole in the atonic heart (agonal) and EMD are usually caused by irreversible myocardial damage and prognosis is very poor.

Management of Electromechanical Dissociation

- Commence CPR
- Intravenous line
- Epinephrine (1-mg IV bolus)
- Intubate
- Assess for cardiac rupture and tamponade
- Search for extracardiac causes of EMD
- Inadequate ventilation, including intubation of right main stem bronchus and tension pneumothorax
- Poor perfusion—hypovolemia [jugular venous pressure (JVP) decreased] gives fluid challenge. If the JVP is markedly elevated, suspect cardiac tamponade or massive pulmonary embolism
- Severe acidosis or hyperkalemia.

Cardiopulmonary resuscitation should be continued with the hope that one of these factors may be correctable. Mobitz Type 2 block and complete heart block must be managed with ventricular pacing. If there is asystole or severe bradycardia unresponsive to atropine continue CPR, give 1 mg epinephrine IV or endotracheal. If there is no response, consider pacing. For severe hypotension with mild bradycardia, dopamine is advisable.

Because most cardiac arrests occur at home unwitnessed, CPR and AEDs have limited effectiveness on reducing overall mortality that occurs in more than 3 million individuals worldwide. The rate of survival to hospital discharge in the United States, with the best CPR and use of AEDs, is only 9–10%.

Prevention involves suppression of atheroma formation, plaque erosion, or rupture that leads to coronary thrombosis. Most individuals who succumb to cardiac arrest have known or undetected CAD. Risks of individuals age approximately 40 should be determined. Those at high risk are usually known CAD, or family history of MI, diabetics hyperlipidemic, and other conditions known to increase risk should be prescribed drugs known to prevent sudden death.

Table 11.1 indicates that we should be prescribing a lipophilic beta 1 beta 2 beta-blockers—timolol or propranolol and not atenolol; metoprolol and bisoprolol are advisable for those with chronic obstructive pulmonary disease (COPD). Carvedilol is not advisable because of alpha1 activity. Physician must now recognize that all beta blockers are not alike (Khan 2005).

- Importantly, low-density lipoprotein cholesterol (LDL-C) is the most important generator for atheroma formation. The evidence relating to LDL-C and atheroma is vast and proven—lower is better; thus, a statin and aspirin must be key medications for all at moderate or high risk. Statin use has not been shown to prevent sudden cardiac deaths.
- In Heart Outcomes Prevention Evaluation-3 (HOPE-3), at more than 5 years follow-up in 13,000 subjects, there was no mention of sudden deaths and total mortality was not decreased in patients claimed to be at intermediate risk. HOPE-3 studied low risk patients.

PERCUTANEOUS CORONARY INTERVENTION

During a study period (2004-2013), 958 patients with an emergent cardiac arrest were investigated. Among them 695 of 958 (73%), mostly male (76%), and average 60 years of age had no evidence of ST-segment elevation MI (STEMI) on the postresuscitation electrocardiography (ECG). Dumas et al. 2016, a percutaneous coronary intervention (PCI) was deemed necessary in 199 of 695 (29%). A favorable outcome was observed in 87 of 200 (43%) in patients with PCI compared with 164 of 495 (33%) in patients without PCI (p = 0.02). After adjustment, PCI was associated with a better outcome [adjusted odds ratio—1.80 (95% confidence interval—1.09-2.97); p = 0.02]. The other predictive factors of favorable outcome were a shorter resuscitation length (<20 min), an initial shockable rhythm, and a lower dose of epinephrine during resuscitation (p <0.001) was the sole independent indicator for PCI requirement (Dumas et al. 2016).

A culprit coronary lesion requiring PCI was found in nearly one-third of patients without STEMI. In these patients, emergent PCI was associated with a nearly twofold increase in the rate of favorable outcome. These findings support the use of an invasive strategy in these patients, particularly in those resuscitated from a shockable rhythm (Dumas et al. 2016).

BIBLIOGRAPHY

1. Davies MJ. Anatomic features in victims of sudden coronary death. Circulation. 1992;85(suppl I):1-19.
2. Dumas F, Bougouin W, Geri G, et al. Emergency PCI in Post-Cardiac Arrest Patients Without ST-Segment Elevation Pattern Insights From the PROCAT II Registry. J Am Coll Cardiol Interv. 2016;9(10):1011-8.
3. Finocchiaro G, Papadakis M, Robertus JL, et al. Etiology of Sudden Death in Sports: Insights From a United Kingdom Regional Registry. J Am Coll Cardiol. 2016;67(18):2108-15.
4. Hagihara A, Hasegawa M, Abe T, et al. Prehospital epinephrine use and survival among patients with out-of-hospital cardiac arrest. JAMA. 2012;307(11):1161-8.
5. Hüpfl M, Selig HF, Nagele P. Chest-compression-only versus standard cardiopulmonary resuscitation: a meta-analysis. Lancet. 2010;376(9752):1552-7.
6. Idris AH, Guffey D, Aufderheide TP, et al. Relationship between chest compression rates and outcomes from cardiac arrest. Circulation. 2012;125(24):3004-12.
7. Koster RW. Continuous or interrupted chest compressions for cardiac arrest. N Engl J Med. 2015;373:2278-29.
8. Kudenchuk PJ, Brown SP, Daya M, et al. Amiodarone, Lidocaine, or Placebo in Out-of-Hospital Cardiac Arrest. N Engl J Med 2016;374:1711-22.
9. Lewis RJ, Gausche-Hill M. Airway Management During Out-of-Hospital Cardiac Arrest. JAMA. 2018;319(8):771-2.
10. Kudenchuk PJ. The Resuscitation Outcomes Consortium Amiodarone, Lidocaine or Placebo Study. Am Heart J. 2014;167(5):653-9.e4.
11. Stiell IG, Callaway C, Dan Davis, T, et al. Resuscitation Outcomes Consortium (ROC) PRIMED Cardiac Arrest Trial Methods Part 2: Rationale and Methodology for "Analyze Later" Protocol. Resuscitation. 2008;78(2):186-95

12. Rottenberg EM. Continuous or Interrupted Chest Compressions during CPR. N Engl J Med. 2016;374:1194-7.
13. Sanders AB, Ewy GA. Cardiopulmonary resuscitation in the real world: when will the guidelines get the message? JAMA. 2005;293:363-5.
14. Stecker EC, Reinier K, Marijon E, et al. Public health burden of sudden cardiac death in the United States. Circ Arrhythm Electrophysiol. 2014;7(2):212-217.
15. Svensson L, Bohm K, Castrèn M, et al. Compression-only CPR or standard CPR in out-of-hospital cardiac arrest. N Engl J Med. 2010;363(5):434-42.
16. The Public Access Defibrillation Trial Investigators. Public-access defibrillation and survival after out-of-hospital cardiac arrest. N Engl J Med. 2004;351:637-46.
17. Viskin S, Belhassen B. Idiopathic ventricular fibrillation. Am Heart J. 1990;120(3):661-71.
18. Wellens HJ, Lemery R, Smeets JL, et al. Sudden arrhythmic death without overt heart disease. Circulation. 1991;85(Suppl I):192-7.
19. Wenzel V, Krismer AC, Arntz HR, et al; European Resuscitation Council Vasopressor during Cardiopulmonary Resuscitation Study Group. A comparison of vasopressin and epinephrine for out-of-hospital cardiopulmonary resuscitation. N Engl J Med. 2004;350:105-13.

CHAPTER 12

Cardiomyopathy

INTRODUCTION

Cardiomyopathy is defined as heart muscle disease of unknown cause. Cardiomyopathies are classified as—hypertrophic, dilated, and restrictive.

Heart muscle disease from known causes, particularly infiltrative or systemic disease, formerly termed secondary cardiomyopathy, is currently referred to as specific heart muscle disease and is discussed at the end of this chapter.

HYPERTROPHIC CARDIOMYOPATHY

Hypertrophic cardiomyopathy (HCM) refers to a condition in which massive ventricular hypertrophy occurs in the absence of any definite cause. This is mainly a disease of young adults.

- The term HCM is preferred because not all affected patients have idiopathic hypertrophic subaortic stenosis or features of hypertrophic obstructive cardiomyopathy.
- Approximately 33% of patients have no significant left ventricular (LV) outflow tract gradient at rest or on provocation.
- The myofibrillar disarray commonly seen in HCM is believed to be caused by an aberration of catecholamine function in the heart of the embryo. Familial cases show an autosomal dominant trait linked to chromosome 14q1.

Pathophysiology

- Most patients show asymmetric hypertrophy of the septum and a hypertrophied nondilated left and/or right ventricle. But the septum may be diffusely hypertrophied or only in its upper, mid, or apical portion. Hypertrophy extends to the free wall of the left ventricle.
- Decreased compliance and incomplete relaxation of the left ventricle cause impedance to diastolic filling.
- Rapid powerful contraction of the hypertrophied left ventricle expels most of its contents in the first half of systole. This hyperdynamic systolic function is apparent in most patients with HCM.

- The anterior leaflet of the mitral valve is displaced toward the hypertrophied septum. Mitral regurgitation (MR) is virtually always present in the obstructive phase of the disease. Therefore, the sequence of events is—eject, obstruct, and leak. A variable LV outflow pressure gradient at rest occurs in approximately 35% of patients. A further 25% develop a similar gradient precipitated by conditions that ↑ myocardial contractility or ↓ ventricular volume. Thus, diuretics and other causes of hypovolemia and preload-reducing agents that ↓ the volume of the small ventricular cavity may increase gradients.
- Fibrosis and occlusive disease in small coronary arteries and arterioles may occur. The major coronary arteries are wide and patent unless occlusive atherosclerotic coronary disease occurs as a chance association.

Clinical Hallmarks

- Dyspnea caused by raised LV end diastolic pressure
- Angina resulting from reduced diastolic coronary perfusion
- Presyncope or syncope during exercise, normal activities, or at rest, not simply related to failure to ↑ cardiac output on exercise
- May present with palpitations or symptoms and signs of congestive heart failure (CHF).

Table 12.1 gives the predominant symptoms and signs and their approximate incidence. General physique is usually normal and well developed. The palpable left atrial beat preceding the LV thrust is a most important sign, since it can occur in the absence of gradient or murmur. The murmur has typical features:

- Crescendo-decrescendo starts well after the first heart sound and ends well before the second. It is best heard between the apex and left sternal border
- Radiates poorly to the neck.
- Intensity increases with maneuvers or drugs that ↓ preload (Valsalva, standing, and amyl nitrate) and decreases in intensity with an increase (↑) in afterload (squatting, hand grip, and phenylephrine)
- Easy to distinguish from aortic valvular stenosis, in which the murmur starts soon after the first heart sound and radiates well to the neck.

An MR murmur is often heard in the last half of the systole with radiation to the axilla. It is usually associated with an outflow tract gradient. A mitral diastolic rumble may be detected.

It must be emphasized that the physical examination may be relatively unremarkable in HCM; attention is necessary to elucidate three subtle signs—(i) rapid carotid upstroke, (ii) abnormal cardiac impulse, and (iii) gallop sounds.

Table 12.1: Clinical hallmarks of hypertrophic cardiomyopathy		
Symptoms and signs	Approximate incidence (%)	Factors
Dyspnea	80	Diastolic dysfunction
Angina	60	Decreased coronary reserve, small vessel disease, or associated CHD
Presyncope	50	Even at rest
Syncope	20	Postexertional and normal activities
Sudden death/annual Adult Children	— 2.5 6	— Mainly arrhythmic —
Annual mortality	4	
Brisk carotid upstroke	90	
Atrial fibrillation	15	
Left atrial beat	50	
Left ventricular thrust	60	
fourth heart sound	50	
third heart sound	30	
Systolic murmur, late onset crescendo-decrescendo	90	Begins well after S1 Little or no radiation to neck or axilla, outflow gradient
Mitral systolic murmur	50	Mitral regurgitation, radiates to axilla

(CHD, coronary heart disease)

Hypertrophic cardiomyopathy causes a brisk carotid upstroke because of the dynamic LV emptying, giving an ill-sustained quality, whereas aortic valvular stenosis produces a slow-rising pulse, with a delayed carotid upstroke.

Supraventricular arrhythmias occur in 20–50% of patients, and ventricular arrhythmias occur in almost all patients.

Warning Symptoms or Signs

- Dizziness and lightheadedness
- Fainting, syncope, or presyncope during exercise or during normal activities
- Exercise increases the LV outflow tract gradient.

Unfortunately, the pathophysiologic mechanism of sudden death remains unresolved. Patients presumed to be at risk for sudden death include those who:

- Are less than 20 years of age at time of diagnosis

- Are less than 20 years of age and have a family history of HCM and sudden death
- Have potentially lethal ventricular arrhythmias, sustained ventricular tachycardia (VT), nonsustained VT, and frequent multiform ventricular ectopics
- Have a history of syncope
- Have severe exertional dyspnea or orthopnea in association with ventricular arrhythmias.

Studies indicate that death cannot be predicted adequately by the following conventional criteria.

The presence of sustained, or nonsustained, VT, or of multiform ventricular ectopy reflects a high risk, but in childhood, the absence of potentially lethal ventricular arrhythmias on 48-hour Holter monitoring must not be interpreted as a lowered risk. Mildly symptomatic or asymptomatic patients who die suddenly have marked LV hypertrophy (LVH). Some evidence indicates that mildly symptomatic patients who have HCM with mild LVH have a low incidence of sudden cardiac death (SCD). The commencement of atrial fibrillation (AF) with loss of atrial function may precipitate pulmonary edema or hypotension.

- Atrial fibrillation occurs in approximately 15% of patients with HCM. The loss of atrial systole with a fast ventricular response may precipitate pulmonary edema and occasionally, severe hypotension. The outcome for patients with HCM and AF is not as bleak as envisaged in the 1970s and 1980s, however. The outlook is not significantly worse for patients with AF and failure to convert than it is for patients with sinus rhythm. Functional class does deteriorate with the onset of AF, but it improves with conversion and control of ventricular response or when chronic AF with controlled ventricular response is achieved
- The chest X-ray may be normal but often shows some left atrial enlargement; the left ventricle ranges from normal to severe enlargement. Aortic valve calcification is absent in HCM, but annular calcification of the mitral valve occurs.

Electrocardiography Findings

- Virtually always abnormal (95%) in patients with significant symptomatic HCM and about 80% abnormal in asymptomatic patients. AF in 15%; an additional 33% have paroxysmal episodes. Other supraventricular and ventricular arrhythmias, nonsustained VT is common, but sustained VT occurs in approximately 3%.
- The electrocardiography (ECG) may be abnormal even when echocardiography is reported normal.
- Deep, narrow Q waves in about 30% in leads II, III, and AVF, V5–V6 or in I, AVL V5–V6, and rarely V1–V3, which may mimic infarction. Intraventricular conduction delay in more than 80%. High QRS voltage

LVH. Diffuse T wave changes in some patients or T waves of LVH. Giant inverted T waves, very high precordial QRS voltage with apical HCM. ST segment depression in some. PR interval occasionally short; pre-excitation may be seen.
- Examples of ECG abnormalities are given in Figures 12.1 and 12.2.

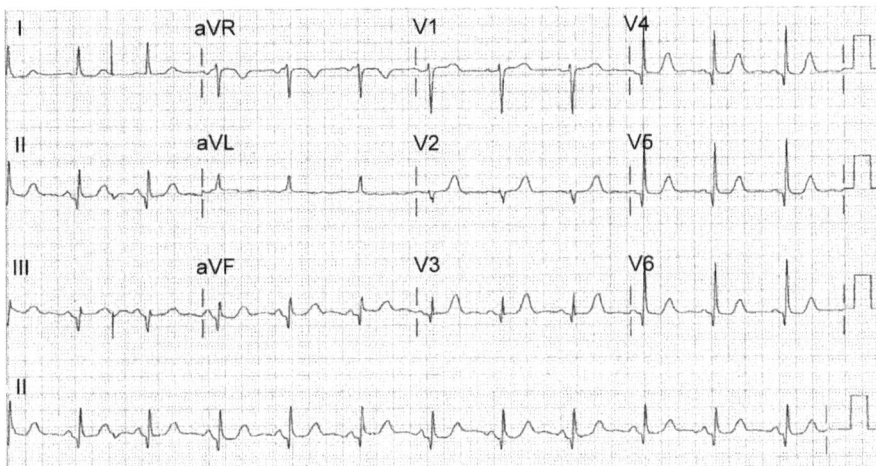

Fig. 12.1: Female age 68 with mild hypertrophic cardiomyopathy. Confirmed by echocardiography at age 45. Note the significant pathologic Q waves in V4–V6, and leads II, III, and arteriovenous fistula (aVF). Incorrectly interpreted by computer as old inferolateral myocardial infarction (MI).
Source: Khan GM. Rapid ECG Interpretation, 3rd edition. United States: Humana Press;2008 pp. 326.

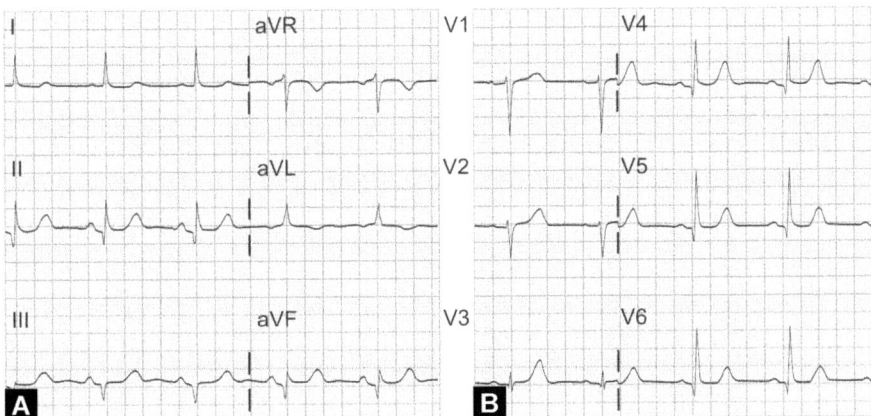

Figs. 12.2A and B: (A) Deep, wide pathologic Q waves in leads II, III, and aVF in a 52-year-old woman with known hypertrophic cardiomyopathy; (B) Same patient as in (A). Wide, deep pathologic Q waves in leads V4 through V6.

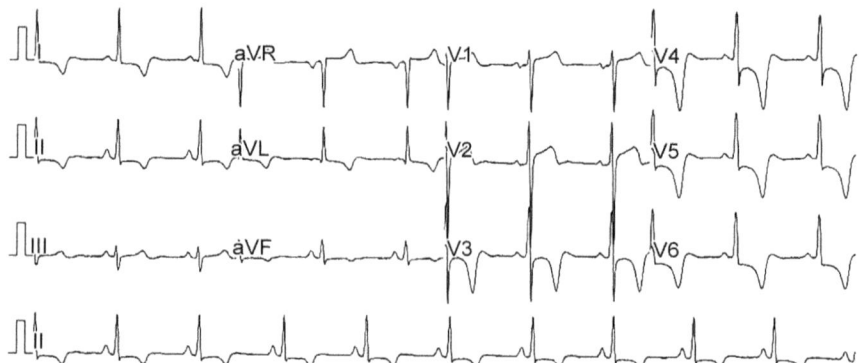

Fig. 12.3: Giant T-wave inversion leads V3–V6 in a patient with apical hypertrophic cardiomyopathy.

Electrocardiography of a 25-year-old man with severe HCM; note ST abnormal elevation V1–V5 can be misdiagnosed as acute myocardial infarction (MI). Note deepest S wave in any lead + S wave in V4 is more than 3 mV, (30 mm) or S wave in lead V1 plus R wave in V6 more than 35 mm (3.5 mV) fills diagnostic criterion for LVH.

At age 20, asymptomatic played soccer, rugby, and hockey for the past 5 years. Routine physical revealed a grade II systolic murmur. Echocardiogram—asymmetric hypertrophy; marked septal hypertrophy—septal thickness 36 mm. 1 year later needed an implantable cardioverter-defibrillator (ICD) (normal <11 mm) (Fig. 12.3).

Echocardiography

- Two-dimensional echocardiography observation of a LV myocardial segment of more than or equal to 1.5 cm thickness in a normal-sized adult is considered diagnostic, if there is no other evident cause (Box 12.1 gives echocardiography hallmarks). Asymmetric hypertrophy is supporting evidence. Myocardial mass increases with age and size. Continuous-wave Doppler echocardiography defines the degree of LV outflow-tract gradient.

Box 12.1: Echocardiography hallmarks of hypertrophic cardiomyopathy.
- Disproportionate septal thickness, septum to posterior wall ratio >1.5
- Left ventricular myocardial segment >1.5 cm in thickness
- Poor septal contraction, hypercontractile free posterior wall
- Systolic anterior motion of the mitral valve when outflow tract gradient >30 mm Hg
- Mid systolic aortic valve closure
- Small left ventricular cavity, typically with virtual elimination in systole
- Mitral regurgitation frequently present
- Left ventricular outflow tract gradient at rest in about 35% of patients

Holter Monitoring

- A 48-hour Holter monitor is necessary because a 24-hour study detects less than 50% runs of nonsustained VT. Repeated studies may be required. Where facilities exist, a signal-averaged ECG is advisable, especially in younger patients. In this subgroup, an abnormal signal-averaged ECG appears to be a marker for sudden death. Further studies are necessary to confirm the role of the signal-averaged ECG in patients with HCM.

Therapy

A decrease in ventricular volume or increase in ventricular contractility increases the outflow gradient. Thus, dehydration and the use of preload-reducing agents, such as diuretics and nitrates should be avoided or used with caution when needed.

Management of the patient with HCM includes counseling and entails screening of all first-degree relatives of newly diagnosed cases. An ECG, chest X-ray, and echocardiogram should usually suffice to identify affected individuals, but cases can still be missed. Holter monitoring and/or examination of relatives is important

- Patients must be instructed to avoid strenuous competitive exercise because it can cause sudden death. A ↓ in ventricular volume or ↑ in ventricular contractility increases the outflow gradient. Thus, dehydration and the use of preload-reducing agents, such as diuretics, nitrates, or angiotensin-converting enzyme (ACE) inhibitors, should be avoided
- Beta-agonists ↑ contractility and are contraindicated
- Digoxin increases contractility and its use should be avoided, except in the management of chronic AF, a fast ventricular response uncontrolled by amiodarone, beta-blockers, or verapamil. Also useful in patients with end-stage disease with CHF (Table 12.2).

Table 12.2: Pharmacologic and surgical interventions for the obstructive and end-stage phase of hypertrophic cardiomyopathy.

Intervention	Obstructive phase	End stage
Negative inotropes	—	—
Beta-blockers	Yes (especially with latent obstruction)	Small dose considered
Verapamil	Yes	Contraindicated
Disopyramide	Yes	Contraindicated
Digoxin	Contraindicated	Needed and useful
Diuretics	Contraindicated	Needed and useful
Afterload-reducing agent: ACE inhibitors	Contraindicated	Of some benefit in patients with ventricular dilatation and heart failure
Surgery	Myectomy	Transplant

(ACE, angiotensin-converting enzyme)

Beta-Blocker Use

It is most important to use a beta-blocker with both beta 1 and 2 activity; propranolol and timolol are advisable. Beta-blockers have subtle and important clinical effects (Table 12.3).

Table 12.3: Total deaths and sudden deaths in beta-blocker randomized control trials of postmyocardial infarction and heart failure patients.

	Control	Drug	% Decrease
Propranolol*			
Total sudden death	78	60	64
5 am–11 am	31	11	64
Total deaths	188/1,460	138/1,456	26
Timolol**			
Total sudden death^	95	47	50
Instant, within seconds	38	11	71
Total deaths	117/718	67/670	42
Metoprolol#			
Total sudden death	21	9	57
Total deaths	31/147	25/154	19##
*MERIT-HF^*			
Total sudden death	132	79	
Total deaths	217/2,001	145/1,990	
Bisoprolol (CIBIS)***			
Total sudden death	83	48	42.2
Total deaths	228/1,320	156/1,327	31.6

(MERIT-HF: Metoprolol CR/XL Randomised Intervention Trial in Congestive Heart Failure; CIBIS: Cardiac Insufficiency Bisoprolol Study)
*BHAT study, AM sudden death (Peters et al. 1989) follow-up 25 months, 120–240 mg daily.
**Timolol Norwegian MI study; mean duration 17 months. Follow-up: 10 mg twice daily.
#*Metoprolol:* A very small study of only approximately 150 patients in each group followed for 3 years.
##"This reduction in cardiac mortality did not reach statistical significance, as was to be expected from our sample size" (Olsson et al. 1985).
^In (MERIT-HF), there were fewer sudden deaths in the metoprolol CR/XL group than in the placebo group [79 vs 132, 0.59 (0.45–0.78); $p = 0.0002$] and deaths from worsening heart failure [30 vs 58, 0.51 (0.33–0.79); $p = 0.0023$].
***Bisoprolol in CIBIS; significant decrease in deaths and sudden deaths

Propranolol

- This remains the beta-blocker of choice.
- *Dosage*: 40 mg three times daily, increased slowly to 240 mg daily. A slow buildup of the dosage to 320 mg may be required.

Timolol

This remarkable drug has been largely discarded in the Americas. It caused a stunning 67% reduction in SCDs in the Norwegian Myocardial Infarction Trial (1981). No other drug can claim such. A major problem with HCM is sudden death.
- *Dose*: 10–15 mg twice daily.
- Atenolol is not recommended. Carvedilol has alpha activity and is not advisable.

Avoid atenolol because it is a relatively ineffective beta-blocker. Atenolol has failed in several randomized controlled trials (RCTs) because of low brain concentration and thus effectiveness. The author strongly advises clinicians to stop prescribing this poorly effective beta-blocker. It is a much prescribed beta-blocker worldwide.

- Drugs that ↓ myocardial contractility or produce myocardial relaxation, particularly beta-blockers, play a major role in the control of symptoms
- Patients without significant obstruction with moderate MR and end-stage disease with CHF and ventricular dilatation may benefit from the judicious use of ACE inhibitors.

Clinical trials have documented the role of beta-blockers in the management of HCM. Beta-blockers and verapamil are equally effective for the management of symptoms, but beta-blockers generally are safer and therefore are considered first-line therapy. Beneficial effects of beta-adrenergic blocking drugs include the following:

- ↓ in myocardial contractility causes a ↓ in "Venturi" effect and therefore less gradient
- Relief of dyspnea in about 40% of patients
- Significant relief of angina in 33–66% of patients
- The heart rate (HR) should be maintained between 55 beats/min and 60 beats/min; this results in an improvement in coronary filling because of prolongation of the diastolic interval
- Improvement in diastolic dysfunction
- Partial control of supraventricular and ventricular arrhythmias.

Angiotensin Converting Enzyme Inhibitors

These were shown to be ineffective in a RCT INHibition of the renin angiotensin system in HCM and the Effect on hypertrophy—a Randomized

Intervention Trial (INHERIT) 132 patients with HCM treated with losartan 100 mg daily for 12 months did not show significant effect on LV mass, thickness or fibrosis for ACE inhibitor therapy compared with placebo in patients with overt HCM
- This result is not surprising because these agents reduce preload and afterload. Drugs that decrease after load are not advisable; this includes dihydropyridine calcium antagonists.

Calcium Antagonists

Verapamil enhances LV diastolic filling by improving ventricular relaxation, actions similar to those produced by beta-adrenergic blockade. Considerable experience with verapamil is now available, but the initial high expectations have not materialized and the drug has caused deaths. Verapamil decreases dyspnea and increases exercise capacity in some patients but does not appear to improve survival; it is contraindicated in patients with end-stage disease associated with ventricular dilatation and CHF.
- *Dosage:* 40 mg tid or 80 mg bid, ↑ slowly over weeks to 120 bid under close observation. Preferably, administration of the drug is begun in the hospital setting.
- *Adverse Effects:* High-grade atrioventricular (AV) block, asystole, sinus arrest, acute pulmonary edema, and hypotension.
- *Contraindications:* Orthopnea or paroxysmal nocturnal dyspnea (PND) (deaths have occurred in these patients as a result of verapamil use); CHF and/or end-stage disease; sick sinus syndrome; AV block and conduction defects.
- *Interactions:*

Amiodarone has gained widespread acceptance as a major advance in the management of patients with AF and, in others, to reduce the incidence of ventricular arrhythmias and sudden death where the risk is assessed to be high. See Chapter 6 for indications, dosage, and adverse effects.

Sotalol is a useful alternative to amiodarone. Dosage—80 mg bid increasing to 240 mg/day if needed.

Anticoagulants are indicated in all patients with AF, to prevent embolism at the time of direct current (DC) conversion, and when waiting for amiodarone to produce conversion. Patients who remain in AF while on amiodarone should receive anticoagulants, but with careful monitoring of international normalized ratio (INR) or prothrombin time since amiodarone enhances the activity of coumarins and life-threatening bleeding can be precipitated.

Surgery or septal resection and mitral valve surgery—indications include the following:
- Patients who have had adequate trials of beta-blockers, verapamil, or amiodarone plus beta-blocker and remain severely symptomatic with angina and dyspnea

- Outflow gradient more than 50 mm Hg at rest
- Moderate or severe MR
- Very thick ventricular septum
- High LV end diastolic pressure.

Sequential AV pacing reduces symptoms and improves hemodynamics. Surgery, which is only palliative, causes an 8% early and about 12% late mortality but depends on the expertise of the surgical team. When surgery is indicated, a septal myotomy or myectomy is performed. Surgery does not reduce mortality, but a significant number of patients obtain relief from anginal symptoms. The Dusseldorf experience shows an encouraging ↓ in sudden death and syncope following successful myotomy or myectomy. Mitral valve replacement is indicated only for severe MR. Transplantation may be considered for intractable symptoms.

The Euro-alcohol septal ablation (ASA) registry demonstrated low periprocedural and long-term mortality after ASA. This intervention provided durable relief of symptoms and a reduction of LV outflow tract obstruction in selected and highly symptomatic patients with obstructive HCM. The short-term potential arrhythmia risk associated with ASA is approximately equal to 10%.

DILATED CARDIOMYOPATHY

A diagnosis of dilated cardiomyopathy (DCM) should be considered in a patient with CHF, documented global hypokinesis and dilation of the left and/or right ventricles, and reduced systolic function in the absence of evidence of CHD, congenital, specific valvular, hypertensive, or specific heart muscle disease, and chronic excessive alcohol consumption. DCM is not due to alcohol but can be exaggerated by it.

Clinical Hallmarks

- Progressive dyspnea on exertion appears over weeks or months, culminating in orthopnea, PND, and edema, which are common features. Physical signs of right and LV failure are prominent in late cases. The extremities tend to be cool and pale due to vasoconstriction.
- The apex beat is displaced downward and outward to the left due to LV dilatation.
- Left lower parasternal lift or pulsation indicates right ventricular (RV) dilatation.
- The jugular venous pressure (JVP) may be elevated and may show a systolic wave of tricuspid regurgitation.
- A soft Grade I-II/VI systolic mitral murmur and a soft tricuspid systolic murmur are commonly present because of mitral and tricuspid regurgitation as a result of dilation of the ventricles and valve rings as well as papillary muscle dysfunction.

- S4 and S3 are constantly present, as well as sinus tachycardia; thus, a summation gallop is a frequent finding.
- The loud S3 is present in virtually all cases and is often heard when CHF is absent. This hallmark serves to differentiate DCM from a Class 4 ventricle due to CHD where a soft S3 is heard during episodes of CHF, but is frequently absent or quite soft when the individual is assessed not to be in CHF, and in the absence of LV aneurysm.
- Blood pressure is frequently low; hypotension carries a poor prognosis.

  Aortic systolic or diastolic murmurs are usually absent and serve to exclude specific valvular heart disease as a cause of the severe CHF but aortic regurgitation occasionally occurs in DCM. These are signs of advanced disease. Echocardiographic diagnosis can be made before overt CHF has developed.
- Electrocardiography features include—sinus tachycardia and flat or inverted T waves. Modest LVH may be masked by low voltage. AF occurs in about 25%; left bundle branch block (LBBB) is observed in a significant minority. Poor R wave progression (V2-V4) or Q waves of pseudoinfarction may suggest an incorrect diagnosis of ischemic heart disease.
- *Chest X-ray:* The heart is enlarged and four-chamber enlargement is commonly present. There is usually evidence of a raised left atrial pressure in the pulmonary vascular pattern. Pleural effusions may be present.

Echocardiography

- Echocardiographic features include—severe dilation of both ventricles; global hypokinesis and commonly paradoxical movement of the septum; increased end systolic and end diastolic dimensions; ejection fraction (EF) usually less than 35%; EF 10-30% in the presence of CHF; atrial enlargement and ventricular thrombi; and a small pericardial effusion.
- *Endomyocardial biopsy:* Used as a research tool to exclude suspected known heart muscle disease and to detect evidence of myocarditis or viral particles
- Holter monitoring carried out for 48 hours helps define patients with potentially lethal ventricular arrhythmias.

Therapy

- The most important aspect of DCM management is the prevention and control of CHF, arrhythmias, and embolization. The standard management for CHF should be instituted—bed-to-chair rest for several days; oxygen and a sedative at night to allow restful sleep, which adds to the patient's comfort and reduces the workload of the failing myocardium; and salt restriction. Avoidance of alcohol is necessary in all patients with CHF

and especially in the patient with a Class 3 or 4 ventricle, because alcohol decreases the EF. Patients should be assessed for the presence of macro-ovalocytes, decreased platelet counts, and increased levels of gamma-glutamyl transferase, which may indicate alcohol damage.
- Digoxin provides some benefit in CHF patients in sinus rhythm and is indicated for AF with uncontrolled ventricular response. The dose should be adequate, but care is needed to avoid digitalis toxicity. In patients with refractory CHF, intravenous (IV) dobutamine may cause temporary "improvement".
- Diuretics play a vital role in the relief of symptoms. The three groups of drugs—(i) diuretics, (ii) digoxin, and (iii) ACE inhibitors—are complementary.
- Angiotensin-converting enzyme inhibitors have made a major contribution to survival of patients with CHF; however, diastolic dysfunction in patients with DCM tends to worsen with ACE inhibitor therapy. The dosage and pharmacologic profile of ACE inhibitors have been explained in detail in the other chapter.

Beta-adrenergic Blockers

Judicious use of beta-blockers appears, however, paradoxically, to benefit some patients with DCM, especially individuals with resting sinus tachycardia and/or diastolic dysfunction. Removal of sympathetic drive on myocytes and restoration toward normal of the downgrading of beta-adrenergic receptors in CHF appear to provide benefits.

Reduction in HR decreases myocardial O_2 demand and also improves coronary blood flow. Prevention of arrhythmias, with even modest ↓ in sudden deaths, is a potential benefit of careful beta-adrenergic blockade. Clinical trials have shown mixed results, however, and large-scale trials are underway.

Warfarin is advisable in most patients to prevent embolization from atrial and ventricular thrombi; it is essential if there is AF. Pulmonary embolism and systemic embolization occur fairly frequently and worsen the dismal prognosis. In addition, immobilization during periods of CHF predisposes deep vein thrombosis and pulmonary emboli.

RESTRICTIVE CARDIOMYOPATHY

This major abnormality is a restriction of ventricular filling, thus an ↑ in filling pressures. Restrictive cardiomyopathy (RCM) is a member of the group of diastolic CHF in which diastolic function is impaired earlier and more severely than systolic function. The usual abnormality is impaired relaxation and compliance. Restrictive pathophysiology may occur at the pericardial, myocardial, or endomyocardial level.

The most common cause of RCM is endomyocardial fibrosis, especially in tropical regions. Myocardial involvement by amyloid, not associated with multiple organ involvement, is the most common cause of RCM in the Western world. Cardiac disease resulting from amyloid-associated multiple organ involvement, sarcoid, hemochromatosis, eosinophilic syndromes, scleroderma, Adriamycin toxicity, and infectious agents, including tuberculosis, causing restrictive physiology is considered specific heart muscle disease. HCM may produce diastolic abnormalities similar to those in RCM.

Clinical Hallmarks

- Intermittent fever, shortness of breath, cough, palpitations, edema, and tiredness
- Hypereosinophilia with abnormal eosinophil degranulation is seen in temperate climates (hypereosinophilic heart disease)
- Hypereosinophilia is less severe in tropical endomyocardial fibrosis
- Symptoms and signs of CHF and of moderate-to-severe mitral and tricuspid regurgitation due to involvement of the papillary muscles serve to differentiate RCM from constrictive pericarditis, as does the greater degree of cardiac enlargement on chest X-ray in the former condition.
- During the early stages, endomyocardial fibrosis may mimic the hemodynamic and clinical features of constrictive pericarditis. Hemodynamic differences are found, but with significant overlap.
- The chest X-ray in patients with endomyocardial fibrosis may show calcification of the right or LV apical myocardium
- Echocardiogram shows obliteration of the apices of the ventricles by echogenic masses. Also, myocardial calcification may be detected, and in later stages, mitral and tricuspid regurgitation may require echocardiography assessment.
- The idiopathic endocardial fibrosis and associated thrombus may progressively obliterate the left or RV cavities. Severe enlargement of the right atrium may occur.

Therapy

- Steroids may be helpful in the early acute inflammatory phase associated with hypereosinophilia, but medical therapy is unrewarding
- Anticoagulants are necessary because thromboembolism is common
- Restriction to filling does not respond to digoxin, diuretics, or vasodilators, and all three medications are relatively contraindicated. Arrhythmias may respond to small doses of beta-blockers, and potentially lethal arrhythmias may require amiodarone therapy

- Resection of masses of obliterating endocardial tissue with valve repair has produced apparent relief in some patients with endomyocardial fibrosis for a few years
- Cardiac transplantation may require consideration in intractable cases.

SPECIFIC HEART MUSCLE DISEASE

- Specific heart muscle disease usually produces a dilated form of cardiomyopathy with impaired systolic function
- Restrictive physiology is seen with amyloid, sarcoid, neoplasm, radiation, scleroderma, hemochromatosis, and eosinophilic endomyocardial disease, in which eosinophilia is usually present. Rarely, myocardial tuberculosis is present with restrictive features. Amyloid heart disease and endomyocardial fibrosis are usually considered examples of RCM, but when cardiac involvement is associated with multiple organ disease, they qualify as specific heart muscle disease
- The findings of systemic disease of other organs, especially the liver, lymph nodes, and skin, which can be easily submitted to biopsy, assist in defining the underlying cause. Endomyocardial biopsy is often required but may not be helpful in patchy disease such as sarcoid
- Treatment should be directed at the underlying disease. Occasionally, cardiac pacing is required for the management of complete heart block due to involvement of conduction tissue by sarcoid, scleroderma, or hemochromatosis
- *Other heart muscle diseases include involvement due to infectious disease*: Chagas due to *Trypanosoma cruzi* is transmitted by a triatoma bug. The disease is prevalent in South America but does occur in the southern United States
- The incidence of human immunodeficiency virus (HIV) is increasing, and myocarditis with pericardial effusion and cardiac tamponade is now surfacing in victims of acquired immunodeficiency syndrome (AIDS). Myocardial involvement might be due to the HIV virus; although this is unproven, involvement by Kaposi, opportunistic infections, and effects of medications must also be excluded
- Rare involvement of cardiac muscle is seen with alcohol abuse, polymyositis, progressive muscular dystrophy, Friedreich's ataxia, and Fabry's disease.
- Deficiency disorders, such as beriberi or selenium deficiency
- Drugs, especially cocaine and toxins, may affect the myocardium; known toxins include cobalt (beer), chloroquine and emetine, phenothiazines, methysergide, and cancer chemotherapeutic agents (adriamycin,

daunorubicin, doxorubicin, and cyclophosphamide); also, methyldopa and phenindione rarely cause a hypersensitivity myocarditis. Overdose with toxic doses of acetaminophen or cocaine may cause myocardial necrosis and arrhythmias, including torsades de pointes.
- Treatment of these disorders involves removal and treatment of the infective agent or toxin where possible.

Takotsubo Stress Cardiomyopathy

- Ballooning out of the apex of the heart with preserved function of the base fostered the name takotsubo syndrome ("takotsubo", Japanese for octopus trap)
- Takotsubo cardiomyopathy causes severe chest pain but can present with mild-to-moderate chest pressure and thus mimics the symptoms of acute MI.

Precipitants

- Panic, fright, caught in a disaster, earthquake, storm, or similar
- Grief from the death of a spouse, other loved one, or relative
- Heated arguments relationship disagreements, domestic abuse, and arguments with spouse or partner
- Catastrophic medical diagnoses, devastating financial, or gambling losses
- Even fear from public speaking, coitus; and also delirium tremens.

Physical triggers include heart attack, stroke, status asthmaticus, and even surgery.

Echocardiography

Most useful during an attack of chest pain because it is virtually always abnormal and prevents a misdiagnosis of acute MI and rush to unneeded angiograms.

It shows transient myocardial stunning—transient left apical ballooning markedly hypokinetic mid ventricular segments, with preserved basal segments—a pattern not observed with coronary artery anatomy.

Electrocardiography

The ECG is abnormal showing nonspecific ST-T changes; ST segment depression or elevation (Fig. 12.4).

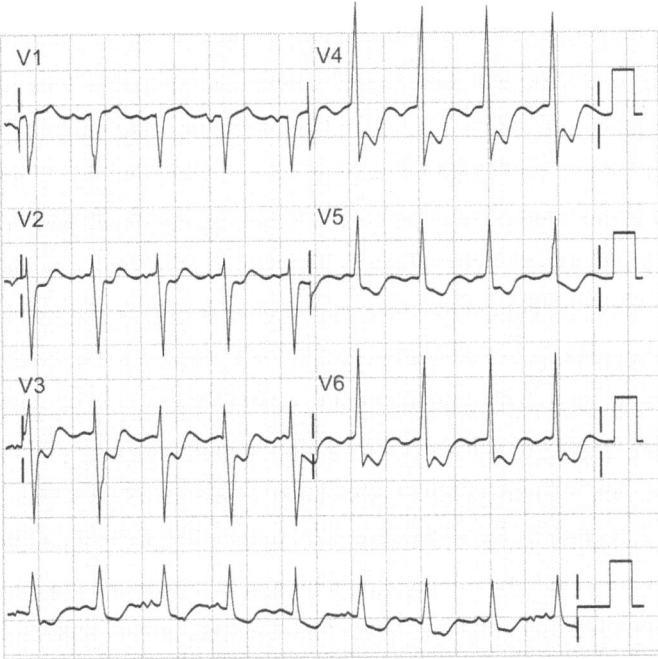

Fig 12.4: Takotsubo stress cardiomyopathy simulating non-Q wave infarction. ECG from a 37-year-old female with acute chest pain during coitus. Marked downsloping ST segment depression V1–V6, no associated Q waves. Coronary angiograms normal.
Source: Khan GM. Practical Cardiology. New Delhi, India: Jaypee Brothers Medical Publishers (P) Ltd.; 2018.

BIBLIOGRAPHY

1. Akashi YJ, Goldstein DS, Barbaro G, et al. Takotsubo cardiomyopathy: a new form of acute, reversible heart failure. Circulation. 2008;118(25):2754-62.
2. Olivotto I, Ashley EA. INHERIT trial (INHibition of the renin angiotensin system in HCM and the Effect on hypertrophy—a Randomised Intervention Trial). Glob Cardiol Sci Pract. 2015;2015:7.
3. Khan GM. Practical Cardiology. New Delhi, India: Jaypee Brothers Medical Publishers (P) Ltd.; 2018.
4. Khan MG. Rapid ECG Interpretation, 3rd edition. New York, Totowa: Humana Press; 2008.
5. Maron BJ, Gardin JM, Flack JM, et al. Prevalence of hypertrophic cardiomyopathy in a general population of young adults: echocardiographic analysis of 4111 subjects in the CAR-DIA Study. Circulation. 1995;92:785.
6. Maron BJ. Contemporary insights and strategies for risk stratification and prevention of sudden death in hypertrophic cardiomyopathy. Circulation. 2010;121(3):445-56.
7. Maron BJ. Sudden death in young athletes. N Engl J Med. 2003;349:1064-75.
8. Nishimura RA, Schaff HV. Evolving Treatment for Patients With Hypertrophic Obstructive Cardiomyopathy. J Am Coll Cardiol. 2015;66(15):1697-9.
9. Veselka J, Jensen MK, Liebregts M, et al. Long-term clinical outcome after alcohol septal ablation for obstructive hypertrophic cardiomyopathy: results from the Euro-ASA registry.Eur Heart J. 2016;37(19):1517-23.

CHAPTER 13

Syncope

INTRODUCTION

Syncope (transient loss of consciousness as a result of inadequate cerebral blood flow) is a common problem representing less than or equal to 1% of medical admissions to general hospitals and less than or equal to 3% of emergency room diagnoses. Its causes are often elusive; the following points deserve attention:

- An obvious cardiac cause can be defined by the history, physical examination, electrocardiogram (ECG), and Holter monitoring in approximately 10% of cases (Flowchart 13.1 and Table 13.1).
- Vasodepressor (vasovagal) syncope, the common form being the simple faint, accounts for more than 35% of cases of syncope. It is therefore most important to exclude this benign problem.
- Unexplained syncope constitutes a large group of cases (>35%), but in patients who have structural heart disease and unexplained syncope, electrophysiologic (EP) testing helps identify a significant number of cardiac cause and ↑ the total cardiac cause of syncope to approximately 22%.
- In patients with unexplained syncope, if structural heart disease is not present, EP testing is rarely diagnostic; the head-up tilt test is useful (*see* Flowchart 13.1).
- Syncope may be the clue to possibly life-threatening underlying cardiac diseases.
- Cardiac syncope carries a 24% incidence of sudden death in 1 year; the incidence is less than 2% in the remaining 78% of individuals. One-year mortality of patients with cardiac syncope is 15–30%, versus less than 2% for individuals with unexplained syncope and without structural heart disease.
- Flowchart 13.1 shows an algorithmic approach to the diagnosis of syncope.
- Dizziness is often a feature of presyncope and has several causes that are difficult to determine. Flowchart 13.2 indicates steps to consider.
- Postural hypotension is an important cause of syncope. It commonly occurs because of an ↓ in preload and often occurs in patients on

Flowchart 13.1: Algorithm for the assessment of syncope.

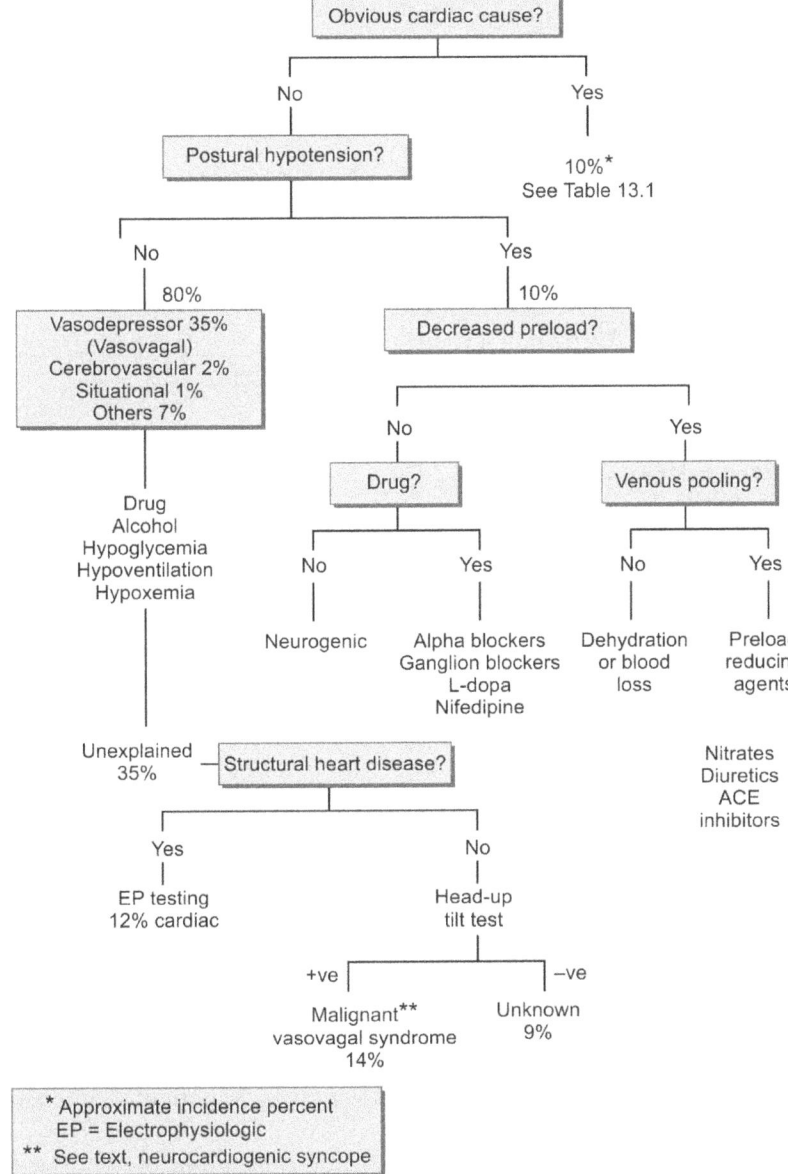

cardiac medications that cause venous pooling. Less often, syncope has a neurogenic cause, being a troublesome feature of autonomic neuropathy (Table 13.2).

It must be re-emphasized that head-up tilt testing has a role in defining the cause of unexplained syncope in patients without structural heart disease. The result may be expedited by the simultaneous administration

Table 13.1: Obvious cardiac causes of syncope and approximate incidence.	
Causes	Approximate incidence

Tachyarrhythmias
  Sustained and nonsustained VT
  Torsades de pointes
  Atrial fibrillation
  Supraventricular tachycardia
  Long QT syndrome
  Wolff–Parkinson–White (WPW) syndrome
  Pacemaker mediated
	45%

Bradyarrhythmias
  Sinus node dysfunction
  (Sick sinus syndrome)
  Atrioventricular (AV) block second and third degree
  Drug induced
	35%

Carotid sinus syncope	3%

Obstruction to stroke volume
  Aortic stenosis
  Hypertrophic cardiomyopathy
  Tight mitral stenosis
  Atrial myxoma or thrombus
  Cardiac tamponade
  Prosthetic valve dysfunction
  Pulmonary embolism
  Pulmonary hypertension
  Pulmonary stenosis
	10%

Others
  Mitral valve prolapse
  Myocardial infarction
  Severe ischemic heart disease
  Coronary artery spasm
  Pacemaker syndrome
  Aortic dissection
  Fallot's tetralogy
	7%

of intravenous (IV) edrophonium; in patients younger than age 50 years, isoproterenol is used in some centers, but a study by Kapoor et al. questions the low specificity of this test.

These intensive investigations result in the prevention of some of the deaths associated with syncope, although syncope remains unexplained in a minority of patients.

The management of syncope entails the elucidation of the cause so that appropriate advice, medications, or corrective measures may be employed to prevent bodily injury or threat to life. Since most cardiac causes pose a threat to life, it is important to use a methodical approach to solving the cause of syncope in a given individual. This medical solution calls for sound

Flowchart 13.2: Algorithm for evaluating patients with dizziness.

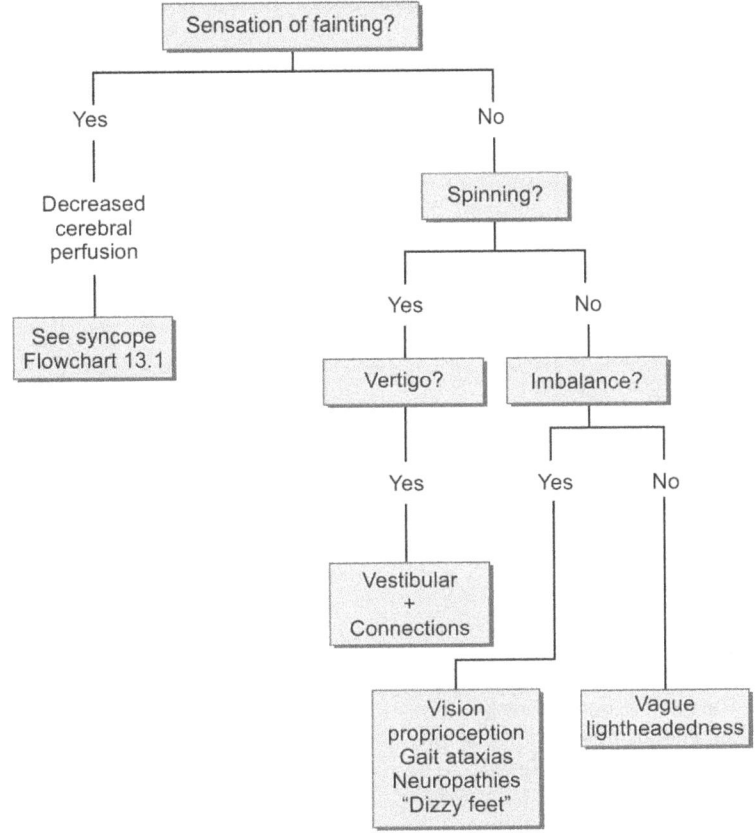

knowledge of basic internal medicine and cardiology and should commence with a detailed history and physical examination. Who should be admitted to a hospital?
- Patients with suspected cardiac cause
- Patients with significant bodily injury
- The elderly patient in whom a readily identifiable cause is lacking
- Recurrent syncope of undetermined etiology
- Recurrence of syncope while awaiting investigation.

HISTORY AND PHYSICAL EXAMINATION

A detailed relevant history and physical examination are mandatory.
- Check the blood pressure (BP) on the patient recumbent for greater than 3 minutes and then on standing, to elicit postural hypotension
- Determine the BP in the arms and legs
- Listen for bruits over the subclavian and carotid arteries

Table 13.2: Noncardiac causes of syncope.

Causes	Approximate incidence
• Vasodepressor (vasovagal)	35%
• Postural hypotension	10%
▪ Decrease preload	
– Venous pooling, caused by extensive varicose veins, postexercise vasodilation venous angioma in the leg. Drugs: nitrates, diuretics, ACE inhibitors	
– Decreased blood volume: blood loss; dehydration: vomiting, diarrhea, excessive sweating, Addison's disease	
▪ Drug induced	
– Alpha-blockers	
– Ganglion blockers	
– Bromocriptine	
– L-dopa	
– Nifedipine	
▪ Neurogenic decrease autonomic activity	
– Bed rest	
– Neuropathies/diabetes	
– Shy Drager syndrome	
– Idiopathic	
▪ Mastocytosis	
• Cerebrovascular disease	2%
▪ Transient ischemic attack	
▪ Subclavian steal	
▪ Basilar artery migraine	
▪ Cervical arthritis, atlanto-occipital dislocation compression vertebral artery	
• Situational	1%
▪ Cough, sneeze, micturition, defecation	
• Others	7%
▪ Drugs/alcohol	
▪ Hypoglycemia	
▪ Hypoxemia	
▪ Hypoventilation	
▪ Hysterical	
• Unexplained	35%
▪ Malignant vasovagal syndrome (neurally mediated syncope) 30–60% of otherwise unexplained	

- Look for finger clubbing and cyanosis as signs of congenital cyanotic heart disease
- Perform a full cardiovascular examination. Check for left ventricular hypertrophy (LVH), presence of thrills, the murmur of aortic stenosis, hypertrophic cardiomyopathy (HCM), mitral stenosis, mitral valve prolapse, and the presence of prosthetic heart valve (*see* Table 13.1).
- Assess for tachyarrhythmias and bradyarrhythmias.

The history should exclude the most common cause of faint, i.e. vasodepressor syncope. All known causes of syncope should be methodically excluded (*see* Flowchart 13.1). After exclusion of postural hypotension, vasodepressor syncope, and cerebrovascular and situational causes, request the following:
- Complete blood count (CBC), electrolytes, blood urea, serum creatinine, and serum calcium (Ca). These routine tests are not usually helpful
- Chest X-ray—low yield
- ECG—low yield
- Echocardiogram—low yield
- 24- or 48-hour Holter monitoring is advisable but has a low yield.

CAUSES

Vasodepressor (Vasovagal) Syncope

The simple faint is the most common cause of syncope and is easily recognized.
- Vasodepressor syncope virtually never occurs in a patient in the recumbent position. Precipitating circumstances are almost always present and typically occur in young individuals and occasionally in older patients in the setting of exhaustion, hunger, prolonged standing or sitting in a hot crowded room, and sudden severe pain or trauma, venipuncture, fright, and sudden emotional stress.

The simple faint usually gives a warning of seconds to minutes: a feeling of weakness, nausea, vague upper abdominal discomfort, diaphoresis, yawn, sighing, hyperventilation, unsteadiness, blurring of vision, an awareness prior to fainting. Importantly, vertigo is not a symptom associated with a simple faint. Thus, a good history identifies the faint and may save expensive and time-consuming investigations.

The constant findings in vasodepressor syncope are:
- A sudden marked fall in total peripheral resistance, resulting in a drastic fall in BP
- Decreased cerebral perfusion, causing loss of consciousness
- Loss of consciousness usually occurs within 10 seconds of onset of diminished perfusion.
- Return of consciousness in seconds to minutes if the individual remains flat with the legs elevated.
- Injuries are most uncommon with vasodepressor syncope.

The exclusion of epilepsy is relatively easy, but occasionally syncope may be confused with akinetic seizures. Bradycardia in association with seizures has been described. The aura, if any, in epilepsy is transient but tells a story. Injuries, including lip and tongue biting, and incontinence with a prolonged postictal state are not seen with vasodepressor syncope.

- Because cardiac sympathetic overstimulation, vigorous left ventricular (LV) contraction, and stimulation of intramyocardial mechanoreceptors (C fibers) appear to be important underlying mechanisms in the genesis of unexplained syncope without structural heart disease, beta-blockers have been given as rational therapy and have proven successful in some patients with this disabling form of syncope, known as malignant vasovagal syndrome, neurocardiogenic syncope, or neurally mediated syncope.
- Metoprolol (100 mg) daily may produce a salutary response.
- Esmolol IV may be used to predict the outcome of oral beta-blocker therapy.

Postural Hypotension

Several cardiac medications may cause orthostatic hypotension, particularly in the elderly. Assess the following:
- Check the BP with the patient recumbent for greater than or equal to 3 minutes and then on standing; an ↓ in systolic pressure of greater than or equal to 20 mm Hg represents orthostatic hypotension.
  - Check for evidence of ↓ in preload, which may manifest itself by venous pooling that may occur on sudden standing after vigorous exercise or because of extensive varicose veins. Preload-reducing agents, particularly nitrates, angiotensin-converting enzyme (ACE) inhibitors or alpha-1 blockers may be implicated. Blood loss and dehydration are obvious causes, but an occult cause of the latter is Addison's disease.
- If conditions causing an ↓ in preload are not present, inquire about the use of medications that cause arterial dilation (particularly alpha-1 adrenergic blockers such as prazosin and labetalol), ganglion-blocking drugs, L-dopa, bromocriptine, and rarely nifedipine.
- If drug use is excluded, postural hypotension may be caused by autonomic imbalance or neurologic diseases. Complete bed rest and a lack of leg exercise, plus an ↓ in autonomic activity, commonly result in postural hypotension. Neuropathy, especially due to diabetes, Shy Drager, and other neurologic problems must be excluded.

Standing from a recumbent or sitting position causes immediate pooling of blood in the lower limbs and a consequent fall in BP that normally triggers a baroreceptor response, sympathetically mediated vasoconstriction, and an increase (↑) in heart rate (HR). As indicated above, conditions that impair baroreceptor function and ↓ sympathetically mediated alpha-1 vasoconstriction may precipitate postural hypotension.
- Orthostatic hypotension as a consequence of autonomic neuropathies and autonomic failure is difficult to treat successfully. It may respond to

increased sodium (Na) intake or fludrocortisone (Florinef), 0.1–0.2 mg qd. The management of orthostatic hypotension caused by autonomic failure can be successfully managed in properly selected patients with midodrine (Amatine), a selective peripherally acting postsynaptic alpha-1 adrenergic agonist. Salutary effects are caused by an ↑ in arterial and venous tone; venous pooling is prevented. Initial dosage: 2.5 mg tid with monitoring of supine BP, then increased in 2.5-mg increments at weekly intervals to a maximum of 10 mg tid.

- Caution is needed because the action of midodrine is identical to that of other alpha-adrenergic receptor stimulants such as methoxamine or phenylephrine; an ↑ in total systemic resistance may cause supine hypertension that can precipitate congestive heart failure (CHF), myocardial ischemia, infarction, or stroke in susceptible individuals. Supine hypertension is more common during the initiation of midodrine therapy; during the titration period, adverse effects include supine hypertension, which may cause headaches and pounding in the ears. Reflex bradycardia may occur, and caution is needed when the drug is combined with agents that cause bradycardia (digoxin, beta-blockers, diltiazem, and verapamil). Urinary retention is an important adverse effect in elderly males.
- The drug is contraindicated in patients with significant coronary heart disease (CHD), CHF, renal failure, urinary retention, thyrotoxicosis, and pheochromocytoma. Midodrine is renally excreted, and care is necessary to ↓ the dose and ↑ the dosing interval in patients with renal dysfunction.

In patients who are not responsive to midodrine or fludrocortisone and have sustained injuries, atrial pacing with a HR of 100/minute may afford some amelioration if combined with increased salt intake, fludrocortisone, elevation of the head of the bed during sleep, and full-length leotards to enhance venous return.

A release of histamine, prostaglandin D, and other vasodilators from mast cell proliferation (mastocytosis) causes vasodilation, and is a rare cause of postural hypotension.

Instruct the patient to change posture slowly and to engage in calf muscle flexion prior to standing. Elevating the head of the bed and gradually changing posture may provide a salutary response.

Aortic Arch Syndrome

Pulseless disease (Takayasu's disease) is an arteritis-producing occlusion of the aortic arch vessels, and syncope may result. The BP is lower in the arms than the legs.

Tachyarrhythmias

The major determinant in cardiac syncope is an ↓ in cardiac output due to reduced HR or ineffectual cardiac contractions secondary to arrhythmia. A diagnosis of cardiac syncope connotes a guarded prognosis with a mortality of less than or equal to 24% in 1 year, although this varies greatly according to the mechanism of the arrhythmia. Early diagnosis with appropriate therapy is lifesaving. Obvious causes of cardiac syncope are listed in Table 13.1.

Sustained rapid ventricular tachycardia (VT) (i.e. VT duration >30 seconds) or symptomatic nonsustained VT commonly causes syncope. When VT is not apparent on the ECG rhythm strip or Holter monitoring, the underlying mechanism may be revealed by EP testing.

Atrial fibrillation (AF) or other supraventricular tachycardia (SVT) with fast ventricular rates may cause syncope, especially in the elderly, or when rapid rates supervene in patients with Wolff-Parkinson-White (WPW) Syndrome.

Aortic Stenosis, Hypertrophic Cardiomyopathy

Syncope in aortic stenosis is typically exertional and suggests significant disease with life expectancy of 1-3 years. With HCM, syncope may be precipitated by exercise but can occur with normal activities or at rest.

Sinus Node Dysfunction, Sick Sinus Syndrome

Severe bradycardia (30-40/minute), sinus arrest, and brady- or tachyarrhythmias may cause lightheadedness, dizziness, confusion, memory loss, or presyncope. More than or equal to one of these associated symptoms usually produce a 1- to 10-second warning prior to syncope; however, syncope can occur without warning in this category of patients, and injuries may occur.

The setting is usually ischemic heart disease (IHD) with old infarction. The ECG may be normal or show evidence of old infarction, bradycardia, or sinus arrest. A 48-hour Holter gives about a 70% chance of detecting a significant arrhythmia, with symptoms noted in the patient's diary, as opposed to less than 48% with a single 24-hour Holter monitoring. Fairly often, repeat 48-hour Holter monitoring is necessary once or twice over a couple of weeks to identify a bradyarrhythmia that is symptomatic. Treatment of sinus node dysfunction is given in other chapter. Sinus node dysfunction and severe bradycardia causing presyncope or syncope may be due to drug therapy that inadvertently depresses sinus node function. Verapamil, diltiazem, digitalis, beta-blockers, Class 1 antiarrhythmic agents, amiodarone, and especially their combinations may cause severe bradycardia, Atrioventricular (AV) block, and asystole in susceptible individuals. Discontinuation of the causative agent or agents is unfortunately rarely practical, and pacing is usually indicated.

Atrioventricular Block, Stokes–Adams Attacks

- Patients with Mobitz type II or third-degree AV block may suddenly have an occurrence of transient asystole or ventricular fibrillation (VF) with complete cessation of cerebral blood flow. Since VF is instantaneous, the cerebral circulation is suddenly deprived of perfusion, resulting in loss of consciousness usually without warning.
- Episodes can happen on sitting, lying, or walking. The unconscious patient appears very pale and, on arousal, becomes flushed as blood rushes to the head. When a patient is assessed hours or days later, ECG may show manifestations of Mobitz type II or complete AV block, right bundle branch block (RBBB) or left bundle branch block (LBBB), or bilateral disease. Cardiac pacing should be instituted.

Prolonged QT Syndrome

- Recurrent syncope in children and young adults with a positive family history may be due to prolonged QT syndrome.
- Episodes of life-threatening arrhythmias appear to be precipitated by increased sympathetic stimulation.
- Thus, beta-blockers have a role in management, despite a tendency for bradycardia in many of these patients. Propranolol in doses of 80–160 mg qd or a similar noncardioselective beta-blocker without agonist activity is preferred.

When recurrent syncope is uncontrolled by beta-blockers, combined pacing and beta-blocker therapy may be required. In uncontrolled cases, excision of the left stellate ganglion may be a last resort.

ELECTROPHYSIOLOGIC STUDY

A provocative EP study is useful in revealing a cardiac cause in approximately 12% of patients with unexplained syncope. Approximately 21% of these patients with negative studies are subsequently diagnosed as having intermittent high-degree AV block or sinus node disease. Caution is therefore necessary because an EP study is not a sensitive test to expose symptomatic bradycardia.

Electrophysiologic studies have been shown to initiate sustained monomorphic VT in approximately 18% of patients and nonsustained VT in approximately 23%. Nonsustained VT, especially if only for a few seconds duration, carries a minimal risk in patients with syncope and requires no arrhythmia therapy. Patients with syncope and sustained monomorphic VT do not appear to benefit from antiarrhythmic therapy, and the incidence of syncope is not reduced except when amiodarone is used as therapy.

Electrophysiologic studies appear to be justifiable in patients who have a high probability of induction of sustained monomorphic VT.
- Post-myocardial infarction (MI) patients with unexplained syncope
- Left ventricular ejection fraction (LVEF) less than 30%
- Left ventricular aneurysm
- Complex ventricular ectopy on Holter.

HEAD-UP TILT TESTING

This test is not advisable if proper thinking is used: it has a low yield and has precipitated stroke, albeit rarely.

PACING

- During vasovagal syncope, bradycardia (cardioinhibitory response) and/or hypotension (vasodepressor response) may occur, decreasing cerebral blood flow and causing transient loss of consciousness.
- Bradycardia is not necessarily the cause of and can occur distinctly after a faint due to a vasovagal reflex (Flowchart 13.1). Therefore, pacing alone may have little, if any, effect.

BIBLIOGRAPHY

1. Bennett MT, Leader N, Krahn AD. Recurrent syncope: differential diagnosis and management. Heart. 2015;101:1591-9.
2. Khan MG. Practical Cardiology. New Delhi, India: Jaypee Brothers Medical Publishers (P) Ltd.; 2018.
3. Olshansky B. Vasovagal syncope: to pace or not to pace. J Am Coll Cardiol. 2017;70(14):1729-31.

CHAPTER 14

Bronchodilators: Asthma–COPD

BRONCHODILATORS

- Bronchodilators are available in several different *dosage* forms—aerosol, oral, and intravenous (IV).
- Proper aerosol technique is most important.

For patients with significant recurrent asthma or episodes of bronchoconstriction in individuals with chronic obstructive pulmonary disease (COPD) to do as follows:

- When a steroid inhaler is prescribed, it is best not to use one combined with a beta-agonist; use separately—it is most important to first use a rapid acting beta-agonist, (salbutamol) 3 puffs; with 5–7 min for the drug to take effect to open the airways, then use the steroid puffer.
- When used as a combination in patients with bronchoconstriction the steroid fails to reach the lower bronchial tree.
- Many chest physicians prescribe a combination product that is effective mainly in individuals with mild disease.
- Compared with inhaled long-acting beta-agonists (LABA) combined with corticosteroids, long-acting muscarinic antagonists (LAMA) combined with inhaled LABA may be associated with a lower risk of COPD exacerbation and with greater improvement in expiratory volume in 1 second (FEV_1) without differences in the incidence of serious severe adverse events or quality of life.
- The study is flawed if the LABA was used with corticosteroid as a combination product.
- Some patients have bronchiolitis that trigger asthmatic episodes. As soon as sputum is noted to be yellowish, it is advisable to give a 7-day treatment with amoxicillin (if not allergic to penicillin)
- Azithromycin was shown to be beneficial in a controlled study of patients with persistent uncontrolled asthma. 420 patients [median age 60 years (interquartile range (IQR) 50–60), 40% males] with uncontrolled persistent asthma despite a maintenance treatment with medium-to-high dose inhaled corticosteroids plus a long-acting bronchodilator [LABA (98%); long-acting muscarinic antagonist (17%)] were randomly assigned to receive azithromycin 500 mg or placebo three times per

week for 48 weeks. Azithromycin significantly reduced the rate of total asthma exacerbations compared with placebo [1.07 exacerbations per patient-year vs 1·86 exacerbations per patient-year; incidence rate ratio (IRR) 0.59 (95% CI 0·47–0·74)) as well as the rate of severe exacerbations (requiring treatment with systemic corticosteroids or hospitalization; azithromycin improved asthma-related quality of life across all domains of the Asthma-specific Quality of Life Questionnaire. Additionally, azithromycin use was associated with improved asthma control; reduced the number of patients reporting a respiratory tract infection, and lowered the rate of antibiotic courses for respiratory indications.
- In this trial, azithromycin was generally safe and well tolerated, though
- Diarrhea was more frequent in users of azithromycin than placebo (34% vs 19%).
- There was a nonsignificant increase in azithromycin-resistant bacteria in surveillance sputum cultures of patients treated with azithromycin.

But caution—watch for interacting drugs that increase QT interval. The drug may precipitate arrhythmias.
- A large randomized, double-blind, and placebo-controlled trial of azithromycin in adult patients with persistent uncontrolled asthma in Australia. 420 patients [median age 60 years (IQR 50–60), 40% males] with uncontrolled persistent asthma despite a maintenance treatment with medium-to-high dose inhaled corticosteroids plus a long-acting bronchodilator [LABA (98%); long-acting muscarinic antagonist (17%)] were randomly assigned to receive azithromycin 500 mg or placebo three times per week for 48 weeks.
- This landmark study has many strengths. First, the large number of patients and the long duration of treatment provided sufficient power to unequivocally show that add-on therapy with azithromycin in adult patients with uncontrolled asthma reduced exacerbation rates and improved quality of life in this study.
- Second, since asthma is a heterogeneous disease, it is of benefit that all study patients were well phenotyped, including assessment of the asthma inflammatory phenotypes using induced sputum, the gold standard. Unexpectedly, azithromycin reduced exacerbations in both eosinophilic patients with both eosinophilic and noneosinophilic asthma. Add-on therapy with azithromycin is effective and safe in adult patients with uncontrolled asthma despite treatment with inhaled corticosteroids and LABA.
- The effects of long-term therapy with macrolides on community microbial resistance remain a public health concern.
- A large well-conducted trial involving children that was mandated by the Food and Drug Administration (FDA) and that shows no excess

Box 14.1: Patient instruction for optimal MDI use.
- Remove cap from inhaler:
  - Shake inhaler for a few seconds
  - Hold inhaler upright and tilt head back slightly
  - Place inhaler between lips* or approximately 2 cm in front of open mouth. Alternatively, a spacer device can be used
  - Take a deep breath and exhale completely
  - Begin inhaling slowly and immediately press down on top of inhaler to deliver aerosol medicine
  - Complete inhalation and hold breath for 5–10 seconds
- Wait at least 2–3 minutes then repeat above for subsequent puffs

(MDI, metered-dose inhaler)
*Recommended for anticholinergic drug, ipratropium bromide, to avoid contact with eyes, or use a spacing device

of serious asthma events in children receiving a combination inhaler containing fluticasone propionate and salmeterol.
- A trial involving adults, there was some evidence of efficacy in terms of secondary outcomes for LABAs (Box 14.1).

The bronchodilators discussed in this chapter will be grouped according to the following classifications:
- Beta-adrenergic agonists
- Anticholinergic agents
- Methylxanthines.

A comparison of various bronchodilators is presented in Table 14.1.

Beta$_2$-adrenergic Agonists

Beta-agonists provide the foundation for acute reversal therapy of obstructive airway disease. The rapidity with which they work makes them the first choice of physicians and patients. The beneficial effects of epinephrine in the treatment of asthma were described early in the 20th century.

Subsequently, numerous other agents similar in structure but more beta$_2$-selective have been developed and tried by several routes with variable degrees of success. The greatest benefit of the beta$_2$-selective agonists may not be in the bronchodilatory capabilities but rather in the diminution of the adverse cardiac side effects. With the advent of beta$_2$-selective agonists, the use of nonselective beta-agonists, such as isoproterenol, metaproterenol, and isoetharine has become inadvisable.
- Short-acting beta-agonists give rapid relief from bronchospasm, but their overuse is a factor in asthma-related deaths, and the less-selective agents have been associated with epidemics of patients dying during acute asthma attacks. In children with uncontrolled asthma.

Table 14.1: Comparison of bronchodilators.

	Beta-adrenergic agonists	Anticholinergics*	Methylxanthines#
Etiology of asthma			
Allergic	++++	+ +/−	+ +/−
Emotional	++	++++	+/−
Exercise-induced	++++	+/−	+ +/−
Intrinsic	++++	+/−	+ +/−
Irritant-induced	++++	+++	+ +/−
Chronic obstructive pulmonary disease			
Emphysema	+/−	+++	+ +/−
Bronchitis	+++	+++	+ +/−
Action			
Onset	Fast (5 minutes)	Slow (1–2 hours)	Variable
Duration	Variable	Variable	Long
Adverse effects			
Arrhythmia-potential	+++	+/−	++++
Hypokalemia	++	−	+/−
Nausea	++	−	++++
Tachycardia	++++	+/−	++
Tremor	+++	−	+++

*Ipratropium bromide will be compared as it is the safest and most frequently prescribed.
#Oral preparations will be compared.

Pharmacology and Mechanisms of Action

- Beta-agonists are structural analogs of norepinephrine
- Modification of the ring constituents generally results in prolongation of action, while modification of the terminal amine confers beta-selectivity
- Aerosolized $beta_2$-agonists have a relatively short time to onset of action, generally within 15 minutes. Oral formulations have an onset of action in the range of 30 minutes to 1 hour, which depends on gastrointestinal (GI) absorption. The duration of action depends on the formulation of the ring constituent and varies with each compound
- $Beta_2$-agonist stimulation of bronchial smooth muscle results in relaxation, and consequently, bronchodilation. This effect is believed to be mediated by ↑ intracellular cyclic adenosine monophosphate (AMP) levels. Increased cyclic AMP leads to a ↓ in cytosolic Ca and smooth muscle relaxation. Virtually all beta-receptors in the bronchial smooth muscles are of the $beta_2$-subtype
- Both $beta_1$- and $beta_2$-agonists ↑ mucus secretion from submucosal glands. $Beta_2$-agonist stimulation increases ion transport in epithelial

cells which, in turn, leads to ↑ water secretion, beta-receptor stimulation may thereby improve mucociliary clearance
- The secretion of histamine and other mast cell mediators appears to be modulated by $beta_2$-adrenergic stimulation, as is pulmonary vasoconstriction
- Lastly, beta-adrenergic receptors are found throughout the alveolar walls. Approximately, two-thirds are of the $beta_2$-subtype. While stimulation of these alveolar beta-receptors results partly in stimulation of surfactant secretion by type II pneumocytes, the function of beta-receptors in other cell populations is not yet clearly defined

Adverse effects are much more prevalent when nonspecific beta-agonists are used
- Common $beta_1$ side effects include tachycardia, palpitations, and muscle tremors
- Hypokalemia may also result from beta-agonist use. This appears to be mediated by $beta_2$-receptor stimulation of a membrane-bound Na/K ATPase. This hypokalemic response has been implicated in the development of cardiac arrhythmias and is speculated to have a role in sudden death in patients with asthma. It would be prudent, therefore, to closely monitor serum K in those patients given frequent high-dose $beta_2$-agonists concomitantly with K-losing diuretics. This would be especially true of patients at risk for cardiac arrhythmias, such as those with congestive heart failure (CHF) or ischemic heart disease (IHD).

Dosages of $beta_2$-selective agonists are given in Table 14.2. The recommendations in Table 14.2 are intended for use in mild-to-moderate obstructive airway disease. More frequent dosing intervals of the shorter-acting $beta_2$-selective agonists (salbutamol and terbutaline) are indicated in more severe obstructive disease, specifically status asthmaticus. In this case, the dosing intervals may be decreased to q 30–60 min, although this should be done only in hospitalized and monitored patients. Some clinical situations require reductions in dosage and dosing interval, most notably in patients with heart disease or those receiving monoamine *oxidase* inhibitors and/or tricyclic antidepressants.

Clinical Applications

- $Beta_2$-agonist therapy is most effective in the treatment of asthma and in the prevention of exercise-induced (and other forms of) bronchospasm. $Beta_2$-agonists are the cornerstone of emergent therapy for the management of acute asthma and exacerbations of COPD. The role of regular $beta_2$-agonist use in chronic stable asthma is less certain. As needed, administration of agonists in conjunction with inhaled corticosteroids is preferable therapy in patients with stable disease

Table 14.2: Beta$_2$ agonist preparation.

Beta$_2$ agonist	Formulation	Dosage
Albuterol (USA)	Tablet; 2 mg	Up to 4 mg qid
Salbutamol (Canada, UK) Ventolin (USA, Can, UK) Proventil (USA) Aerolin (UK) Salbulin (UK)	Tablet; 24 mg Syrup; 2 mg/5 mL Repetabs; 4 mg (ext. release) MDI; 90 µg/puff Solution; 0.25% Solution; 0.5% Rotocaps; 200 µg	Up to 4 mg qid Up to 4 mg qid Up to 16 mg bid 2 puffs q 4–6 h 2.5 mg/3 mL q 4–6 h 2.5 mg/3 ml q 4–6 h 200 µg q 4–6 h
Bitolterol Tomalate (USA)	MDI; 350 µg/puff	2–3 puffs q 4–6 h
Fenoterol Berotec (Canada, UK)	MDI; 180–360 µg/puff	1–2 puffs q 6–8 h
Pirbuterol Maxair (USA) Exirel (UK)	MDI; 200–400 µg/puff	1–2 puffs q 6 h
Reproterol Bronchodil (UK)	MDI; 500 µg/puff	1 puff q 6 h
Rimiterol Plumadil (UK)	MDI; 400–600 mg/puff	1 puff q 6 h
Terbutaline Brethaire (USA) Brethine (USA) Bricanyl (USA, Can, UK)	Tablet; 2.5 mg Tablet; 5 mg Solution; 1 mg/mL MDI; 200 µg/puff	2.5–5 mg q 6–8 h not >15 mg/day Nebulizer 1–2 mg q 4–6 h Subcutaneous—0.25 mg repeated in 15–30 min Not >0.5 mg q 4 h IV—Not recommended 2 puffs q 4–6 h

- There is data suggesting beneficial effects in chronic airflow obstruction with less reversibility. These beneficial effects include improvements in objective measurements of airway function, improvements in exercise capacity, and improvements in overall subjective quality of life measurements. However, while beta$_2$-agonists are clearly superior to anticholinergics in asthma, anticholinergics have equivalent, if not greater, effects in most patients with chronic bronchitis and emphysema. This is particularly true for patients with "fixed" obstructive airway disease.

Anticholinergics

Two forms of anticholinergic bronchodilators are most commonly used—atropine (as SO_4 and methonitrate salts) and ipratropium bromide.

Pharmacology and Mechanism of Action

- Anticholinergic bronchodilators act through antagonism of the muscarinic receptor.
- Stimulation of these receptors is believed to be responsible for "resting" bronchomotor tone.
- Muscarinic receptors are found predominantly in the larger, central airways, and the anticholinergics are believed to exert their greatest bronchodilatory effects on these airways.
- Anticholinergics appear to mediate the bronchoconstrictive effects of certain stimuli, including cholinergics (carbachol and methacholine), cold air, and psychogenic stimuli.
- Anticholinergic bronchodilators have little or no effect on those bronchoconstrictive effects believed to be the result of inflammatory mediators, e.g. histamine. This makes them theoretically less effective for antigen-induced bronchoconstriction, as is frequently seen in asthma.
- Compared to beta-agonists, the anticholinergics have a delayed onset of action, with maximal response occurring in 1–2 hours. However, the duration of action is longer, with the effects being maintained for less than or equal to 6 hours.

Adverse effects of anticholinergic alkaloids are easily predicted and result from their antagonism of the muscarinic receptor.

- Inhalation of atropine may result in mouth dryness, dry skin, mydriasis, tachycardia, urinary retention, flushing, GI disturbances, and visual blurring. These symptoms are dosage dependent. Higher doses (>5 mg) result in central nervous system (CNS) excitement, fever, headache, weakness, slurred speech, bowel and bladder dysfunction, delirium, and eventually coma.
- There have also been reports of decreased mucociliary clearance secondary to the use of atropine. The mechanism of this effect is multifactorial.

Adverse effects do not seem to be a problem with ipratropium bromide, whose use is much less frequently associated with side effects, even in large doses. It has been estimated that dosages 100 times more than currently used for bronchodilatory effects would be necessary to produce significant side effects.

- The most common complaints associated with ipratropium bromide use are a bitter taste, mouth dryness, and throat or tracheal irritation. These are usually well tolerated, and the incidence is significantly decreased when a spacer device is used.
- One adverse effect that is clinically significant is mydriasis after inadvertent aerosol delivery to the eyes. This can result in acute angle closure glaucoma, in addition to unnecessary diagnostic evaluation by individuals not aware of this side effect.

The difference in the side effect profiles of the two anticholinergics is the result of structural differences. Atropine is a tertiary ammonium compound with a neutral charge, while ipratropium bromide is a quaternary ammonium compound with a positive charge. The charge difference makes ipratropium bromide relatively lipid insoluble, resulting in markedly decreased systemic absorption of ipratropium bromide as compared to atropine. With the advent of ipratropium bromide in most markets, the use of atropine salts has waned.

Ipratropium bromide: Dosage—2-4 puffs via metered dose inhaler q 6 hours. Each actuation of the MDI contains 40 μg of ipratropium. Higher doses have been shown to be beneficial in patients with COPD with essentially no ↑ in adverse effects. An inhalant solution (250 μg/mL) is available in Europe and Canada for use as a wet aerosol with a recommended dose of 100–500 μg q 4 hours. This agent is often given in combination (salbutamol 0.5 mL in 2 mL ipratropium q 4-6 hours).

Clinical Applications

- In diseases, such as chronic bronchitis and emphysema, the use of ipratropium bromide may result in therapeutic effects comparable to or even more than those of the beta-adrenergic agonists.
- In addition, the combined effect of ipratropium bromide and $beta_2$-agonists appears to be better than either drug alone. This synergistic effect appears to be active in asthma as well. Ipratropium bromide also appears to act synergistically with methylxanthines. The three agents together have also been shown, in some instances, to be more effective than any single agent or combination of agents.
- In patients with fixed obstructive pulmonary disease unresponsive to beta-agonist therapy (specifically emphysema), ipratropium use may not show an improvement in FEV_1 but it results in an ↑ in vital capacity, with subsequent decreased work of breathing and hence symptomatic improvement.
- Tachyphylaxis does not appear to develop with ipratropium therapy in contrast to beta-agonist therapy.
- Older patients with obstructive airway disease appear to have a better clinical response to ipratropium than to beta-agonists.
- The effects of ipratropium bromide have a longer duration of action when compared to the presently available agonists, although longer-acting $beta_2$-agonists are currently undergoing trial (*see* Table 14.1).
- While the effects of ipratropium bromide in asthma are less clear, there currently exists a considerable amount of data to support its use in asthmatic patients. Specifically, in those patients whose symptoms are not controlled by $beta_2$-agonist or theophylline therapy, a trial of ipratropium bromide is indicated as an adjunct to these therapies.

Theophylline

Theophylline is a methylxanthine and has been in use in obstructive airway disease since the early 20th century. Its use has decreased since its time of greatest popularity in the 1970s and 1980s.

Pharmacology and Mechanisms of Action

The precise mechanism of action of bronchodilation by methylxanthines is not well defined, but the primary effect appears to be relaxation of smooth muscle in the bronchial walls:
- Initial research was concentrated on the inhibition of phosphodiesterase. However, other phosphodiesterase inhibitors currently in use in clinical medicine (e.g. dipyridamole) do not result in bronchodilatory effects similar to those of theophylline.
- Other proposed mechanisms of bronchodilatory action have included antagonism of adenosine receptors, prostaglandin antagonism, altered metabolism of smooth muscle, and stimulation of catecholamine release.
- In addition to its bronchodilatory effects, theophylline may ↑ diaphragmatic contractility and reduce diaphragmatic fatigue.
- There is evidence of improved biventricular cardiac performance as well
- Theophylline may stimulate hypoxic ventilatory drive, enhance mucociliary clearance, inhibit mast cell mediator release, and ↓ posteroanterior (PA) vasoconstriction.
- There are data to suggest an anti-inflammatory mechanism of theophylline in the therapy of asthma. It appears to be effective in blunting the late asthmatic response to bronchial challenge. This action of theophylline requires further definition.

Most theophylline preparations are primarily hepatically metabolized, with the exception of dihydroxypropyl theophylline, which is excreted unchanged in the urine. Unlike other bronchodilators, theophylline use is best guided by serum concentrations.
- Multiple studies have shown that the bronchodilatory effects are relatively insignificant in most patients at a serum level of less than 10 μg/mL (10 mg/L or 55 μmol/L).
- At levels more than 20 μg/mL (20 mg/L or 110 μmol/L), toxic effects often emerge.
- Thus, it is recommended that serum concentrations of 10–20 μg/mL (10–20 mg/L or 55–110 μmol/L) define the therapeutic endpoints.
- Benefit may be observed in some patients at lower serum theophylline concentrations, in the range of 6–10 μg/mL (6–10 mg/L or 35–55 μmol/L). This is seen predominantly in patients who receive theophylline in addition to beta-agonist therapy. The benefits deal primarily with

subjective measures of improvement, such as patient's perception of disease activity, quality of life, and decreased hospital admissions.

Adverse effects are generally dose related and are much more prevalent at plasma concentrations more than 20 µg/mL (20 mg/L or 110 µmol/L)
- The most common side effects include abdominal discomfort, nausea, vomiting, diarrhea, headache, tremor, and restlessness
- A mild diuretic effect and ↑ gastric acid secretion may also occur
- Insomnia and other disturbances of sleep pattern have been reported
- While these symptoms are bothersome to patients and may result in noncompliance, they are rarely life-threatening
- However, theophylline, even at therapeutic concentrations, has been associated with cardiac dysrhythmia, including atrial and ventricular premature contractions (VPCs), atrial fibrillation (AF), and perhaps most commonly, multifocal atrial tachycardia. At higher concentrations, seizures and more malignant cardiac arrhythmias may occur, which can be lethal, albeit rare

Side effects can be evident in some patients at any serum concentration but are distinctly more common with levels more than 30 µg/mL (30 mg/L or 165 µmol/L). Adequate monitoring and maintenance of theophylline levels in the therapeutic range lessens these adverse drug manifestations.

Dosage: A partial list of available oral formulations is shown in Table 14.3. While dosage must be individualized for the patient and the underlying illness, rough estimates of oral dosing are as follows:
- *Oral loading dose:* 5 mg/kg ideal body weight
- *Oral maintenance dose*: 10 mg/kg ideal body weight/day, divided into three doses, depending upon formulation

Oral dosage must be adjusted to maintain serum level of 10–20 µg/mL (10–20 mg/L or 55–110 µmol/L).

Intravenous dosing estimates and clinical scenarios requiring dosage adjustment are given in Table 14.3. Theophylline drug interactions are listed in Table 14.4.

Clinical Applications

- Although it has little effect on the airways of normal individuals, theophylline ameliorates bronchoconstriction in individuals with asthma.
- The bronchodilatory effects add to those of beta-agonists and anticholinergics, but theophylline is a less effective bronchodilator than either agent alone.

There is a subset of patients with asthma who experience symptoms during the nocturnal hours and have disrupted sleep secondary to these symptoms. In these patients, there has been some improvement in symptoms and sleep with bedtime dosing of a 24-hour theophylline preparation.

Table 14.3: Dosing guidelines for intravenous theophylline.

Intravenous dosage:
- 5–6 mg/kg ideal body weight given over 20–30 minutes if no theophylline preparation used in the last 24 hours
- 2–3 mg/kg ideal body weight given over 20–30 minutes if a theophylline preparation used in the last 24 hours
- Maintain an infusion rate of 0.4–0.6 mg/kg ideal body weight per hour with the following adjustments in dosing due to other clinical circumstances:

Increase dosage 0.6–0.8 mg/kg/hr:	Decrease dosage 0.3–0.4 mg/kg/hr:
• Children	• Elderly
• Cigarette smoker	• Hepatic insufficiency
• Hyperthyroidism	• Hypothyroidism
• Marijuana use	• Congestive heart failure
• High protein diet	• Febrile illness
• Medications	• Medications

Note: Serum theophylline concentration should be determined approximately 6 hours after initial infusion and dosage adjusted accordingly. A general rule is adjustment of dose by 25% to achieve an increment or decrement of 5 µg/mL (5 mg/L or 27.5 µmol/L) in serum theophylline concentration.

The beneficial effects of theophylline in patients with chronic bronchitis and emphysema are less clear. There does appear to be subjective symptomatic improvement in patients with chronic bronchitis, but objective improvement in airflow is lacking

Theophylline should be considered for use in patients with asthma and chronic bronchitis who have failed optimal inhalation therapy prior to the initiation of systemic steroids. However, the decision to begin theophylline therapy versus steroid therapy should include a knowledge of possible drug interactions and underlying disease states that alter theophylline pharmacokinetics. In some cases, the toxicity of short-term systemic steroids will be less than the toxicity of theophylline and may therefore be the preferred alternative.

ASTHMA

Asthma is a disease of the airways characterized by ↑ responsiveness of the trachea and bronchi to a wide range of stimuli. Intermittent symptoms of cough, chest tightness, and wheezing usually alter in severity, either spontaneously or due to treatment. The widespread airway narrowing results from a combination of smooth muscle contraction, inflammation, edema, and mucous secretion. *Airway inflammation is present in virtually all patients with asthma* and, with widespread mucous plugging of airways, is a constant finding in patients who have died of status asthmaticus.

Table 14.4: Theophylline interactions.

Drug	Effect	Response
Allopurinol	Decrease theophylline clearance	Decrease dose of theophylline
Barbiturates	Increase theophylline clearance	Increase dose of theophylline
Carbamazepine	Increase theophylline clearance	Increase dose of theophylline
Corticosteroids	Variable metabolic effects	Monitor theophylline levels
Coumarins	Interferes with assay method for serum level resulting in falsely low values	No adjustment in dose necessary
Diltiazem	Slight decrease in theophylline clearance	Possible decrease in theophylline dose
Erythromycin	Decrease theophylline clearance	Decrease dose of theophylline
Estrogens	Decrease theophylline clearance	Decrease dose of theophylline
H_2 Blockers Cimetidine Ranitidine Famotidine	– Decrease theophylline clearance No effect No effect	– Decrease dose of theophylline No adjustment No adjustment
Influenza Vaccine	Decrease theophylline clearance	Decrease dose of theophylline
Interferon	Decrease theophylline clearance	Decrease dose of theophylline
Isoniazid	Decrease theophylline clearance	Decrease dose of theophylline
Isoproterenol	Increase theophylline clearance	Increase dose of theophylline
Lithium	Increase lithium clearance	Increase dose of lithium
Mexiletine	Decrease theophylline clearance	Decrease dose of theophylline
Nicorette	No effect	No response
Oral contraceptives	Decrease theophylline clearance	Decrease dose of theophylline
Pancuronium	Decrease pancuronium responsiveness	Increase dose of pancuronium
Phenytoin	Increase theophylline clearance	Increase dose of theophylline
Quinolones	Decrease theophylline clearance	Decrease dose of theophylline

Contd...

Contd...

Drug	Effect	Response
Tobacco smoking	Increase theophylline clearance	Increase dose of theophylline
Troleandomycin	Decrease theophylline clearance	Decrease dose of theophylline
Verapamil	Decrease theophylline clearance	Decrease dose of theophylline
Vidarabine	Decrease theophylline clearance	Decrease dose of theophylline

The complex forces that combine to cause asthma result in certain macroscopic and microscopic features that are common to those who have died from this disease:
- Overinflated lungs that do not deflate upon opening the thoracic cavity
- Widespread airway plugging with thick mucus
- Airway wall thickening
- Upper lobe bronchiectasis (sometimes)
- Little evidence of emphysema
- *Infiltration of airway walls by inflammatory cells, particularly eosinophilic infiltration*
- Epithelial desquamation
- Smooth muscle hypertrophy
- Basement membrane thickening; subepithelial deposition of collagen.

Other features of asthma include mucus gland hyperplasia and ↑ goblet cell numbers. Patients with asthma who are asymptomatic appear to have varying degrees of the abnormalities noted above.

Asthma Triggers

Allergens

Allergic asthma depends upon immunoglobulin E (IgE) response modulated by B and T cell lymphocytes and the interaction of mast-cell-bound IgE with antigen. Small amounts of antigen reach distal airways, where mast cells interdigitate with epithelial cells. There is usually an immediate response, resulting in bronchoconstriction, followed in some patients by a late-phase response 6–10 hours later. Once contracted, the mast cells and other cells release mediators that cause constriction, edema, and vascular congestion.
- Major airborne allergens include house dust, mites, and pollens.
- Asthmatics who respond to allergens usually have a fair number of antigens that can trigger their disease.

- The role of different foods (Cow's milk, monosodium glutamate, preservatives, food coloring agents, etc.) are not clearly defined, although some individuals may react strongly.
- Symptoms can be continual or seasonal, depending on the antigen.

Pharmacologic agents that trigger asthma include drugs such as aspirin, tartrazine dye, beta-blockers, and sulfating agents.

- Nasal polyps, rhinorrhea, and asthma comprise a syndrome that has been associated with aspirin use in some patients
- Sulfating agents such as potassium bisulfite and sodium bisulfite, sulfur dioxide, and others are widely used in the fresh-food industry and may cause symptoms in some.

Environmental and Air Pollution

Climatic conditions can ↑ the concentration of allergens and cause exacerbation of asthma. Occupational asthma refers to patients who develop symptoms while in the work place in response to some specific trigger. These symptoms will often improve when the patient is out of the offending environment, but chronic problems can also occur. Specific agents include:
- Wood and vegetable dusts, such as western red cedar
- Metal salts, such as platinum, chrome, and nickel
- Pharmaceutical agents, including antibiotics, piperazine, and cimetidine
- Industrial chemicals and plastics, such as toluene, isocyanate, phthalic acid, ethylenediamine, and others
- Biologic enzymes, including detergents
- Animal and insect dusts, serums, and secretions.

The underlying mechanisms for airway obstruction in occupational asthma include the formation of specific IgE, the direct release of factors causing bronchoconstriction by the offending agent, and direct airway stimulation.

Infections

Respiratory infections by viruses and bacteria are the most common causes of asthma exacerbation. Respiratory syncytial and parainfluenza virus are major offenders in children, while rhinovirus and influenza virus are *most* common in adults. The reason that viruses induce asthma is unclear, but bronchial hyperresponsiveness may last less than 8 weeks. *Bacteria* are less common than viruses as triggers of asthmatic exacerbation but can superinfect a prior viral process.

Exercise and Stress

Physical exertion can worsen asthma, and the first episode often occurs with exercise in children. This acute process may be due to thermal changes in the intrathoracic airways as heat and water are transferred from tracheal mucosa to the inspired air. High ventilation may lower airway temperature further, especially in colder, dryer air, and worsen symptoms. Hence, ambient temperatures and the level of exertion may correlate with the degree of obstruction. Activities such as cross-country skiing or ice skating usually produce more symptoms than swimming. Objective *evidence* suggests that psychological features play a role in asthmatic symptoms. These interactions are complex but may be *related* to vagal efferent activity mediating airway caliber. The extent of the influence of psychological factors on asthma is unclear.

The six predominant causes of asthma-related death are:
- Lack of access to healthcare or failure to seek timely professional help
- Lack of personal action plans
- Underuse of glucocorticoids
- Overuse or inappropriate use of bronchodilators
- Underestimation of asthma severity by treating doctors and by parents
- Lack of objective measures of airway obstruction and nonadherence to the regimen.

For the unusual child with asthma who needs more than low-dose inhaled glucocorticoids to control the disease or who has persistent, objectively documented, and variable airflow obstruction, the present trial provides reassuring evidence that combination inhalers containing a LABA and an inhaled glucocorticoid are safe.

Among adolescents and adults with predominantly moderate-to-severe asthma, treatment with budesonide–formoterol was associated with a lower risk of asthma exacerbations than budesonide and a similar risk of serious asthma-related events.

Diagnosis

Symptoms and signs include:
- *Symptoms:* These include dyspnea, chest tightness, wheezing and cough, exercise intolerance, rhinitis, sinusitis, nasal polyposis, and atopic dermatitis. The hallmark of asthma is the variable nature of respiratory symptoms that are caused by the changing degree of airway obstruction. The marked variability in degree of airway obstruction is the main factor distinguishing asthma from other forms of chronic obstructive lung disease. Typically, symptoms in asthma are episodic. In some cases, the patient's clinical history may be so characteristic of asthma that a presumptive diagnosis of asthma can be comfortably made on the history alone. It is important to remember, however, that "not all that wheezes is asthma" and, in most cases, it will be necessary to have objective data to support a clinical diagnosis. Other features of medical history include—positive family history for allergies or asthma (50%), aspirin sensitivity (5-10%), and frequent association with sinusitis.

- *Pertinent findings of the physical examination:* These include nasal polyps and scattered or diffuse wheezes with prolonged expiration in the chest.
- *Differential diagnosis of asthma:* It includes emphysema, bronchitis, CHF, pulmonary emboli, foreign body in airway, aspiration, carcinoid syndrome, bronchiectasis, laryngeal edema, hyperventilation syndrome, factitious wheezing, and cystic fibrosis.

Clinical data indicating severe asthma include:
- Previous intensive care unit (ICU) admission, frequent emergency room visits, or hospital stay more than 4 days for treatment of documented severe asthma.
- Recent oral corticosteroid use for exacerbation
- Brittle asthma
- Extreme dyspnea with inability to speak more than a few words
- Pulsus paradoxus more than 18 mm Hg
- Use of accessory muscles and paradoxical thoracoabdominal motion
- Diaphoresis
- Inability to lie supine
- Heart rate (HR) more than 120 beats/minute
- Respiratory rate more than 30
- Absence of audible wheezing in a patient with severe exacerbation of asthma
- Partial pressure of oxygen (PaO_2) less than 60 mm Hg
- Partial pressure of carbon dioxide ($PaCO_2$) more than or equal to 40 mm Hg
- Peak expiratory flow rate (PEFR) or FEV_1 less than 30% of predicted for adults
- Failure of PEFR to improve more than or equal to 10% after initial treatment.

Pulmonary function testing may be normal in patients with asthma, if they are in remission at the time of testing. When patients are symptomatic, however, abnormalities in pulmonary function should be present.
- *Expiratory volume in one second:* ↓
- *Expiratory volume in one second or forced vital capacity (FVC):* ↓
- Typically, a more than or equal to 20% ↑ in FEV_1 is noted after administration of an inhaled bronchodilator
- *Total lung capacity*: Normal or ↑
- *Residual volume*: ↑
- Normal or ↑ diffusion capacity (transfer factor).

Arterial blood gases (ABGs) may be normal, if the patient is in remission at the time of testing. If the patient is symptomatic, however, ABGs will demonstrate abnormalities, the pattern of abnormalities indicating the disease severity. The ABGs may be useful, therefore, in determining the aggressiveness of treatment and the need for close monitoring of patients in the hospital or in the ICU (Table 14.5).

Table 14.5: Changes in the arterial blood gases.				
Severity of attack	Mild	Moderate	Severe	Very severe
pH	↑	↑	normal	↓
PaO_2	normal	↓	↓	↓
$PaCO_2$	↓	↓	normal	↑

(PaO_2, partial pressure of oxygen; $PaCO_2$, partial pressure of carbon dioxide)

Chest X-ray is generally of little value in making a diagnosis of asthma. In asthmatics presenting with an acute attack, the chest X-ray generally appears normal or demonstrates hyperinflation. The main value of the chest X-ray is to rule out densities and/or atelectasis secondary to mucus plugging and other diagnostic possibilities, such as pneumothorax or pneumonia.

Therapy of Asthma

The available agents can be classified as bronchodilators, functioning primarily to directly reduce bronchoconstriction, or as anti-inflammatory agents (corticosteroids or cromolyn), *decreasing airway inflammation, which is the primary stimulus for bronchoconstriction and bronchial hyperresponsiveness.* Inhaled corticosteroids are *listed* in Table 14.6. Some patients with chronic and stable asthma have symptoms even with multi-drug treatment (inhaled steroids, beta$_2$-agonists, theophylline, cromolyn, or ipratropium). In these patients, oral corticosteroids have a role (Table 14.7).

Asthma Clinical Trial

- It is well established that a low-dose inhaled glucocorticoid if taken regularly through an appropriate device, should control most children with asthma.
- If asthma is not controlled, check the adequacy of technique with the medication-delivery device.
- A combined inhaler as first-line preventive therapy in children is not advisable and is commonly done.
- Monotherapy with a LABA in a child is improper therapy.
- For those who require more than low-dose inhaled glucocorticoids to control the disease or have persistent, objectively documented, variable airflow obstruction, combination inhalers containing a LABA, and an inhaled glucocorticoid are recommended safe.

Leukotriene Receptor Antagonists for Asthma can save Millions, Says NICE

A leukotriene receptor antagonist is very inexpensive and should be offered before a combination inhaler in patients with poorly controlled asthma.

Table 14.6: Inhaled corticosteroids*: aerosol metered dose inhaler.		
Product	Supplied	Dosage†
Beclomethasone		
Beclovent	50 µg/puff	2 puffs 2–4 times daily
Vanceril	100–200 µg/Rotacap	
Becloforte	250 µg/puff	1–2 puffs 2 times daily
Becotide (UK)	50 µg/puff	2 puffs 2–4 times daily
	200 µg/puff	1–2 puffs 2–4 times daily
	100–200 µg/Rotacaps	2–4 times daily
Budesonide		
Pulmicort	100–400 µg/puff	1–2 puffs 2–3 times daily
Turbuhaler‡	250 µg/puff	1–2 puffs 2 times daily
Flunisolide		
Bronalide		
Bronkolid		
Aerobid	100 or 200 µg/puff	2–4 puffs 2 times daily
Triamcinolone acetate§		

*Not recommended for acute attacks
†Dose inhaled 10–20 minutes after beta$_2$-agonist inhalation. Dose more than 1,500 fig/daily; risk adrenal suppression and osteoporosis
‡Pulmicort chlorofluorocarbon-based inhaler replaced by Pulmicort Turbuhaler (nonchlorofluorocarbon) in some countries
§High dosage of fluorinated agents may rarely cause myopathy.

Table 14.7: Treatment of chronic and stable asthma.	
Patient type	Agents recommended
• Only occasional dyspnea, such as with exercise • Chronic cough without airway obstruction • Frequent or prolonged episodes of dyspnea • Asthma not controlled by inhaled steroids and beta$_2$-agonists	• Beta$_2$-agonist inhaled as needed • Inhaled steroid regularly • Inhaled steroid regularly and beta$_2$-agonist as needed • Consider cromolyn and adding ipratropium

Status Asthmaticus

It refers to an asthmatic episode that does not respond to usual initial therapy and is severe enough to threaten life. This form of asthma is a medical emergency and requires intensive treatment and monitoring. The history is usually one of poorly controlled asthma that progresses over days or weeks, although in some cases there will be a more abrupt onset. Initial treatment in the emergency room for patients with acute, severe asthma should include inhaled beta$_2$-agonists and IV corticosteroids; for status asthmaticus ipratropium is added with aminophylline given consideration.

Beta$_2$-agonists and Beta$_2$-selective agents should be given frequently by inhalation, e.g. q 20 minutes over the 1st hour.
- *Inhaled beta$_2$-agonists:* Albuterol (salbutamol) 2.5–5 mg (0.5–1 mL of 0.5% solution)
- *Subcutaneous beta-agonists*: Epinephrine (1:1000) 0.3–0.5 mL, avoid in older asthmatics (>40) and anyone with a history of heart disease; terbutaline 0.24–0.50 mg.

Corticosteroids

In patients with severe asthma, early use of IV corticosteroids is warranted. The optimal dose of corticosteroids is not known, but doses of 80–125 mg of methylprednisolone repeated q 6–8 hours have been recommended. Patients who have responded to IV steroids can be safely switched to comparable doses of oral steroids. Because oral doses of steroids are frequently significantly lower than IV doses, however, it is wise to carefully monitor the clinical response of the patient during the switch from IV to oral steroids. Following discharge from the hospital, oral steroids should be tapered carefully with frequent determination of PEFR to monitor for any deterioration in pulmonary function. Inhaled steroids are not useful in the treatment of acute and severe asthma, but should be used to aid in the weaning process of oral steroids. Inhaled steroids have a role in patients with asthma requiring fj$_2$ agonists more than three times daily for control.

Corticosteroids ↑ the effectiveness of p$_2$ agonists and have been shown to induce the formation of new p$_2$ receptors in the human lung.

Anticholinergics

Several studies have demonstrated some benefit from adding nebulized ipratropium bromide to treatment with inhaled beta$_2$-agonists in acute and severe asthma. Given the safety and lack of significant side effects associated with the use of ipratropium, it is a reasonable adjunct to treatment in patients who have demonstrated a limited clinical response to beta$_2$-agonists and corticosteroids.

Dosage: Ipratropium (via nebulizer) 500 µg/2 mL unit; administer 2 mL q 4 hours; in severe asthma, give q 2 hours for 4 doses then 4–6 hours under supervision. When the patient has been stabilized, a metered-dose inhaler (20 µg puff, 1–4 puffs three to six times daily) may be required.

Methylxanthines

There is little objective evidence that addition of methylxanthine therapy adds any significant benefit to patients treated with beta$_2$-agonists and IV or oral corticosteroids. IV aminophylline therapy is controversial. Some studies have demonstrated that although there was no therapeutic benefit, a significant ↑ in treatment toxicity (including nausea and palpitations) was associated with the addition of methylxanthine therapy. There appears to still be a role for methylxanthines in chronic treatment of asthma, but it appears that these agents do not have a clear role in the treatment of acute and severe asthma. In patients who are being treated chronically with methylxanthines and present with acute and severe asthma, it is reasonable to obtain a serum theophylline level and, if subtherapeutic, administer aminophylline, or theophylline to bring serum levels to a safe therapeutic range (10–15 μg/mL, *United* States; 10–20 mg/L, UK; and 55–110 μmol/L, Canada).

Supplemental Oxygen

This should generally be provided by nasal cannula to these patients. Oxygenation should be monitored by pulse oximetry; O_2 flow rates can then be titrated to maintain O_2 saturation more than 90%. In some cases, a higher inspired concentration of O_2 provided by a high-flow face mask may be required. In severely obstructed patients, it is important to obtain frequent *ABGs*, in addition to following oximetry, to determine whether there are progressive increases in arterial CO_2 that would indicate impending ventilatory failure.

Mechanical Ventilation

Endotracheal intubation and mechanical ventilation of patients in status asthmaticus are last-resort treatments indicated in patients with impending ventilatory failure. Indications for intubation include:
- Inability to maintain airway control, resulting in progressive ↑ in arterial CO_2 tension to elevated levels (particularly >50 mm Hg)
- Altered mental status
- Clinical evidence of respiratory muscle fatigue (paradoxical movement of diaphragm)
- Refractory hypoxemia, acidemia, or seizures.

Mechanical ventilation of asthma patients may be complicated by very high airway pressures, which may lead to barotrauma. Mortality associated with mechanical ventilation for status asthmaticus has been reported to be relatively high (5–23%). Controlled hypoventilation, which uses lower tidal volumes and a lower respiratory rate and tolerates some hypercarbia while maintaining oxygenation, may result in a lower mortality. In general, the tidal volume and respiratory rate should be adjusted to maintain peak airway pressures at less than 50 cm H_2O.

Outpatient Management of the Severe Asthmatics

Optimal outpatient management of patients with severe asthma should include routine assessment of PEFR, as the presence or absence of symptoms may not accurately reflect lung function. The patient should possess, and learn to use, a peak flow meter. Appropriate adjustments in inhaled medications or in oral corticosteroids should be made if the PEFR falls significantly. Patients should be instructed to obtain emergency medical assistance, if the PEFR falls dramatically (<150 L/min). Monitoring PEFR on a regular basis will help limit any delay in initiating treatment for bronchospasm. This approach may help reduce mortality that may result from delayed initiation of treatment for bronchospasm in some asthmatics.

Features that characterize patients at ↑ risk for asthma-associated death include:
- Age more than 55 years
- Prior history of ICU admission, intubation, or respiratory acidosis
- Hospitalization for asthma in last year
- Recent withdrawal from systemic steroids
- Psychological or psychosocial problems
- Lack of access to healthcare
- Inadequate medical management.

CHRONIC OBSTRUCTIVE PULMONARY DISEASE

Chronic obstructive pulmonary disease is a generic term used to describe the condition of patients with expiratory airflow obstruction. The diseases usually included under COPD are chronic bronchitis and emphysema, which both have varying degrees of expiratory airflow obstruction.

Chronic Bronchitis

The definition of chronic bronchitis is based on a clinical symptom complex—cough with sputum production for 3 months of the year over 2 consecutive years in the absence of other causes with or without expiratory airflow obstruction. The pathophysiology is described as chronic excessive secretion of mucus with hypertrophy of the subepithelial tracheobronchial mucous glands. The goblet cells are another source of excessive mucous secretion. Studies have demonstrated that the mucous glands are ↑ in size. The Reid Index, or ratio of gland to bronchial wall thickness, is the most common means of measuring mucous gland enlargement.
- The ↑ bronchial smooth muscle present in chronic bronchitis has been determined to result from smooth muscle hyperplasia. A correlation has been demonstrated between ↓ FEV_1 and ↑ amounts of smooth muscle in the major airways, ↑ amounts of smooth muscle are related neither to bronchodilator response nor to methacholine responsiveness in surgically resected lung.
- Bronchoscopy and bronchoalveolar lavage performed on patients with chronic bronchitis demonstrated ↑ inflammation of the tracheobronchial tree compared to that of asymptomatic smokers or normal individuals. Bronchial samples of the lavage demonstrated ↑ neutrophils. Airway

neutrophilia was associated with sputum production, airway obstruction, and cigarette smoking.
- Bronchial walls are thickened with encroachment on the airway lumen. Patients with severe obstruction had double the bronchial wall width internal to the cartilage or lumenal diameter of that in patients without obstruction. Most series have reported that the ↑ in bronchial wall thickness resulting from mucous gland hypertrophy is minimal.

Emphysema

Emphysema is defined as the abnormal, permanent enlargement of the airspace distal to the terminal (nonrespiratory) bronchioles with concomitant destruction of their walls without obvious fibrosis. Emphysema can be classified as follows:
- *Centriacinar emphysema*: This form of emphysema involves the respiratory bronchioles with scarring and focal dilation of the bronchiole and adjacent alveoli, and exists as centrilobular and focal emphysema. Centrilobular emphysema is most frequently associated with prolonged cigarette smoking. It usually involves the posterior upper lobes and is the most common clinically expressed form of emphysema. Focal emphysema is associated with exposure to biologically inactive dust and is uniformly distributed throughout the lung.
- *Panacinar emphysema*: This form of emphysema involves dilation of all the respiratory airspaces and of the secondary lung lobule with either diffuse or focal involvement. The diffuse form may be associated with deficiency of protease inhibitors (alpha$_1$-antitrypsin deficiency), and the lung bases are involved more often than the upper lobes.

Risk Factors

- *Cigarette smoking:* Smoking is by far the most important single factor associated with, the development of COPD. Only a portion of chronic smokers, however, show an accelerated decline in FEV_1. Chronic cough and sputum occur independently of the development of airflow obstruction.
- *Air pollution*: Exposure to particulate matter is related to symptoms of chronic bronchitis and ↓ in pulmonary function. Exposure to irritants can lead to cellular changes and acute respiratory infection or may enhance allergic response.
- *Occupational exposure*: Exposures to both organic and inorganic dust may lead to symptoms of chronic bronchitis. Any effect that such exposure may have on the development of airflow obstruction has been difficult to demonstrate in cross-sectional studies; however, most longitudinal studies show the accelerated decline in indices typical of

an airflow associated with chronic dust exposure. The effect is more pronounced in smokers.
- *Atopy*: The role of immunologic response and airway hyperresponsiveness in the development of COPD is important. The immunologic precursors to COPD are in part genetically determined. Bronchial reactivity may be a precursor to obstructive airway disease. A relationship exists between COPD prevalence and serum IgE levels.
- *Heredity*: Hereditary factors, such as deficiency of protease inhibitors (alpha$_1$-antitrypsin deficiency), have been related to the development of emphysema. Prevalence of this deficiency has been shown by blood donor studies to be 350 per 1,000,000. Nonsmoking patients may remain asymptomatic with little abnormality of lung function through their 6th-7th decades of life; however, smokers with protease inhibitor deficiencies may experience severely limited respiratory function by age 40.

Diagnosis

- Dyspnea or acute chest illness with cough, sputum production, *chest* tightness, and wheezing may be of sufficient magnitude to bring the patient to seek medical attention. This condition usually occurs in the 6th-7th decade of life. Chronic bronchitis and emphysema often coexist and are reviewed together in the remaining sections.
- The dyspnea is usually of insidious onset.
- Smoking of more than 20 cigarettes/day for more than 25 years is often present. Hemoptysis may occur and, if so, is usually associated with the development of purulent sputum in a lower respiratory tract infection. Recurrent symptoms of cough, ↑ and/or purulent sputum, wheeze, and dyspnea are common.
- Active accessory muscles (scalenes and sternomastoids) are a consistent finding with significant airflow obstruction because of the inability of the diaphragm to produce the force required for inspiration.
- Pursed lip expiration is a common feature in patients with severe airflow obstruction.
- Examination of patients with emphysema often demonstrates a barrel chest, caused by air trapping, and thus a prominent sternal angle, horizontal ribs, and an ↑ anteroposterior diameter. Also seen is a low diaphragm with limited motion or decreased excursion. Normal diaphragmatic excursion is approximately 5-6 cm.
- Indrawing of the intercostal space is a sign of hyperinflation of the chest
- Paradoxical abdominal and diaphragmatic movement during respiration indicates diaphragmatic fatigue or weakness. Patients with exacerbations of COPD who manifest this sign are more likely to require ventilator assistance.

- Hoover's sign (paradoxical inward movement of the lateral costal margin) may be observed and is caused by horizontal rather than vertical (downward) diaphragmatic contraction that results from the flat position of the diaphragm. Hoover's sign is not a sign of diaphragmatic fatigue.
- Tracheal tug (the downward movement of the thyroid cartilage and trachea with each inspiration) may be observed.
- Wheezes (rhonchi), which are musical sounds produced by the rapid passage of air through a bronchus that is narrowed to the point of closure, may be heard. The walls of the bronchus oscillate between closed and barely open positions and generate audible sound. Wheezes are typically expiratory but may occur in both inspiration and expiration. Although wheezes vary in pitch, inferences as to the size of the airways involved cannot be made from the pitch.
- Cardiac dullness is decreased.
- Reduction in breath sounds is marked.
- Central cyanosis and signs of cor pulmonale—jugular venous distension, hepatojugular reflux, hepatomegaly, and pedal edema—are apparent.
- Signs of hypercapnia (asterixis, chemosis, and fundal vessel dilation), usually without papilledema, are important indicators of elevated $PaCO_2$.
- A forced expiratory time of more than 6 seconds indicates airflow limitation. This maneuver is performed by placing the stethoscope over the trachea and requesting the patient to expire from full inspiration to full expiration. Normally, the patient should be able to expire completely in less than 6 seconds.
- Finger clubbing is not a feature of COPD and, if present, should alert the physician to other possible causes, such as bronchiectasis and carcinoma.

The chest X-ray may reveal the marked and persistent overdistension of the lungs that is strongly suggestive of emphysema; however, the sensitivity of chest radiography for the detection of emphysema is poor. The diaphragms are often low and flattened in emphysema. An enlarged retrosternal airspace (>3.5 cm) and a deep anteroposterior diameter of the chest may be present.

- Hyperinflated, hypertransradiant lungs, as well as a large and small bullae are seen.
- Excessively rapid tapering of the vascular shadows, with narrow-angle branching and general oligemia resulting from loss of pulmonary vessels, is apparent.
- A narrow, seemingly elongated heart is not uncommon.
- The chest X-ray of the patient with chronic bronchitis may be normal or may demonstrate accentuation of the normal bronchovascular markings.
- Heart size is not a sensitive indicator of cor pulmonale.

The chest X-ray may be suggestive of emphysema if air trapping, hyperinflation, vascular deficiency, and bullae are present, but these findings are often not present until late in the course of the disease.

Pulmonary function testing reveals:
- The FEV_1 is ↓. An FEV_1 less than 70% of that predicted for age-, sex-, and height-matched controls is abnormal and indicates airflow obstruction.
- The ratio of FEV_1 to FVC of less than 70% with incomplete reversibility indicates an airflow obstruction. Moderate airflow obstruction is evidenced as an FEV_1/FVC ratio of less than 65%, whereas severe airflow obstruction is evidenced as an FEV_1/FVC ratio of less than 60% with a markedly ↓ FEV_1 (<0.75 L).
- The FVC may be normal or may ↓ in proportion to any ↑ in the residual volume.
- The diffusing capacity for carbon monoxide (DLCO) is usually ↓ in emphysema and often remains near normal in chronic bronchitis.
- The ABGs may be normal or may show varying degrees of hypoxemia or hypercapnia, depending on the type of disease and the point in its natural course. Patients with predominant chronic bronchitis typically develop hypoxemia and hypercapnia earlier in the progression of airflow obstruction than do patients with predominant emphysema, who may have normal or near-normal ABGs despite severe airflow obstruction (FEV_1 <0.75 l). In such patients, development of hypercapnia is often a preterminal sign.

Therapy

Therapy should be directed at:
- Improvement of reversible airflow obstruction
- Treatment of complications in COPD
- Oxygen therapy
- Pulmonary rehabilitation
- Prevention
- Home care.

Improvement of reversible airflow obstruction involves treatment of bronchospasm, mucosal inflammation, and infection and control of abnormal and excessive mucoid or mucopurulent secretions that occur with varying degrees of clinical significance at different times in the same patient. A careful clinical assessment of the patient and examination of the sputum often provide hints as to which of these components of airway obstruction is contributing most to the current exacerbation.

Salutary effects of pharmacological therapy are obtained in most patients with the use of bronchodilators. Occasionally, pulsed corticosteroids are used in combination with antibiotics during exacerbations when bacterial infection is deemed present. The use of antibiotics in an exacerbation of COPD has been demonstrated in various studies to be both beneficial and of little benefit. The initial infection in most patients with an acute exacerbation of COPD is most commonly viral. Because of impaired mucociliary clearance, bacterial superinfection occurs in a substantial proportion of patients.

Accurately differentiating those patients whose course will be improved by antibiotics from those who will receive no benefit is difficult or impossible. The administration of a broad-spectrum antimicrobial agent to a patient who is producing purulent, copious sputum during an exacerbation is a reasonable addition to therapy.

Sputum culture is not helpful or necessary in most exacerbations. If the patient fails to improve with first-line therapy, culture should be obtained because the emergence of drug-resistant organisms, especially *Pseudomonas*, may occur after repeated courses of antibiotics. Choice of antibiotics when drug-resistant organisms are present should be guided by sensitivity testing.

As potent anti-inflammatory drugs, corticosteroids may be useful in the treatment of active bronchial inflammation. Judicious use is mandatory because of the well-known deleterious side effects of long-term, high-dose corticosteroids.

- Hospitalized patients with acute exacerbations causing respiratory failure should receive high-dose IV methylprednisolone, 250–500 mg/24 hours. *Supplied*— vials, 40 or 125 mg; convenient to give 80–125 mg q 6 hours. After 48 hours, the dose may be halved daily until a dose of 40–60 mg is reached. The patient is then changed to oral prednisone, and the dosage is tapered.
- Outpatients with exacerbations associated with acute, purulent bronchitis often benefit from a short, pulsed dose of oral prednisone. A dose of 40–60 mg/day for 5 days without tapering is frequently successful in accelerating improvement in airflow obstruction. If obstruction flares when corticosteroids are stopped, a tapering schedule may be needed.
- Patients with severe airflow obstruction (FEV_1 <1 L) deserve 1 controlled trial of corticosteroids to determine whether they are 1 of the approximately 20% who show substantial improvement in airway obstruction. Prednisone administered 40–60 mg/day for 2–4 weeks is an adequate trial (Table 14.8). The trial must be controlled by baseline and post-therapy measurements of FEV_1. A response is determined by improvement in airflow obstruction. Most patients show subjective improvement because of the euphoric effect of the drug. Maintenance of a therapeutic response requires chronic corticosteroid therapy.
- Inhaled corticosteroids are commonly ineffective in patients with COPD, even in those who improve with systemic therapy. The lack of effect is probably caused by poor peripheral aerosol distribution.
- Patients requiring chronic corticosteroid therapy to maintain improved airway function should be tapered to the lowest possible single daily dose or tried on alternate-day administration (1 dose q 48 hours) to minimize side effects. Measures to prevent weight gain, hyperglycemia, and osteoporosis are important.

Table 14.8: Corticosteroids and bronchodilators

Name	Preparation	Route of administration
Methylprednisolone (Solu-Medrol)	80 to 125 mg q 6 hr	Intravenous
Prednisolone (Medrol)	Variable (initial 20-40 mg qd)	Oral
Dexamethasone (Decadron)	4-10 mg qd to qid	Intravenous, oral
Prednisone	Variable (40-60 mg qd to bid)	Oral
Anticholinergic agents:		
Atropine	1-3 mg q 6 hr	Nebulized aerosol
Ipratropium bromide (Atrovent)	2-4 putts qid	Metered dose inhaler
Beta-2 agonist:		
Albuterol epinephrine (*see* Table 14.2)		Nebulized Subcutaneous
Methylxanthines:		
Theophylline (*see* Table 14.4)	10–15 µg/mL	Intravenous

- Efficacy of single-inhaler combination of an extrafine formulation of beclometasone dipropionate, formoterol fumarate, and glycopyrronium bromide (BDP/FF/GB) in COPD.
- TRILOGY was a randomized, parallel group, double-blind, and active-controlled study done in 159 sites across 14 countries.
- Findings; TRILOGY provides evidence for the clinical benefits of stepping up patients with COPD from an inhaled corticosteroid or long-acting beta$_2$-agonist combination treatment to triple therapy using a single inhaler.

Treatment of Complications

Acute Exacerbations

The patient has ↑ dyspnea, chest tightness, and wheezing usually accompanied by ↑ cough and sputum production. The most common cause is acute lower respiratory infection, usually viral. Exposure to respiratory irritants may also cause an exacerbation. Treatment depends on the severity of the baseline disease and of the exacerbation. Severity is best judged by peak flow measurement, spirometry, and/or ABGs in addition to symptoms. An increasing order of intensity of therapy involves:
- ↑ frequency of inhaled bronchodilators
- Antibiotic administration
- Use of pulsed corticosteroids

- Oxygen if PaO$_2$ less than 55 mm Hg
- Mechanical ventilation for ventilatory failure with consideration of the patient's and the family's wishes.

Pulmonary Thromboembolism

An estimated 20–40% of patients with exacerbation of COPD experience acute pulmonary thromboembolism.

Pneumothorax

Spontaneous pneumothorax rarely causes the exacerbation of COPD and is most often secondary to the rupture of a bulla or bleb. Identification of a pneumothorax can be lifesaving. The chest examination often reveals decreased breath sounds on the side of the pneumothorax. The affected side of the chest is often more hyperresonant than the contralateral side, but this finding is difficult to ascertain clinically. If tension is involved, the trachea may be shifted to the opposite side of the pneumothorax and hemodynamic deterioration may arise emergently.

Respiratory Drive Depression

Neuromuscular abnormalities, sedative or hypnotic medication, narcotic analgesics, and metabolic alkalosis, which may be caused by diuretics that induce hypochloremia and elevated bicarbonate levels, hypocalcemia, hypomagnesemia, and hypophosphatemia.

Oxygen Therapy

The predominant pathophysiologic mechanism leading to hypoxemia and hypercapnia in COPD is ventilation or perfusion mismatching leading to ↑ numbers of gas-exchanging units with low V/Q ratios. In addition, when the work of breathing exceeds respiratory muscle capacity for work, generalized hypoventilation occurs, either acutely or chronically, thus further worsening both hypoxemia and hypercapnia. Hypoxemia may be acutely lethal. Chronic hypoxemia leads to pulmonary hypertension, polycythemia, cognitive impairment, and premature death.

Types of O$_2$ therapy include:

- *Nasal cannula*: The most comfortable, generally most suitable means for O$_2$ therapy in COPD (Table 14.9). Less likely to be removed by patients.
- *Oxygen masks*: Venturi masks achieve the most accurate control of fraction of inspired oxygen (FIO$_2$). Rebreather and nonrebreather masks can achieve FIO$_2$ between 40 and 80%. All masks are somewhat uncomfortable and more likely to be removed.

Table 14.9: FiO$_2$/flow rate equivalents

Nasal cannula flow rate (L/min)	Approximate FiO$_2$(%)
1	23
2	27
3	30
4	33
5	36
6	40

- *Endotracheal intubation with mechanical ventilation:* Can achieve FIO$_2$ of 100%. Necessary when adequate oxygenation cannot be achieved without hypercapnia with respiratory acidosis severe enough to cause somnolence or coma.
- *Oxygen-conservation devices:* Pulsed flow devices and reservoir devices both conserve O$_2$ by avoiding the wasted O$_2$ that does not reach the alveolar level or is delivered during expiration.

Oxygen therapy is indicated during acute exacerbations when the PaO$_2$ is less than 60 mm Hg or the arterial oxygen saturation (SaO$_2$) is less than 90%. The dose of O$_2$ required is generally low unless pneumonia or pulmonary embolism is present:

- In the absence of hypercapnia, the dose of O$_2$ is not critical. A PaO$_2$ more than 65 mm Hg or SaO$_2$ more than 90% is adequate.
- Hypercapnic patients may depend on their hypoxic drive to stimulate respiration. O$_2$ therapy may result in worsening hypercapnia and respiratory acidosis. Many such patients can be successfully treated with carefully controlled FIO$_2$ achieving a PaO$_2$ of 55-65 mm Hg without producing clinically significant respiratory acidosis. A Venturi mask or pediatric O$_2$ flow meter may be used to achieve a more precise FIO$_2$.
- If a PaO$_2$ of 55 mg Hg cannot be achieved without clinically significant respiratory acidosis, mechanical ventilation may be required. Clinically significant respiratory acidosis is best judged by cerebral effects (somnolence, coma, and inability to cooperate with therapy) rather than by any arbitrary level of PaCO$_2$ or pH.
- Hypoxemia can be rapidly lethal or deleterious. Respiratory acidosis can be tolerated for several hours. O$_2$ should never be discontinued in a patient with respiratory failure who has a rising PaCO$_2$.
- The duration of O$_2$ therapy for acute exacerbation is unpredictable. Some patients require several weeks of O$_2$ therapy to restore their previous level of PaO$_2$. If the PaO$_2$ is less than 55 mm Hg at the time of discharge, home administration of O$_2$ should be arranged with a repeat ABG measurement taken in 2-4 weeks to determine when or whether O$_2$ therapy can be discontinued.

Stable patients with COPD who remain hypoxemic despite optimal med with cor pulmonale, pulmonary hypertension or polycythemia:

- Partial pressure of oxygen less than or equal to 55 mm Hg or SaO_2 less than 88% during exercise or sleep.
- *Dose:* O_2 flow sufficient to raise PaO_2 to 65 mm Hg or SaO_2 more than 90%.
- *Duration*: At least 15 hours/day unless only needed during exercise or sleep.

Prevention

Educational and psychosocial measures that lead to a choice not to smoke are the most cost-effective in approaching the problem of COPD. The accelerated rate of decline in FEV_1 that occurs in susceptible smokers appears to return to a normal rate once smoking has stopped, even when early airflow obstruction is present. Surveys of ex-smokers suggest that a physician's advice is the single most important factor leading to smoking cessation. Other adjunctive measures, such as self-help, group counseling, hypnosis, and nicotine substitution, may benefit selected patients. Although far less important than smoking, inhaled irritants and dusts accelerate the normal aging decline in FEV_1, especially in patients who smoke. Measures to control atmospheric and occupational pollution and protection of workers need to be taken.

Patients with COPD should receive an annual vaccination against influenza. Unvaccinated patients may benefit from amantadine during an influenza epidemic. Vaccination with a multivalent pneumococcal vaccine is recommended. Revaccination is now advised after 6 years

In the rare patient with COPD caused by $alpha_1$-antitrypsin deficiency (at 1%), replacement therapy should be considered. When therapy should be started is uncertain, but most clinicians advise beginning when the patient shows early signs of emphysema. Whether the progression of far-advanced disease is affected by replacement is uncertain.

BIBLIOGRAPHY

1. Brusselle G, Pavord I. Azithromycin in uncontrolled asthma. Lancet. 2017;390(10095):629-30.
2. Bush A, Frey U. Safety of Long-Acting Beta-Agonists in Children with Asthma. N Engl J Med. 2016;375(9):889-91.
3. Horita N, Nagashima A, Kaneko. T Long-Acting β-Agonists (LABA) Combined With Long-Acting Muscarinic Antagonists or LABA Combined With Inhaled Corticosteroids for Patients With Stable COPD. JAMA. 2017;318(13):1274-5.
4. Gibson P. Effectiveness trials in asthma: time to SaLSA? 2017;390:2217-8.
5. McCracken JL Veeranki SP, Ameredes BT, et al. Diagnosis and Management of Asthma in Adults: A Review. JAMA. 2017;318(3):279-90.
6. Peters SP, Bleecker ER, Canonica GW, et al. Serious Asthma Events with Budesonide plus Formoterol vs. Budesonide Alone. N Engl J Med. 2016;375:850-60.
7. Pingleton S, khan MK, Bartlett JG, et al. Medical Diagnosis and Therapy. Philadelphia: Lea and Febiger; 1994.

8. Singh D, Papi A, Corradi M, et al Single inhaler triple therapy versus inhaled corticosteroid plus long-acting β2-agonist therapy for chronic obstructive pulmonary disease (TRILOGY): a double-blind, parallel group, randomised controlled trial. Lancet. 2016;388(10048):963-73.
9. Stempel DA, Szefler SJ, Pedersen S, et al. Safety of Adding Salmeterol to Fluticasone Propionate in Children with Asthma. N Engl J Med. 2016;375:840-9.
10. Wise J. Leucotriene receptor antagonists for asthma can save millions, says NICE. BMJ. 2016;355:i6835.

CHAPTER 15

Pneumonias

COMMUNITY-ACQUIRED PNEUMONIA

Microbiologic Cause

- *Streptococcus pneumoniae* (pneumococcus) is the single most important pathogen responsible for community-acquired pneumonia (CAP) in all age groups, accounting for 30-70% of cases. *Mycoplasma pneumoniae* has been implicated as the causative agent in 20-30% of CAP in young adults (< age 35), but accounts for only 1-9% of CAP in older adults.
- *Legionella* and *Chlamydia* species each accounts for 2-6% of CAP, but the incidence of these pathogens has been variable among geographic regions.
- In recent studies, *Haemophilus influenzae* has been the second or third most common pathogen, accounting for 5-18% of CAP in adults.
- Gram-negative bacilli (GNB) (predominantly Enterobacteriaceae) have been implicated in 3-8% of cases in recent series; even higher prevalence rates have been noted in elderly patients, residents of chronic care facilities, or patients with significant underlying diseases.
- *Staphylococcus aureus* accounts for 3-8% of CAP in adults, usually in patients with staphylococcal carriage risk factors [nursing home residence, advanced age, intravenous (IV) drug abuse, and chronic dialysis] or in association with epidemics of influenza.
- *Moraxella (Branhamella) catarrhalis*, which has only recently been recognized as an important pathogen in exacerbations of bronchitis, accounts for 1-2% of CAP.
- Viruses, particularly influenza, parainfluenza, and adenovirus have been implicated in as many as 5-15% of CAP; most cases occur during the winter months.
- No specific pathogen can be identified in 30-60% of CAP.

Clinical and Radiographic Features

Figures 15.1 to 15.8 give examples of pneumonias and other conflicting diagnoses.

- Clinical and radiographic features of CAP may suggest certain pathogens but are not specific. An abrupt onset associated with high fever, a

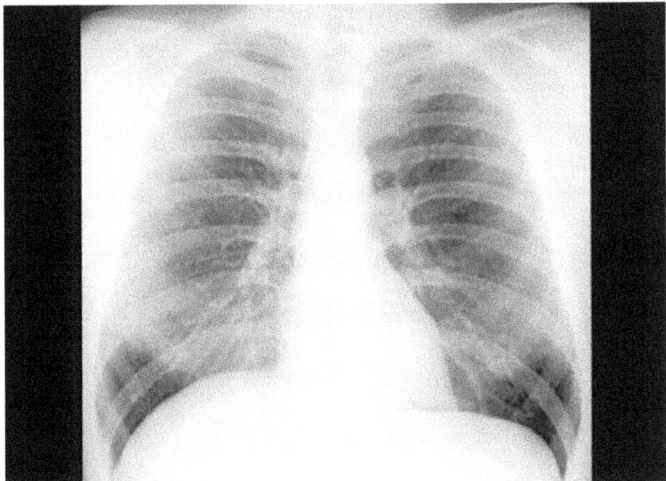

Fig. 15.1: Normal posteroanterior radiograph of the chest.
Source: Khan MG. On Call Cardiology, 3rd edition. Philadelphia: WB Saunders, Elsevier Science; 2006. p. 144.

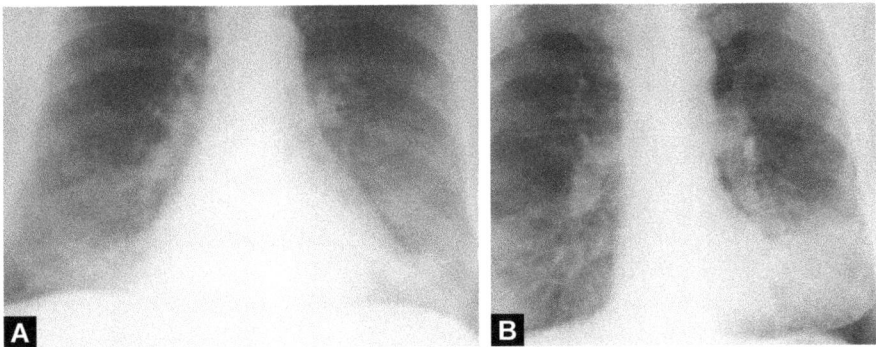

Figs. 15.2A and B: Blurring of the lower aspect of both cardiac borders by pericardial fat.
Source: Khan MG. On Call Cardiology, 3rd edition. Philadelphia: WB Saunders, Elsevier Science; 2006; p. 154.

shaking chill, pleuritic chest pain, and lobar consolidation on physical examination and chest X-ray is highly characteristic of bacteremic infections caused by *S. pneumoniae*. Identical features, however, may be observed with other bacteria, such as *H. influenzae, Escherichia coli, Klebsiella,* or *Legionella* species. Admittedly, this type of presentation is rare with *Mycoplasma* or *Chlamydia*.

- Many of the "classic" features of acute bacillary pneumonia may be absent, particularly in elderly or debilitated patients. Nearly 25% of patients more than 65 years old with pneumonia are afebrile; leukocytosis is present in only 50–70%. Clinical features of pneumonia in this context may be subtle; lethargy, fatigue, nausea, anorexia, or deterioration in

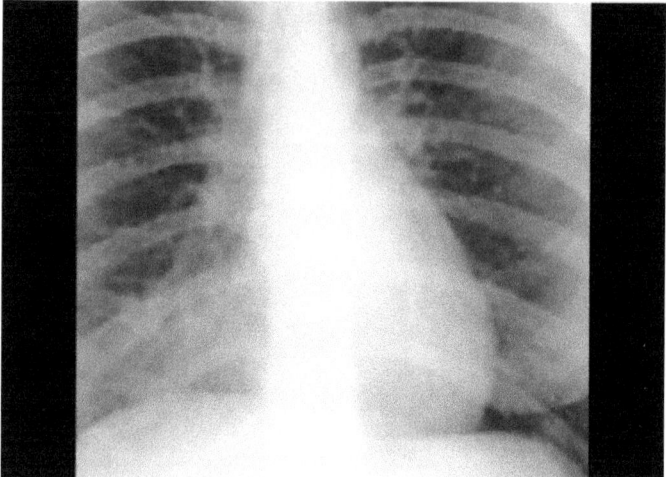

Fig. 15.3: Blurring of the right heart border by consolidation in the medial segment of the middle lobe.
Source: Khan MG. On Call Cardiology, 3rd edition. Philadelphia: WB Saunders, Elsevier Science; 2006; p. 155.

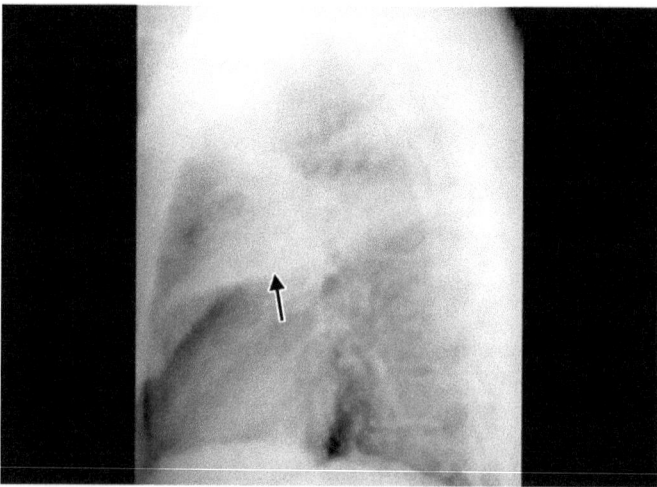

Fig. 15.4: Acute right upper lobe pneumonia showing the sharp inferior margination of the consolidation by the minor fissure (arrow).
Source: Khan MG. On Call Cardiology, 3rd edition. Philadelphia: WB Saunders, Elsevier Science; 2006. p. 15.

overall condition may be the predominant features. Unfortunately, delay in recognition and treatment of pneumonia may be disastrous. Mortality associated with CAP in the elderly population is 10–25%.
- Chest radiographic changes in CAP are variable. Patchy bronchopneumonic infiltrates are most common.

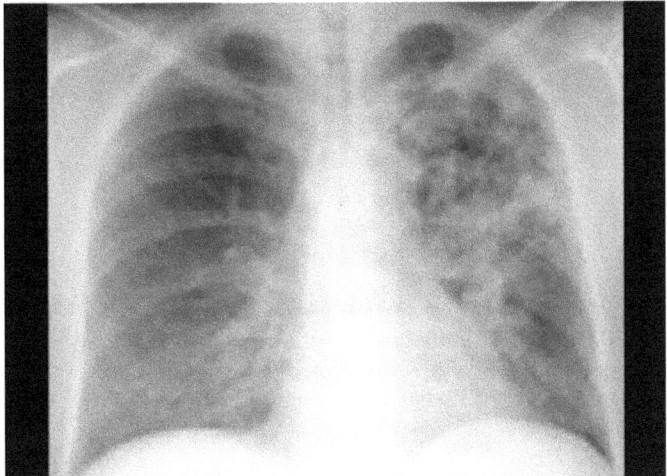

Fig. 15.5: Acute tuberculous pneumonia in the left upper lobe. The disease is poorly marginated and fades imperceptibly into the normal lung.
Sources:
1. Khan MG. On Call Cardiology, 3rd edition. Philadelphia: WB Saunders, Elsevier Science; 2006.
2. Khan MG. Pulmonary Disease Diagnosis and Therapy: A Practical Approach. Baltimore: Williams & Wilkins, 1997; p. 59.

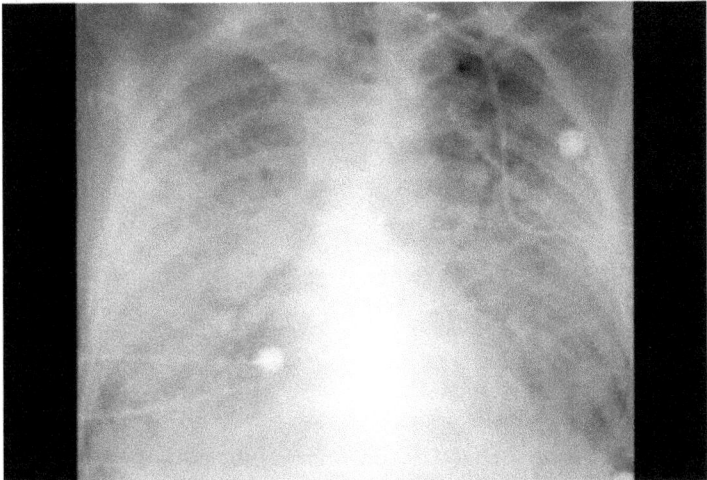

Fig. 15.6: Diffuse bilateral consolidation from combined *Pneumocystis carinii* and cytomegalovirus infection in an AIDS patient.
Sources:
1. Khan MG. On Call Cardiology, 3rd edition. Philadelphia: WB Saunders, Elsevier Science; 2006.
2. Khan MG. Pulmonary Disease Diagnosis and Therapy: A Practical Approach. Baltimore: Williams & Wilkins, 1997; p. 58.

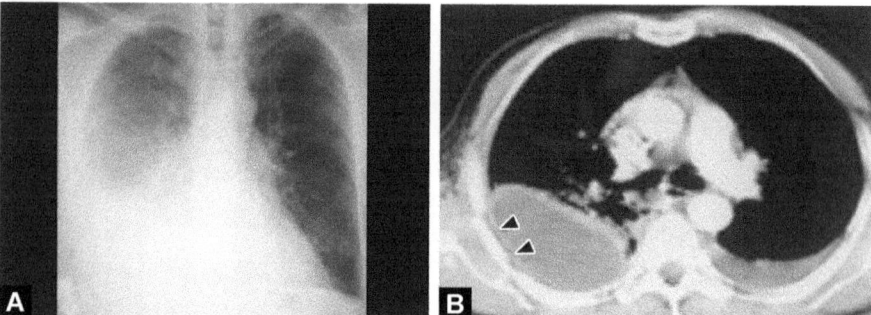

Figs. 15.7A and B: (A) Plain radiograph and (B) CT scan in a man with right-sided streptococcal pneumonia and empyema. Note the lentiform shape of the pleural fluid collection and the thin enhancing pleural wall (arrowheads) on the CT scan, which are characteristic of empyema.
Sources:
1. Khan MG. On Call Cardiology, 3rd edition. Philadelphia: WB Saunders, Elsevier Science; 2006.
2. Khan MG. Pulmonary Disease Diagnosis and Therapy: A Practical Approach. Baltimore: Williams & Wilkins, 1997; p. 104.

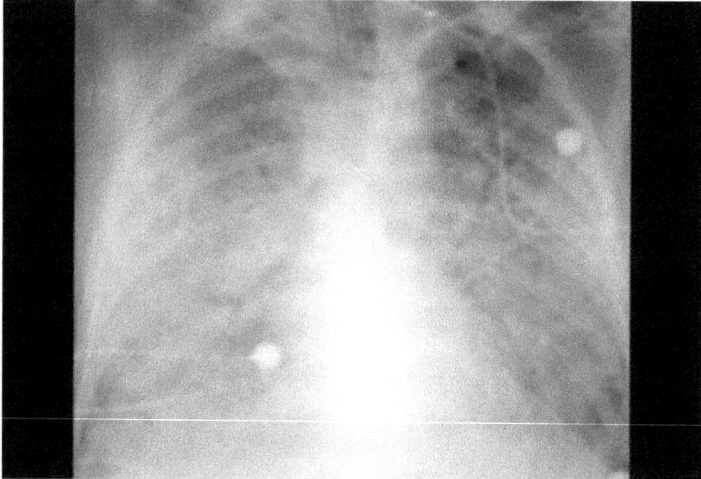

Fig. 15.8: Diffuse bilateral consolidation from combined *Pneumocystis carinii* and cytomegalovirus infection in an AIDS patient.
Sources:
1. Khan MG. On Call Cardiology, 3rd edition. Philadelphia: WB Saunders, Elsevier Science; 2006.
2. Khan MG. Pulmonary Disease Diagnosis and Therapy: A Practical Approach. Baltimore: Williams & Wilkins, 1997; p. 58.

- Dense lobar consolidation with air bronchograms occurs in less than 33% of patients.
- Pleural effusions complicate CAP in 10–25% of patients, and are not etiologically specific.
- Cavitation, rare with *S. pneumoniae*, *Mycoplasma*, or *Chlamydia*, suggests such pathogens as *S. aureus*, *Klebsiella* (or other GNB), anaerobes, or nonbacterial causes, such as mycobacteria, fungi, or neoplasm.
- An air fluid level is most characteristic of an anaerobic or mixed aerobic or anaerobic lung abscess.
- Basilar interstitial or reticulonodular infiltrates suggest *Mycoplasma species*; however, frank lobar pneumonia indistinguishable from bacillary pneumonias may also be seen in as many as one-third of the cases of *Mycoplasma species*. Small (2–3 cm) patchy bronchopneumonic infiltrates have been stated to be characteristic of *M. catarrhalis*, but also may be observed with a wide range of pathogens.
- Radiographic features may favor certain pathogens, but significant overlap exists. Thus, smears and cultures of sputum, blood, or pleural fluid (when present) are important to substantiate a specific microbiologic diagnosis.

Etiologic (Cultural) Diagnosis

Despite a relatively low sensitivity and specificity, sputum smears and cultures should be obtained in all cases of suspected or proven pneumonia. The sputum Gram stain is most useful for distinguishing predominantly gram-negative from gram-positive organisms, but is not specific for a unique organism.

- Sputa demonstrating numerous leukocytes, rare or absent contaminating epithelial cells, uniform morphologic and staining characteristics of microorganisms, and many intracellular organisms within leukocytes may guide therapy. For example, lancet-shaped diplococci in pairs suggest *S. pneumoniae*, clumps of gram-positive cocci suggest *S. aureus*, gram-negative coccobacillary forms in a smoker may suggest *H. influenzae*, and gram-negative rods are characteristic of *Klebsiella* species or other Enterobacteriaceae.
- In most instances, however, mixed gram-negative and gram-positive organisms are observed. Even when a dominant pathogen is noted, the reliability of sputum smears is inexact.
- Caution should be taken when basing initial therapy solely on a sputum Gram stain.
- In bacteremic cases of pneumonia, the pathogen can be isolated in only 40–60% of sputum cultures. Higher rates of isolation can be expected if a "good quality" sputum is obtained, but in clinical practice a pathogen can be isolated from sputum cultures in only 25–50% of cases of pneumonia (including nonbacteremic cases).

- Identification of the microorganisms on sputum cultures may take 2 or 3 days; even longer delays can be expected for antimicrobial susceptibility profiles.
- The value of sputum cultures is further confounded because potential pathogens, such as *S. pneumoniae* and *H. influenzae*, may be part of normal oral flora. Thus, the isolation of a potential pathogen from sputum does not prove that the isolated pathogen is responsible for pneumonia. This inconclusiveness may be particularly true in pneumonia caused by atypical pathogens, *Legionella* species, or anaerobes; in such instances only normal oral flora may be isolated on routine sputum cultures.

In summary, Gram's stain and cultural results may be useful as guides to the diagnosis in some cases, but are frequently nondiagnostic and may even be misleading.

TYPICAL PNEUMONIAS

Streptococcus pneumoniae

- *Streptococcus pneumoniae* remains the most common cause of CAP (accounting for 30–60% of cases) and, with *Legionella* species, has been associated with the most fatalities resulting from CAP. *S. pneumoniae* has been implicated in only 15–30% of CAP in most recent series, but these data underestimate its true frequency, because no causative pathogen was identified in 50–70% of cases. Pneumococcal pneumonia has a predilection for the elderly patient and for patients with preexisting disease, such as ethanol abuse and chronic obstructive pulmonary disease (COPD). It can also affect previously healthy individuals in all age groups.
- *Streptococcus pneumoniae* and *M. pneumoniae* are the two most common causes of CAP in adults less than age 35.
- *Streptococcus pneumoniae* is the leading cause of pneumonia in all age groups (including the elderly). Thus, therapy for CAP (irrespective of age and presence or absence of underlying disease) should always include coverage for *S. pneumoniae*.
- Classic features include a temperature of more than 103°F, drenching sweats, chills, purulent sputum, pleuritic chest pain, and lobar consolidation. These features occur in 50–70% of persons with bacteremic pneumonia caused by *S. pneumoniae*, but do not distinguish pneumococcal pneumonia from other bacillary pneumonias.
- Many of these manifestations are absent in nonbacteremic forms, in the elderly population, or in patients with serious associated diseases.
- A single shaking chill, often stated to be a hallmark for pneumococcal pneumonia, occurs in less than 10% of patients; recurrent chills are more common.
- Blood-tinged sputum occurs in as many as 15% of patients.

- Constitutional symptoms, myalgias, nausea, vomiting, and prostration may be prominent. Headache is a common early feature; stiff neck may reflect meningeal spread. Diarrhea, seen in 20-30% of cases of legionellosis, occurs in less than 10% of cases of pneumococcal pneumonia.
- Bacteremia occurs in 15-30% of patients; higher rates have been noted among patients with dense lobar consolidation and rigors.
  The course of pneumococcal pneumonia is highly variable, but may be fulminant. Mortality in bacteremic cases of pneumococcal pneumonia is 15-30%, and has not changed significantly over the past 3 decades. Multilobar involvement, respiratory failure requiring mechanical ventilatory support, extrapulmonary spread (endocarditis and meningitis), leukopenia, age more than 60 years, and certain serotypes (e.g. type 3 strains) have been associated with even higher mortality rates.
- The demonstration of lancet-shaped, gram-positive diplococci on sputum Gram stain supports the diagnosis, particularly when intracellular forms are present within leukocytes. Sputum cultures are positive in only 40-60% of bacteremic cases. Peripheral blood leukocytosis or left shift on differential count occurs in more than 80% of patients; leukopenia has been noted in less than or equal to 33% of alcoholic or debilitated patients, and has been associated with a worse prognosis.
- Chest X-rays demonstrate lobar consolidation with air bronchograms in 30-60% of patients; patchy bronchopneumonic infiltrates occur as commonly. Pleural effusions have been noted in less than or equal to 20% of patients; empyema occurs in less than 5%.

Therapy

- Penicillin G, 4.8-10 million U IV until clinical improvement and defervescence have been achieved.
- Penicillin VK, 500 mg qid po, then can be substituted for a full 10-14-day *course—alternative therapy*—erythromycin, 500 mg q 6 hours, or doxycycline, 100 mg bid, IV or po; virtually all beta-lactams, clindamycin, and trimethoprim or sulfamethoxazole (TMP or SMX) are active against *S. pneumoniae.*

Despite the lack of firm data supporting efficacy, vaccination with the 23-valent vaccination should be administered to patients at risk for *S. pneumoniae.* Revaccination is now advised after 6 years.

Haemophilus influenzae

- *Haemophilus influenzae* is a pleomorphic gram-negative rod that accounts for 5-15% of pneumonias, both community acquired and hospital acquired. Both typeable (encapsulated and primarily type B)

- and nontypeable (nonencapsulated) strains are capable of causing disease.
- *Haemophilus influenzae* is a common commensal and may be part of normal oral flora; 20-40% of healthy individuals harbor *H. influenzae* in the oropharynx, and colonization rates of 50-70% have been demonstrated among smokers with COPD.
- *Haemophilus influenzae* characteristically affects smokers, or elderly debilitated patients, but may also affect previously normal hosts.
- Clinical features of *H. influenzae* pneumonia are indistinguishable from those of other bacillary pathogens. Lobar or segmental bronchopneumonic infiltrates are characteristic. Mortality rates of 10-20% have been reported with bacteremic pneumonia caused by *H. influenzae*; higher rates have been noted in immunosuppressed or debilitated individuals.
- Pleomorphic gram-negative rods are characteristic on Gram's stain. Because *H. influenzae* is often part of normal oral flora, however, distinguishing infection from colonization may be difficult. The diagnosis of lower respiratory tract infection caused by *H. influenzae* may be further confounded by the fastidious growth requirements of the organism, and other bacteria may overgrow the culture plates. Thus, even in bacteremic cases of *H. influenzae* pneumonia, sputum cultures have been positive for the organism in only 40-60% of patients.

Therapy

- Ampicillin or sulbactam, cefuroxime, and ceftriaxone
- Oral agents (amoxicillin or clavulanate, cefuroxime axetil, and TMP or SMX) may be acceptable for mild infections in young, otherwise healthy individuals or following initial parenteral therapy.

Alternative agents:
- Trimethoprim or SMX, fluoroquinolones, and newer macrolides (azithromycin and clarithromycin)
- Ampicillin, only for beta-lactamase-negative strains; activity of erythromycin is marginal.

Moraxella (Branhamella) catarrhalis

- *Moraxella catarrhalis* (formerly termed *Neisseria catarrhalis* or *Branhamella catarrhalis*) has long been recognized as part of the normal bacterial flora of the upper respiratory tract and as an important pathogen in otitis media and sinusitis (particularly in children); it accounts for 1-3% of CAP, especially in patients with COPD.
- *Moraxella catarrhalis* is of low virulence, and respiratory tract infections caused by *M. catarrhalis* are typically mild, manifesting

as exacerbations of chronic bronchitis or purulent tracheobronchitis. Pneumonia occurs in only 5–20% of cases of *M. catarrhalis* infections and is usually mild.
- Morphologically, *M. catarrhalis* resembles other *Neisseria* species; kidney bean-shaped gram-negative diplococci are characteristic on Gram's stain.

Therapy

- Cefuroxime (po or IV), ampicillin or sulbactam, amoxicillin or clavulanate.

Alternative therapy:
- Trimethoprim or SMX, erythromycin, tetracycline, and quinolones.

ATYPICAL PNEUMONIAS

- Pneumonia caused by *M. pneumoniae*, *Chlamydia pneumoniae* (TWAR), and viruses may be grouped under the term "atypical pneumonias". These pathogens are considered atypical because they lack many of the cardinal features of acute bacterial pneumonia, such as leukocytosis, pleuritic chest pain, rigors, and consolidation findings. Cough is often nonproductive, and extrapulmonary features such as sore throat, arthritis, myalgias, gastrointestinal (GI) symptoms, headache, and viral prodromal symptoms, may dominate the clinical picture. *M. pneumoniae* has a predilection for previously healthy, young individuals; *Chlamydia-TWAR* and viruses affect all age groups. *Mycoplasma* and *Chlamydia* species are usually mild and self-limited; fatalities are rare.
- Bibasilar interstitial infiltrates or small, patchy, and subsegmental infiltrates are characteristic findings on chest X-ray of pneumonia caused by *M. pneumoniae* or *Chlamydia-TWAR*; however, classic lobar pneumonia indistinguishable from bacillary pneumonias may occur in less than or equal to 20% of patients. Although characteristic clinical and radiographic features exist, none reliably discriminates between atypical and typical bacillary pathogens.

Mycoplasma pneumoniae

- *Mycoplasma pneumoniae*, a cell-wall-deficient microbe within the class Mollicutes, is a pathogen of low virulence that accounts for 2–14% of CAP. *M. pneumoniae* has a striking predilection for younger patients and often spares older individuals, thereby suggesting that pre-existing antibody or prior exposure may confer lasting protection.
- *Mycoplasma pneumoniae* has been implicated in 20–30% of pneumonias in adolescents and adults less than age 35. By contrast, *Mycoplasma* accounts for only 2–9% of pneumonias among adults of ages 40–60,

and for only 1–3% of pneumonias among adults more than age 60. Mycoplasma has rarely been implicated as a nosocomial pathogen.
- Epidemics of *Mycoplasma* have been described in university dormitories, military institutions, schools, and families; prolonged close contact is usually necessary for transmission of infection. Pneumonia caused by *M. pneumoniae* occurs in only 3–10% of exposed individuals.
- Despite the frequency of *M. pneumoniae* in certain populations, its importance as a serious pulmonary pathogen is overrated, because pneumonia caused by *M. pneumoniae* is usually mild and rarely life-threatening. Bronchitis and upper airway symptoms are the predominant features of infections from *M. pneumoniae*. Radiographically, evident pneumonia can be demonstrated in only 5–15% of infected individuals and rarely warrants hospitalization.
- The onset of mycoplasmal pneumonia may be insidious, however, and the course may be protracted. Typical features include fever, malaise, headache, and an intractable hacking cough, which may be productive or nonproductive. Features commonly observed in acute bacillary pneumonia, such as pleuritic chest pain, rigors, and lobar consolidation, are uncommon. Rhinorrhea, sore throat, earache, and hoarseness occur in 25–50% of mycoplasmal infections. On physical examination, erythema of the oropharynx and tender cervical lymphadenopathy can be appreciated in 30–50% of patients. Rhonchi and a few scattered crackles may be detected on auscultation; frank consolidation findings are rare. Bullous myringitis, a frequently emphasized feature of mycoplasmal pneumonia, occurs in 3–7% of patients. Nausea, vomiting, diarrhea, myalgias, and arthralgias occur in 20–45% of patients, but do not distinguish mycoplasmal pneumonia from pneumonias caused by bacteria, *Legionella*, or *Chlamydia* species. Skin rashes occur in 10–15% of patients with mycoplasmal pneumonia; diffuse maculopapular rash, petechiae, urticaria, erythema nodosum, and erythema multiforme have been described.
- Rare (1–3% of patients) complications of mycoplasmal infections include encephalitis, neurologic symptoms, myocarditis, pericarditis, and hemolytic anemia.
- Chest X-ray findings are variable. Diffuse or patchy interstitial infiltrates or patchy bronchopneumonia are most characteristic. Frank lobar consolidation with air bronchograms is evident in less than 15% of patients. Cavitation does not occur. Small pleural effusions have been noted in 5–15% of patients. Peripheral blood leukocyte counts are usually normal, but neutrophilia or a left shift in the differential count occurs in 60–80% of patients. Cold agglutinin immunoglobulin M (IgM) antibodies have been demonstrated in 40–70% of patients. Cold agglutinins, however, may be positive in 10–15% of viral or bacterial pneumonias and, thus, are of limited diagnostic value.

- Serum complement fixation (CF) antibody directed against *Mycoplasma* species is the preferred test because of its high specificity and sensitivity. A fourfold titer ↑ from acute to convalescent sera or single titers of more than 1:128 are considered diagnostic of recent or active infection. Indirect fluorescent antibody and enzyme-linked immunosorbent assay (ELISA) methods have been applied to detect IgM antibodies against *M. pneumoniae*; neither technique has been shown to be superior to CF titers.

Therapy

- Erythromycin, 250–500 mg qid po or IV
- Doxycycline, 100 mg bid po or IV; tetracycline, 250 mg qid. *Alternative agents*—fluoroquinolones (e.g. ciprofloxacin and ofloxacin); azalides (e.g. azithromycin); clarithromycin (because *Mycoplasma* species lack a cell wall, beta-lactams and other cell wall-active antibiotics have no significant activity against *Mycoplasma*).

Chlamydia pneumoniae

- Clinical features of *Chlamydia-TWAR* pneumonia are similar to those of *M. pneumoniae*—fever and cough occur in 50–80% of patients; severe sore throat, often with hoarseness, has been noted in more than 33% of patients and may be the presenting feature.
- Chest X-rays typically demonstrate small (2–3 cm), patchy bronchopneumonic infiltrates; dense lobar consolidation is rare. Pleural effusions are rare in young adults but may be observed in less than or equal to 20% of older adults (many of whom may have coexisting organisms). Peripheral blood leukocyte and differential counts are usually normal.
- The illness is usually mild (albeit often protracted). Tetracyclines or erythromycin may shorten the duration of illness.
- Diagnosis of *Chlamydia-TWAR* pneumonia may be made by culture, direct fluorescent antibody (DFA) staining of sputum, or by serologic methods. The microimmunofluorescence (IF) assay measures both IgM and IgG titers and is the most accurate serologic test. IgM antibody titers more than 16 or IgG titers more than 512 suggest recent or active infection; lower titers of IgG antibody suggest previous infection. The micro-IF test has been positive in more than 90% of culturally confirmed cases and is more than 95% specific. Antibodies do not appear until more than or equal to 10 days after the onset of illness, however, titers may peak at 6–12 weeks. CF studies are less sensitive; less than or equal to 30% of patients with culturally confirmed infections have nondetectable CF antibodies. A fourfold ↑ in CF titer, or single antibody titers more than 64, are considered evidence of recent infection.

Therapy

- Doxycycline or tetracycline po for 14-21 days. *Alternative therapy*—erythromycin, 500 mg qid (less effective than tetracyclines); fluoroquinolones and azalides (highly active in vitro, but limited data in vivo). Beta-lactams and aminoglycosides have no significant activity.

Legionella Species

- *Legionella* species are endemic in the community and account for 2-10% of CAP. The prevalence of nosocomial legionellosis appears to be lower, but has been implicated in less than or equal to 10% of pneumonias in some centers.
- Nosocomial acquisition has been linked to contamination by *Legionella pneumoniae* of the hospital water distribution system. Environmental control measures aimed at eradicating *Legionella* species from hospital water supplies have been highly efficacious in limiting nosocomial legionellosis. Advanced age, renal failure, cigarette smoking, ethanol abuse, organ transplantation, and serious underlying disease have been associated with a higher prevalence of legionellosis and a predilection for more severe disease (including respiratory failure and fatalities).
- *Legionella* species have been associated with severe respiratory failure in 20-40% of patients and with fatality rates of 10-30%.
  Clinically, pneumonia caused by *Legionella* species may be indistinguishable from other bacterial pneumonias. Diffuse alveolar infiltrates, patchy bronchopneumonic infiltrates, or lobar consolidation may occur. Pleural effusions occur in less than 10% of patients; cavitation has been described, but is rare chest X-ray.
  Several features that occur more commonly with pneumonia caused by *Legionella* species than with pneumonia caused by other pathogens may provide clues to the diagnosis. These include:
    - Progression of pneumonia while taking antimicrobials (particularly penicillins or cephalosporins)
    - Hyponatremia in 20-50% of patients
    - Neurologic symptoms (confusion, lethargy, and headache) in 20-30% of patients
    - Gastrointestinal symptoms (principally nausea, vomiting, and diarrhea) in 20-40% of patients
    - Elevations in serum transaminases in 20-40% of patients.
  Although characteristic, these features do not distinguish legionellosis from other types of pneumonia:
- *Legionella* species are gram-negative rods but are difficult to visualize on conventional Gram's stains. In addition, *Legionella* species have fastidious growth requirements; thus, specialized media are required for culture. The diagnosis requires demonstration of the *Legionella* organisms

by DFA or cultures of expectorated sputum, tracheal secretions, or bronchoalveolar lavage (BAL). The organisms can be identified also in tissue by using Dieterle silver stains or DFA. Newer diagnostic techniques, such as ELISA or radioimmunoassay for urinary antigen or Gen-Probe detection of *Legionella pneumophila* in respiratory secretions, have been developed, but the role of these adjunctive techniques has not been established. Measurements of serum antibodies against *Legionella* species by the indirect fluorescent technique are invaluable to determine the prevalence of legionellosis in prospective epidemiologic surveys, but are of no value in individual patients, because results may not be available for more than or equal to 2-4 weeks. A single titer of 1:256 or a fourfold or greater ↑ in specific antibody titer is considered diagnostic of acute infection.

Therapy

- Erythromycin, 1 g q 6 hours IV; 500 mg qid po may be substituted once clinical improvement and defervescence have occurred. 21 days of therapy are optimal.
- Rifampin, synergistic in vitro; consider combining with erythromycin in seriously ill or immunocompromised host: *Alternative therapy*—doxycycline, 100 mg bid IV followed by oral administration once patient's condition has improved; ciprofloxacin, ofloxacin, azalides, and *TMP/SMX* (highly active in vitro; limited data in man). Beta-lactams and aminoglycosides are not active against *Legionellae* species.

EMPIRIC (INITIAL) THERAPY

In most cases of pneumonia, therapy is empiric, based on the probability of certain pathogens being involved. Initial treatment for CAP (undertaken while waiting for cultural confirmation) should be sufficiently broad to cover most likely pathogens while avoiding polypharmacy or excessively expensive or toxic antimicrobials. Choice of empiric therapy must be modified based on such clinical features as age, the presence or absence of underlying disease, radiographic appearance, prior use of antimicrobials, and severity of the pneumonic process.

Young, Previously Healthy Adults

Pneumonia in previously healthy young adults (<age 35) can be successfully treated with a variety of agents, including penicillin G, ampicillin, sulbactam, erythromycin, doxycycline, or cefuroxime. *M. pneumoniae* has been implicated in 20-30% of CAP in this population; *S. pneumoniae* has been implicated in 30-60%. *Chlamydia, Legionella* species, and *H. influenzae* each account for 2-6% of cases, viruses for 5-15%, and Enterobacteriaceae

or *S. aureus* for less than 2% of CAP in previously healthy young adults. In view of the limited spectrum of microbes involved in this patient population, relatively narrow spectrum (and less expensive) agents can be considered. The choice of agent depends in part on the clinical and radiographic presentation.

- If a lobar process is evident and a sputum Gram's stain demonstrates predominantly gram-positive cocci within leukocytes, treatment with penicillin G or ampicillin may be adequate. These agents fail to cover atypical pneumonias (e.g. those caused by *Mycoplasma, Legionella*, and *Chlamydia* species), but have excellent activity against *S. pneumoniae* and other streptococci.
- When a sputum Gram's stain or clinical course is nonspecific, treatment with erythromycin or doxycycline to provide coverage against atypical pathogens may be appropriate. These agents are also active against *S. pneumoniae* but provide marginal coverage against *H. influenzae*.
- When atypical pneumonia is unlikely based on clinical grounds, and Gram's stain is nondiagnostic, the use of broader-spectrum agents, such as ampicillin or sulbactam or cefuroxime, is reasonable. These antimicrobials are highly active against *S. pneumoniae, H. influenzae, S. aureus*, and certain Enterobacteriaceae (Flowchart 15.1).

Flowchart 15.1: Antibiotic therapy for community-acquired pneumonia.

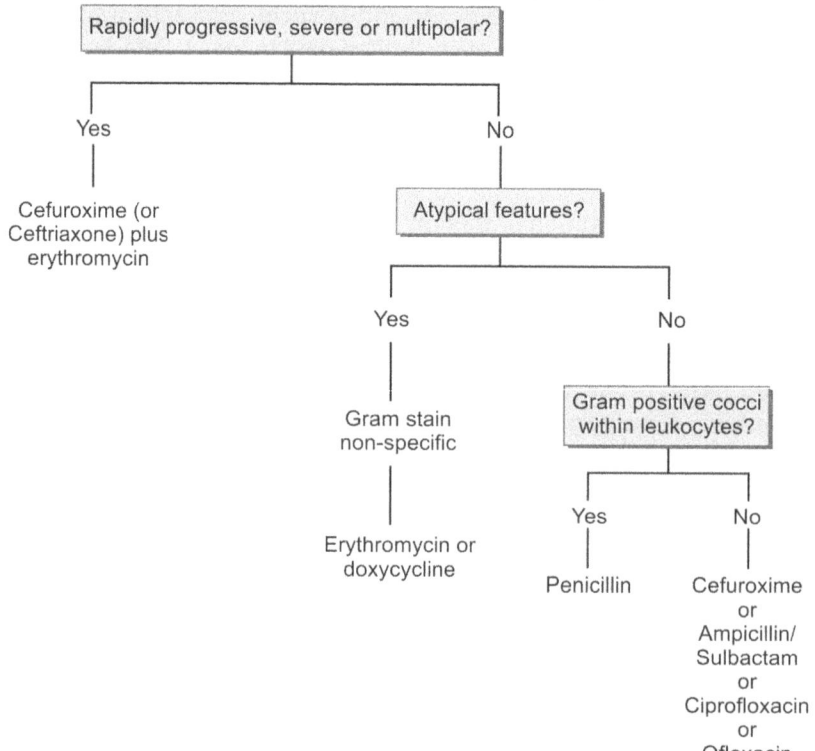

Elderly Patients or Those with Underlying Disease

- In the elderly patient or debilitated patient of any age, enteric GNB and *H. influenzae* may account for more than or equal to 20% of pneumonias. Taken together, GNB, *H. influenzae*, and *S. aureus* cause at least as many cases of CAP in this patient population as does *S. pneumoniae*.
- In these "at-risk" patient populations, treatment strategies must encompass these pathogens.
- Broader-spectrum agents are needed to encompass *S. pneumoniae*, *H. influenzae*, *M. catarrhalis*, and Enterobacteriaceae (principally *E. coli, Klebsiella*, and *Proteus* species).
- Penicillin G and ampicillin do not provide adequate coverage against GNB or *H. influenzae* and are not recommended.
- Ampicillin or sulbactam provides ↑ activity against *H. influenzae, E. coli,* and *Klebsiella* species, but has limited activity against other GNB.
- Cefuroxime (a second-generation cephalosporin) and ceftriaxone (a third-generation cephalosporin) are advisable empiric treatment of pneumonia for these "at-risk" patients.
- Exceptionally broad-spectrum agents, such as antipseudomonal penicillins or imipenem, are efficacious but too expensive to justify as first-line therapy.
- Ciprofloxacin has broad-spectrum activity against GNB and *H. influenzae* and has been used with success in community-acquired and nursing home-acquired pneumonias. The activity of ciprofloxacin against *S. pneumoniae* and anaerobes is marginal, however; thus, this agent should be restricted to patients in whom the presence of these pathogens is unlikely. Specific therapy against *M. pneumoniae* (e.g. erythromycin or doxycycline) is usually not warranted for elderly patients, because less than 2% of cases of CAP in this age group are caused by *Mycoplasma* species.
- For rapidly progressive, multilobar, or severe pneumonias, however, combination therapy with a broad-spectrum beta-lactam, such as cefuroxime or ceftriaxone, to cover *H. influenzae, S. aureus,* and Enterobacteriaceae, together with erythromycin to cover *Legionella* and *Mycoplasma*, is appropriate.

NOSOCOMIAL PNEUMONIA

Microbiology and Pathogenesis

Pneumonia develops in 0.5-2% of hospitalized patients and has been associated with a mortality rate of 30-60%.
- In striking contrast to CAP, *S. pneumoniae* and *M. pneumoniae* account for only 3-8% of pneumonias in hospitalized patients. Enteric GNB are

responsible for 70–85% of nosocomial pneumonias. Enterobacteriaceae (predominantly *Klebsiella* and *Enterobacter* species) have been implicated in 30–50% of nosocomial pneumonias; 15–20% are caused by *Pseudomonas aeruginosa*. *H. influenzae* is responsible for 3–8% of nosocomial pneumonias. A host of other aerobic enteric GNB, such as *Providencia, Citrobacter, Morganella,* and *Acinetobacter* species, may each account for an additional 2–5% of cases. Aerobic gram-positive organisms, such as *Staphylococcus* species (*S. aureus* and *S. epidermidis*) and streptococci account for 10–25% of nosocomial pneumonias. A disproportionate number of gram-positive infections, however, occur in patients with intravascular devices, such as Hickman catheters, arteriovenous (AV) shunts, and hemodialysis shunts, and in neurosurgical patients or patients receiving hyperalimentation via indwelling central lines.
- The dominant mechanism by which nosocomial pneumonia occurs is via aspiration of endogenous oropharyngeal bacilli into the tracheobronchial tree. Oropharyngeal and tracheal colonization with enteric GNB is markedly ↑ed in hospitalized patients and in patients with serious underlying diseases, and is an important precursor of infection.

Diagnosis

The diagnosis of nosocomial pneumonia may be difficult, particularly in intensive care unit (ICU) patients or postoperative surgical patients, because infiltrates on the chest X-ray may be seen with other concurrent disorders, such as congestive heart failure (CHF), atelectasis, pulmonary embolism, or acute respiratory distress syndrome (ARDS). Pneumonia complicates ARDS in 50–75% of patients; persistence or progression of respiratory failure in ARDS may reflect concomitant pulmonary suppuration, which may not be evident clinically:
- The hallmarks of bacterial infection may be lacking in critically ill or debilitated patients unable to mount an adequate host response. Pleuritic chest pain, high fever, and chills are usually lacking; chest X-rays often demonstrate only minimal, and patchy infiltrates that mimic fluid overload or CHF. Frank consolidation with air bronchograms or cavitation, the cardinal findings of suppurative infection, is present in a distinct minority of patients. Thus, a high index of suspicion is required to make a diagnosis of lower respiratory tract infection in a timely fashion.
- The development of unexplained leukocytosis (or left shift) worsening dyspnea, purulent tracheobronchial secretions, or new infiltrates on chest X-ray warrants an aggressive approach.

- A Gram's stain of expectorated sputum or tracheal secretions should be done to assess a predominant organism, but one should avoid over-reliance on sputum or tracheal aspirates, smears, and cultures in dictating therapeutic strategy. Potential pathogens may be demonstrated on culture of tracheal aspirates in 60–100% of pneumonias, but cultures are also positive in most patients without clinical evidence of infection. Thus, specificity is low (<20%).
- Blood cultures should be done, even though only 5–10% of nosocomial pneumonia cases are bacteremic. Unfortunately, in many cases, a precise microbiologic diagnosis is never established, despite appropriate cultures.
- Invasive diagnostic techniques, such as flexible bronchoscope (FB) with a sheathed catheter (PB) and BAL and quantitative cultures have been employed to define more accurately the microbacteriologic aspect of nosocomial pneumonia. A "negative" study does not reliably exclude pneumonia. The routine application of FB with PB or BAL in suspected nosocomial pneumonia and the modification of therapy according to these results have not reduced either morbidity or mortality.

Therapy

Because the diagnostic techniques used to ascertain the microbiologic cause of pneumonia remain inexact, treatment of nosocomial pneumonia often remains empiric. In view of the potentially lethal nature of nosocomial pneumonia, it is advisable to initiate therapy with broad-spectrum parenteral antibiotics pending identification of the responsible organism(s). Selection of antibiotics in this context should take into account findings on sputum Gram's stain, host and environmental factors that may point to specific pathogens, the known frequency of specific isolates in the hospital or ICU setting, and antimicrobial susceptibility patterns within institutions (and individual ICUs). Antimicrobial therapy can be switched to a narrower spectrum agent once a definitive microbiologic diagnosis has been established.

Patients who have recently received parenteral antimicrobial agents are at risk of acquiring highly resistant organisms, such as *P. aeruginosa*, *Acinetobacter*, *Serratia* species, and methicillin-resistant staphylococci. Antibiotic resistance patterns may vary widely within hospitals or even within ICUs within hospitals, depending on previous trends of antibiotic use.

Monotherapy may be as effective as combination therapy in some circumstances, but the efficacy of monotherapy for nosocomial gram-negative pneumonia (particularly when *P. aeruginosa* has been implicated) has not been convincingly established. This area remains controversial.

Empiric Therapy (Prior to Identification of a Specific Organism)

In view of the relatively high prevalence of *P. aeruginosa* as a cause of nosocomial pneumonia in mechanically ventilated patients, initial empiric therapy in this context should include coverage against *P. aeruginosa*.

- Combination therapy with an antipseudomonal broad-spectrum beta-lactam, such as ceftazidime, piperacillin, ticarcillin or clavulanate, or imipenem/cilastatin, and an amino glycoside (typically gentamicin because of its lower cost) is preferred as initial therapy. If contraindications to aminoglycosides exist, monotherapy with ceftazidime or imipenem may be adequate.
- Ciprofloxacin can be substituted for the beta-lactam, if the patient is allergic to penicillin.
- Agents with broad-spectrum gram-negative activity but without antipseudomonal activity, such as ceftriaxone, cefotaxime, and ceftizoxime, may be adequate in noncritically ill, nonventilated patients in whom the risk of infections caused by *Pseudomonas* species is lower. First- or second-generation cephalosporins, ampicillin, or sulbactam are not adequate for the initial empiric treatment of nosocomial pneumonia. Aminoglycosides alone are not adequate for the treatment of gram-negative bacterial pneumonia.

Modification of Antimicrobial Therapy

The initial (empiric) antimicrobial therapy should be reassessed once cultural results are available (usually by 48–72 hours) and the clinical course has been clarified. The appropriate agent (s) depends on the suspected (or confirmed) organism (s) and the microbiologic susceptibility results for each individual patient (Table 15.1). For infections caused by *P. aeruginosa*, combination therapy with an extended-spectrum penicillin (e.g. piperacillin or ticarcillin), ceftazidime, or imipenem or cilastatin plus an aminoglycoside is warranted. Other third-generation cephalosporins, such as cefotaxime, ceftizoxime, and ceftriaxone, extended-spectrum penicillins, or imipenem or cilastatin provide excellent activity against most other enteric GNB. First- or second-generation cephalosporins may be substituted for more expensive agents, if a specific organism has been isolated and shown to be susceptible. If highly susceptible pathogens, such as *E. coli*, *Klebsiella*, and *Proteus* species, are isolated and the patient is improving, the aminoglycoside may be discontinued. For highly virulent strains, such as *P. aeruginosa*, *Serratia*, *Acinetobacter*, and *Enterobacter* species, the synergistic microbiocidal activity achieved with combination therapy is important to maintain for the duration of therapy.

Preferred combination therapy for specific pathogens is given in Table 15.1. Irrespective of the agent (s) utilized, duration of therapy for nosocomial pneumonia must be adequate to avoid recrudescent infection. Treatment is usually necessary for a minimum of 10 days; a more prolonged course (extending for ≥21 days) may be appropriate for more virulent pathogens, such as *P. aeruginosa*, or for complicated, severe, or protracted cases.

Table 15.1: Therapy for specific pathogens causing nosocomial pneumonia.

Specific pathogens	Preferred therapy
Acinetobacter calcoaceticus	• TMP or SMX, antipseudomonal penicillins, imipenem or cilastatin, ceftazidime, aminoglycosides, and the fluoroquinolones are usually highly active (choice of agent depends on results of susceptibility testing) • Combine with an aminoglycoside to confer synergistic killing
Enterobacter species	• Imipenem (combine with aminoglycoside) • Antipseudomonal penicillin (combine with aminoglycoside)
Escherichia coli	• Ampicillin or sulbactam, cefuroxime, or cefotetan (these agents are highly effective and less expensive than third-generation cephalosporins, imipenem, or aztreonam) • Ampicillin (only for beta-lactamase-negative strain). *Alternative agents*: TMP or SMX, ciprofloxacin, aztreonam, and imipenem
Klebsiella pneumoniae	Second- or third-generation cephalosporins (monotherapy is adequate) *Alternative agents*: Imipenem, Ciprofloxacin, aztreonam, and TMP or SMX
Serratia marcescens	Third-generation cephalosporin (combine with aminoglycoside). *Alternative Agents*: Imipenem, aztreonam, Ciprofloxacin, and TMP or SMX
Pseudomonas aeruginosa	• Piperacillin or ceftazidime (combine with aminoglycoside) • Imipenem (reserve for resistant strains; combine with aminoglycoside). *Alternative agents*: Ciprofloxacin, aztreonam
Pseudomonas cepacia	• TMP or SMX, ciprofloxacin: Aztreonam (depending on susceptibility) • Aminoglycosides may confer synergistic killing in some strains. *Alternative agents*: Ceftazidime, chloramphenicol (virtually all isolates are resistant to imipenem)

Contd...

Contd...

Specific pathogens	Preferred therapy
Xanthomonas maltophilia	TMP or SMX (ciprofloxacin also acceptable). *Alternative agents*: Antipseudomonal penicillins ceftazidime (only a minority are susceptible). Addition of aminoglycosides does not confer
Streptococci (other than enterococcus)	• Penicillin G or ampicillin • Combined with aminoglycoside for life-threatening infections. *Alternative agents*: Third-generation cephalosporins, imipenem (highly active but expensive) • Erythromycin, clindamycin, and vancomycin for patients allergic to penicillin
Group 0 Streptococci (enterococci)	Ampicillin (or vancomycin) combined with an aminoglycoside (cephalosporins are uniformly resistant)
Staphylococcus aureus	• Oxacillin or cloxacillin (only for methicillin-susceptible strains) • Vancomycin (uniformly active for both methicillin-susceptible and methicillin-resistant strains) • *Alternative agents*: Clindamycin, imipenem, and cefazolin
Methicillin-resistant Staphylococcus aureus	Vancomycin. *Alternative* agents: TMP or SMX, clindamycin, and imipenem
Coagulase-negative staphylococci (Staphylococcus epidermidis)	• Vancomycin • Nafcillin (only for susceptible strains)

(TMP, trimethoprim SMX, sulfamethoxazole)

ANAEROBIC PLEUROPULMONARY INFECTIONS

Epidemiology

Aspiration of many oropharyngeal bacilli may lead to a spectrum of pleuropulmonary manifestations, including acute pneumonitis, necrotizing pneumonia with cavitation, lung abscess, and empyema. The predominant oropharyngeal anaerobes include *Bacteroides melaninogenicus, Fusobacterium nucleatum, Peptococcus, Peptostreptococcus,* and microaerophilic streptococci. *Bacteroides fragilis* and species within the *B. fragilis* group (e.g. *B. ovatus, B. vulgatus,* and *B. thetaiotaomicron*) account for 10-15% of isolates. Anaerobes have been implicated as either sole or concomitant pathogens in 60-97% of aspiration pneumonias or primary lung abscesses and in 6-15% of pneumonias in the community.

Clinical Features

Aspiration pneumonia should be considered in patients with primary neurologic or esophageal disease; common associated conditions include ↓ed level of consciousness, alcohol or drug abuse, general anesthesia, previous strokes, seizures, periodontal disease, and the presence of nasogastric (NG), endotracheal, and tracheostomy tubes. Aspiration pneumonia preferentially involves the dependent segments of the lung (posterior segments of the upper lobes and superior segments of the lower lobes) as a result of gravitational forces; however, basilar infiltrates may also occur. Community-acquired aspiration pneumonia often exhibits an indolent course, evolving over 1–3 weeks. Cough, sputum production, and low-grade fever are characteristic. The hallmarks of acute bacillary pneumonias, such as chills, rigors, pleuritic chest pain, and consolidation findings, are usually lacking. In fact, constitutional signs, such as weight loss, anemia, and generalized weakness, may be the presenting features. The course of aspiration pneumonitis may be more fulminant, however, particularly when *S. aureus* or enteric GNB are present concomitantly. Chest X-rays typically demonstrate patchy infiltrates without clear evidence for consolidation; persistence of the pneumonic infiltrate may lead to necrosis and cavitation. An air-fluid level indicates a lung abscess.

Microbiology

Clarification of the microbiologic cause of aspiration pneumonia (or lung abscess) is usually difficult. Expectorated sputum cultures often grow only normal oral flora because concomitant upper respiratory tract flora usually overgrow any anaerobes that may be present. Foul-smelling, putrid sputum is a clue to the presence of anaerobes but is only present in one-third of patients. Gram's stain of expectorated sputum or empyema fluid may demonstrate a mixture of both gram-negative (e.g. *Bacteroides* species, *F. nucleatum*) and gram-positive (e.g. streptococci and peptococci) organisms; however, these findings are nonspecific and of limited value. Only percutaneous needle aspiration, transtracheal aspirates, or thoracentesis can be considered reliable sources for anaerobic cultures. Because of the invasive nature of percutaneous needle aspiration or transtracheal aspiration, however, these procedures are not recommended for microbiologic diagnosis of aspiration pneumonia or lung abscess. Pioneering studies in the early 1970s by Gorbach, Finegold, and Bartlett (using transtracheal aspirates) elegantly delineated the organism (s) responsible for aspiration pneumonia or primary lung abscess in the community. Of primary lung abscesses, 50% were caused by pure anaerobes; 47% by a mixture of anaerobes and aerobes, and 3% predominantly by aerobes.

Therapy

Antibiotic therapy is almost always sufficient for management of anaerobic pneumonitis or lung abscess; drainage of abscess cavities usually can be accomplished by expectoration of sputum and local percussion and drainage. Progression of the infection to the pleural space may result in empyema; in such cases, aggressive drainage (employing a surgical empyema tube) in addition to antibiotics is required.

The decision as to initial therapy must be individualized. In view of its lower cost, penicillin G 8-12 million U daily is a reasonable first choice for patients with mild disease. Clindamycin is preferred for seriously ill patients with lung abscess or for patients who have failed initial therapy with penicillin. Metronidazole (Flagyl) has exquisite activity against anaerobes (including *B. fragilis*) in vitro, but has been associated with a high failure rate when used as monotherapy for pulmonary anaerobic infections and is not recommended.

Alternative agents: Cefotetan, antipseudomonal penicillins, or imipenem (may be particularly useful when infection with enteric GNB coexists).

Antimicrobial Agents

Beta-lactams

This class of agents includes penicillins, cephalosporins, carbapenems, and monobactams; the 4-membered beta-lactam ring (usually fused to a second ring) is integral to the structure. Modifications or substitutions of the beta-lactam ring may alter antimicrobial activity or resistance to beta-lactamases.

Penicillins: Since the introduction of penicillin for clinical use in 1941, the penicillin group of antibiotics has remained key to the treatment of pulmonary infections. Penicillins have excellent bactericidal activity and relatively low toxicity. The basic structure of the penicillin group of antimicrobials consists of a beta-lactam ring fused to a 5-membered thiazolidine ring; modification of the side chains attached to the beta-lactam ring may alter the antimicrobial spectrum, beta-lactamase, stability, and pharmacokinetics. Many of the newer penicillins are modifications of ampicillin. Substitution of a carboxy group for an amino group on ampicillin produced the carboxypenicillins, carbenicillin, and ticarcillin. Substitution of an ureido group for the carboxy group produced the ureidopenicillins (piperacillin, mezlocillin, and azlocillin).

- Mechanism of action: Penicillins interfere with bacterial cell wall (peptidoglycan) synthesis and activate endogenous autolytic enzymes, inducing cell lysis. Killing of GNB requires that penicillins penetrate outer portions of the bacterial cell wall and combine with key penicillin-binding proteins (PBPs) on the inner membrane of the bacteria.

- Antimicrobial resistance: The most common mechanism of resistance to penicillins is via beta-lactamases. Beta-lactamases are produced by both gram-negative and gram-positive bacilli and hydrolyze the beta-lactam ring, thereby inactivating penicillin.
- Toxicity: Adverse effects include maculopapular rash, eosinophilia, drug fever (particularly with ampicillin and methicillin), bleeding disorders with high doses of carbenicillin and ticarcillin, and seizures when in high doses (particularly in presence of renal failure).

Benzyl-penicillin (Penicillin G): Antimicrobial spectrum—outstanding activity against *S. pneumoniae* (pneumococci). *S. pyogenes* (group A), all other beta-hemolytic streptococci. Most *S. viridans*, and group D streptococci (*Enterococcus* species). More than 80% staphylococci are resistant. Anaerobes (with exception of beta-lactamase [+] strains of *B. fragilis*) are exquisitely sensitive. Active against gram-negative cocci, such as *Neisseria meningitidis* and *N. gonorrhoeae*. No significant activity against *H. influenzae* or enteric GNB. No activity against *Mycoplasma*, *Chlamydia*, and *Legionella* species; most *M. catarrhalis* are now resistant.

- Dosage: 4.8-10 million U of aqueous crystalline penicillin G IV qd in 4-6 divided doses; oral penicillin [the K salt of phenoxymethyl penicillin (Penicillin VK)] can be substituted in a dose of 500 mg qid once clinical response and defervescence have occurred.
- Indications: Drug of choice for pneumonia caused by *S. pneumoniae* and most other streptococci—one of the choices for empiric therapy for suspected lung abscess (clindamycin may be superior). Therapeutic for infections caused by enterococci (*S. faecalis* and *S. faecium*); however, these streptococci are inhibited but not killed by penicillins alone. Thus, must be combined with either rifampin or an aminoglycoside.

Because of its limited spectrum, penicillin G is not suitable as empiric therapy for CAP except when *S. pneumoniae* is strongly suspected from a compatible clinical picture and confirmatory Gram's stain Penicillin G has no therapeutic role for nosocomial pneumonia.

Antistaphylococcal penicillins: The semisynthetic penicillins were developed for treatment of beta-lactamase-producing staphylococci resistant to penicillin G; the addition of an acyl side chain prevented disruption of the beta-lactam ring by beta-lactamases. The three semisynthetic penicillins available for parenteral use are methicillin (staphcillin and celbenin), nafcillin (Nafcil and Unipen), and oxacillin (Prostaphlin).

- Antimicrobial spectrum: Active against most staphylococci, including beta-lactamase-producing strains. Not active against methicillin-resistant staphylococci. Less active than penicillin G against streptococci and other penicillin-susceptible organisms. No significant activity against anaerobes. No activity against GNB, *Chlamydia*, *Mycoplasma*, or *Legionella* species.

- Toxicity: Similar to that of penicillin, but also includes interstitial nephritis. Intensely irritating to veins (phlebitis).
- Dosage: 1-2 g IV q 4-6 hours; oral antistaphylococcal penicillins (cloxacillin or dicloxacillin) can be substituted in some patients when clinical response has occurred (dose, 250-500 mg qid).
- Indications: In view of their limited spectrum of activity, the antistaphylococcal penicillins should be reserved for patients with pneumonia caused by susceptible strains of staphylococci. Other agents are preferred for other pathogens. Nafcillin, oxacillin, and methicillin are equivalent in efficacy, but side effects (particularly interstitial nephritis) are most frequent with methicillin. Thus, nafcillin and oxacillin are preferred agents.

Aminopenicillins: The aminopenicillins (ampicillin and amoxicillin) were the first of the penicillins to have activity against GNB. Ampicillin (the first of the aminopenicillins) was developed by adding an amino group to the benzylpenicillin molecule; other agents (amoxicillin and bacampicillin) were later developed. These agents have significant activity against *H. influenzae* and selected enteric GNB. Ampicillin and amoxicillin have no activity against *Klebsiella pneumoniae* and indole-positive *Proteus* species, and can no longer be considered reliable against *H. influenzae* or *E. coli*. Antimicrobial resistance to these agents has ↑ed dramatically over the past decade, even among isolates that previously were highly susceptible, such as *H. influenzae*, *M. catarrhalis*, and *E. coli*. These factors have relegated ampicillin and amoxicillin to secondary roles in the treatment of pneumonia.

- Antimicrobial spectrum: Excellent activity against gram-positive cocci (including *S. pneumoniae*, other streptococci, and enterococci) and anaerobes (comparable to penicillin G). Active against *Neisseria* species, beta-lactamase-negative strains of *Haemophilus* species (not against beta-lactamase-producing *H. influenzae*, which comprise 10-20% of isolates), 60-70% of *E. coli*, and *Proteus mirabilis*. Fails to cover l3-lactamase-producing strains of *M. catarrhalis*. No significant activity against *Klebsiella*, *Enterobacter*, *Serratia*, indole-positive *Proteus*, or *Pseudomonas* species. No activity against *Chlamydia*, *M. pneumoniae*, or *Legionella* species.
- Toxicity: Similar to that of penicillin G except higher incidence of diarrhea and GI symptoms (10-15%) and skin rash (3-5%).
- Dosage: Ampicillin 1-2 g IV q 6 hours; in some patients, oral ampicillin 500 mg qid (or amoxicillin 500 mg tid) can be substituted once a clinical response to IV therapy has been demonstrated.
- Indications: Pneumonia caused by a susceptible strain of *H. influenzae*, *E. coli*, or *Proteus mirabilis*. Infections caused by enterococci (combine with an aminoglycoside). Because of the limited spectrum of ampicillin and amoxicillin, other agents are preferred for empiric therapy of CAP or nosocomial pneumonia.

Beta-lactamase inhibitors: Clavulanate and sulbactam inhibit beta-lactamases produced by certain gram-positive and gram-negative bacteria (e.g. *H. influenzae*, *K. pneumoniae*, and staphylococci), but lack intrinsic antibacterial activity. The addition of these beta-lactamase inhibitors to the parent compound (ticarcillin, ampicillin, and amoxicillin) extends the spectrum of activity of these agents to include beta-lactamase-producing strains resistant to the parent compound alone. Clavulanate and sulbactam do not improve the activity of the parent compound for beta-lactamase-negative strains or bacteria that are resistant by mechanisms other than beta-lactamase production. In addition, neither clavulanate nor sulbactam affects beta-lactamases of the type 1 Richmond–Sykes classification produced by *P. aeruginosa*, *Enterobacter*, *Morganella*, and *Serratia* species. These agents are not adequate for infections caused by methicillin-resistant *S. aureus* (MRSA).

Ampicillin or sulbactam: The addition of sulbactam to ampicillin extended the spectrum of ampicillin to include beta-lactamase-producing strains of *S. aureus*, *M. catarrhalis*, *H. influenzae*, *B. fragilis*, *Klebsiella*, *E. coli*, *Proteus*, and *Acinetobacter* species. Ampicillin or sulbactam is less active against Enterobacteriaceae than are third-generation cephalosporins.

- Antimicrobial spectrum: Excellent activity against gram-positive bacteria (including *S. aureus*, streptococci, and enterococci) and anaerobes (inhibiting more than 95% of strains, including *B. fragilis*). Active against and *Proteus mirabilis*. Not active against *P. aeruginosa*, *Serratia*, *Enterobacter* species, or difficult-to-treat gram-negative infections.
- Dosage: Supplied as 3-g or 1.5-g vials for IV use in fixed 2:1 ratio of ampicillin to sulbactam; dose, 1.5–3 g q 6 hours (pharmacokinetics similar to those of ampicillin).
- Indications: Most useful for polymicrobial infections including anaerobes. Reasonable as empiric therapy for CAP in nonimmunocompromised hosts. Less useful for nosocomial pneumonia because of its lack of activity against *P. aeruginosa* and limited spectrum of activity against gram-negative bacteria. Excellent for pelvic and abdominal infections.

Amoxicillin or clavulanate: This combination was the first of the penicillin or beta-lactamase inhibitors available for clinical use), it is available only in oral form.

- Antimicrobial spectrum: Spectrum of ampicillin or amoxicillin plus beta-lactamase-producing strains of *H. influenzae*, *E. coli*, *Proteus*, *Klebsiella*, *M. catarrhalis*, and *S. aureus*. No activity against *P. aeruginosa*, *Serratia*, *Enterobacter*, *Citrobacter*, and MRSA
- Toxicity: Similar to that of ampicillin or amoxicillin
- Dosage: 250–500 mg tid
- Indications: Useful as oral empiric therapy for mild CAP (in patients at low risk for more resistant gram-negative bacteria) or following initial therapy with a parenteral agent.

Antipseudomonal penicillins: Carbenicillin, a carboxypenicillin produced by substituting a carboxyl group for the amino group on ampicillin, extended the gram-negative spectrum of ampicillin and was the first of the penicillins with significant activity against *P. aeruginosa*. Substitutions on carbenicillin resulted in ticarcillin, which had even broader gram-negative activity. Attachment of ureido groups to the acyl side chain of ampicillin led to the "ureidopenicillins," which include piperacillin, mezlocillin, and azlocillin. Antipseudomonal penicillins are effective in the treatment of CAP, nosocomial pneumonias, and serious nosocomial sepsis, and as empiric treatment of sepsis in immunocompromised and granulocytopenic hosts.

- Antimicrobial spectrum: Antipseudomonal penicillins are broad-spectrum agents active against most GNB, including beta-lactamase-negative *H. influenzae*, most Enterobacteriaceae, indole-positive *Proteus, Providencia, Morganella*, and *P. aeruginosa*. The activity of antipseudomonal penicillins against *E. coli* is less predictable (only 80–90% of isolates susceptible) than that of third-generation cephalosporins. As many as 20–40% of *Enterobacter* species are resistant. The carboxypenicillins (ticarcillin and carbenicillin) are not reliable against *Klebsiella, Serratia* species, or enterococci; the ureidopenicillins, particularly piperacillin, have generally good activity against these pathogens. Piperacillin and mezlocillin have excellent activity against *Klebsiella* species (>80% of isolates susceptible), whereas only 10–30% of *Klebsiella* species are susceptible to carbenicillin, azlocillin, and ticarcillin. Compared to the other penicillins, piperacillin has slightly greater activity [lower minimal inhibitory concentration (MIC)] in vitro, and is the most active agent against *P. aeruginosa*. Whether these in vitro differences result in improved efficacy in vivo has not been established, Timentin represents a fixed combination of 3 g of ticarcillin and 100 mg of clavulanate K (a beta-lactamase inhibitor). The clavulanate binds to beta-lactamases secreted by staphylococci, *B. fragilis, M. catarrhalis, H. influenzae, Klebsiella* species, *Proteus* species, and certain enteric GNB and thus extends the spectrum of activity of ticarcillin to include these beta-lactamase-producing organisms. Clavulanate, however, does not affect type 1 beta-lactamases, such as those released by certain strains of *Pseudomonas, Serratia, Citrobacter*, and *Enterobacter* species. Thus, clavulanate does not improve (and may actually reduce) the activity of ticarcillin against these strains. In addition, clavulanate does not improve the activity of ticarcillin against strains of bacteria resistant by mechanisms other than beta-lactamase production (e.g. changes in the permeability of the cell wall). The activity of ticarcillin or clavulanate is no more than that of ticarcillin alone against susceptible, beta-lactamase-negative strains. Thus, for susceptible organisms, ticarcillin alone is preferable and is less expensive than ticarcillin or clavulanate. Ticarcillin or clavulanate exhibits good activity against staphylococci in vitro (including MRSA), but treatment failures in vivo suggest that it is not adequate for proven infections caused by MRSA (irrespective of in vitro susceptibility data). Ticarcillin or clavulanate has only modest activity against enterococci. Activity of the antipseudomonal penicillins against streptococci and most gram-positive bacteria is good, but less effective than that afforded by penicillin G or ampicillin. None of these agents (except for ticarcillin or clavulanate) is effective against beta-lactamase-producing strains of staphylococci. MRSA are invariably resistant. Anaerobic activity is generally excellent, but is less than the anaerobic activity of metronidazole or clindamycin; beta-lactamase-producing strains of *B. fragilis* may be susceptible only to ticarcillin or clavulanate. The major "holes" in coverage are *E. coli*, *Enterobacter* species (resistance rates in nosocomial settings of 15–30%), and staphylococci (beta-lactamase producing and MRSA).

- Toxicity: Adverse effects include skin rash, hypokalemia, and Na load (particularly with disodium salts carbenicillin and ticarcillin; 4.7 mEq/g of Na for carbenicillin and ticarcillin; only 1.8 mEq/g for mezlocillin and piperacillin). Prolonged bleeding time and abnormalities in coagulation tests, especially in uremic patients, are noted with carbenicillin, which is no longer used.
- Dosage: 3-4 g IV q 4-6 hours (3.1 g q 4-6 hours for ticarcillin or clavulanate)
- Indications: Piperacillin or ticarcillin or clavulanate may be used as first-line agents for empiric therapy of nosocomial pneumonia, serious nosocomial sepsis, or when *P. aeruginosa* is a consideration (e.g. cystic fibrosis, mechanical ventilation, previous antimicrobials, granulocytopenia, and immunocompromised hosts). Ticarcillin or clavulanate has superior gram-positive activity but slightly less gram-negative activity compared to piperacillin; overall, these agents are therapeutically equivalent for serious nosocomial infections. Both agents are superior to mezlocillin or azlocillin in this context. Combination therapy with an aminoglycoside may provide synergy and is recommended. Antipseudomonal penicillins are not recommended for CAP. *P. aeruginosa* is rarely a consideration in this context, and less expensive agents (e.g. cefuroxime, ceftriaxone, and ampicillin or sulbactam) provide adequate coverage against community-acquired respiratory pathogens, including most Enterobacteriaceae.

Cephalosporins:
- Antimicrobial spectrum: Broad-spectrum activity against both gram-negative and gram-positive bacteria. Gram-positive activity (particularly against staphylococci) is best with cefazolin and modest with succeeding generations; ceftazidime has poor activity. Adequate against most streptococci (including *S. pneumoniae*), but generally less active than penicillins; ceftazidime is least active. Anaerobic activity is

modest (only cefoxitin, cefotetan, and moxalactam) and less than that of penicillins. First-generation cephalosporins have marginal activity against *H. influenzae*; the second-generation cephalosporins (cefoxitin and cefotetan) have modest activity. Cefamandole is active only against ampicillin-susceptible strains. Cefuroxime and all third-generation agents are highly active. Activity against enteric GNB improves with each succeeding generation (particularly against Enterobacteriaceae). First-generation cephalosporins are active against most strains of *E. coli, Proteus mirabilis,* and *K. pneumoniae,* but do not typically cover *Enterobacter, Citrobacter, Serratia, Providencia, Proteus vulgaris,* and *Morganella* species. These species are variably sensitive to cefuroxime, cefotetan, and cefoxitin; most are inhibited by third-generation agents. Only ceftazidime and cefoperazone have significant activity against *P. aeruginosa. Acinetobacter calcoaceticus* is usually resistant to all cephalosporins, although some strains are susceptible to ceftazidime. None of the cephalosporins is active against enterococci, MRSA, *Chlamydia, Mycoplasma,* or *Legionella* species.
- *Toxicity:* Adverse effects include hypersensitivity reactions, fever, rash (1-5%), and nonspecific GI symptoms (5-10%). The presence of methylthiotetrazole group in position 3 with cefamandole; cefotetan, cefoperazone, and moxalactam are associated with hypoprothrombinemia. Only moxalactam has been associated with significant risk of clinical bleeding.

First-generation cephalosporins:
- *Mechanism of action:* Cephalosporins bind to PBPs and interfere with bacterial cell wall (peptidoglycan) synthesis.
- Antimicrobial spectrum: The first-generation cephalosporins for parenteral use include cephalothin, cephapirin, cephradine, and cefazolin. Only cefazolin is currently used. Cefazolin has limited activity against *H. influenzae,* and its activity against Enterobacteriaceae (including *K. pneumoniae* and *E. coli*) is inconsistent. The spectrum of oral cephalexin is similarly narrow. First-generation cephalosporins are not recommended for empiric treatment of either community- or hospital-acquired pneumonia. Cefazolin should be restricted to uncomplicated pneumonias caused by an organism that is highly susceptible to this agent.
- Dosage: 1 g q 8 hours.

Second-generation cephalosporins: These agents include cefuroxime, cefamandole, cefonicid, cefoxitin and cefotetan for parenteral use; cefaclor and cefuroxime axetil are available for oral administration. Cefamandole is no longer used, and cefoxitin has largely been replaced by cefotetan, except for antimicrobial surgical prophylaxis.
- Antimicrobial spectrum: Second-generation cephalosporins have broader activity against gram-negative bacteria (including most

E. coli, Klebsiella, Proteus species, and H. influenzae) compared to first-generation agents. Activity against staphylococci is modest, but is excellent against S. pneumoniae and most streptococci (other than enterococci).

Cefuroxime: Cefuroxime, a broad-spectrum agent with excellent activity against common respiratory pathogens, has supplanted cefamandole as the cephalosporin of choice for empiric treatment of CAP. Several features favor the use of cefuroxime over cefamandole: greater beta-lactamase stability; lack of the methylthiotetrazole side chain, which has been associated with prolongation of prothrombin time and risk of bleeding; superior central nervous system (CNS) penetration; and slightly longer half-life (q 8 hours vs q 6 hours dosing).

- Antimicrobial spectrum: Active against S. pneumoniae, S. aureus, H. influenzae, K. pneumoniae, and oral anaerobes.
- Dosage: 0.75–1.5 g IV q 8 hours; can switch to oral formulation, cefuroxime axetil, after an initial response to parenteral cefuroxime.
- Indications: Cefuroxime is excellent for empiric therapy of CAP in adults, including elderly patients and patients with underlying disease. Cefuroxime has excellent CNS penetration. It is not recommended for nosocomial pneumonia (unless a susceptible pathogen is identified) because alternative agents (third-generation cephalosporins, antipseudomonal penicillins, and imipenem) have broader activity against gram-negative bacteria.

Cefuroxime axetil for oral use is more active than cefaclor against M. catarrhalis and H. influenzae and is an ideal agent for completing a course of therapy after an initial brief course of IV cefuroxime (dose of cefuroxime axetil is 500 mg bid).

Cefonicid: It may be comparable to cefuroxime but has been used sparingly for the treatment of lower respiratory tract infections. Few studies have evaluated cefonicid in this context. The antimicrobial activity of cefonicid is no more than that of cefuroxime. Ceftriaxone (a third-generation cephalosporin that has greater gram-negative activity) can also be dosed once daily. Thus, there is little advantage of cefonicid over cefuroxime or ceftriaxone, agents that have been widely used for empiric therapy of CAP. Neither cefuroxime nor cefonicid has any role in nosocomial pneumonias.

- Antimicrobial spectrum: Similar to that of cefuroxime, but slightly less active than cefuroxime against staphylococci, H. influenzae, and Enterobacteriaceae
- Dosage: 1–2 g IV/IM q 24 hours

Cefotetan: Cefotetan, a cephamycin, has superior anaerobic activity as compared to that of other cephalosporins, but less activity against H. influenzae. It is particularly suited for aspiration pneumonias or polymicrobial infections involving anaerobes and enteric GNB.

- Antimicrobial spectrum: Superior anaerobic activity (including beta-lactamase-producing *B. fragilis*); less activity against *H. influenzae* as compared to that of cefuroxime
- Toxicity: Has methylthiotetrazole side chain; theoretic risk for bleeding (low)
- Dosage: 1–2 g q 12 hours
- Indications: Empiric therapy of community-acquired or nursing home-acquired pneumonias in alcoholic patients, patients with esophageal disease, or patients in whom aspiration is suspected (particularly when polymicrobial anaerobic or gram-negative bacillary infections are a consideration).

Third-generation cephalosporins: Within this group, cefotaxime, ceftizoxime, and ceftriaxone have similar antimicrobial spectra and may be therapeutically equivalent. The activity of cefotaxime may be slightly greater against *S. aureus* as compared to that of the other agents; none is active against *P. aeruginosa*. Ceftazidime and cefoperazone are the only cephalosporins with significant activity against *P. aeruginosa*; however, these agents have inferior activity against anaerobes, *S. aureus*, and gram-positive bacteria compared to that of cefotaxime, ceftizoxime, and ceftriaxone. Moxalactam is no longer used because of bleeding complications associated with its use.

- Antimicrobial spectrum: Third-generation cephalosporins extend the gram-negative spectrum of second-generation agents to include *Serratia*, *Morganella morganii*, *Providencia* species, and *Citrobacter* species in addition to *E. coli*, *Klebsiella* species, and *Proteus mirabilis*. Despite wide-spread use over the past decade, the activity of third-generation cephalosporins against *E. coli*, *Klebsiella* species (*K. pneumoniae* and *K. oxytoca*), *Proteus* species, *Serratia*, *Haemophilus* species, *Neisseria*, and *Providencia* has remained excellent (>95% susceptible). All the third-generation agents are extremely active against *H. influenzae* and other *Haemophilus* species, such as *H. parainfluenzae*, including beta-lactamase-producing isolates. Some strains (10–20%) of *Citrobacter freundii* are resistant. *Enterobacter* species (*E. cloacae* and *E. aerogenes*) are a major weakness; 20–40% of strains produce beta-lactamases that hydrolyze cephalosporins. The prevalence of resistant strains of *Enterobacter* species has ↑ dramatically within the past decade, particularly in centers in which use of third-generation cephalosporins is high. Among the cephalosporins, only ceftazidime and cefoperazone have significant activity against *P. aeruginosa*. Activity against *Pseudomonas cepacia* is variable; some strains are inhibited by ceftazidime, but most are resistant to other agents. *Xanthomonas maltophilia* is generally resistant. Activity against *Acinetobacter* species is variable; usually ceftizoxime, ceftriaxone, and cefoperazone exhibit poor activity; some strains are susceptible to cefotaxime or ceftazidime. Third-generation cephalosporins are highly active against *M. catarrhalis*. Gram-positive activity is variable; cefotaxime (and its diacetyl metabolite) is the most active; ceftazidime is the least active. Cefotaxime, ceftizoxime, and ceftriaxone are highly active against streptococci, including *S. pneumoniae*, *S. pyogenes*, hemolytic streptococci, *S. mutans*, *S. milleri*, *S. sanguis*, *S. mitis*, *S. bovis*, and the viridans group of streptococci. These agents are also moderately active against methicillin-sensitive *S. aureus*; ceftazidime exhibits fair to poor activity. MRSA and enterococci (*S. faecalis* and *S. faecium*) are invariably resistant to cephalosporins (irrespective of in vitro susceptibility testing). Anaerobic activity of third-generation cephalosporins is fair. The activity is modest against mouth anaerobes (peptococci, peptostreptococci, and *B. melaninogenicus*), but is fair to poor against the *B. fragilis* group. Moxalactam and ceftizoxime are the most active agents in this class; ceftazidime is the least active.

Cefotaxime: It is an excellent agent for empiric therapy of nosocomial pneumonias because of its broad-spectrum activity, low toxicity, and relatively low cost compared to that of other third-generation cephalosporins. Its lack of activity against *P. aeruginosa* makes it less than ideal for treatment of ICU-acquired pneumonias unless this pathogen has been excluded.
- Antimicrobial spectrum: Broad-spectrum antimicrobial activity comparable to that of ceftriaxone and ceftizoxime; cefotaxime's activity against *S. aureus* may be superior to that of these agents.
- Distinguishing features: The desacetyl metabolite of cefotaxime (desacetyl cefotaxime) has excellent antimicrobial activity similar to that of the parent compound, but has a longer half-life and confers improved activity against staphylococci (including *S. epidermidis*). It is synergistic with cefotaxime against susceptible strains of Enterobacteriaceae. Cefotaxime, ceftriaxone, and ceftizoxime penetrate well into the CSF and can be used to treat meningitis.
- Dosage: 1–2 g IV q 8 hours
- Indications: Cefotaxime is an excellent empiric agent for nosocomial pneumonia arising outside the ICU when *P. aeruginosa* is not a major consideration, and is acceptable treatment for documented pneumonia caused by *E. coli*, *Klebsiella*, *Proteus*, *Serratia*, *H. influenzae*, and other susceptible organisms. Because of its inadequate activity against *P. aeruginosa*, cefotaxime (or ceftriaxone or ceftizoxime) is not recommended for empiric treatment of pneumonia in mechanically ventilated patients suffering from complications and residing in ICUs.

Ceftriaxone: Because of its broad-spectrum antimicrobial activity and prolonged half-life, which permits once-daily dosing, ceftriaxone is one of the most widely used antibiotics, both in the community and nosocomial setting.
- Antimicrobial spectrum: Similar to that of cefotaxime and ceftizoxime
- Toxicity: Ceftriaxone is primarily eliminated by the biliary system. Compared to other cephalosporins, ceftriaxone causes slightly ↑ GI symptoms and diarrhea. High concentrations in bile may lead to biliary sludge (biliary pseudolithiasis) and symptoms resembling cholelithiasis

- Dosage: 1–2 g q 24 hours (q 12 hours dosing is not recommended because any cost advantage achieved with once-daily dosing is negated by more frequent administration; cefotaxime or ceftizoxime is less expensive when administered in a comparable dose q 8 hours).
- Distinguishing features: The prolonged half-life of ceftriaxone allows once-daily dosing; 90% protein binding as compared to 15–35% for ceftizoxime and cefotaxime. Ceftriaxone has excellent penetration into the CSF, as do cefotaxime and ceftizoxime.
- Indications: The antimicrobial spectrum of ceftriaxone is exceptionally broad, and thus this agent may be useful in the empiric therapy of community- or hospital-acquired pneumonias. Because of its prolonged half-life, which permits once-daily dosing, ceftriaxone may be used as initial therapy for CAP in nursing homes or in patients with underlying diseases because coverage is excellent against *S. pneumoniae*, most Enterobacteriaceae, and *H. influenzae*. Intramuscular (IM)-administered ceftriaxone (1 g q 24 hours) may permit outpatient administration in the clinic or emergency department, with follow-up doses at 24 hours. Subsequent therapy can be converted to an oral agent once clinical improvement has occurred. This strategy may limit the need for hospitalization among patients deemed to require parenteral antibiotic therapy. Ceftriaxone may be useful in the nosocomial setting as well, but its lack of significant activity against *P. aeruginosa* makes this agent less appropriate for treatment of ICU-acquired pneumonia.

Cefoperazone: It has broad-spectrum antimicrobial activity and is the only cephalosporin other than ceftazidime to have excellent activity against *P. aeruginosa*. Cefoperazone has been successfully used as empiric therapy for nosocomial pneumonia. Significant gaps in the spectrum exist, however. Cefoperazone is less consistently active against common GNB, such as *E. coli* and *Klebsiella*, as compared to cefotaxime, ceftriaxone, and ceftizoxime, and its activity against *P. aeruginosa* is less than that of ceftazidime. Thus, we rarely use cefoperazone, preferring these other agents (the specific choice depends on suspected or confirmed organisms).
- Antimicrobial spectrum: Excellent activity against *P. aeruginosa* (> that of either ceftriaxone or ceftizoxime but < that of ceftazidime); less consistent activity against some Enterobacteriaceae, including *E. coli* and *Klebsiella* species, and less beta-lactamase stability compared to that of other third-generation cephalosporins. Modest activity against anaerobes and gram-positive bacilli (< that of cefotaxime).
- Toxicity: Contains methylthiotetrazole chain, and thus has potential for bleeding resulting from prothrombin deficiency.
- Dosage: 1–2 g q 8–12 hours
- Distinguishing features: Excreted primarily via biliary route (75%); 90% protein bound.

Ceftazidime: It is the most active cephalosporin against *P. aeruginosa* and has excellent activity against most GNB. Its activity against gram-positive bacilli and anaerobes is less than that of other cephalosporins. This agent is most appropriate when *P. aeruginosa* is a consideration.
- Antimicrobial spectrum: Excellent activity against *P. aeruginosa*; comparable to other third-generation cephalosporins against Enterobacteriaceae and aerobic GNBs; least active of the cephalosporins against staphylococci, gram-positive cocci, and anaerobes.
- Dosage: 1-2 g IV q 8 hours
- Indications: Cornerstone of therapy for pneumonia when *P. aeruginosa* is suspected or documented (e.g. in mechanically ventilated patients, patients in ICU, and patients with cystic fibrosis or neutropenia).

When *P. aeruginosa* is not a prime consideration, less expensive third-generation cephalosporins (e.g. cefotaxime, ceftizoxime, or ceftriaxone) that have better gram-positive and anaerobic activity are preferable to ceftazidime.

Cefixime: It is the only third-generation cephalosporin that can be administered orally. Cefixime is more active than second-generation agents against enteric GNB, but has poor activity against staphylococci and anaerobes and fails to cover *Pseudomonas* species. The role of this agent in the treatment of community-acquired and nosocomial pneumonias has not yet been established.

Carbapenems: The carbapenems represent a new class of beta-lactams that differ from the penicillins by the substitution of a carbon atom for sulfur at position 1 and an unsaturated bond between carbon atoms 2 and 3 in the 5-membered ring. Carbapenems also have unique side chains that confer remarkable resistance to a variety of beta-lactamases and provide antipseudomonal activity.

Imipenem or cilastatin: The only carbapenem currently in clinical use is imipenem. Because imipenem is not stable to renal dehydrogenases and its degradation products may be nephrotoxic, it is administered with a fixed combination of the dehydropeptidase inhibitor, cilastatin.
- Antimicrobial spectrum: Imipenem has the broadest spectrum of activity among all beta-lactams. It is active against most GNB, including multiply resistant *P. aeruginosa*, *Serratia* species, and *Acinetobacter* species, but *Pseudomonas cepacia* and *Xanthomonas maltophilia* are nearly invariably resistant. Imipenem is highly active against gram-positive cocci (including both methicillin-sensitive and MRSA strains); however, the MIC90 for MRSA isolates may be 8-400 times the MIC90 for susceptible strains, and vancomycin is preferred for MRSA. The activity of imipenem against *S. faecium* and methicillin-resistant *S. epidermidis* is inconsistent; anaerobic activity (including *B. fragilis* species) is outstanding.

- Toxicity: Imipenem may induce seizures. Although the risk of seizures is low (<0.5%) among patients with normal renal function and no underlying neurologic disease, considerably higher seizure rates (10-20%) have been noted among patients with renal failure who are receiving conventional dosages or who have underlying CNS disease. In this context, imipenem is not recommended. Superinfection or colonization with *Xanthomonas maltophilia* or *Pseudomonas cepacia* may complicate therapy.
- Dosage: 0.5-1.0 IV q 8 hours. In view of the exquisite sensitivity of most organisms to imipenem, initiate therapy at 500 mg q 8 hours, and reserve higher doses (to a max of 1,000 mg q 6 hours) for serious infections caused by *P. aeruginosa* or pathogens with a relatively high MIC.
- Distinguishing features: The extraordinarily broad antimicrobial spectrum of imipenem may relate to its ability to penetrate well through the outer cell envelope of GNB, its high affinity for PBP targets, and its resistance to a wide variety of beta-lactamases. Imipenem is not hydrolyzed by penicillinases or cephalosporinases, which degrades penicillins, third-generation cephalosporins, and aztreonam. Resistance to *P. aeruginosa* developed in as many as 25% of patients when imipenem was used as monotherapy.
- Indications: Because of its remarkably broad antimicrobial spectrum, imipenem may be useful as empiric therapy for severe nosocomial pneumonias. It is particularly useful in patients with pneumonias and complications in whom regimens have failed, or in patients in whom antimicrobial resistance to more conventional beta-lactams is likely. Because of its expense, CNS toxicity, and potential for selection of resistant organisms, imipenem is not indicated for CAP or uncomplicated nosocomial infections susceptible to other beta-lactams.

Meropenem is a new carbapenem currently being evaluated in clinical trials in the United States, and has an extraordinarily broad spectrum of activity. It appears to be slightly less active than imipenem against gram-positive organisms but may be slightly more active against gram-negative organisms; anaerobic activity is comparable. As with imipenem, *Xanthomonas maltophilia* is usually resistant. Meropenem may have some advantages over imipenem, e.g. meropenem carries no definite risk of seizures, induction of beta-lactamases is less, and it is stable to human renal dehydropeptidases, thus not requiring the concomitant administration of an enzyme inhibitor.

Monobactams: Aztreonam—it is the first of a generation of monobactams within the beta-lactam group. Elimination of the second carbon ring leaves the beta-lactam ring as a monocyclic compound. Although aztreonam is a beta-lactam, the cleavage of the second member of the beta-lactam ring makes this agent structurally dissimilar from other beta-lactams, such as penicillin, cephalosporins, and imipenem or cilastatin. Thus, aztreonam may be used safely in patients who are allergic to penicillins or cephalosporins because cross-reactivity with these agents does not occur.

- Antimicrobial spectrum: Aztreonam is highly active against aerobic GNB, including most strains of *P. aeruginosa*, and is stable against beta-lactamases; however, it has no significant activity against gram-positive organisms or anaerobes. Aztreonam may provide synergy with aminoglycosides; also, synergy may be achieved with aztreonam and other beta-lactams in more than 40% of isolates.
- Toxicity: Uncommon (<1% rash and <2% serious diarrhea)
- Dosage: 1–2 g q 8 hours (lower doses of 1 g q 12 hours may be adequate provided the organism is susceptible with a low MIC (<1 μg/L). Dosage must be ↓ in the presence of impaired renal function.
- Indications: Aztreonam has a greater role in nosocomial infections in which aerobic GNB are suspected or documented. In combination with agents with gram-positive activity, such as clindamycin, vancomycin, or a beta-lactam, it provides exceptional broad-spectrum activity; however, as empiric therapy for serious nosocomial pneumonia. The use of aztreonam may eliminate the need for an amino glycoside in this context. Aztreonam has minimal activity against common pathogens implicated in bronchitis and CAP, such as *S. pneumoniae* and *M. catarrhalis*, and should not be used as empiric therapy in these conditions.

Aminoglycosides

These include gentamicin, tobramycin, and amikacin. The use of aminoglycosides in the treatment of pneumonia is controversial. Several factors argue against the use of these agents—their high toxicity (nephrotoxicity or ototoxicity); their low penetration into bronchial secretions and lung tissue; their inactivation at low pH (conditions that may prevail in infected lung parenchyma); and the availability of alternative broad-spectrum agents with gram-negative activity and less toxicity (e.g. beta-lactams and quinolones). Despite these arguments, aminoglycosides may be useful as adjunct therapy (combined with a broad-spectrum antimicrobial agent, such as beta-lactams or quinolones), primarily to achieve synergistic killing.
- Antimicrobial spectrum: Exceptionally broad spectrum against aerobic GNB; no significant activity against anaerobes. May confer synergistic killing against certain gram-positive organisms, such as enterococci and staphylococci, in combination with beta-1actams.
- Toxicity: Nephrotoxicity and ototoxicity are most important. Synergistic toxicity may occur when aminoglycoside is combined with other nephrotoxic agents, such as vancomycin. Risk factors associated with enhanced nephrotoxicity include old age, prior aminoglycoside use, and preexisting renal disease. The toxicity of tobramycin and gentamicin are comparable; both agents may be slightly more nephrotoxic than amikacin and netilmicin. Netilmicin shows the least ototoxicity. Peak and trough

serum levels are mandatory to limit toxicity. Peak levels more than 6 µg/mL are required for optimal microbiocidal activity; however, trough levels more than 2 µg/mL (2 mg/L) correlate with excessive toxicity.
- Dosage: 3–5 mg/kg/day IV, or IM in divided doses q 8 hours for gentamicin or tobramycin; 15 mg/kg/day for amikacin (two- to threefold higher dosage are required in patients with cystic fibrosis because of the rapid clearance of aminoglycosides in this patient population). Dose adjustment may be required (need peak and trough serum levels). Higher serum levels are achieved with single daily dosing, thus suggesting that bactericidal activity may be enhanced. Single dosing would be cost-saving because less pharmacy and nursing time would be required. Single-dose regimens, however, have not been studied in humans; thus, the safety and efficacy of this practice have not been established.
- Indications: Aminoglycosides are inadequate as single agents for pulmonary infections. The addition of an aminoglycoside to a broad-spectrum antimicrobial should be considered in the following circumstances to provide synergistic killing: as initial empiric therapy for serious sepsis or nosocomial pneumonias caused by suspected or proven gram-negative enteric bacteria; as therapy for pneumonia caused by highly virulent pathogens, such as *Pseudomonas* species, *Enterobacter* species, *Serratia*, and *Acinetobacter* species (continue aminoglycoside for duration of therapy); and to treat infections caused by enterococci (combine with penicillin or vancomycin).

Macrolides: The macrolides represent a class of antimicrobials characterized by substituted 14-, 15-, or 16-member rings. Macrolides penetrate into tissues better than do beta-lactams. Erythromycin (a 14-member macrolide) has been the only antibiotic of this class in clinical use in the United States for the past 2 decades. Several newer 14-member macrolides with a spectrum of activity similar to that of erythromycin but with more resistance to acid hydrolysis have been synthesized; these include roxithromycin, clarithromycin, dirithromycin, erythromycin, and flurithromycin. Clarithromycin is the only one of these newer macrolides currently available in the United States.

Erythromycin is active against *S. pneumoniae*, *M. catarrhalis*, *Mycoplasma*, and *Legionella* species, and has been used extensively for community-acquired bronchitis and pneumonia. Penicillins and cephalosporins, however, have a much broader spectrum of activity and are the preferred agents for most CAP. Erythromycin is not consistently reliable against *H. influenzae*, has no significant activity against GNB, and is less active than penicillins against streptococci, staphylococci, and anaerobes. Thus, erythromycin should be reserved primarily for CAP in young healthy adults who are at low risk for resistant pathogens or in patients in whom *Mycoplasma*, *Chlamydia*, or *Legionella* species are suspected.

- Mechanism of action: Interferes with microbial protein synthesis at the ribosomal level (binds to 50S ribosome subunit).
- Antimicrobial spectrum: Effective against *S. pneumoniae*, other streptococci (except enterococcus), and *M. catarrhalis*; not reliable against *S. aureus* or *S. epidermidis* (10-40% of strains are resistant). Only 40-70% of *H. influenzae* are susceptible. Anaerobic coverage is modest (10-20% of oral anaerobes and 30-40% of *B. fragilis* are resistant). No significant gram-negative activity. Excellent against *Legionella* and *Mycoplasma* species; less active than tetracyclines against *Chlamydia* species.
- Toxicity: GI side effects (principally nausea, epigastric distress, diarrhea, and vomiting) are common (>20%) and limit its usefulness. IV erythromycin is intensely irritating to veins and may cause phlebitis. Hepatotoxicity (cholestatic hepatitis) is a rare complication (primarily with the estolate form) that usually resolves with cessation of therapy.
- Dosage: 500-1,000 mg q 6 hours IV; 250-500 mg q 6 hours po. The active component is the erythromycin base. Oral forms include an acid-resistant enteric coated tablet, erythromycin stearate (a salt), erythromycin ethyl succinate (an ester), and erythromycin estolate (an ester salt). These salts and esters confer more stability against gastric acids than does the parent compound. Erythromycin lactobionate and erythromycin gluceptate are available for IV use (oral absorption is not consistently reliable). IV administration is recommended as initial therapy for serious infections (e.g. *Legionella* species); oral therapy may be substituted once a clinical response has occurred.
- Indications: Erythromycin provides excellent coverage against common pathogens acquired in the community, including *S. pneumoniae*, *Legionella*, *Chlamydia*, and *Mycoplasma* species, and may be used as first-line therapy among young, previously healthy adults with CAP in whom potentially resistant pathogens, such as *S. aureus* and enteric GNB, are rarely problematic. In view of its limited spectrum of activity against GNB and marginal activity against *H. influenzae*, however, erythromycin is not adequate as monotherapy for CAP in patients at risk for infections with these pathogens (e.g. age >55, ethanol abuse, cigarette smoking, or any preexisting underlying disease). Erythromycin has no role in the treatment of nosocomial pneumonias, except as adjunctive therapy when *Legionella* species are suspected.

Clarithromycin is the first of the newer macrolides to be introduced into the United States. Clarithromycin retains the antimicrobial activity of erythromycin, but also extends its spectrum to include *H. influenzae* and some Enterobacteriaceae. Clarithromycin is as effective as cefaclor, cefuroxime axetil, and cefixime for mild-to-moderate lower respiratory tract infections (bronchitis and pneumonia).

- Toxicity: Much less than erythromycin; significant GI symptoms complicate its use in only 3-6% of cases.
- Dosage: 250-500 mg bid for 7-14 days.

Azalides

The addition of a nitrogen atom to the macrolide ring (resulting in a 15-member ring) results in compounds (azalides) that are far more resistant to acid hydrolysis than are macrolides. Azalides have greater penetration into tissues, a larger volume of distribution, and a longer half-life (>2 days) compared to macrolides, beta-lactams, or quinolone antibiotics. Azithromycin is the first azalide to be developed for clinical use, although several other agents are currently being studied.

Azithromycin extends the spectrum of erythromycin to cover *H. influenzae* and some Enterobacteriaceae and has few side effects.
- Mechanism of action: Inhibits protein synthesis at 50S ribosomal level
- Antimicrobial spectrum: Azithromycin is highly active (comparable to erythromycin) against *Chlamydia*, *Mycoplasma*, and *Legionella* species. It is bactericidal against *S. pneumoniae* and erythromycin-sensitive strains of streptococci and staphylococci, but is less active than erythromycin against these organisms. Azithromycin has no activity against erythromycin-resistant strains of streptococci or staphylococci; MRSA and enterococci are usually resistant. Activity against anaerobes is slightly superior to that of erythromycin. Most oral anaerobes, such as peptococci, peptostreptococci, and *B. melaninogenicus*, are readily inhibited; activity against *B. fragilis* is marginal. Azithromycin is much more active against GNB than are the 14-member-ring macrolides. Azithromycin is bactericidal against *H. influenzae*, *Neisseria* species, and *M. catarrhalis*. Activity against Enterobacteriaceae is inconsistent, but some strains of *E. coli*, *Klebsiella*, *Enterobacter*, and *Citrobacter* species are susceptible. Most isolates of *Serratia* or *Acinetobacter* species are resistant; activity is insignificant against *Pseudomonas* species or *Xanthomonas maltophilia*.
- Toxicity: Minor, primarily GI
- Dosage: 500 mg initial dose, then 250 mg once daily for 2–5 days
- Distinguishing features: Azithromycin is more acid stable and better absorbed following oral administration than is erythromycin. It also has a much longer biologic half-life. A unique property of azithromycin is its ability to be concentrated in phagocytes and tissues; phagocytes continue to concentrate azithromycin intracellularly for as many as 24 hours. The preferential distribution of the drug in tissues and its slow release result in high concentrations of active drug at sites of infection for prolonged periods despite low serum concentrations. Levels of azithromycin in sputum, bronchial mucosa, and alveolar macrophages may exceed the MIC for most common respiratory pathogens for 2–4 days following a single 500-mg oral dose.
- Indications: In view of its excellent activity against common respiratory pathogens (*S. pneumoniae*, *H. influenzae*, *M. catarrhalis*, *Chlamydia*, *Mycoplasma*, *Legionella*), prolonged half-life (permitting once-daily

dosing), and low incidence of side effects, azithromycin may be a logical agent for CAP among nonimmunocompromised hosts in whom the risk of serious gram-negative pathogens is low. Data evaluating azithromycin for moderately severe or severe pneumonias are limited. Studies in Europe and the United States, however, have shown oral azithromycin to be superior or equivalent to amoxicillin or cefaclor for the treatment of sinus and lower respiratory tract (primarily bronchitis) infections. The role of azithromycin as empiric therapy for CAP in moderately ill patients at risk for gram-negative pathogens (e.g. patients with ethanol abuse, diabetes mellitus, age >65 years, residence in chronic care facility, COPD, and serious underlying diseases) needs to be studied. Currently, cefuroxime or ceftriaxone are preferred in this context. Azithromycin is not appropriate treatment for nosocomial pneumonia.

- Caution—do not use with drugs that prolong the QT interval.
- Clarithromycin extended-release tablets should be taken with food.
- Do not crush, chew, or break an extended-release tablet. Swallow it whole.
- The drug may cause liver problems.
- *QT prolongation warning:* Clarithromycin may cause the heart rhythm problem QT prolongation. Do not take with drugs that cause QT prolongation.
- *Diarrhea warning:* Almost all antibiotics, including clarithromycin, can cause *Clostridium difficile*-associated diarrhea.

Tetracyclines

Tetracyclines, derived from *Streptomyces* species, were isolated in the early 1950s. Substitutions on the hydro-naphthacene 4-ringed nucleus differentiate the derivatives tetracycline hydrochloride, oxytetracycline, chlortetracycline, doxycycline, and minocycline. Tetracyclines (particularly doxycycline) are inexpensive and relatively effective agents for uncomplicated bronchitis, but have a limited role as therapeutic agents for pneumonia.

- Mechanism of action: Bind to 30S subunit of bacterial ribosomes.
- Antimicrobial spectrum: Tetracyclines are active against *S. pneumoniae*, modest against other *Streptococcus* species, and generally not adequate for *S. aureus* or enterococci. Anaerobic activity is modest (*E. fragilis* species are resistant); marginal against *H. influenzae*; and not active against most enteric GNB. It is the drug of choice for *Chlamydia* and *Rickettsia* species; acceptable for *Mycoplasma* and *Legionella* species.
- Toxicity: GI (nausea, emesis, and GI distress) common; photosensitivity (doxycycline or minocycline; discoloration of teeth or depression of bone growth in infants and children; and vertigo. Outdated tetracyclines may cause renal tubular acidosis. Fatal hepatotoxicity has been described but is rare.
- Dosage: 250–500 mg po qid for tetracycline, oxytetracycline, and chlortetracycline; doxycycline and minocycline 100 mg bid (po or IV).

Food binds the drug and impairs absorption; tetracyclines need to be taken on empty stomach. This effect is less problematic with doxycycline and minocycline.
- Distinguishing features: Doxycycline (Vibramycin) has a prolonged half-life (permitting twice-daily dosing) and is less affected by food; activity is as good as that of other tetracyclines, and it is the preferred agent.
- Indications: Tetracyclines are the drug of choice for pulmonary infections caused by *Chlamydia* and *Mycoplasma* species and are acceptable alternatives to erythromycin for legionella infections.

Fluoroquinolones

Fluoroquinolones are derivatives of nalidixic acid and include ciprofloxacin; norfloxacin, ofloxacin, lomefloxacin, enoxacin, and pefloxacin the last two not being available in the United States. Norfloxacin is recommended only for urinary sepsis, whereas both ciprofloxacin and ofloxacin may have important roles in the treatment of lower respiratory tract infections, including serious gram-negative bacillary pneumonias. Lomefloxacin, a fluoroquinolone released in 1992, has only marginal activity against *S. pneumoniae* and is less active than ciprofloxacin or ofloxacin against GNB (particularly *P. aeruginosa*).
- The Food and Drug Administration (FDA) has updated the labels of systemic fluoroquinolones (e.g. ciprofloxacin and levofloxacin) to emphasize that they are associated with numerous serious and potentially irreversible adverse effects that can occur simultaneously. For patients with sinusitis, bronchitis, or uncomplicated urinary tract infections, the agency says, these antibacterials should be used only when there are no alternative options.
- Disabling side effects may include tendinitis, tendon rupture, muscle pain, muscle weakness, joint pain, joint swelling, peripheral neuropathy, and central nervous system effects (e.g. depression and psychosis).
- Adverse reactions may begin within hours or weeks of treatment initiation; data suggest that such reactions last, on average, 14 months after stopping treatment.
- Antimicrobial spectrum: Excellent potency against aerobic GNB, including most Enterobacteriaceae, *H. influenzae*, *Neisseria* species, *M. catarrhalis*, and *P. aeruginosa*. Less active against *P. cepacia* or *Xanthomonas maltophilia*. Good activity against *S. aureus* and *S. epidermidis*, but less active against streptococci (including *S. pneumoniae*). Minimal activity against anaerobes.
- Features: Fluoroquinolones (with the exception of norfloxacin) exceed most other antibiotics in their ability to penetrate the lower respiratory tract. Ciprofloxacin and ofloxacin penetrate into the bronchial lining and achieve high concentrations in the lung, bronchial mucosa, and sputum; concentrations in the lung typically exceed serum concentrations. The concentration of quinolones in macrophages and polymorphonuclear leukocytes may enhance clinical efficacy.

- Mechanism of action: Antagonizes bacterial DNA gyrase (interferes with DNA replication)
- Antimicrobial resistance: Resistance can be mediated by mutations affecting DNA gyrase, drug permeability, or both; plasmid-mediated resistance has not been observed. Resistance to *P. aeruginosa* may require multiple mutations, whereas a single-step mutation may be sufficient to induce resistance against *S. aureus*.

Ciprofloxacin: Ciprofloxacin was released in the United States in 1987 as the first oral antibiotic with activity against *P. aeruginosa*. It has excellent activity against common respiratory pathogens implicated in CAP, such as *H. influenzae, M. catarrhalis, Chlamydia,* and *Legionella*. Oral or IV ciprofloxacin has been associated with cure rates more than 80% in community-, nursing home-, and hospital-acquired pneumonias. Significant gaps in the spectrum of ciprofloxacin exist, however. Despite its excellent gram-negative activity, ciprofloxacin has only modest activity against *S. pneumoniae*, other gram-positive organisms, and anaerobes. Ciprofloxacin is less than optimal therapy for infections caused by *S. pneumoniae*. Thus, it is not generally recommended as first-line therapy for CAP nor should it be used for anaerobic or aspiration pneumonias. IV ciprofloxacin appears comparable to broad-spectrum beta-lactams, including ceftazidime, for hospital-acquired pneumonias or sepsis in neutropenic patients, and may be suitable for suspected or documented gram-negative bacillary infections. Unrestricted use of ciprofloxacin, however, may lead to ↑ed antimicrobial resistance; thus, alternative agents (penicillins and cephalosporins) are preferred as first-line therapy.

- Antimicrobial spectrum: Exceptionally broad activity against aerobic gram-negative organisms (including *P. aeruginosa, H. influenzae,* and Enterobacteriaceae). Excellent against *S. aureus*, including MRSA. Marginal activity against *S. pneumoniae* and group A streptococci. Poor anaerobic activity. Excellent against chlamydia, *Legionella* species, and *M. catarrhalis*.
- Toxicity: Uncommon; GI symptoms most common (3–6%); colitis rare. CNS effects (headache, dizziness, and sleep disturbance) occur in 1–2%; rash in 0.5–2%. Do not use in pregnancy because fetal deaths and skeletal abnormalities have been noted in animals in utero.
- Dosage: 200–400 mg IV q 12 hours; po, 500–750 mg bid
- Indications: Because oral bioavailability is excellent, oral ciprofloxacin may be adequate for nursing home-acquired or hospital-acquired pneumonias provided the pathogen is susceptible and *S. pneumoniae* has been reasonably excluded. More importantly, oral ciprofloxacin may be substituted in hospitalized patients receiving more expensive parenteral agents, such as beta-lactams, for documented infections caused by susceptible pathogens. The substitution of an effective oral agent may markedly reduce drug costs and shorten the hospital stay. IV

ciprofloxacin IV (400 mg q 12 hours) combined with an aminoglycoside is a reasonable option for the treatment of nosocomial pneumonia in patients unable to tolerate beta-lactams or with organisms resistant to beta-lactams. Antimicrobial resistance, particularly among *S. aureus* and *P. aeruginosa*, may develop quickly when ciprofloxacin is used alone. Thus, when ciprofloxacin is used for serious nosocomial pneumonias, *P. aeruginosa* infections, or sepsis in neutropenic patients, it is advisable to combine this agent with an aminoglycoside. Ciprofloxacin is not recommended as first-line empiric therapy for nosocomial pneumonia because beta-lactams are usually efficacious (ciprofloxacin is not suitable for infections caused by streptococci or anaerobes).

- Antimicrobial resistance: Although ciprofloxacin remains highly active against aerobic GNB, and has broad-spectrum activity, data from Europe suggest that increasingly drug-resistant strains of *P. aeruginosa* and *S. aureus* have been associated with the liberal use of ciprofloxacin. Emergence of resistance may be particularly common for infections in which many organisms are present, such as in cystic fibrosis, or for infections in sequestered areas where tissue penetration of the antibiotic may be inadequate, such as osteomyelitis. Within 3 years of the introduction of the drug to the United States, 4–6% of strains of *P. aeruginosa* and *S. aureus* were resistant; higher rates of resistance (10–15%) have been observed in some institutions. This potential for rapid induction of antimicrobial resistance has led to concerns about using ciprofloxacin as first-line therapy. Whether combining ciprofloxacin with an additional antibiotic limits or reduces the emergence of resistance is not known; however, combination therapy appears ineffective in limiting resistance against *P. aeruginosa* in patients with cystic fibrosis. Notwithstanding these concerns, ciprofloxacin remains an excellent drug, particularly for the treatment of gram-negative pneumonia with pathogens displaying broad resistance to other antimicrobials.

Ofloxacin (Floxin): Ofloxacin represents an attractive agent for empiric treatment of CAP because its spectrum covers most common respiratory pathogens, including streptococci, staphylococci, *H. influenzae*, Enterobacteriaceae, *Chlamydia*, *Mycoplasma*, and *Legionella*. In a recent multicenter trial, Sanders and associates reported that oral ofloxacin (400 mg q 12 hours) was as effective as parenteral antibiotic therapy (specific antimicrobial agents were selected by individual investigators) for patients hospitalized for CAP. Among 69 patients receiving oral ofloxacin, 56 were cured and 13 were improved. In that study, patients with neutropenia, rapidly fatal illnesses, or severe renal failure were excluded.

- Antimicrobial spectrum: Similar to that of ciprofloxacin. Excellent activity against *H. influenzae* (both ampicillin-sensitive and ampicillin-resistant strains), *Neisseria*, *E. coli*, *M. catarrhalis*, and most Enterobacteriaceae. Less active in vitro against *P. aeruginosa* as compared to ciprofloxacin;

studies in vivo in cystic fibrosis exacerbations suggest both agents may be comparable. Modest gram-positive activity; less active than penicillins against streptococci, including *S. pneumoniae* (comparable to ciprofloxacin). Moderate activity against staphylococci (including *S. epidermidis* and MRSA). Anaerobic activity fair to poor. Active against *Chlamydia*, *Mycoplasma*, and *Legionella* species.
- Toxicity: Similar to that of ciprofloxacin; few serious adverse effects. Unlike ciprofloxacin, no effect on theophylline.
- Dosage: Oral 400 mg q 12 hours (98% bioavailability); IV 400 mg q 12 hours
- Antimicrobial resistance: As with other fluoroquinolones, development of resistance, particularly by *P. aeruginosa* and *S. aureus*, may be problematic with ofloxacin. Susceptibility to ofloxacin, however, has been demonstrated in some strains exhibiting high-grade resistance to ciprofloxacin.

Other Agents
Chloramphenicol

The recognition that aplastic anemia and the "grey baby syndrome" were complications arising from its use led to a dramatic decline in prescriptions for this agent in the 1960s. Currently, chloramphenicol should be restricted to infections resistant to alternative agents.
- *Mechanism of action:* Binds to 50S subunit of the 70S bacterial ribosome (blocks the attachment of aminotransfer RNA to the ribosomes)
- *Antimicrobial spectrum:* Broad-spectrum agent, but other antimicrobials preferred for common pathogens. Excellent activity against unusual pathogens that exhibit resistance to most antimicrobials (e.g. *Rickettsia*, *Pseudomonas pseudomallei*, *P. cepacia*, and *Salmonella typhi*).
- *Toxicity:* Aplastic anemia (<1:20,000 cases); dose-related myelosuppression; hemolytic anemia; grey baby syndrome in infants; and reversible neurologic dysfunction.

Trimethoprim/Sulfamethoxazole

- *Mechanism of action:* TMP and SMZ interfere with bacterial cell replication by inhibiting sequential enzymes involved in the formation of tetrahydrofolic acid. TMP inhibits dihydrofolate reductase; SMZ competitively inhibits synthesis of dihydrofolic acid from para-aminobenzoic acid. The inhibition of differing enzyme steps improves antimicrobial activity and confers synergistic killing.
- *Antimicrobial spectrum:* Active against more than 99% of *S. pneumoniae* and *M. catarrhalis*; excellent activity against most gram-positive organisms, including streptococci and staphylococci (including MRSA); not adequate against group A streptococci or enterococci. Active again more

than 80% of strains of *H. influenzae* (including ampicillin-resistant strains). Anaerobic activity is limited; most isolates, including *Bacteroides* species, are susceptible in vitro, but clinical efficacy has not been established. TMP or SMX has excellent activity against Enterobacteriaceae, and emergence of resistance has been rare. Consistently high activity against *E. coli, Proteus mirabilis*; active against most strains of *P. vulgaris, Klebsiella,* and *Serratia* species; *P. aeruginosa* is usually resistant. TMP or SMX is usually active against *P. cepacia, P. pseudomallei, Xanthomonas maltophilia, Citrobacter, Enterobacter cloacae,* and *Acinetobacter* species (pathogens that are often resistant to third-generation cephalosporins). Excellent activity against *Legionella* species in vitro and in animal models of legionellosis; data in man are lacking, however.
- *Toxicity:* Skin rash (3%) (usually minor); exfoliative dermatitis (Stevens-Johnson syndrome) or erythema multiforme rare (<1:10,000) excessive fluid when administered IV in high doses; nausea, GI distress (3–10%); diarrhea (<1%); may contribute to marrow toxicity in patients with hematologic neoplasia or underlying marrow disorder; substantial ↑ in incidence and severity of side effects in patients with AIDS.
- *Dosage:* Regular strength tablets (80 mg TMP; 400 mg SMZ) or double strength (160/800); for parenteral use, 1 ampoule (5 mL) contains 80 mg TMP and 400 mg SMX/mL. Doses of 20 mg/kg/day for TMP component in 4 divided doses for *Pneumocystis carinii*; lower doses q 8–12 hours may be adequate for bacterial infections.
- *Indications:* TMP or SMZ is a reasonable option for both CAP and nosocomial pneumonias in patients with hypersensitivity reactions to penicillins or beta-lactams. TMP or SMZ is less expensive than third-generation cephalosporins or antipseudomonal penicillins, and may be given orally following a favorable response to parenteral therapy (60–75% bioavailable). Despite an excellent in vitro susceptibility profile, clinical experience with TMP or SMX in the treatment of pneumonia has been limited. TMP or SMX, however, has been successfully used in nosocomial infections caused by staphylococci (including MRSA) and in each other.

Clindamycin

- *Antimicrobial spectrum:* Highly active against anaerobes, including *Fusobacterium* species, peptostreptococci, peptococci, clostridia, and *Bacteroides* species (including *B. fragilis*); excellent activity against *S. pneumoniae*, most streptococci, and methicillin-sensitive *S. aureus*; enterococci, and MRSA are resistant. No significant activity against aerobic gram-negative rods. Does not cover *Mycoplasma, Chlamydia,* or *Legionella* species.

- *Toxicity:* Skin rash (5-10%); diarrhea (2-10%); pseudomembranous colitis no more common with clindamycin than with many other antibiotics commonly prescribed; and metallic taste in mouth with parenteral administration (4%).
- *Dosage:* 150-450 mg tid (po); maximal IV dose 900 mg q 8 hours, but 600 mg q 8 hours is probably adequate even for serious infections; and dose must be ↓ed in renal failure.
- *Indications:* Primary therapy for community-acquired anaerobic lung abscess or aspiration pneumonia (penicillin G is an alternative, but clindamycin may be more efficacious). Combination of clindamycin with aztreonam may provide outstanding empiric therapy for nosocomial pneumonia in patients allergic to beta-lactams in whom penicillins, cephalosporins, and imipenem are contraindicated.

Vancomycin

Vancomycin, a complex glycopeptide initially isolated from *Streptomyces orientalis* has been in use since 1956 primarily for treatment of staphylococcal infections. The use of vancomycin declined following the introduction of methicillin, but interest in this agent has surged over the past decade concomitant with an ↑ed incidence of awareness of methicillin-resistant staphylococci, the increasing prevalence of gram-positive infections among patients with granulocytopenic cancer, and its efficacy against *Clostridium difficile* colitis.

- *Mechanism* of *action:* Multiple mechanisms of action include inhibition of bacterial cell wall synthesis (interferes with glycopeptide synthesis); occurs at an earlier step than penicillins; interferes with RNA synthesis; alters permeability of bacterial cell membrane.
- *Antimicrobial spectrum:* Vancomycin is exceptionally active against aerobic gram-positive cocci but has a narrow spectrum. It is bactericidal against aerobic gram-positive organisms (*S. epidermidis* and *S. aureus*, including MRSA), diphtheroids (e.g. corynebacteria), streptococci, pneumococci, and clostridia, but is only bacteriostatic against enterococci. No significant activity against gram-negative organisms, anaerobes, *Mycoplasma, Chlamydia,* or *Legionella* species.
- *Toxicity:* Phlebitis (>10% in some series); maculopapular or erythematous rash (4-5%); hearing loss, particularly with high serum levels; and "red man's syndrome" (erythematous flushing of the torso, neck, and face associated with pruritus, hypotension, and rarely cardiac arrest, agents such as penicillins. Because of its narrow spectrum, vancomycin is not adequate as single-agent empiric therapy for pneumonia. Vancomycin is bactericidal against MRSA and other gram-positive organisms that exhibit resistance to penicillins (e.g. pathogenic *Corynebacterium* species, *S. epidermidis*) and is the drug of choice for these pathogens.

Effective against infections caused by enterococci but need to combine with gentamicin for bactericidal activity.
- *Special considerations*: Antimicrobial resistance to vancomycin rarely (if ever) develops during therapy; no cross-resistance occurs between vancomycin and unrelated antibiotics. Thus, vancomycin remains exceptionally reliable against traditionally susceptible organisms (gram-positive cocci) even with widespread use.

BIBLIOGRAPHY

1. Clinical guidance for bronchiolitis. Lancet. 2017;389(10065):128.
2. Lynch J, Toews G. In: Khan MG, Bartlett JG, Chopra S, Topol EJ (eds). Medical Diagnosis and Therapy. Philadelphia: Lea and Febiger: 1994.pp.288-320.
3. Schuetz P, Wirz P, Mueller B. Procalcitonin testing to guide antibiotic therapy in acute upper and lower respiratory tract infections. JAMA. 2018;319(9):925-6.

CHAPTER 16

Pulmonary Embolism

INTRODUCTION

Pulmonary embolism (PE) is a common condition. The diagnosis of PE is often missed; however, because symptoms are not specific, and investigations other than lung scan and angiography are nondiagnostic. The mortality rate of patients with massive PE is more than 40%.

Questions to analyze:
- Is the patient stable or in severe distress?
- What are the vital signs?
- Is acute dyspnea associated with central chest pain or pleuritic pain?
- Is the patient tachypneic?
- Did syncope, presyncope, or dizziness occur with the dyspnea?
- Has the patient had surgery within past weeks?

Consider the following causes of PE. Strongly consider PE, if one or more of the following scenarios discussed below is present.

DIAGNOSIS

- Acute, unexplained dyspnea lasting only a few minutes to several hours (i.e. sudden dyspnea) not due to:
  - An obvious cardiac cause
  - An obvious pulmonary lesion
- Acute cor pulmonale and cardiogenic shock
  - If more than 70% of the pulmonary vascular cross-sectional area is obliterated acutely by emboli, acute pulmonary hypertension at more than 40 mm Hg results. Right ventricular failure occurs, and death results often within the 1st hour of the onset of acute dyspnea or cardiogenic shock.
  - Massive or submassive PE poses an immediate threat to life.
- With massive PE, pain is usually central, oppressive, and nonpleuritic. Presyncope, syncope, marked apprehension, signs of cardiogenic shock, cough, and features that may simulate an acute exacerbation of chronic obstructive pulmonary disease (COPD) are hallmarks.
- Chronic cor pulmonale in patients with recurrent PE

- Increasing dyspnea owing to pulmonary hypertension
- Signs of right ventricular failure without an obvious cardiac cause.

Probability from Clinical Assessment

The physician must devise a system to evaluate the probability for the presence of PE based on a systematic clinical assessment that includes:
- A rapid but relevant history is crucial for determining a probability from clinical assessment (PCA).
  - *History of thromboembolic disease*: Deep venous thrombosis (DVT) present or recent:
    - Hemoptysis
    - Acute unexplained shortness of breath with distress.
  - Prolonged anesthesia associated with surgery.
  - Surgery or injury to the lower extremities or hip.
  - Surgical treatment triggers an increase in factor VIII and a decrease in protein C activity and an increase in platelet adhesiveness.
  - Immobilization for more than 24 hours after a fracture, major or minor surgery, myocardial infarction (MI), heart failure (HF), or stroke.
  - Pregnancy, particularly in the early postpartum phase and also the use of estrogen-containing compounds.
  - Malignancy, tumor cells appear to interact with thrombin and plasmin-generating systems; some cancer causes a decrease in platelet antithrombin and antithrombin III activities and cause an increase in fibrinogen.
  - Street drugs that increase platelet count and adhesiveness.
  - Hypercoagulable diathesis, protein C, S, or antithrombin III deficiency, polycythemia vera, AND Thrombocythemia are implicated in less than 15% of cases of deep vein thrombosis; rarely, high levels of factor, V or factor VII may be underlying factors.
  - Patients with primary or secondary antiphospholipid syndrome.
  - Prolonged air travel less than 6 hours is a common cause for embolism, and preventive measures can significantly reduce the prevalence of DVT and embolism.
- Selective physical signs
- Chest X-ray
- Electrocardiogram (ECG)

The analysis of these four assessments should result in a PCA. The Wells score is redundant.

At the Bedside: Quick-look Test

- Does the patient look relatively well, sick (uncomfortable or distressed), or critical (about to die)? Suspect massive embolism and immediate therapy
- Airway and vital signs

- What is the blood pressure?
- Cardiogenic shock may occur as a result of PE. The blood pressure may be in the normal range; however, with significant embolism.
- Tachycardia is common but is nonspecific.

Selective History

Rapidly assess the following:
- *The quality of pain:* Central chest pain with acute dyspnea, apprehension, and sinus tachycardia in the absence of pulmonary diseases, a history of unstable angina, and ECG signs of acute MI suggest PE.
- Pleuritic chest pain and hemoptysis in a patient without symptoms and signs of pneumonia or chest infection. If these symptoms are associated with an infiltrate or right-sided pleural effusion or with oligemic lung in a patient with a predisposing factor, such as a postoperative state, the PCA is high.
- History of presyncope or syncope within the past few hours
- Predisposing causes or risk factors for thromboembolism:
  - Postorthopedic surgery; incidence of PE 40–70%
  - All other surgical interventions with immobilization of more than 1 day; incidence of PE 15–20%
  - Past history of thromboembolism or previous DVT
  - Congestive HF
  - Malignancy
  - Birth control pill use in a smoker more than 25 years old
  - Hypercoagulable diathesis.

The presence of risk factors and unexplained chest pain or unexplained dyspnea or syncope in a patient with a normal chest X-ray strongly suggests a diagnosis of PE.

Selective Physical Examination

Clinical findings are nonspecific and require rapid documentation.
- Tachypnea and tachycardia are the most frequent signs.
- Increased P_2 sound
- S_4 gallop caused by right ventricular dysfunction
- A systolic murmur at the left lower sternal border that increases with inspiration indicates tricuspid regurgitation caused by acute pulmonary hypertension.
- Crackles (crepitations)
- Pleuritic friction rub over the area of pain
- Deep venous thrombosis present.

The differential diagnosis includes pneumonia, exacerbation of asthma or COPD, MI, pulmonary edema, anxiety, dissecting aneurysm, pericardial tamponade, pneumothorax, and musculoskeletal pain.

Diagnostic Testing

D-dimer

- This test should be done on all patients suspected to have PE.
- Plasmin digests cross-linked fibrin from pulmonary emboli; degradation products containing D-dimers are released and can be detected in the plasma by monoclonal antibodies.
- A D-dimer enzyme-linked immunosorbent assay more than 500 ng/mL is abnormal and is present in more than 90% of patients with PE.
- The test is highly sensitive but not specific for the diagnosis of PE.
- *Specificity is improved if other causes of abnormal results are excluded:* MI, congestive HF, and N-terminal pro–B-type natriuretic peptide (NT-proBNP) less than 300 pg/mL strongly exclude the presence of acute HF.
- Pneumonia, cancer, and postsurgery. But these should be easy to rapidly exclude.
- D-dimer alone cannot exclude or confirm the presence of PE.
- A D-dimer concentration of less than 500 µg/L measured using a high-sensitivity assay system is a robust means of excluding PE in patients with a low pretest probability of PE, as determined by a validated clinical prediction rule, obviating the need for imaging [e.g. computed tomography (CT) pulmonary angiography] in such patients (Flowchart 16.1).
- The positive predictive value of D-dimer values above this threshold; however, is less robust. D-dimer concentrations more than or equal to 500 µg/L.

D-dimer cutoffs for further evaluation are:

- Age multiplied by 10 in patients 50 years and older (e.g. in a 78-year-old patient, the age-adjusted cutoff would be 780 µg/L). A cutoff of 500 µg/L was retained for patients younger than 50 years.
- The combination of D-dimer, partial end tidal carbon dioxide (PetCO$_2$) less than or equal to 28.5 mm Hg and the clinical probability could improve diagnostic accuracy in patients with suspected PE.
- *A normal D-dimer result gives reassurance* in more than 90% of cases that PE is not present. In one study using a whole-blood agglutination assay (SimpliRed), the test yielded a negative predictive value of 99%.
- A rapid latex-agglutination test is not recommended because it is inaccurate.

Radiation

The adverse effects of contrast in people undergoing CT remain a major concern. Thus several algorithms have evolved including D-dimer testing to arrive at a diagnosis and avoid radiation CT. With careful thinking and

Flowchart 16.1: Pulmonary embolism probability from clinical assessment.*, **

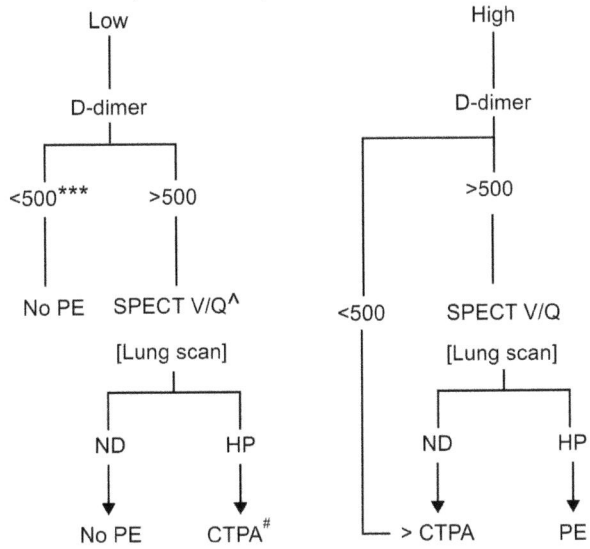

(CTPA, computed tomography pulmonary angiography; HP, high probability; ND, non-diagnostic lung scan; PE, pulmonary embolism; SPECT V/Q, single photon emission computed tomography ventilation/perfusion)
*Gabriel Khan, Joseph P Lynch. Pulmonary disease diagnosis and therapy: A practical approach; 1997.
**Khan MG. On Call Cardiology, 3 edition. Philadelphia: Elsevier Health Sciences; 2006. (Figure 16.1)
***(≥500 µg/L) 500 micrograms/L patients age <50—multiply by 10 for those over age 50
^Lung scan is safe, and remains useful in developing countries; decreases use of CTPA
#CT pulmonary angiography is the preferred diagnostic test but high radiation remains a concern; caution, contrast use in renal dysfunction.
Spiral CT is most useful in patients with renal dysfunction or women over age 50. But all CTs carry radiation risks. Algorithms do not cover all scenarios; clinical correlation is required.

D-dimer testing, it appears that avoidance of CT may be achieved in in approximately 15% of patients presenting with symptoms and signs that suggest PE.

It appears that a new diagnostic work-up algorithm for patients suspected of having a PE could substantially reduce the need for chest CT scans and could eliminate as many as 14% of the CT scans ordered when patients come to the emergency room complaining of chest pain.

The algorithm could replace the somewhat complicated Wells rule or revised Geneva score.

With the standard algorithm, the decision tree on whether
- To order a CT pulmonary angiography to look for pulmonary emboli begins with the clinician's own thoughts on whether the patient is having a PE event (PCA; *see* Flowchart 16.1)
- If that probability is low, a D-dimer test is performed, and if the test is negative, no CT is performed. If it is positive then a CT scan is done, and standard treatment follows if the CT finds an embolism.

- When the clinician believes that a PE is likely, then the patient proceeds to a CTA.
- Caution in females less than age 50 and in patients with renal dysfunction to avoid contrast nephropathy.

Arterial Blood Gas

Findings are nonspecific. Acute respiratory alkalosis is the most common finding. Carbon dioxide retention may occur with massive PE. The absence of acute respiratory alkalosis should not be taken as evidence against the diagnosis of PE. In medicine, a positive finding supports the diagnosis; a negative finding should not significantly alter diagnostic probabilities. The finding of hypoxemia and hypocapnia in the absence of conditions listed in the differential diagnosis with a normal chest X-ray increases the PCA, but these findings are nonspecific. A normal blood gas result does not decrease the PCA.

Chest X-ray

The chest X-ray may be normal. Subtle signs may be apparent on close scrutiny. The radiologic signs are nondiagnostic (Fig. 16.1) but can be used in conjunction with the clinical findings and arterial blood gas results to assess the PCA (Fig. 16.1).
- *Atelectasis:* Platelike or small segmental atelectases
- Pleural effusion
- "Infiltrate" or pleural-based consolidation; a peripheral wedge-shaped density above the diaphragm (Hampton's hump)
- Pulmonary artery enlargement and abrupt vessel cutoff (Fig. 16.1)
- An enlarged right descending pulmonary artery (Palla's sign)
- Oligemic, hyperlucent lung, and distal to the abrupt cutoff of the pulmonary artery—focal oligemia (Westermark's sign)
- Elevated hemidiaphragm
- Dilation of azygos vein.

Electrocardiography

The ECG may be normal, but subtle, transient abnormalities should alert suspicion.
- Sinus tachycardia without an obvious cause
- T wave inversion in leads V_1-V_4 is one of the most common abnormalities.
- S_1, S_2, and S_3 heart sounds
- S_1, Q_3, and T wave inversion in lead III with lead, II ST segment and T wave normal and similar to lead I, rather than to lead III (i.e. finding is in contrast to acute MI—leads II, III, and aVF are involved with MI).

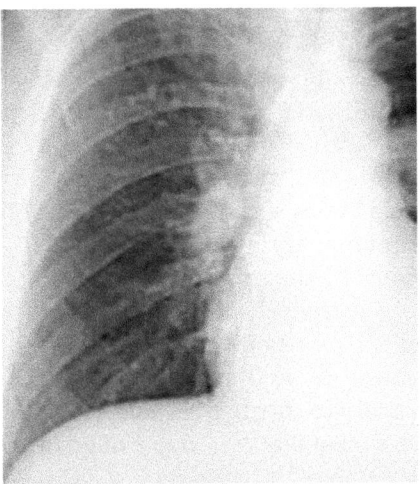

Fig. 16.1: Enlargement of the right hilum from distention of the descending right pulmonary artery from a massive pulmonary embolus. The transverse diameter of the pulmonary artery is 22 mm. The distention is the result not of increased pulmonary artery pressure proximal to the clot, but of distention by thrombus. Note the abrupt change of caliber in the descending pulmonary artery, which is accompanied by diminished vascularity in the lower lobe.
Source: Khan M Gabriel. On Call Cardiology, 3rd edition. Philadelphia: WB Saunders, Elsevier Science; 2006. p. 150.

- *Right ventricular strain pattern*: T wave inversion in leads V_1-V_3; S wave in leads V_5 and V_6
- Sudden right axis deviation compared with previous reading
- Transient right bundle branch block
- Nonspecific ST-T changes, including T wave inversion in leads V_5 and V_6, occurring for a few hours only.

Computed tomography pulmonary angiogram (CTPA) has effectively become the first-line imaging test for the evaluation of PE. Patients with a high-quality negative CTA do not require further examination or treatment for suspected PE.

- Spiral CT has a definite role except in women less than age 50; it is most often diagnostic. Use of multidetector CTPA was associated with significant radiation exposure that potentially increases risk of secondary malignancies. This is particularly a concern for young women given the risk of breast cancer.

Spiral CT—in developing countries, spiral CT may not be available. CTA is gold standard but is a more complex investigation requiring staff; renal dysfunction or allergy to dye is concerns. Thus lung scan has a role in some countries.

Lung Scan

Outcome studies have supported the use of single photon emission computed tomography (SPECT) ventilation/perfusion (V/Q) as the first imaging test in patients with suspected acute PE, since false-negative rates are close to 1%, which is similar to the rate for CTA. In addition, reports from outside the United States strongly advise that SPECT further improves the performance of pulmonary scintigraphy; SPECT V/Q, has a role for follow-up examinations of patients, to avoid unjustified radiation exposure and added costs from multiple CT studies.

- A low PCA along with a negative highly sensitive D-dimer essentially rules out a diagnosis of venous thromboembolism. A low PCA but positive D-dimer calls for further testing—CT (single or multidetector CT depending on availability and departmental preferences) or CTPA or lung scan.
- There has been a fortunate resurgence of experts appropriately recommending the use of V/Q lung scan, preferably SPECT V/Q scintigraphy. If positive, PE is confirmed.
- If negative, and D-dimer is negative. PE is excluded.
- Request a V/Q scan as soon as the clinical impression suggests a diagnosis of PE for patients without unexplained acute shortness of breath, and not in distress.
- A lung scan is the first-line investigation in some countries except for patients suspected of having a massive PE, which is indicated by acute cor pulmonale or cardiogenic shock. A lung scan should be interpreted as one of the following:
  - Normal
  - Nondiagnostic (intermediate and low-probability scans)
  - High probability.

  A normal scan in a patient with a normal D-dimer and low PCA indicates an absence of PE in more than 99% of cases.
- A high-probability scan is indicated by multiple, segmental perfusion defects without corresponding ventilation or chest X-ray abnormalities. A high-probability scan is 98% specific for PE but lacks sensitivity.

Echocardiography

Right ventricular hypokinesis is present in approximately 40% of patients with PE; this finding is associated with a doubling of the mortality rate in 2 weeks, and it triples in 1 year. A typical feature is regional right ventricular dysfunction in which apical wall motion remains normal despite hypokinesis of the free wall (McConnell's sign). Diastolic and systolic bowing of the septum into the left ventricle reflects right ventricular volume and pressure overload.

Venous Ultrasonography

Venous ultrasonography is accurate in patients with symptomatic DVT, but detection of DVT is much lower if symptoms and signs are absent; a normal result does not exclude DVT or PE. More than 20% of patients with normal ultrasonography results have proven PE.

A combination of tests can resolve diagnostic difficulties—positive ultrasonography of the veins of the lower limbs and right ventricular hypokinesis on echocardiography are virtually diagnostic of PE. A normal lung scan and normal D-dimer virtually exclude PE.

Pulmonary Angiography

- As an emergency procedure in patients suspected of having a massive embolism requiring immediate embolectomy.
- In patients with nondiagnostic lung scan and a negative femoral venogram but a high PCA.
- In patients with a high-probability scan and a high risk of bleeding.

MANAGEMENT

- *Heparin:* If there is no contraindication to heparin, start intravenous (IV) heparin, 5,000–10,000-U bolus, and a simultaneous infusion of heparin, 1,520 U/hr in patients without known risks of bleeding and 1,200 U/hr in patients with risk of bleeding. Request the partial thromboplastin time 6 hours later, and adjust the infusion to maintain a partial thromboplastin time of 1.5–2.3 times the patient control.

Contraindications to heparin include:
  - A bleeding disorder or a very low platelet count
  - Recent bleeding from a peptic ulcer
  - Recent intracranial bleeding.

Heparin is advised for 5–7 days, depending on departmental policies. For submassive embolism, 5 days of heparin therapy should suffice. Assess platelet count on day 3 of heparin therapy, then daily to detect heparin-induced thrombocytopenia. The complications of heparin-induced thrombocytopenia may be life-threatening.

- *Oral anticoagulants:* Warfarin (Coumadin), 5 mg, is started on day 2 of heparin therapy. The initial dose should not exceed 5 mg. A larger loading dose used to be recommended but may precipitate venous gangrene of the limbs, albeit rarely. This dose is repeated the next day; subsequent doses of warfarin depend on the international normalized ratio or prothrombin time. Heparin is continued until the international normalized ratio is in the desired range of 2–3 or prothrombin time is 1.3–1.5 times the control for at least 2 days. For submassive embolism,

5 days of IV heparin decreases hospital costs. Oral anticoagulants are continued for 3–6 months.
- Assess for hypercoagulable state in selected cases. Test for:
  - Factor V Leiden mutation
  - Hyperhomocysteinemia, which, if present, can be treated with B vitamins and folic acid.
  - The presence of antiphospholipid antibodies (lupus anticoagulant or anticardiolipin antibodies), which demands more intensive anticoagulation.

BIBLIOGRAPHY

1. Anderson DR, Kahn SR, Rodger MA, et al. Computed tomographic pulmonary angiography vs ventilation-perfusion lung scanning in patients with suspected pulmonary embolism: a randomized controlled trial. JAMA. 2007;298:2743-53.
2. Bonderman D, Lang IM. End-tidal CO_2 for exclusion of suspected pulmonary embolism: a new partner for Wells? Eur Respir J. 2010;35(4):723-4.
3. Freund Y, Cachanado M, Aubry A, et al. Effect of the Pulmonary Embolism Rule-Out Criteria on Subsequent Thromboembolic Events Among Low-Risk Emergency Department Patients The PROPER Randomized Clinical Trial. JAMA. 2018;319(6):559-66.
4. Hemnes AR, Newman AL, Rosenbaum B, et al. Bedside end-tidal CO2 tension as a screening tool to exclude pulmonary embolism. Eur Respir J. 2010;35:735-41.
5. Konstantinides S. Acute pulmonary embolism. N Engl J Med. 2008;359:2804-13.
6. Le Gal G, Righini M, Roy PM, et al. Prediction of pulmonary embolism in the emergency department: the revised Geneva score. Ann Intern Med. 2006;144:165-71.
7. Miles S, Roges KM, Thomas P, et al. A comparison of Single-Photon Emission CT Lung Scintigraphy and CT Pulmonary Angiography for the diagnosis of pulmonary embolism. Chest. 2009;136:1546-53.
8. Palmer LP, Khan M Gabriel. Pulmonary embolism. In: Khan M Gabriel (Ed). Cardiac and pulmonary management. Philadelphia, PA: Lea and Febiger; 1993. p. 894.
9. Stein PD, Fowler SE, Goodman LR, et al. Multidetector computed tomography for acute pulmonary embolism. N Engl J Med. 2006;354:2317-27.
10. Stein PD, Woodard PK, Weg JG, et al. Diagnostic pathways in acute pulmonary embolism: recommendations of the PIOPED II Investigators. Radiology. 2007;242:15-21.
11. Stein EG, Haramati LB, Chamarthy M, et al. Success of a safe and simple algorithm to reduce use of CT pulmonary angiography in the emergency department. Am J Roentgenol. 2010;194:392-7.
12. Stein PD, Freeman LM, Sostman HD, et al. SPECT in Acute Pulmonary Embolism. J Nucl Med. 2009;50(12):1999-2007.

CHAPTER 17

Pleural Diseases: Pleural Effusions

INTRODUCTION

Anytime a patient with an abnormal chest X-ray is evaluated, and the possibility of a pleural effusion should be considered. Increased densities on the chest X-ray are frequently attributed to parenchymal infiltrates, although they actually represent pleural fluid. The earliest radiologic sign of a pleural effusion is blunting of the posterior costophrenic sulcus on lateral X-ray. If this angle is blunted, bilateral decubitus chest X-rays should be obtained to ascertain whether free pleural fluid is present.

(Dr Light provided most of this chapter and now gives an excellent N Engl J Med review article.)

The presence of pleural fluid can be documented by one of the following:
- Bilateral decubitus X-rays of the chest
- Computed tomography (CT) scan of the chest
- Ultrasonic examination of the chest.

PHYSIOLOGY OF PLEURAL FLUID FORMATION

Fluid can enter the pleural space from:
- Capillaries in the parietal pleura
- Capillaries in the visceral pleura
- Interstitial spaces of the lung.

Pleural fluid accumulates when the rate of fluid formation more than the rate of fluid absorption. This situation can be caused by either an increase (↑) rate of formation or a ↓ rate of absorption. Rate of formation is normally 0.01 mL/kg/hr, whereas capacity for absorption is 0.20 mL/kg/hr.
- Absorption is almost exclusively via the lymphatics in the parietal pleura
- Lymphatics in the visceral pleura do not communicate with the pleural space; little fluid exits the pleural space via capillaries.

Fluid entry into the pleural space from the capillaries follows Starling's equation. The following factors ↑ the rate of pleural fluid formation from the capillaries:
- Increased hydrostatic pressure in the capillaries in either the visceral or the parietal pleura
- Decreased pressure in the pleural space

- Decreased oncotic pressure in the blood
- Increased oncotic pressure in the pleural fluid.

The rate of fluid entry into the pleural space from the interstitial spaces of the lungs ↑ when interstitial fluid is ↑; the lymphatics that normally drain the lung become disrupted, such as occurs with lung transplantation.

- *Symptoms of pleural effusion*: Dyspnea on exertion; chest tightness; and pleuritic chest pain
- *Signs of pleural effusion*: Dullness to percussion absent tactile fremitus ↓ breath sounds.

APPROACH TO PATIENTS WITH PLEURAL EFFUSION

Pleural effusions can occur as complications of many different diseases (Box 17.1). The vigor with which various diagnoses are pursued depends on the likelihood that the individual has that particular disease. Rough estimates as to the incidence of the most common causes of pleural effusions are provided in Table 17.1.

Box 17.1: Differential diagnosis of pleural effusions
1. Transudative pleural effusions
    a. Congestive heart failure
    b. Cirrhosis
    c. Peritoneal dialysis
    d. Nephrotic syndrome
    e. Superior vena cava obstruction
    f. Fontan procedure
    g. Urinothorax
    h. Myxedema
    i. Pulmonary emboli
2. Exudative pleural effusions
    a. Neoplastic diseases
        - Metastatic disease
        - Mesothelioma
    b. Infectious diseases
        - Bacterial infections
        - Tuberculosis
        - Fungal infections
        - Viral infections
        - Parasitic infections
    c. Pulmonary embolization
    d. Gastrointestinal diseases
        - Acute pancreatitis
        - Chronic pancreatic pleural effusion
        - Esophageal perforation
        - Intra-abdominal abscesses
        - Diaphragmatic hernia
        - Postabdominal surgery
        - Endoscopic variceal sclerotherapy

Contd...

Contd...
  e. Collagen vascular diseases
     - Rheumatoid pleuritis
     - Lupus erythematosus
     - Churg–Strauss syndrome
     - Familial Mediterranean fever
     - Immunoblastic lymphadenopathy
  f. Drug-induced pleural disease
     - Nitrofurantoin
     - Dantrolene
     - Methysergide
     - Bromocriptine
     - Procarbazine
     - Amiodarone
  g. Asbestos exposure
  h. Postcardiac injury syndrome
  i. Pericardial disease
  j. Postcoronary artery bypass surgery
  k. Uremia
  l. Yellow nail syndrome
  m. Sarcoidosis
  n. Trapped lung
  o. Meigs' syndrome

Table 17.1: Approximate annual incidence of various types of pleural effusions in the United States.

Causes	Incidence (reported cases)
Congestive heart failure	500,000
Pneumonia (bacterial)	300,000
Malignant disease	200,000
Lung	60,000
Breast	50,000
Lymphoma	40,000
Other	50,000
Pulmonary embolization	150,000
Viral disease	100,000
Cirrhosis with ascites	50,000
Gastrointestinal disease	25,000
Collagen vascular disease	6,000
Asbestos exposure	2,000
Mesothelioma	1,500
Tuberculosis	1,000

When a patient has a pleural effusion that measures more than 10 mm on the decubitus X-ray, a diagnostic thoracentesis usually should be performed. If the patient has obvious congestive heart failure (CHF), consideration can be given to postponing the thoracentesis until the CHF is treated. The characteristics of pleural fluid change little with diuresis over several days. If, however, such a patient is febrile or has pleuritic chest pain, or if the effusions are not of comparable size on both sides, a thoracentesis should be performed without delay.

Figures 17.1 to 17.4 give radiologic features of pleural effusions.

Performing a Diagnostic Thoracentesis

This procedure is usually performed while the patient sits upright. A table should be available for the patient to rest his arms upon. The patient's back should remain relatively vertical, for if the patient leans forward too far, the lowest part of the hemithorax may move anteriorly and no fluid will remain posteriorly. Insert the needle posteriorly where the ribs are easily palpable and where the fluid gravitates. Make the first attempt one interspace below the level where the tactile fremitus is lost. Most unsuccessful thoracentesis procedures result from attempting to perform the thoracentesis at a level that is too low. Insertion of the needle at a low level is dangerous because

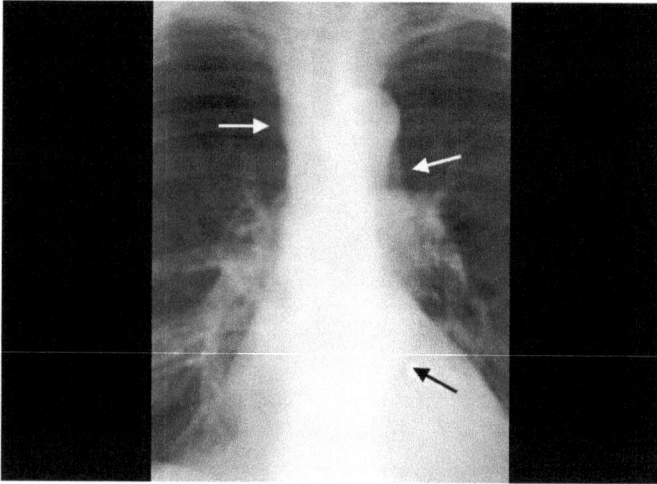

Fig. 17.1: The left paravertebral soft-tissue shadow behind the left side of the heart (black arrow) could be mistaken for a paravertebral soft-tissue swelling if the continuity of the margin with the upper descending aorta (white arrow above black arrow) is not recognized. Note also the right paratracheal bulge and loss of the paratracheal stripe from enlarged nodes (white arrow).
Source: Khan M Gabriel. On Call Cardiology, 3rd edition. Philadelphia: WB Saunders, Elsevier Science; 2006. p. 158.

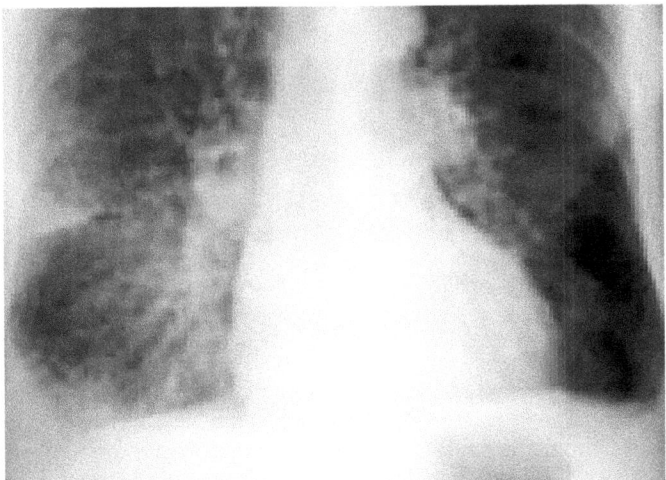

Fig. 17.2: Bilateral pleural effusions in a patient with metastatic nodules scattered throughout both lungs, primary unknown. There is a small left pleural effusion obliterating the left costophrenic angle, with an ill-defined margin. There is a larger right pleural effusion, also with an ill-defined margin, extending along the axillary margin of the lung. There is a little atelectasis in the anterior segment of the right upper lobe, abutting on the outer aspect of the lesser fissure.
Sources:
1. Khan M Gabriel. On Call Cardiology, 3rd edition. Philadelphia: WB Saunders, Elsevier Science; 2006.
2. Khan M Gabriel. Pulmonary Disease Diagnosis and Therapy: A Practical Approach. Baltimore: Williams & Wilkins, 1997. p. 36.

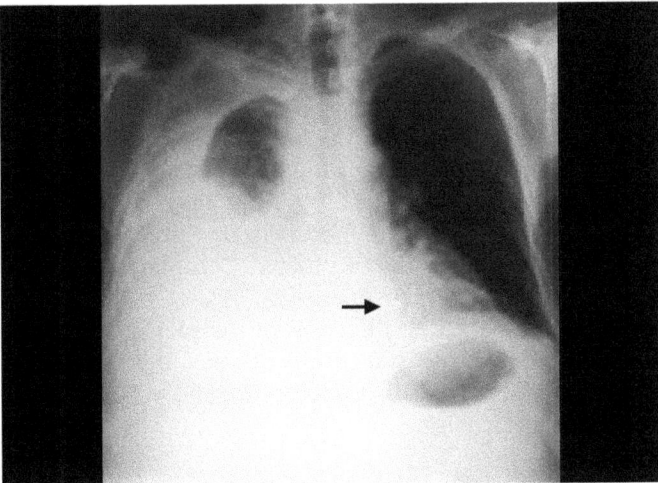

Fig. 17.3: Massive right pleural effusion, extending over the apex of the lung onto the mediastinal aspect of the upper lobe. There is no mediastinal shift because of the complete collapse of the middle and lower lobes. The left paravertebral opacity (arrow) is the result of right pleural effusion bulging the azygoesophageal recess to the left of the midline.
Source: Khan MG. On Call Cardiology, 3rd edition. Philadelphia: WB Saunders, Elsevier Science; 2006. p. 159.

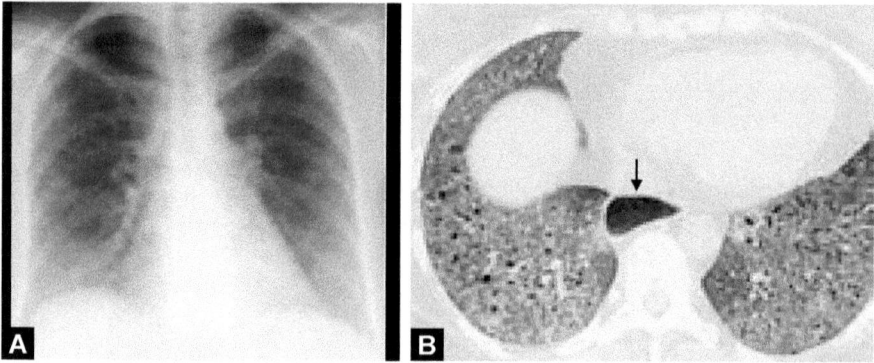

Figs. 17.4A and B: (A) Plain radiograph of a patient with CREST syndrome showing basilar reticulonodular disease; (B) HRCT shows that the pattern is actually one of small cysts or honeycombing. Note: The dilated air-filled esophagus (arrow).
Source: Khan MG. On Call Cardiology, 3rd edition. Philadelphia: WB Saunders, Elsevier Science; 2006.

the spleen or liver may be lacerated. Evaluate with ultrasound if fluid is not obtained after two or three attempts.
- Thoroughly cleanse the skin over the site
- Anesthetize the skin with lidocaine using a short 25-gauge needle
- Anesthetize the periosteum of the underlying rib and the parietal pleura by performing the following steps with a 22-gauge needle 1.5 inches long. Move the needle up and over the rib with frequent injections of small amounts (about 0.1 mL) of lidocaine. Once superior to the rib, slowly advance the needle toward the pleural space, with aspiration followed by the injection of 0.1–0.2 mL lidocaine q 1–2 mm. Once pleural fluid is obtained through the anesthetizing needle, withdraw the needle
- Withdraw the fluid by using a second 22-gauge needle attached to a 50–60-mL syringe that contains 0.5–1.0 mL heparin. Slowly insert the needle along the same tract with constant aspiration until pleural fluid is obtained. Continue aspiration until the syringe is filled
- Withdraw the needle.

If more than 60 mL of pleural fluid is to be removed, a plastic catheter rather than a sharp needle should be utilized. Complications of thoracentesis include—pneumothorax, which occurs in 10% of patients (20% of these patients require a chest tube); infection of the pleural space; hemothorax from laceration of an intercostal artery or vein, the spleen, or the liver; seeding of the needle tract with tumor cells; and vasovagal reaction with bradycardia and hypotension.

Separating Transudative from Exudative Pleural Effusions

The first question to be answered with a diagnostic thoracentesis is whether the patient has a transudative or an exudative pleural effusion. An exudative effusion results from disease of the pleural surfaces, a transudative effusion results from alterations in the systemic factors that influence the formation and reabsorption of pleural fluid.

This differentiation can be made by simultaneous analysis of the protein and lactate dehydrogenase (LDH) levels in the pleural fluid and in the serum. Exudative pleural effusions meet more than one of the following criteria, whereas transudative pleural effusions meet none:
- Ratio of pleural fluid to serum protein more than 0.5
- Ratio of pleural fluid to serum LDH more than 0.6
- Absolute level of pleural fluid LDH more than two-thirds upper normal limit for serum.

If none of the above criteria is met, the patient has a transudative pleural effusion, and the pleura itself can be ignored while the CHF, cirrhosis, or nephrosis is treated. Remember, however, that transudative pleural effusion can result from pulmonary embolization.

If a transudative pleural effusion is probable, the most cost-effective use of the laboratory is initially to measure only the pleural fluid protein and LDH levels. Other diagnostic tests, such as cytology, cell count, and differential, amylase, glucose, and cultures, are obtained only if the patient is proved to have an exudative pleural effusion.

TRANSUDATIVE PLEURAL EFFUSIONS

Congestive heart failure is the disease most responsible for pleural effusions. The accumulation of pleural fluid in patients with CHF appears to be more related to left ventricular (LV) than to right ventricular (RV) failure. LV failure leads to ↑ interstitial fluid, which then traverses the visceral pleura to enter the pleural space. In animal experiments, approximately 25% of pulmonary edema fluid moves directly from the lung into the pleural space. Patients with pleural effusions secondary to CHF usually have other signs and symptoms (*see* Chapter 5).

Hepatic Hydrothorax

Pleural effusions sometimes develop in patients with cirrhosis, particularly if ascites is present. The incidence of pleural effusion is approximately 6% in patients with cirrhosis and ascites, but is less than 1% in patients with cirrhosis with hypoalbuminemia but without ascites. The predominant mechanism is the movement of the ascitic fluid directly from the peritoneal cavity through the diaphragm into the pleural space. Small pores in diaphragm have been demonstrated.

The pleural effusion with hepatic hydrothorax tends to be large because of the large reservoir of fluid in the peritoneal cavity that can flow directly into the pleural space with its lower pressure. Usually, tense ascites is present, but occasionally the ascites is subclinical. A large effusion may produce severe dyspnea. The pleural effusions are usually right sided (67%), but may be left sided (16%) or bilateral (17%).

In a patient with cirrhosis, tense ascites, and a pleural effusion, the diagnosis is easy.
- Both a paracentesis and a thoracentesis should be performed to ascertain that both fluids are transudates. The pleural fluid protein level, although usually slightly higher than the ascitic fluid protein level, is still less than 3.0 g/dL.
- Patients with hepatic hydrothoraces are prone to develop bacterial infections of the pleural space.
- Primary treatment is geared toward treatment of the ascites because the hydrothorax is an extension of the peritoneal fluid. A low-salt diet is recommended and diuretics should be administered judiciously. Serial therapeutic thoracenteses are not indicated because the pleural fluid rapidly reaccumulates and the thoracenteses deplete the patient of body protein.

If the pleural effusion persists despite optimal therapy directed toward the ascites, three therapeutic options, none of which is ideal, are available:
- Tube thoracostomy followed by the injection of a sclerosing agent; however, electrolyte depletion can lead to death.
- Implantation of a peritoneal-to-venous shunt; however, these shunts frequently do not control the effusion.
- Thoracotomy with surgical repair of the diaphragmatic leak; however, thoracotomy is a major surgical procedure.

Peritoneal Dialysis

Large pleural effusions occasionally complicate peritoneal dialysis:
- Dialysate appears to move directly through the diaphragm.
- Incidence is 10% in those on continuous ambulatory peritoneal dialysis
- The effusion is almost always on the right side.
- The pleural fluid has biochemical characteristics between those of the dialysate and of the serum.
- Treat with chemical pleurodesis combined with a short period of small-volume, intermittent peritoneal dialysis.

Nephrotic Syndrome

Pleural effusion occurs in approximately 20% of patients with nephrotic syndrome:
- Effusions are usually bilateral transudates because of the low oncotic pressure in the serum.
- Pulmonary embolus must be ruled out in this situation because emboli are common in patients with nephrotic syndrome.
- Primary treatment is aimed at treating the nephrotic syndrome, but chemical pleurodesis occasionally may be performed.

Superior Vena Caval Syndrome

Pleural effusions are not present in most patients with superior vena caval obstruction. Pleural effusions do occur in neonates with superior vena caval thrombosis, however.

Fontan Procedure

This procedure is used to treat infants and children with hypoplastic right ventricles. The right ventricle is bypassed with an anastomosis between the superior vena cava, the right atrium, or the inferior vena cava and the pulmonary artery (PA). Almost all patients develop postoperative bilateral pleural effusions, which are frequently large and clinically significant. With refractory effusions, consider chemical pleurodesis or a pleuroperitoneal shunt.

Urinothorax

Pleural fluid can accumulate in the presence of retroperitoneal urinary leakage secondary to urinary obstruction, trauma, or retroperitoneal inflammatory or malignant processes.
- Effusion develops within hours of the precipitating event.
- Pleural fluid looks and smells like urine.
- Diagnosis is confirmed by demonstrating a higher creatinine level in the pleural fluid than in the serum.
- Effusion resolves once urinary tract obstruction is relieved.

Myxedema

Pleural effusions occasionally occur as a complication of myxedema—incidence is probably less than 5%. Pleural fluid may have biochemical characteristics of either a transudate or an exudate.

Miscellaneous Causes

About 20% of the pleural effusions secondary to pulmonary embolism are transudative. Although pleural effusions secondary to Meigs' syndrome and sarcoidosis have been described as transudative, this is probably not the case.

EXUDATIVE PLEURAL EFFUSIONS

Pneumonia, malignant disorders, and pulmonary embolization account for most exudative pleural effusions (Table 17.1).

Tests on Pleural Fluid

The following tests should be performed on the pleural fluid from a patient with an exudative pleural effusion of unknown origin—glucose level, amylase level, LDH level, differential cell count, microbiologic studies, and cytology. In selected patients, other tests on the pleural fluid, such as the pH, antinuclear antibody (ANA) level, adenosine deaminase (ADA) level, rheumatoid factor level, and lipid analysis, may be of value.

Appearance

The gross appearance of the pleural fluid should always be described and its odor noted:
- *Bloody fluid*: Obtain hematocrit. If hematocrit is more than 50% that of peripheral blood, hemothorax is present and tube thoracostomy should be considered.
- *Cloudy fluid*: Centrifuge fluid. If supernatant is clear, the initial cloudiness was caused by cells or debris. If supernatant is cloudy, the initial cloudiness was caused by high lipid levels and the patient has chylothorax or pseudochylothorax.
- Putrid odor indicates bacterial infection (probably anaerobic) of the pleural space.
- Urine-like odor strongly suggests urinothorax.

Glucose

Measurements of the pleural fluid glucose level are indicated, because a ↓ level [<60 mg/dL (3.4 mmol/L)] narrows the diagnostic possibilities to the following seven conditions—(i) parapneumonic effusion, (ii) malignant effusion, (iii) tuberculous effusion, (iv) rheumatoid effusion, (v) hemothorax, (vi) Churg-Strauss syndrome, and (vii) paragonimiasis.

Amylase

Measurement of the pleural fluid amylase level is indicated because an ↑ level (above the upper normal limit of serum) indicates that the patient has one of the following three diseases—(i) esophageal perforation (important to establish diagnosis early because mortality is high, if not properly treated), (ii) pancreatic disease (patients with chronic pancreatic pleural effusions often appear to have cancer), or (iii) pleural malignancy (salivary-type amylase in this situation).

Lactate Dehydrogenase

The pleural fluid LDH level is not used in the differential diagnosis of exudative pleural effusion. Nevertheless, a pleural fluid LDH level should be measured every time a diagnostic thoracentesis is performed because it is a good indicator of the degree of inflammation in the pleural space. Increasing levels with serial thoracenteses indicate that the degree of inflammation is worsening and that the diagnosis should be pursued more aggressively.

White Blood Cell Count and Differential

The absolute pleural fluid white blood cell count has limited utility:
- Counts more than 10,000/mm^3 are most common with parapneumonic effusions, but are also seen with pancreatitis, pulmonary embolism, collagen vascular disease, malignant disorders, and tuberculosis.
- The differential cell count on the pleural fluid is of more utility than is the absolute cell count.
- Presence of predominantly polymorphonuclear leukocytes indicates an acute disease process, such as pneumonia, pulmonary embolization, pancreatitis, intra-abdominal abscess, or early tuberculosis.
- Presence of predominantly mononuclear cells indicates a chronic disease process, such as malignant disease, tuberculosis, or a resolving acute process.
- Presence of predominantly small lymphocytes indicates that the patient probably has tuberculosis or a malignant disease.
- Presence of more than 10% eosinophils usually indicates that the patient has had either blood or air in the pleural space. If neither air nor blood is present in the pleural space, several unusual diagnoses should be considered—benign asbestos pleural effusions, pleural effusions caused by drug reactions, paragonimiasis, or the Churg-Strauss syndrome. Diagnosis is never determined for approximately 20% of exudative pleural effusions, and, interestingly, pleural fluid eosinophilia is found in approximately 40% of these effusions.
- The presence of more than 5% mesothelial cells in the pleural fluid basically rules out a diagnosis of pleural tuberculosis.

Cytology

Pleural fluid cytology is useful in establishing the diagnosis of malignant pleural effusion:
- Cytologic results are positive in 40-90% of malignant pleural effusions and depend on the type of tumor (difficult with lymphomas), the amount of fluid submitted (more fluid and higher yield), and the skill of the cytologist
- Immunohistochemical tests using monoclonal antibodies are complementary to cytology.
- Flow cytometry can demonstrate abnormal numbers of chromosomes in approximately two-thirds of patients with malignant pleural effusions. The number of chromosomes is normal in benign cells.
- Diagnosis of malignancy can be facilitated via electron microscopy.

Culture and Bacteriologic Stains

The following pleural fluid cultures should be obtained on patients with undiagnosed exudative pleural effusions—aerobic and anaerobic bacterial cultures plus a Gram's stain; mycobacterial cultures; and fungal cultures and fungi.

pH

The pleural fluid pH is most useful in determining whether chest tubes should be inserted in patients with parapneumonic effusions.
- If the pleural fluid pH is less than 7.00, tube thoracostomy should be instituted.
- If the pleural fluid pH is more than 7.20, the patient probably does not require tube thoracostomy.

The ↓ of pleural fluid pH to less than 7.20 can occur with nine other conditions:
- Systemic acidosis (pleural fluid pH approximates blood pH normally)
- Esophageal rupture (caused by concurrent infection)
- Rheumatoid pleuritis
- Tuberculous pleuritis
- Malignant pleural disease (if tumor burden is large)
- Hemothorax
- Paragonimiasis
- The Churg-Strauss syndrome (the patient also has asthma)
- Urinothorax (protein and LDH levels may be low).

When the pleural fluid pH is used as a diagnostic test, the pleural fluid must be measured with the same care as arterial pH:
- The fluid should be collected anaerobically in a heparinized syringe.
- The fluid should be placed in ice between collection and analysis.
- The analysis should be performed with a blood gas machine.

Immunologic Studies

Patients with systemic lupus erythematosus (SLE) or rheumatoid arthritis may have a pleural effusion during the course of their disease:
- The best screening test for lupus pleuritis is the pleural fluid ANA titer. With lupus pleuritis, the pleural fluid ANA titer is more than or equal to 1:160 or more than or equal to the serum titer. The test is both sensitive and specific.
- Only patients with rheumatoid pleuritis have a pleural fluid rheumatoid factor titer more than or equal to 1:320 or more than or equal to the serum titer.

Other Diagnostic Tests

Several other tests are useful at times in the differential diagnosis of pleural effusions:

- *Pleural fluid ADA levels*: Levels more than 70 U/L are virtually diagnostic of tuberculous pleuritis, whereas levels less than 40 U/L virtually rule out this diagnosis.
- *Pleural fluid lipid analysis*: A pleural fluid triglyceride level more than 110 mg/dL is diagnostic of chylothorax. With pseudochylothorax, the pleural fluid cholesterol level is elevated.
- Perform lipoprotein analysis of the pleural fluid in confusing cases. The demonstration of chylomicrons in the pleural fluid establishes the diagnosis of chylothorax.
- Measurements that have not been unequivocally demonstrated to be of value in the differential diagnosis of pleural effusions are carcinoembryonic antigen, hyaluronic acid, lysozyme, alkaline, and acid phosphatase.

Invasive Tests for Undiagnosed Exudative Effusions

In most patients, the cause of the pleural effusion is apparent after the initial clinical assessment and a diagnostic thoracentesis. If the diagnosis is not apparent, the following invasive tests might be considered—needle biopsy of the pleura, pleuroscopy, bronchoscopy, and open biopsy of the pleura. Because pulmonary embolism is one of the leading causes of pleural effusion, this diagnosis should be considered in all patients with an undiagnosed pleural effusion. A diagnosis is never established for approximately 20% of the exudative pleural effusions that resolve spontaneously leaving no residua. Three factors should influence the vigor with which one pursues the diagnosis in patients with undiagnosed exudative effusions:
- *The symptoms and clinical course of the patient*: If the symptoms are minimal or improving, a less aggressive approach is indicated.
- *The trend of the pleural fluid LDH level*: If the pleural fluid LDH tends to ↑ with serial thoracenteses, a more aggressive approach is indicated because the process is getting worse.
- *The attitude of the patient*: If the patient is desperate to know why a pleural effusion has developed, an aggressive approach should be taken.

Needle Biopsy

With special needles, small specimens of the parietal pleura can be obtained relatively noninvasively:
- Useful mainly to establish the diagnosis of malignant or tuberculous pleural effusion.
- The initial biopsy is positive for granulomas in 50-80% of patients with pleural tuberculosis. The demonstration of granulomas on the pleural biopsy is virtually diagnostic of tuberculous pleuritis. Culture of a portion of the pleural biopsy specimen for mycobacteria ↑ the diagnostic yield.

- The initial biopsy is positive in about 40% of patients with malignant pleural disease.
- Overall, the yield from pleural fluid cytology is higher than that obtained by needle biopsy.
- When malignant disease is strongly suspected, pleural biopsy should be performed only if initial cytology is nondiagnostic.

Pleuroscopy

With this procedure, also called thoracoscopy, a rigid scope or a fiberoptic scope is introduced through the chest wall into the pleural space after a pneumothorax has been induced on the side of the pleural effusion.
- Excellent results are obtained when the procedure is done by experienced personnel.
- In this country, only a few physicians are well trained in pleuroscopy.
- This procedure is nearly as invasive as open pleural biopsy.
- Diagnoses of benign disease are rarely made.
- The open biopsy procedure is generally preferable unless personnel experienced in pleuroscopy are available.

Bronchoscopy

The procedure is recommended for undiagnosed pleural effusions in the following situations:
- Parenchymal infiltrate is apparent on chest X-ray or CT scan.
- Presence of hemoptysis
- Diagnostic yield should exceed 70% in these two situations.

Open Biopsy

Thoracotomy with direct biopsy of the pleura is the most invasive procedure used to diagnose pleural effusion:
- Open biopsy provides the best visualization of the pleura and the best biopsy specimens.
- The procedure does not provide a definitive diagnosis in a substantial percentage of patients.
- Open biopsy should be done in conjunction with pleural abrasion to prevent recurrence.

MALIGNANT PLEURAL EFFUSIONS

The annual incidence of malignant pleural effusions is approximately 200,000 in the United States. The three tumors that cause approximately 75% of all malignant pleural effusions are (i) lung carcinoma (30%), (ii) breast carcinoma (25%), and (iii) tumors of the lymphoma group (20%). The

initial step in the development of pleural metastases is the embolization of the tumor to the lung and/or visceral pleura—parietal pleura is involved via secondary seeding from the visceral pleura or the pleural fluid. Direct mechanisms include the following:
- Pleural metastases can ↑ the permeability of the pleural surfaces so more fluid is formed.
- Lymphatic involvement can lead to ↓ pleural fluid clearance.
- The thoracic duct can be interrupted, thereby leading to a chylothorax.
- Bronchial obstruction can lead to markedly ↓ pleural pressure and a pleural effusion.
- Pericardial involvement with a malignant tumor is frequently associated with the accumulation of pleural fluid.

Indirect mechanisms:
- Hypoproteinemia can ↓ the serum oncotic pressure and lead to pleural effusion.
- Patients with a malignant disorder have a higher incidence of pulmonary embolism, which may cause a pleural effusion.
- The postobstructive pneumonia secondary to bronchogenic carcinoma may cause a parapneumonic effusion.
- The therapy for the tumor (radiation or chemotherapy) may itself cause the effusion.

The most common symptom reported by patients with malignant pleural effusions is dyspnea, which occurs in about 50% of patients.
- Only about 25% of patients with malignant pleural effusions have chest pain. The pain is usually dull and aching rather than pleuritic in nature.
- Symptoms attributable to the tumor itself are frequent, e.g. weight loss in 32%, malaise in 21%, and anorexia in 14%.
- The pleural fluid is an exudate.
- The ratio of pleural fluid to serum protein level is less than 0.5 in about 20% of patients with pleural malignancy, but the LDH ratio is more than 0.60, or the absolute pleural fluid LDH meets exudative criteria in this 20%
- The fluid may be serous or bloody.
- The predominant cells can be lymphocytes, other mononuclear cells, or polymorphonuclear leukocytes.
- Pleural fluid eosinophilia is uncommon.
- The pleural fluid glucose level is reduced to less than 60 mg/dL in 15-20% of malignant pleural effusions, thereby indicating that the patient has a high tumor burden. Mean survival is less than 2 months (the pleural fluid pH is also reduced in most patients with a low glucose malignant pleural effusion).

The diagnosis of a malignant pleural effusion is established by demonstrating malignant cells in the pleural fluid or in the pleura itself:
- Diagnosis is most commonly established with pleural fluid cytology, which is positive in approximately 60% of patients.

- Needle biopsy of pleura is positive in 40% of patients.
- Immunohistochemical tests using monoclonal antibodies directed against various antigens are useful in differentiating malignant from benign pleural effusions and adenocarcinomas from mesotheliomas.
- Chromosomal abnormalities demonstrated by flow cytometry are highly suggestive of malignant disease.
- Pleuroscopy effectively establishes the diagnosis, as does open biopsy.

Treatment

The initial step is to identify the location of the primary tumor:
- The clinician must determine whether the tumor is of a type that is responsive to chemotherapy. Small-cell lung carcinoma, lymphomas, leukemias, and rarely germ-cell tumors may have an associated pleural effusion and respond to chemotherapy.
- Obliteration of the pleural space via a pleurodesis, or removal of fluid via a pleuroperitoneal shunt, should be considered if the patient is symptomatic (dyspnea at rest or during exercise) from the presence of the pleural fluid and the dyspnea is relieved with a therapeutic thoracentesis.
- Pleurodesis should not be attempted, if the mediastinum is shifted toward the side of the effusion.
- Tetracycline, the most commonly used sclerosing agent for the past decade, is no longer available. The following five agents are reasonable alternatives—minocycline 300 mg intrapleurally; doxycycline 500 mg intrapleurally; bleomycin 60 IU intrapleurally (cost exceeds $700); mitoxantrone hydrochloride (Novantrone) 30 mg intrapleurally (cost exceeds $600); and talc (an excellent sclerosing agent but must be used in conjunction with pleuroscopy or open biopsy).
- The goal of a chemical pleurodesis is obliteration of the pleural space so that room is not available for the pleural fluid to reaccumulate.
- Intense inflammatory response results in fusion of the visceral and parietal pleurae and obliteration of the intervening space.
- A chest tube should be inserted
- Systemic sedation and local anesthesia (4 mg/kg lidocaine) should be given because the procedure at times is painful.
- The sclerosing agent should be injected only if the underlying lung has expanded.
- After injection, the patient is repositioned frequently and the chest tube is clamped for 1-2 hours.
- Suction is maintained for more than 48 hours and until the pleural drainage is less than 150 mL/day.

Pleurodesis effectively controls the pleural effusions in 80-90% of properly selected patients. Most failures occur because of poor patient selection; either the mediastinum is shifted toward the side of the pleural effusion or the lung does not expand after the chest tube is inserted.

PARAPNEUMONIC EFFUSIONS AND BACTERIAL INFECTIONS OF THE PLEURAL SPACE

A parapneumonic effusion is any pleural effusion associated with bacterial pneumonia, lung abscess, or bronchiectasis. Parapneumonic effusions are probably the most common exudative pleural effusions in the United States. Approximately, 40% of the 1.2 million individuals who develop a bacterial pneumonia in the United States each year have a pleural effusion. The subcategories of parapneumonic effusions are:
- Complicated parapneumonic effusions, which require tube thoracostomy for their resolution.
- An empyema, which is an exudative effusion on which the Gram's stain of the pleural fluid is positive.

The evolution of a parapneumonic effusion can be divided into three stages that represent a continuous spectrum:
- The exudative stage is the first stage and is characterized by the collection of sterile fluid in the pleural space. The pleural fluid in this stage is an exudate with primarily polymorphonuclear leukocytes, a normal glucose level, and a normal pH level. Appropriate antibiotic therapy effects resolution of both the pneumonic process and the pleural disease.
- The fibropurulent stage is the next stage and is characterized by infection with the offending bacteria of the previously sterile pleural fluid. The pH and glucose levels of the pleural fluid become progressively lower while the LDH level of the pleural fluid becomes progressively higher. As this stage progresses, the pleural space becomes loculated as the result of the formation of fibrin membranes.
- The organization stage is the final stage and is characterized by fibroblasts growing into the exudate from both the visceral and the parietal pleural surfaces to produce an inelastic membrane called the pleural peel. This peel encases the lung and renders it nearly functionless.

Prior to the antibiotic era, *Streptococcus pneumoniae* or hemolytic streptococci were responsible for most empyemas. At present, anaerobic organisms, aerobic organisms, and mixed infections with aerobes and anaerobes each account for about one-third of culture-positive parapneumonic effusions.

The clinical picture depends on whether organisms are aerobic or anaerobic:
- If aerobic, an acute febrile illness with chest pain, sputum production, and leukocytosis ensues.
- If anaerobic, a subacute illness with weight loss, anemia, and leukocytosis ensues. Most patients also have a history of an episode of unconsciousness or some other factor that predisposes them to aspiration and anaerobic pneumonia.

The possibility of a parapneumonic effusion should be considered whenever a patient with a bacterial pneumonia is initially evaluated:
- Obtain bilateral decubitus chest X-rays if either of the posterior costophrenic angles is blunted on the lateral chest X-ray or if either diaphragm is not visible throughout its length.
- Semiquantitate the amount of pleural fluid by measuring the distance between the inside of the chest wall and the outside of the lung. If the thickness of the fluid is less than 10 mm, the effusion is not clinically significant and a thoracentesis is not indicated. If the thickness of the fluid is more than 10 mm, a diagnostic thoracentesis should be performed immediately.

Treatment

One can identify a complicated parapneumonic effusion only by examining the pleural fluid. A diagnostic thoracentesis should be performed as soon as the presence of a significant amount of pleural fluid is demonstrated.
- Aliquots of the pleural fluid should be sent for measurement of the pleural fluid glucose, LDH, amylase and protein levels, pH, a differential and total white blood cell count, Gram's stain, and aerobic and anaerobic bacterial cultures.
- Usually, the fluid also is submitted for mycobacterial and fungal smears and cultures, as well as for cytologic studies.

At the time of the initial evaluation, the pleural effusion of some patients with parapneumonic effusions is already loculated.
- Ultrasonic examinations of the pleural space are quite effective in distinguishing loculated fluid from pneumonic infiltrates.
- Perform thoracentesis with ultrasonic guidance.
- Loculated fluid by itself is not an indication for tube thoracostomy.

The decision whether to initiate tube drainage of the pleural space must be made and an appropriate antibiotic must be selected.
- Individuals who require tube thoracostomy must be identified immediately. A delay of even 24 hours ↑ morbidity and mortality.
- Indications for chest tube insertion are the presence of gross pus in the pleural space, organisms on the pleural fluid Gram's stain, pleural fluid glucose less than 60 mg/dL, and pleural fluid pH less than 7.00.

Even when none of these criteria is met, tube thoracostomy should still be considered if the pleural fluid pH is less than 7.20 or if the pleural fluid LDH is >1,000 IU/L.
- In borderline cases, serial thoracenteses at 12–24-hour intervals are quite useful in deciding whether to place chest tubes. If the pleural fluid LDH tends to ↓ and the pleural fluid pH and glucose levels tend to ↑ with serial thoracenteses, the patient is improving and tube thoracostomy is not indicated. Alternatively, if the LDH is ↑ and the pH and glucose levels are ↓, tube thoracostomy should be performed without delay.

A relatively large chest tube should be utilized (small tubes are likely to become obstructed with fibrin and debris):
- Position tube in the most dependent part of the effusion.
- Leave tube in place until the volume of the pleural drainage is less than 50 mL/24 hours and until the draining fluid becomes clear yellow.
- If no clinical and radiologic improvement occurs within 24 hours, either the pleural drainage is unsatisfactory or the patient is receiving the wrong antibiotic—review culture results.
- If drainage is inadequate, check position of chest tube and consider facilitating drainage with intrapleural streptokinase (SK) or urokinase.

Certain factors can help to predict whether closed tube drainage will be sufficient therapy for a complicated parapneumonic effusion. In general, when a patient has a purulent empyema that is loculated, chest tubes alone usually are not sufficient therapy. The following scheme is a useful classification of complicated parapneumonic effusions:
- *Class I, low pH pleural effusion*: Pleural fluid pH is less than 7.20, but pleural fluid cultures are negative. Tube thoracostomy by itself is usually successful.
- *Class II, classic empyema*: Pleural fluid cultures are positive, but no loculations. Patient may need thrombolytic therapy in addition to chest tubes.
- *Class III, complicated empyema*: Multiple loculations on chest X-ray, initially or subsequently, or trapped lung. Almost all patients require thrombolytic therapy and many require decortication or open drainage procedure.

Tuberculous Pleural Effusions

In many parts of the world, the most common cause of an exudative pleural effusion is tuberculosis. Such pleural effusions, however, are relatively rare in the United States, with an annual incidence of 1,000 cases.

Tuberculous pleural effusions are thought to result when a subpleural caseous focus in the lung ruptures into the pleural space.
- Delayed hypersensitivity is responsible for pleural effusion.
- Tuberculous pleuritis can appear as an acute or a chronic illness. The acute presentation is characterized by cough and chest pain; the chronic presentation is characterized by low-grade fever, weakness, and weight loss.
- The effusion is almost always unilateral and is usually small-to-moderate in size, although at times it may be massive. One-third of patients have concurrent parenchymal infiltrates.
- When untreated, the effusion resolves, but most patients subsequently develop tuberculosis.
- Pleural fluid is an exudate with predominantly small lymphocytes.
- The diagnosis is established by needle biopsy of the pleura demonstrating granuloma or positive mycobacterial cultures of the pleural fluid or pleural biopsy specimen. Elevated levels of ADA or gamma-interferon in the pleural fluid are suggestive of the diagnosis.

- Appropriate therapy is the administration of two antituberculous drugs for 9 months. All patients with an undiagnosed exudative pleural effusion and a positive purified protein derivative (PPD) should be treated.

Pleural Effusions in Patients with AIDS

- Pleural effusions are uncommon in patients with acquired immunodeficiency syndrome (AIDS).
- The most common cause is Kaposi's sarcoma. Diagnosis is difficult, and open biopsy usually is required.
- Parapneumonic effusions are the second most common cause, followed by tuberculosis, cryptococcosis, and lymphoma.
- Effusions are unusual with *Pneumocystis carinii* infection.
- Patients with AIDS and pleural effusion should undergo diagnostic thoracentesis. If no diagnosis, a needle biopsy of pleura is performed if fluid is exudative. If still no diagnosis, one should consider treatment for tuberculosis. If the patient is symptomatic, a pleuroperitoneal shunt should be implanted or chemical pleurodesis should be attempted.

Pleural Effusions Caused by Pulmonary Embolization

Although pulmonary embolism is one of the most common causes of pleural effusion (Table 17.1), it is frequently not considered in the differential diagnosis of pleural effusion.

- Effusion may be either a transudate or an exudate with any cell type. Pleural fluid may or may not be bloody.
- Patients have usual symptoms of pulmonary embolization.
- Parenchymal infiltrate is also apparent in 50% of patients.
- The initial diagnostic study is usually a perfusion lung scan. If the perfusion scan is abnormal, a ventilation lung scan should be obtained. If doubt still exists after these tests, a pulmonary arteriogram should be performed.
- The treatment is the same as that for any patient with a pulmonary embolus. If effusion enlarges during treatment, thoracentesis should be repeated to rule out infection or hemothorax.

Pleural Effusions Caused by Diseases of the Gastrointestinal Tract

Several different gastrointestinal (GI) diseases may have an associated pleural effusion.

Pancreatitis

Approximately 20% of patients with acute pancreatitis have an exudative pleural effusion:

- The effusion probably results from diaphragmatic inflammation.
- Occasionally, chest symptoms dominate the clinical picture.
- The pleural fluid is an exudate with predominantly polymorphonuclear leukocytes and an elevated amylase.
- The effusion does not alter the treatment plan for a patient with acute pancreatitis.

Chronic Pancreatic Pleural Effusion

The possibility of a chronic pancreatic pleural effusion should be considered in all patients who seem to have a malignant pleural effusion but in whom the pleural fluid cytologic results are negative.
- Results from a sinus tract leading from the pancreas through the aortic or esophageal hiatus into the mediastinum.
- Clinical picture is dominated by chest symptoms such as dyspnea, cough, and chest pain.
- Effusion is usually very large and recurs rapidly after a therapeutic thoracentesis.
- Markedly elevated pleural fluid amylase level is key to the diagnosis.
- Usually therapy requires abdominal exploration with ligation or excision of the sinus tract and drainage or partial resection of the pancreas.

Esophageal Perforation

This diagnosis should be considered in all acutely ill patients with exudative pleural effusions, because if this condition is not treated rapidly and appropriately, the mortality approaches 100%.
- Usually follows instrumentation of esophagus, but may occur spontaneously.
- Severe symptoms result from intense infection of the mediastinum.
- Pleural fluid amylase level is a good screening test. The amylase level is markedly elevated because saliva, with its high amylase content, enters the mediastinum through a hole in the esophagus. The diagnosis is confirmed with contrast studies of the esophagus.
- The treatment of choice for esophageal perforation is exploration of the mediastinum with, primary repair of the esophageal tear and drainage of the pleural space and mediastinum.

Intra-abdominal Abscess

Approximately 80% of subphrenic abscesses, 40% of pancreatic abscesses, 30% of splenic abscesses, and 20% of intrahepatic abscesses have an accompanying pleural effusion.
- Effusion results from diaphragmatic irritation.
- The possibility of an abscess should be considered strongly in any patient with an undiagnosed exudative pleural effusion containing predominantly polymorphonuclear leukocytes when pulmonary parenchymal infiltrates are absent.

- The diagnosis of intra-abdominal abscess is best established with abdominal CT scanning.
- Treatment consists of drainage of the abscess.

Pleural Disease Caused by Collagen Vascular Diseases

Rheumatoid Pleuritis

Approximately 5% of patients with rheumatoid arthritis develop a pleural effusion in the course of their disease.
- The pleural effusion usually develops only after the arthritis has been present for several years.
- Most patients are male, more than 35 years, and have SQ nodules.
- The pleural fluid is characterized by a glucose level less than 30 mg/dL, an LDH level more than 700 IU/L, a pH less than 7.20, and a rheumatoid factor titer more than 1: 320.
- No treatment has proved effective for rheumatoid pleuritis.

Lupus Pleuritis

The incidence of pleural effusion with either systemic or drug-induced lupus erythematosus is about 40%:
- Arthritis or arthralgias is usually present before effusion develops.
- Almost all patients with lupus pleuritis have pleuritic chest pain, and most are also febrile.
- Many different drugs have been incriminated for producing drug-induced lupus erythematosus. Hydralazine, procainamide, isoniazid, phenytoin, and chlorpromazine are most commonly indicted. The presenting signs, symptoms, and radiographic abnormalities are similar to those of spontaneous lupus.
- The pleural fluid is an exudate that may have predominantly polymorphonuclear leukocytes or lymphocytes. The pleural fluid glucose level is usually more than 60 mg/dL, the LDH level is less than 500 IU/L, and the pH is more than 7.20.
- Measurement of the level of ANA in the pleural fluid is the best test for lupus pleuritis. With lupus, the ANA titer is more than or equal to 1:160 or the pleural fluid to serum ANA ratio is more than or equal to 1.
- Oral corticosteroids are effective therapy for lupus pleuritis.

Pleural Effusions Caused by Drug Reactions

Administration of the following drugs has been associated with the development of a pleural effusion:
- Nitrofurantoin, the urinary antiseptic
- Dantrolene, the muscle relaxant

- Methysergide, the antimigraine drug
- Bromocriptine, the anti-Parkinson's drug
- Procarbazine, the antineoplastic drug
- Amiodarone, the antiarrhythmic drug.

Individuals with drug-induced pleural effusions may appear with acute, subacute, or chronic illnesses—concomitant pulmonary infiltrates are sometimes present. Characteristics of fluid are poorly described, but it is frequently eosinophilic.

BIBLIOGRAPHY

1. Feller-Kopman D, Light R. Pleural Disease. N Engl J Med. 2018;378(8):740-51.
2. Khan GM. Medical Diagnosis and Therapy. Philadelphia: Lea and Febiger; 1994.
3. Light RW. Pleural Diseases. In: Khan MG, Bartlett JG, Chopra S, Topol EJ (Eds). Medical Diagnosis and Therapy. Philadelphia: Lea and Febiger; 1994.
4. Light RW. Pleural Diseases, Pleural Effusions. In Khan M Gabriel (ED). Cardiac and Pulmonary Management. Philadelphia: Lea and Febiger; 1993.

CHAPTER 18

Gastrointestinal Diseases

IRRITABLE BOWEL SYNDROME

- The irritable bowel syndrome (IBS) is a chronic, distressing, and common functional bowel disorder.
- It can be disabling disturbing work and sleep.
  Diagnosis is not perfect—Ford et al. provide a review of this common perplexing disorder.
- Recurrent abdominal pain related to defecation or with a change in frequency of stool or form. Some patients also experience bloating.
- These symptoms must occur at least once per week, on average, in the previous 3 months, over a period of 6 months to qualify as IBS.
- No abnormal structural intestinal abnormalities are present.
- Irritable bowel syndrome occurs with diarrhea, or constipation; in some constipation and diarrhea occur.
- Loose or watery stools and in some hard or lumpy stools or a combination occur.
- About 25% with the diarrheal subtype of IBS has evidence of bile acid diarrhea and a therapeutic trial of a bile acid sequestrant may be an alternative diagnostic approach.
- In patients with these subtypes of IBS, measurement of the fecal calprotectin level can distinguish between IBS and inflammatory bowel disease (IBD) (high sensitivity and specificity).
  Dietary measures are helpful:
   - Fermentable oligosaccharides, disaccharides, and monosaccharides and polyols (FODMAPs), are present in stone fruits, (apples, pears, peaches, nectarines, and others] legumes, lactose-containing foods, and artificial sweeteners, exacerbate symptoms in some patients because they cause fermentation that results in osmotic effects and osmotic explosive expulsion of massive amounts of loose often floating stools.
   - The recognition of fermentation and osmotic effects that certainly occur in some with IBS has fostered the use of a low-FODMAP diet that has been shown to be helpful in this subset of IBS.

- One randomized trial showed a good effect; two other trials comparing a diet—eating smaller meals, avoidance of insoluble fiber, fatty foods, and caffeine showed little difference, but significantly greater improvements in abdominal pain, bloating, stool frequency, and consistency, were noted in one trial.

FODMAPs—fermentable, oligosaccharides, disaccharides, and polyols (sorbitol and mannitol) include fructose (when in excess of glucose), fructans, galacto-oligosaccharides (GOS), lactose, and polyols (e.g. sorbitol and mannitol).

Low FODMAP foods include:

Caution: A small to medium amount of the food listed under low content contain low concentration but a large helping example more than 25% of an avocado results in high amounts and most so termed low FODMAP are rated high

Alfalfa, avocado—1/8 whole avocado, 20 g, bamboo shoots, and bean sprouts. Beetroot, canned and pickled, pak choi, and broccoli—1 cup, brussels sprouts—1 serving of 2 sprouts, butternut squash—1/4 cup, cabbage, common and red up to 1 cup, callaloo, carrots celery—less than 5 cm of stalk, chicory leaves chick peas, canned—1/4 cup, (half cup is high) chilli, red or green, chives, corn or sweet corn—1/2 cob, cucumber, green beans, green pepper or green bell pepper, ginger, lettuce, okra, olives, parsnip, pickled onions, large—2 onions, potato, pumpkin radish, red peppers or red bell pepper

High FOODMAP foods include—very ripe banana, blackberries, blackcurrants, cherries, currants, black eyed peas, broad beans, butter beans, cassava, and cauliflower.

Medications

It is difficult for patients to try medications daily that are partially effective to ameliorate a problem that occurs three to four times or month. Some patients may have one episode per month, 1/week then relief for 4-6 weeks.

In general several medications have shown small benefit and not sufficiently effective in small trials and shown in meta-analysis.

The following were somewhat useful in some subsets of IBS:
- *Peppermint oil* has antispasmodic properties due to smooth-muscle relaxation through blockade of calcium channels. It was shown in a meta-analysis, to be more effective than placebo. Sustained release peppermint oil is available.
- *Alosetron*—acts on 5-hydroxytryptamine (HT) type 3 receptors to slow colonic transit. In a meta-analysis, the drug was more effective than placebo in patients who had IBS with diarrhea, for both reductions of global symptoms. In reasonably large randomized trials, reduction of

abdominal pain or discomfort was noted. But adverse events included constipation and, rarely ischemic colitis.
- *Ondansetron*, used as an antiemetic agent for 30 years, has a well-established safety profile. In a crossover randomized trial involving 98 patients, treatment with ondansetron did not reduce abdominal pain but cause significant improvements in stool consistency, with a response rate of 80 as compared with 41% on placebo.
- *Probiotics*: These are attenuated bacteria or bacterial products bifidobacterium (*Lactobacillus plantarum:* strain DSM 9843) species may be of modest benefit and is probably worth a trial for some patients; proof of significant efficacy is lacking.

PEPTIC ULCER DISEASE

Peptic ulcer refers to either gastric or duodenal, duodenal being more common than gastric.

An ulcer is a breach in the mucosa that extends through the muscularis mucosa into the submucosa or deeper.

"Peptic" signifies that proteolysis by pepsin is important in the development of this lesion (in contrast, an erosion is defined as a superficial hole that extends into the mucosa but does not penetrate the muscularis mucosa).

Erosions are frequently encountered in patients taking aspirin or nonsteroidal anti-inflammatory drugs (NSAIDs), or in the setting of stress gastritis.

Etiology

- Heredity
- Gastric acid hypersecretion
- The use of aspirin or NSAIDs
- Smoking
- *Helicobacter pylori*
- Approximately 40% of patients with duodenal ulcers have more than or equal to one family member with the disease.
- The secretion of acid alone does not appear to be a sufficient cause of peptic ulcer disease.
- Most patients with gastric ulcer have normal or ↓ acid secretion.
- Gastric ulcers almost always occur in the nonacid-secreting mucosa.
- Nonsteroidal anti-inflammatory drugs—these drugs produce both gastritis and peptic ulceration. The major damage is felt to be secondary to inhibition of endogenous prostaglandin production.
- The risk of gastric ulcer and duodenal ulcer is ↑ tenfold in individuals taking 1 g of aspirin on a daily basis.

- Gastric ulcer is also more likely in patients who take NSAIDs, occurring in 2-4% per patient-year. More importantly, NSAIDs are associated with ulcer complications, notably perforation and bleeding.
- Smoking—individuals who smoke are more likely than nonsmokers to develop ulcers. In addition, ulcers appear to heal more slowly in smokers and to recur sooner.
- Cigarette smoking ↑ the likelihood that surgical treatment will be required for peptic ulcer disease, and aggravates the operative risk.
- Physiologic effects related to smoking include an ↑ in the rate of gastric emptying, a ↓ in pancreatic bicarbonate secretion, and a ↓ in gastric mucosal blood flow and prostaglandin synthesis
- *Helicobacter pylori* is a gram-negative, microaerophilic, and S-shaped rod that has been proven to cause active antral gastritis in humans. This organism evokes both a local response [immunoglobulin A and M (IgA and IgM) antibodies to *H. pylori* is present in the gastric juice] and a systemic one (IgG and IgA antibodies to *H. pylori* is present in the serum). *H. pylori* is found in the antrum of more than 95% of patients with duodenal ulcer disease and about 75% of those with gastric ulcer disease.
- This organism is also found in 50% of patients with nonulcer dyspepsia and in approximately 20% of normal volunteers. It is estimated that less than 5% of individuals harboring *H. pylori* develop peptic ulceration.
- *H. pylori* is associated with hypergastrinemia that reverses when the *H. pylori* is eradicated. Several studies have demonstrated that eradication of *H. pylori* leads to a significant ↓ in the recurrence of symptomatic ulcer disease (Chopra and Waxman).
- Peptic ulcer disease occurs in one of three kinds of settings:
  - Acid hypersecretion (patients with gastrinoma, g-cell hyperplasia, and some patients with duodenal ulcer disease)
  - The use NSAIDs
  - In association with *H. pylori*.

Diagnosis

- Ulcer pain is epigastric; gnawing; relieved by foods, antacids, or H_2 blockers; and recurs 2-3 hours after eating. Although it may interrupt sleep, the pain is virtually never present when the patient first awakens, unless the patient has gastric outlet obstruction (Chopra and Waxman).
- Importantly, ulcer pain may bear no relationship to meals.
- It may occur within an hour of eating and may actually worsen after eating.
- Approximately 90% of ulcer patients report nocturnal pain relieved by antacids or H_2 blockers.
- More than 30% of patients with chronic abdominal pain not due to an ulcer also report this feature. It is usually not possible to distinguish

between duodenal ulcer and gastric ulcer based on symptoms, and it should be noted that the disappearance of symptoms does not always signal that the ulcer crater has disappeared.
- Duodenal ulcer disease is rare before the age of 15. Symptoms most commonly occur between the ages of 25 and 60. Gastric ulcer usually appears between 40 and 65.
- Sites of chronic peptic ulcer disease include the duodenal bulb and stomach. Sometimes ulcers occur in the postbulbar duodenum. In such patients, one should exclude acid hypersecretory states, such as Zollinger–Ellison syndrome (gastrinoma) and antral G-cell hyperplasia. Peptic ulcers may also occur in the ileum in patients with Meckel's diverticulum and in the jejunum in patients after a gastrojejunostomy. Peptic ulcers occurring in the esophagus are most unusual, with the exception of ulcerations that occur in acquired columnar epithelium, a condition referred to as Barrett's esophagus.

Complications

The major complications of peptic ulcer disease are—hemorrhage (20%), perforation (5-10%), and gastric outlet obstruction (5%). Complications are more frequent in patients with gastric ulcers.

Diagnostic Investigations

Peptic ulcer disease includes upper gastrointestinal (UGI):
- Upper GI series is accurate in detecting ulcers in approximately 85% of cases.
- Endoscopy, assessment of acid secretion
- Measurement of serum gastrin.
- Benign and malignant gastric ulcers can be ascertained in 90% of patients, based on radiographic criteria.
- However, endoscopy of gastric ulcer is necessary advisable in most cases of gastric ulcer disease in order to obtain adequate specimens for biopsy and brush cytology.

Endoscopy should be performed in patients with persistent dyspepsia despite a normal UGI series. In patients who have undergone gastric surgery, the UGI series is notoriously unable to distinguish surgical deformity from active peptic ulcer disease. Endoscopy is also indicated in patients with UGI bleeding.

Therapy

- Accomplish pain relief pain
- Accelerate healing of the ulcer crater
- Prevent complications and recurrences

- Special diets offer no advantage
- Eat three meals a day
- Acid secretion is the same whether coffee is decaffeinated or regular since the critical factor is an increment in serum gastrin associated with the peptide present in the roasted grain from which the coffee is made.
- Quit smoking cigarettes and avoid taking aspirin or NSAIDs.

HYDROGEN POTASSIUM ATPASE (PROTON PUMP) INHIBITORS

Proton Pump Inhibitors

- These agents are proven to heal peptic ulcers. Caution is necessary as long-term treatment may rarely cause renal dysfunction and may increase risk of bone fracture in the hip, wrist, or spine, and B12 deficiency. These effects are ill defined but have been noted.
- Caution if severe liver disease, low magnesium levels, lupus, osteoporosis, or taking methotrexate.
- Omeprazole may reduce the effects of clopidogrel, used after coronary stenting.

Lansoprazole

- *Dosage:* Take in the morning approximately 30 minutes before breakfast.
- Do not crush, chew, break, or open a delayed-release capsule. Swallow the capsule whole.

Pantoprazole

Dosage: 40 mg twice daily

Omeprazole

Drug may increase your risk of severe diarrhea. This may be caused by an infection in your intestine caused by the bacteria *Clostridium difficile*.

Several doses of a proton pump inhibitor drug, such as omeprazole, every day for a year or longer may have an increased risk of bone fractures.

Omeprazole can cause cutaneous lupus erythematosus (CLE) and systemic lupus erythematosus (SLE).

Dosage: Active duodenal ulcer—20 mg taken once per day for up to 4 weeks. Some people may need more than 4 weeks of treatment.
- This drug is not advised.

Surgical Treatment

Surgery is indicated for complications such as persistent or recurrent GI bleeding, obstruction, or perforation. In patients with nonhealing ulcer disease prior to surgery, a concerted effort should be made to exclude surreptitious use of aspirin or NSAIDs. In addition, gastrinoma should be excluded (Chopra and Waxman).

Surgical procedures include subtotal gastrectomy, vagotomy with antrectomy, vagotomy with pyloroplasty, vagotomy with gastrojejunostomy, and superselective (parietal cell) vagotomy. Postoperative complications include early satiety, bilious vomiting, diarrhea, malabsorption, dumping, anemia, osteoporosis, and osteomalacia.

Zollinger–Ellison Syndrome

The classic triad consists of severe peptic ulcer disease, gastric acid hypersecretion, and a non-p-cell tumor of the pancreas. The term "gastrinoma" is preferred. Fewer than 0.1% of patients with duodenal ulcer disease will have gastrinoma. Some patients are diagnosed at an early stage with abdominal pain (about 80%) and diarrhea (about 30%). In 20% of patients, the syndrome is associated with the MEN type I syndrome.

Diagnosis is based on evidence of acid hypersecretion and an elevated serum gastrin. Other rare causes of acid hypersecretion and hypergastrinemia include the retained antrum syndrome and antral G-cell hyperplasia. The secretin test is positive in patients with gastrinoma. A positive test is defined as an increment in serum gastrin of more than 200 pg/mL above baseline following IV administration of secretin. Radiologic clues on a UGI series include prominent gastric folds, evidence of acid hypersecretion (a "wet-looking stomach"), postbulbar ulcers, and multiple ulcers.

Candidates for surgical resection can be identified by:
- Excluding those with the MEN type I syndrome
- Performing abdominal computed tomography (CT) or magnetic resonance imaging (MRI) to exclude hepatic metastases
- Performing selective venous sampling or intraoperative ultrasound to localize the tumor.

Removal of the gastrinoma is successful in 10% of patients. Associated hyperparathyroidism should be treated. If no tumor is found at the time of exploratory laparotomy, parietal cell vagotomy may be considered. This procedure can significantly facilitate medical control of the acid hypersecretion. Omeprazole at the starting dose of 60 mg per day usually results in control of acid hypersecretion, healing of ulcers, and resolution of the diarrhea and steatorrhea (Chopra and Waxman).
- *Antacids:* Antacids are superior to placebo and comparable to H_2 receptor antagonists in healing duodenal ulcers. Liquids are more potent than tablets. The dose is 30–60 mL 1 hour and 3 hours after meals, and

as needed. Side effects include constipation (aluminum-containing antacids), diarrhea (magnesium-containing antacids), and acid rebound (Ca-containing antacids). In some cases the Na+ load of the antacids may be clinically significant.
- *Histamine H_2 receptor antagonists*
  - Cimetidine:
    - Inhibits basal acid secretion by 80–95%, and meal-stimulated acid secretion by 60%. The dose is 400 mg bid, or 800 mg at bedtime. Although this drug has been used by millions of patients, toxic effects are rare.
    - One potentially significant side effect is its ability to interact with other drugs by virtue of its inhibition of the cytochrome p-450 mixed oxidase system. Occasionally, mental confusion has been noted, particularly in elderly patients with liver disease or renal insufficiency.
  - Ranitidine:
    - Ranitidine is more potent and has a longer duration of action than cimetidine.
    - The oral dose is 150 mg bid or 300 mg at bedtime.
    - Side effects are probably less common with ranitidine.
    - There is no interaction with hepatic microsomes, no bone marrow suppression, no antiandrogen effect, and less central nervous system (CNS) toxicity.
  - Famotidine: This drug is 32 times more potent than cimetidine and nine times more potent than ranitidine.
    - Randomized controlled trials (RCTs) show that famotidine 20 mg bid or 40 mg at bedtime is as effective as ranitidine for healing duodenal ulcers.
    - 40 mg at bedtime appears to heal benign gastric ulcers.

A bedtime dose of 20 mg is usually effective in preventing duodenal ulcer relapse.
  - Sucralfate: This is a basic aluminum salt of sucrose octasulfate. At a pH of less than or equal to 4.0, it becomes a viscous gel that tenaciously adheres to ulcerated mucosa. Sucralfate neutralizes acid, binds bile salts, and inhibits peptic activity. In addition, it offers cytoprotection by releasing endogenous prostaglandins. It is as effective as H_2 receptor antagonists in the treatment of duodenal ulcer. The dose is 1 g qid or 2 g bid. Side effects include constipation and the potential to bind to other orally administered drugs.
- Do not take concomitant proton pump inhibitors and/or H_2 antagonists.

Diarrhea in Adults

Acree and Davis provide a JAMA review article on Acute Diarrheal Infections in Adults.

The human GI tract handles about 9 liters of fluid on a daily basis. Most of the fluid is absorbed in the small bowel; only 1-1.5 liters enters the colon, where most of it is absorbed, leaving 100-150 mL of fluid to be excreted in the feces. When the water content of the stool is more than 150 mL or the total weight of the stool is more than 250 g, the bowel secretion is usually perceived by the patient as diarrhea.

Mechanisms of diarrhea:

- *Secretory*: Large volume (>1 L q 24 hours; persists during fasting)
- *Osmotic*: volume >1 L/d; diarrhea abates when the patient fasts or no longer ingests the poorly absorbed solute; positive osmotic gap in stool [stool osmolality-stool $(Na^+ + K^+) \times 2 = >50$ mOsm] in patients with carbohydrate malabsorption, the stool is often acidic (pH 5-6; normal pH is 7.0).
- *Dysmotility*: Volume may vary, usually associated with systemic disorder.
- *Exudative*: Less than 1 L q/d; if longstanding, hypoalbuminemia and anemia can be present; tenesmus and urgency are present with rectal bleeding (Chopra and Waxman).

Common Etiologies

- Norovirus is the most common cause of gastroenteritis and is associated with 26% of cases of diarrhea in emergency departments, with 90% of *Norovirus* deaths occurring in people aged 65 years or older.
- Immunocompromise and abnormal gastrointestinal physiology also increase the risk of severe diarrhea.
- Bacterial infections potentially amenable to antibiotics (*Shigella, Salmonella,* and *Campylobacter* species, Shiga toxin–producing *Escherichia coli* strains, *Vibrio parahaemolyticus,* and enterotoxigenic *E. coli*) were identified in only 9% of acute diarrhea in a multicenter, emergency department-based study of adults.
- *Secretory*: Infectious (enterotoxin-mediated like Cholera, *E. coli, Bacillus cereus*); neuroendocrine tumors (gastrin and vasoactive intestinal peptide); miscellaneous (bile salt malabsorption).
- *Osmotic*: Lactase deficiency; magnesium-containing drugs; and sorbitol ingestion (chewing gum diarrhea)
- *Exudative*: Infectious and IBD
- *Dysmotility*: Rapid transit time like hyperthyroidism, carcinoid, pyloroplasty, and IBS; delayed transit time, scleroderma, and amyloidosis
- *Malabsorption*: Lymphatic obstruction, pancreative disorders, and mucosal disease

Usually more than 1 pathophysiologic process is involved (Chopra and Waxman).

Acute Diarrhea

- *Acute diarrhea*: Less than 3 weeks

- *Etiology*: infections—viral; bacterial; and parasitic. Drugs—antacids, antibiotics, alcohol, digitalis, quinidine, propranolol, colchicine, lactulose, and laxatives
- *Evaluation*: Complete history, including recent travel and recent antibiotic therapy
- *Management*: Correction of fluid and electrolyte disturbances; treatment of specific underlying disease if warranted; and antidiarrheal agents.

Specific Etiologic Agents
Bacterial and Viral Infections
Most patients with infectious diarrhea have a mild and self-limited course. It usually does not require stool culture or specific treatment. The presence of high fever (>103°C), systemic illness, tenesmus, bloody diarrhea, or dehydration warrant further diagnostic studies and treatment. Infectious diarrhea is classified into:
- Toxigenic (enterotoxin mediated), i.e. *E. coli, Vibrio cholera, Bacillus cereus, Aeromonas* species
- Invasive (organism penetrates mucosal barrier), i.e. *Shigella, Campylobacter, Salmonella*, and *Yersinia* (Chopra and Waxman)
- Parasitic infections—amebiasis is caused by *Entamoeba histolytica*. Manifestations range from asymptomatic carrier to fulminant colitis. Diagnosis is made by coproparasitoscopic examination of 3-6 fresh stool specimens. Recommended treatment is—asymptomatic intestinal infection: Iodoquinol 650 mg po tid for 20 days; mild-to-moderate intestinal disease: Metronidazole 750 mg po tid for 10 days or paromomycin 25-35 mg/kg/d in three doses for 7+ days. Iodoquinol 650 mg po tid for 20 days.

  Giardiasis is caused by *Giardia lamblia*. Manifestations range from mild diarrhea to malabsorption and steatorrhea. Diagnosis can be made by stool examination, but as many as 50% of stool specimens may not contain the parasite, requiring mucosal biopsy, or duodenal aspiration. Treatment of choice is quinacrine 100 mg po tid for 7 days or metronidazole 250 mg po tid for a week.

Chronic Diarrhea
- Need to differentiate between functional and organic categories according to four features—(i) weight loss, (ii) bloody diarrhea, (iii) nocturnal diarrhea, and (iv) incontinence. The presence of any of these suggests an organic source.
- In addition, the history may suggest the etiology—the presence of tenesmus or urgency would place the process in the distal colon.

- Periumbilical pain and bulky and large-volume stools suggest a small bowel source.
- A history of greasy or oily stools, or of stools that stick to the bowl, requiring repeated flushing, may suggest steatorrhea and point to the small bowel or pancreas as the cause of the problem.
- Surreptitious laxative abuse should be kept in mind in the differential diagnosis of chronic unexplained diarrhea; alkalization of the stool with sodium hydroxide is a simple way to confirm the presence of phenolphthalein-containing laxatives (by turning the sample to a pink or red color).
- *Clinical management*: Request fecal leukocytes; stool cultures and ova and parasites; and stool specimen for anal or rectal swab. An etiologic agent will be identified in 50% of cases. If no etiology is found, consider colonoscopy, upper endoscopy, and small bowel biopsy, which may raise the yield to 80% (Chopra and Waxman).
- *Therapy*: Supportive therapy includes correction of fluid and electrolyte disturbances, antidiarrheal agents, treatment of specific pathogens, and in refractory cases using somatostatin analogs.

Diarrhea in Acquired Immunodeficiency Syndrome

Diarrhea is very common (>50%) in patients with acquired immunodeficiency syndrome (AIDS). Three clinical syndromes can be described:

- *Enteritis (crampy periumbilical abdominal pain, weight loss, large-volume diarrhea, and/or steatorrhea)*: Cryptosporidiosis, *Isospora belli*, microsporidiosis, *Mycobacterium avium-intracellulare* complex, *Mycobacterium tuberculosis*, *Salmonella*, *Shigella*, *Campylobacter*, *Giardia*, cytomegalovirus (CMV), Kaposi's sarcoma (KS), lymphoma, idiopathic [human immunodeficiency virus (HIV) enteropathy]
- *Proctocolitis (small-volume diarrhea and lower quadrant abdominal pain)*: Campylobacter, Shigella, Salmonella, Amebiasis, C. difficile, Chlamydia [lymphogranuloma venereum (LGV)], CMV, and *Blastocystis hominis*
- *Proctitis (tenesmus, hematochezia, and small-volume diarrhea)*: Herpes simplex virus, *Neisseria gonorrhoea*, Chlamydia, CMV, *Treponema pallidum*, lymphoma, and trauma (Chopra and Waxman).

MALABSORPTION SYNDROMES

Malabsorption syndromes are characterized by weight loss and steatorrhea. It may be generalized or highly selective.

Pathophysiologic Mechanisms

- *Impaired intraluminal digestion*: Pancreatic disorders like chronic pancreatitis, pancreatic cancer, and biliary obstruction

- *Altered mucosal absorption*: Celiac sprue and abetalipoproteinemia
- *Impaired transport from the mucosa to systemic circulation*: Lymphatic obstruction.

Diagnosis and Work-up

- Initial laboratory studies should try to establish the presence of malabsorption. A quick screening test for fat malabsorption is a qualitative fecal fat test or Sudan III stain. In the presence of moderate steatorrhea (>15 g/d of stool fat), the test has a sensitivity and specificity of 90-95%. The gold standard remains a 72-hour collection of stool for fecal fat analysis after the patient has been on a 100 g fat/d diet for 48 hours. Massive steatorrhea (80-100 g fat/d in stool) is highly suspicious for pancreatic insufficiency. A D-xylose absorption test helps rule out small intestine disease. If the D-xylose absorption is abnormal, a small bowel biopsy either via endoscopy or by a suction tube (Rubin tube) is indicated. A small bowel aspirates to rule out the presence of *Giardia* should be done simultaneously. Serum Ca^{++} and magnesium should be measured as well as complete blood count (CBC), prothrombin time (PT), vitamin B_{12}, and folate, which may be abnormal in malabsorptive states (Chopra and Waxman).
- Determination of the physiopathologic category will help tailor further work-up.
- By far the most common causes of malabsorption in the Western world include—pancreatic insufficiency, bacterial overgrowth in association with GI surgery or dysmotility disorders (blind loop syndrome, ileal resection, small bowel diverticulosis, and scleroderma), giardiasis, and lactose intolerance. A history and physical exam may provide clues (ingestion of unfiltered water, surgical history or abdominal scars, dietary history, etc.). Treatment is aimed at correcting specific disorders and nutrient deficiencies.

INFLAMMATORY BOWEL DISEASE

Ulcerative Colitis

Ulcerative colitis is a recurrent inflammatory process of unknown etiology involving the mucosa and submucosa of the colon.
- The disease may be limited to the rectum, involve the left side of the colon, or extend in a continuous fashion to the cecum. Ungaro et al. provide an excellent Lancet seminar—most cases start between the ages of 15 and 40; nevertheless.
- Clinical features include diarrhea with watery stools, rectal bleeding, and abdominal pain. Clinical presentation is variable.
- The disease is characterized by periods of remission and exacerbation.

- It is classified, according to symptoms, into mild, moderate, and severe.
- Patients with mild IBD usually have distal colonic or rectal involvement, often with mild diarrhea or insidious rectal bleeding, tenesmus, and mild cramping.
- Patients with moderate symptoms usually have less than or equal to 10 bowel movements a day, frequent bleeding, mild anemia, and abdominal pain.
- Patients with severe or fulminant symptoms usually have pancolitis, more than 10 bowel movements a day, bleeding requiring transfusion, severe abdominal pain, and fever.

Diagnosis

Ungaro et al. presented a Lancet seminar and indicated that the pathogenesis is multifactorial, involving genetic predisposition, epithelial barrier defects, dysregulated immune responses, and environmental factors.
- Mucosal inflammation usually starts in the rectum and can extend continuously to proximal segments of the colon.
- Ulcerative colitis usually presents with bloody diarrhea and is diagnosed by colonoscopy and histological findings.
- Treatments for this disease include 5-aminosalicylic acid (ASA) drugs, steroids, and immunosuppressants. Some patients can require colectomy for medically refractory disease or to treat colonic neoplasia.
- Endoscopy with biopsies is the only way to establish the diagnosis of ulcerative colitis.
- Colonoscopy with intubation of the terminal ileum is recommended for patients with suspected IBD.
- After routine stool cultures have ruled out infectious processes, flexible sigmoidoscopy, and biopsy readily establish the diagnosis, given that the disease *always* affects the rectum. Mucosal change includes edema, friability, loss of vascular pattern to macro-ulceration, and pseudopolyps (Chopra and Waxman).

Therapy

- *Sulfasalazine:* Efficacious in approximately 80% of patients with mild-to-moderate IBD. Also has a prophylactic role in patients in remission; 75% of patients maintained on sulfasalazine stay in remission for less than or equal to 3 years. 5-ASA drugs have also been shown to be effective at maintaining remission, and patients who achieve remission with 5-ASA should continue on the same medication. Patients with proctitis should be treated initially with 5-ASA suppositories since they directly target the site of inflammation and appear to be more effective than oral 5-ASA (Ong et al).

Sulfasalazine consists of sulfapyridine linked to 5-ASA by an azo bond. Intestinal bacteria cleave the bond, releasing two metabolites. Sulfapyridine is largely absorbed, metabolized by the liver, and excreted in the urine. The 5-ASA is mostly unabsorbed, stays in contact with the diseased mucosa, and is excreted in the feces. Most of the drug's side effects—such as headaches, nausea, and allergic reactions—can be traced to the sulfa moiety.
- *Dosage:* Starting dose is 0.5 mg po bid advancing as tolerated less than or equal to 2-4 g in four divided doses. Optimum maintenance dose is 2 g/d.

In left-sided colitis, 5-ASA should be administered as an enema instead of a suppository in order to reach the splenic flexure. For patients with left-sided or extensive disease, it is recommended that oral 5-ASA be used in combination with topical 5-ASA to induce remission.
- *Side effects*: Less than or equal to one-third of patients may develop side effects. Headaches, nausea, malaise, and abdominal pain are the most common and are dose related. Idiosyncratic reactions include hemolytic anemia, aplastic anemia, hepatitis, pulmonary dysfunction, agranulocytosis, skin rash, fever, and occasionally Steven-Johnson syndrome. The drug should not be restarted in patients with hypersensitivity reactions.
- *Mesalamine:* Mild-to-moderate colitis.
  - *Dosage:* 1.2-2.4 g/d in three divided doses. Mesalamine enemas also available for distal colitis.
- *Olsalazine:* Maintenance of remission.
  - *Dosage:* 1-2 g po qd in two divided doses. Although these newer agents are as efficacious as sulfasalazines, and have fewer side effects, they are more costly.
- *Glucocorticoids:* Successful in treating moderate-to-severe disease. Disease limited to the rectum and distal colon can be treated with glucocorticoid enemas (100 mg hydrocortisone Qhs, or 20 mg of methylprednisolone qd) for several weeks. More extensive disease should be treated with oral prednisone in doses of 40-60 mg qd. In patients responding promptly, withdrawal should be gradual at rates not exceeding a 5-mg ↓ q 3-7 days. If no improvement appears after 2-3 weeks of oral steroids, parenteral therapy should be considered. In the severely ill patient, hydrocortisone 50-100 mg intravenous (IV) q 6 hours or prednisolone 100 mg in divided doses or by continuous infusion is recommended. Failure to improve after 2 weeks of therapy should indicate colectomy.

Ungaro et al. advised the following in a lancet Seminar:
- Corticosteroids are advisable for patients who do not respond or do not achieve remission on 5-ASA drugs.
- Rectal corticosteroids can be tried as a second-line add-on therapy to induce remission in proctitis or left-sided ulcerative colitis.

- Topical 5-ASA is superior to topical corticosteroids at inducing, but clinical and endoscopic improvement could be higher when combining rectal 5-ASA and corticosteroids. Foam formulations of rectal corticosteroids can be administered and are often better tolerated than enemas with active distal ulcerative colitis.
- Oral corticosteroids are needed to induce remission in patients with mild-to-moderate disease who are not benefiting from 5-ASA treatment.
- Oral steroids with minimal systemic activity (due to high first-pass liver metabolism) such as budesonide-multimatrix and prolonged release beclomethasone dipropionate are effective at inducing remission in ulcerative colitis. Given the lower risk for systemic side-effects, these drugs should be considered as alternative first-line induction drugs for mild-to-moderate ulcerative colitis, failing 5-ASA (Ungaro et al.).
- *Azathioprine*: Patients with moderate-to-severe colitis should be managed with thiopurines or biological drugs, or both. Thiopurines (azathioprine or 6-mercaptopurine) can be used in patients with steroid-dependent moderate-to-severe disease to maintain remission (Ong et al.); the drug has a limited role in ulcerative colitis. Should be considered in patients who are refractory to conventional medical therapy and not surgical candidates. May also be used to ↓ the glucocorticoids maintenance dose in patients who cannot undergo surgery. The effects may not be apparent for less than or equal to 3 months.
  - *Dosage:* 1.5 mg/kg/d orally with frequent CBC follow-up.

New Medication

- Vedolizumab blocks the gut-homing α4β7 integrin.
  - The drug is approved for moderate-to-severe ulcerative colitis, refractory to standard medications.
- *Antidiarrheals*: Agents like diphenoxylate, loperamide, and tincture of opium must be used cautiously in patients with chronic IBD since they may precipitate ileus and even toxic megacolon in patients with active disease. Their use is contraindicated during an exacerbation.
- *Nutrition*: No specific diet has been shown to help in this disorder—a low-roughage diet may provide symptomatic relief by decreasing stool weight. Lactose intolerance should be considered as possibly contributing to the symptoms. Total parenteral nutrition (TPN) is indicated to improve and maintain nutritional status but has not been shown to affect the cause of the disease for patients with disease so severe they require hospitalization.
- *Total colectomy:* Surgery is indicated in patients with refractory disease or complications (perforation, high-grade dysplasia, or severe toxic megacolon). Absolute indications for surgery include uncontrolled hemorrhage, perforation, and colorectal carcinoma.

Complications

- Toxic megacolon occurs in less than or equal to 10% of patients with ulcerative colitis.
- Clinical presentation is characterized by fever, abdominal pain, distention, and malaise.
- Physical examination reveals an ill-appearing patient with fever, dehydration, tachycardia, hypoactive bowel sounds, abdominal distention, and localized or diffuse rebound tenderness. Leukocytosis, anemia, and hypoalbuminemia are common laboratory findings.
- On plain abdominal radiography, dilation (usually by >7 cm) of the mid-transverse colon diameter is the most conspicuous finding.

Treatment

- Careful correction of fluid and electrolyte deficits. Particular attention should be paid to hypokalemia. 100 mEq of KCl may be needed during the first 24 hours.
- Blood transfusions should be given to correct anemia and hypovolemia in the presence of colonic bleeding.
- Nasogastric (NG) suction to prevent further bowel distention should be instituted.
- Intravenous glucocorticosteroids such as hydrocortisone 100 mg IV q 6 hours should be started.
- Parenteral antibiotics to cover for intra-abdominal sepsis should be administered.
- Anticholinergics and opiates should be withdrawn.
- Early surgical consultation is mandatory.
- Total colectomy should be considered for patients who deteriorate or fail to improve within 48 hours after aggressive medical therapy has been instituted.

Colonic cancer—patients with ulcerative colitis have 10 times the risk for adenocarcinoma of the colon depending on the duration, extent, and severity of their IBD. The highest risk is in those with pancolitis and those who have had the disease for more than 10 years. Colonoscopy with biopsy surveillance for dysplasia is indicated. In patients in whom high-grade dysplasia or carcinoma is found, colectomy is indicated.

Crohn's Disease

Joana Torres et al. provided an excellent Lancet seminar:
- All segments of the gastrointestinal tract can be affected.
- The most common being the terminal ileum and colon
- Inflammation is typically segmental, asymmetrical, and transmural.

- Most patients present with an inflammatory phenotype at diagnosis, but over time complications (strictures, fistulas, or abscesses) will develop in half of patients, often resulting in surgery Joana Torres et al.
- The disease usually occurs in the 2nd to 4th decade of life.
- Most often occurs in a patient at age 20–45 presenting with right lower quadrant abdominal pain, chronic diarrhea, and weight loss.
- About 50% of patients present with skin, joint, or eye extraintestinal manifestations that can precede diagnosis.
- The disease is characterized by periods of clinical remission alternating with periods of recurrence Joana Torres et al. affect any portion of the GI tract. About one-third of patients have only small intestine involvement, with most of these cases occurring in the distal ileum; 20% may have only colonic involvement. In contrast to ulcerative colitis, Crohn's disease is a transmural process in which the inflammatory reaction extends through all layers of the bowel wall. On the serosal surface, mesenteric fat becomes hyperemic and edematous and encases the bowel wall ("creeping fat").

Clinical Manifestations

- Diarrhea
- Crampy abdominal pain
- Gastrointestinal bleeding—in rare instances, massive
- Small bowel obstruction due to strictures
- *Fistulas:* Enterovesical (pneumaturia), enterocutaneous, and anorectal
- Bowel perforation.

Diagnosis

- *Colonoscopy*: Very useful when Crohn's colitis is suspected. Findings include focal segmental colitis with aphthoid ulcerations in between normal mucosa.
- *Small bowel X-rays*: Remain the mainstay in the diagnosis of Crohn's disease of the small intestine. Radiologic features include nodularity, ulceration, stricture formation, and separation of bowel loops (due to small bowel thickening). In biopsy specimens, granulomas can be found in less than 30% of cases.

Treatment

Joana Torres and colleagues provided a lancet seminar:
- The most widely used drugs in Crohn's disease are corticosteroids and immunosuppressants [thiopurines (azathioprine and mercaptopurine) and methotrexate] (Joana Torres).
- Biologicals [antitumor necrosis factor (TNF) (infliximab, adalimumab, and certolizumab pegol] and antiadhesion molecules (vedolizumab) have an expandingrole. (Joana Torres).

- Joana Torres et al. indicated that investigators have shown that thiopurines and methotrexate should be considered only for maintenance therapy.
- Several studies have reported that thiopurine use in Crohn's disease is associated with reduced need for surgery and has modest benefit in maintaining remission.
- Two controlled trials of early Crohn's disease failed to show that azathioprine has the potential for disease modification. Furthermore, an increased risk of malignancies (lymphoma, nonmelanoma skin cancers, myeloid disorders, and urinary tract cancers) is associated with these drugs.
- Thiopurines should be used with caution in young men (aged <35 years) and in older people who are at increased risk of developing malignancy
- *Sulfasalazine:* In doses of less than or equal to 1 g po qid, is effective in mild-to-moderate disease, including colonic or ileocolic disease. Not helpful in ileal disease per se. No role for maintenance therapy.
- *Mesalamine:* Can be used in mild-to-moderate Crohn's disease, but no advantage over sulfasalazine has been reported. *Dosage*—1.2–2.4 g po qd in three divided doses.
- *6-Mercaptopurine:* May be used in patients refractory to steroids or for steroid-sparing effect. Serious side effects include bone marrow suppression and pancreatitis. Careful follow-up CBCs are mandatory
- *Glucocorticoids:* Prednisone is beneficial in acute exacerbations. Dose is 20–40 mg po qd. In severe disease, IV glucocorticoids should be used, i.e. hydrocortisone 50–100 mg IV q 6 hours.

Three anti-TNF agents (infliximab, adalimumab, and certolizumab pegol) are effective to induce and maintain remission in Crohn's disease (see appendix for response and remission rates). Certolizumab is only available in North America, Switzerland, and a few other countries. Anti-TNF drugs are the most potent agents available to treat Crohn's disease, but their use is restricted to patients who have not responded to treatment with steroids or thiopurines according to drug labeling. Infliximab has been the only anti-TNF drug to show efficacy for the treatment of RCT.

New Biological Drugs

- Vedolizumab is an intravenously administered monoclonal antibody that blocks α4β7 integrin, resulting in gut-selective anti-inflammatory activity. It is effective in the induction and maintenance of clinical remission in refractory and luminal Crohn's disease.
  - Vedolizumab has been approved by the European Medicines Agency and the US Food Drug Administration in adults with moderately to severely active Crohn's disease who have had an inadequate response with anti-TNFs or immunosuppressants, lost response to anti-TNFs or immunosuppressants, or were intolerant to anti-TNFs or immunosuppressants, or who had an inadequate response with corticosteroids, were intolerant to corticosteroids, or showed dependence on corticosteroids. Its efficacy is lower in patients in whom previous anti-TNF therapy was unsuccessful.

- Ustekinumab is a monoclonal antibody directed against interleukin 12 and interleukin 23 through their common p40 subunit.
- After an IV infusion for induction, it is administered subcutaneously every 8 weeks for maintenance therapy. RCTs in patients with moderate-to-severe Crohn's disease have shown that ustekinumab is superior to placebo in anti-TNF naive and refractory patients. It is less effective in patients in whom anti-TNF therapy has failed. The safety profile of both drugs looks favorable, but long-term safety needs to be formally investigated in postmarketing studies.

As several biologicals are in the process of being approved for the treatment of Crohn's disease, choice among available agents is likely to become challenging in the future:

- *Antibacterials*: Metronidazole 250 mg po tid or ciprofloxacin have been shown to be effective in colonic disease and should be considered in patients intolerant of other agents.
- *Antidiarrheals*: Can be used for mild exacerbation.
- *Nutrition*: Specific replacement of B_{12} or folate may be necessary in patients with extensive ileal disease. Oxalate nephrolithiasis can be a problem; therefore, a low-oxalate diet is indicated.
- *Surgery*: Reserved for complications such as obstruction, fistulae, perforations, or abscess.

Complications

- *Intestinal obstruction*: May occur at a strictured segment. Treatment is supportive and consists of NG suction, IV fluid replacement, and IV corticosteroids aimed at decreasing edema. Avoidance of seeds and indigestible foods (nuts and popcorn) should be recommended.
- *Fistulae*: Medical management includes TPN, metronidazole (Flagyl), and perhaps 6-MP, which some studies have suggested may be useful although recurrences are high. Surgical evaluation should be obtained.
- *Perianal disease*: Flagyl 250 mg po or IV tid may be useful.

Pseudomembranous Colitis

Syndrome characterized by fever, diarrhea, and abdominal cramping that develops within 10 weeks of antibiotic therapy. Most of the cases are associated with *C. difficile*.

Clinical Manifestations

Nonbloody diarrhea, but blood may be present in less than 10% of cases; fever; leukocytosis; fecal leukocytes in 50% of cases; rebound tenderness in 10–20% of cases; and although usually left-sided, 10% of cases may involve the right colon.

Diagnosis

Proctosigmoidoscopy: Pseudomembranes seen in 85–90% of cases. Positive *C. difficile* toxin in less than or equal to 90% of cases.

Treatment

- Vancomycin 125 mg po q 6 hours for 7 days
- Metronidazole 250 mg po q 6 hours for 7 days
- Intravenous metronidazole 500 mg q 6 hours should be given to patients with ileus or where questionable oral absorption is suspected
- Relapses usually respond to repeated courses of the above agents.

Diverticular Disease

Diverticula are herniation of colonic mucosa and submucosa through the bowel wall. It is thought to be due to ↓ in dietary fiber, which causes ↓ transit time, ↓ stool bulk, ↑ straining at stool, and ↑ colonic segmentation, which ↑ intracolonic pressure. In Western countries, 5% of the population is affected by age 40, increasing linearly to 50% by age 80. Shah and Adam provide an excellent JAMA review.

Clinical Manifestations

- Asymptomatic diverticulosis
- Spastic diverticular disease (constipation, left lower quadrant pain, and postprandial distention; no fever or peritoneal signs present)
- Diverticulitis (left lower quadrant pain, fever, and leukocytosis; may have sign of peritoneal irritation)
- Diverticular bleeding
- *Complications*: Abscess formation, perforation, and fistulae to bladder or skin

Treatment

For spastic diverticular disease, management includes reassurance of the patient and ↑ dietary fiber. Metamucil 2 tsp bid may be required for complete relief of constipation. Antispasmodic drugs like dicyclomine 20 mg po qid can be used for painful episodes. For very mild diverticulitis, a clear liquid diet with an oral antibiotic (ampicillin, tetracycline, or a cephalosporin) may be given. Standard therapy for acute diverticulitis consists of bowel rest with nil per os (NPO). If abdominal distention is present, consider NG suction. Antibiotic therapy to cover intra-abdominal sepsis is indicated.

GALLSTONES

Epidemiology

- It is estimated that 20 million Americans have gallstones and that 1 million new cases develop each year. Gallstones can be divided according to composition into cholesterol and pigment stones. Cholesterol stones, which account for 80–90% of gallstones, are mostly radiolucent, solitary, tan or clay-colored, and larger than pigment stones, which are multiple, small, and black or brown. Chemical dissolution therapy is only effective on cholesterol stones.
- *Risk factors for cholesterol gallstones*: Female gender, pregnancy, estrogen therapy, age, ileal disorders, obesity, and gallbladder stasis (patient receiving TPN or somatostatin).
- *Risk factors for pigment gallstones*: Hemolytic disorders and cirrhosis.

Clinical Presentation

- *Asymptomatic*: Prophylactic cholecystectomy is recommended only for children and patients with sickle cell disease.
- *Biliary pain*: Recurrent right upper quadrant or epigastric pain is steady, lasts several hours, and self-resolves. Irradiates to right scapula or right shoulder.
- *Acute cholecystitis*: Severe abdominal pain, nausea, vomiting, fever, and leukocytosis.
- *Choledocholithiasis*: Present with biliary pain. Can be associated with cholangitis (infection of the bile ducts) or gallstone pancreatitis.

Diagnosis

- Ultrasonography can detect stones more than 1–2 mm in size
- Oral cholecystography
- *Nuclear cholescintigraphy*: Permits rapid evaluation of gallbladder function when cholecystitis is suspected.

Treatment

Cholecystectomy laparoscopic or surgical is the best treatment for recurrent symptomatic cholelithiasis and acute cholecystitis. It can be performed in standard fashion or via a laparoscope. No studies comparing both techniques are available, but shorter hospital stay and rapid recovery time has made laparoscopic cholecystectomy very popular.

Oral Dissolution Therapy

- This is an alternative option. Ursodeoxycholic acid 300 mg po bid or in combination with chenodeoxycholic acid 375 mg qd for symptomatic

cholelithiasis can achieve complete dissolution of small cholesterol stones in patients who refuse or are not candidates for surgery. Dissolution rate is 1 mm per month. Recurrence after dissolution is approximately 43% after 4 years.
- *Indications and criteria for treatment*: Radiolucent stones, patent cystic duct, stones less than 2 cm in diameter, and floating stones. Not indicated for the management of acute cholecystitis or complicated biliary disease (choledocholithiasis or gallstone pancreatitis).
- *Side Effects:* Diarrhea and reversible elevation of aminotransaminases.
- Contact dissolution therapy requires percutaneous catheter into the gallbladder or an endoscopically placed nasobiliary catheter.
- *Methyl tert-butyl*: Instillation can achieve dissolution in 24 hours. If contact with duodenum is severe, mucosal irritation can be seen. Recurrence is a significant problem.
- *Extracorporeal biliary lithotripsy*: Uses focused high-amplitude sound waves to fragment stones. Experience with this technique is limited and, in available series, only 25–30% of referred patients were suitable candidates. Long-term concomitant oral dissolution therapy may be required, and the abnormal gallbladder remains in place.
- *Choledocholithiasis*: Endoscopic retrograde cholangiopancreatography (ERCP) with sphincterotomy and stone removal is an extremely valuable alternative to open common bile duct exploration for treatment of symptomatic choledocholithiasis (cholangitis or gallstone pancreatitis). In a recent study of patients with cholangitis and bile duct stones, emergency endoscopic biliary drainage was associated with less morbidity and mortality than immediate surgery.

PANCREATITIS

Acute Pancreatitis

- Conditions associated with pancreatitis include—alcoholism, gallstones, drugs (e.g., azathioprine, thiazides, valproic acid, and pentamidine), hyperlipemia, hypercalcemia, and trauma.
- *Clinical manifestations*: Severe unremitting epigastric pain that frequently radiates to the back and is usually accompanied by nausea and vomiting.
- Physical examination in patients with mild pancreatitis reveals epigastric tenderness and guarding. Bowel sounds are hypoactive or absent. In severe disease, signs of vascular collapse may be present, with tachycardia and hypertension. A mass may be palpable in the epigastrium. Tachypnea may be present secondary to pulmonary complications from pancreatitis [pleural effusion and acute respiratory distress syndrome (ARDS)]. Mild fever (37.5–38.5°C) is commonly seen.

Diagnosis

- Serum amylase elevation twofold or more
- Elevation of serum lipase helpful in patients who present late in the clinical course (remains elevated longer than amylase) or when diagnosis unclear.
- Dynamic CT scan is very useful in confirming diagnosis and evaluating complications.

Management

- Mainly supportive. Specific therapy treats complications.
- *Narcotic analgesics*: Meperidine is the most commonly used agent that has no significant effect on the sphincter of Oddi.
- Patient should be kept NPO until pain and nausea resolve. NG suction is indicated in patients with recurrent vomiting or symptomatic abdominal distention from an ileus.
- Aggressive fluid resuscitation with lactate ringer or normal saline with careful monitoring of input or output
- Antibiotics have no proven role in the management of acute pancreatitis
- Serum Ca^{++}, Mg, glucose, triglycerides, and hematocrit should be monitored and corrected as necessary
- Patients with prolonged bowel rest should be started on TPN.

Complications

- *Infection*: Infected phlegmon or abscess is suspected when high, spiking fever with an elevated white blood cell (WBC) occurs more than or equal to 7 days into the course of the illness. A CT scan of the pancreas with a "skinny needle" aspiration of peripancreatic fluid collection may show bacteria on Gram's stain which suggests the diagnosis. Treatment includes surgical damage and in very selected cases percutaneous damage via CT-guided catheter placement with parenteral broad-spectrum antibiotics.
- *Pseudocysts*: Should be suspected in the presence of persistent pain or hyperamylasemia. Most acute pseudocysts will subside spontaneously within several weeks. Large (>5 cm) pseudocysts that persist for more than 6 weeks should be treated surgically or percutaneously, as they may become infected or bleed.
- *Pulmonary complications*: Include pleural effusions, atelectasis, or ARDS in the severely ill patient.
- *Renal insufficiency*: May be due to prerenal azotemia or acute tubular necrosis (ATN). Careful monitoring of fluid balance, serum creatinine, and blood urea nitrogen (BUN) are necessary. Occasionally, patients require peritoneal dialysis or hemodialysis support.

- *Surgery*: Indicated in complicated pancreatitis, i.e. abscess, hemorrhagic pancreatitis, or persistent pseudocyst.
- *Endoscopic therapy*: In patients with gallstone pancreatitis, ERCP with sphincterotomy may have a role in removing obstructing gallstones and decompressing the biliary tree.

Chronic Pancreatitis

- Alcohol is the leading cause of chronic pancreatitis. Other conditions include hereditary pancreatitis, cystic fibrosis, hemochromatosis, and tropical obstructive pancreatitis (India, Southern Africa, and Indonesia).
- Clinical manifestation includes chronic pain and exocrine and endocrine insufficiency manifested by diabetes, steatorrhea, and weight loss. It should be suspected in any patient with abdominal pain, diabetes, steatorrhea, or jaundice.

Diagnosis

- Less than or equal to 30% of patients have pancreatic calcifications on plain abdominal X-rays.
- Stool sample for Sudan III staining
- *Bentiromide test*: After an overnight fast, 500 mg of N-benzoyl-L-tryosila-para-aminobenzoic acid (NBT-PABA) is given and a 6-hour urine collection performed. If the PABA ↑ in the urine is less than 50%, the probability of severe pancreatic insufficiency is significant.
- Computed tomography scan may reveal pancreatic calcification, ductal dilation, or the presence of pseudocysts.
- Endoscopic retrograde cholangiopancreatography may show specific roentgenographic changes of chronic pancreatitis and can help in differentiating pancreatitis from pancreatic cancer.

Management

- *Pain*: Narcotics are frequently needed. Large meals, fatty foods, and alcohol should be avoided. The role of pancreatic enzymes in pain management remains controversial. Celiac plexus block may give initial relief in less than 70% of patients, but by 6 months only 50% continue to show benefit.
- Surgery should be reserved until no other modalities are available. Drainage procedures are indicated when dilated ducts are present, and they can relieve pain in less than or equal to 70% of cases. The role of pancreatic resection in patients without ductal dilation is more controversial.
- *Exocrine insufficiency*: Treatment consists of a low-fat diet (<50 g/d) and oral pancreatic supplement. A variety of agents is available; a nonenteric coated medication with a total lipase content of 20,000–40,000 U per

meal is adequate. Enzyme replacements should be taken 30 minutes before the meal and at bedtime. If no improvement occurs, 650 mg of sodium bicarbonate or an H_2 receptor antagonist can be given before meals to prevent degradation by gastric acid. If switching to an enteric coated preparation, the bicarbonate or H_2 receptor antagonist should be discontinued.
- *Endocrine insufficiency*: Pancreatic diabetes usually requires insulin therapy.

GASTROINTESTINAL BLEEDING

The initial approach to the bleeding patient depends on the site, extent, and rate of bleeding.
- Maintaining adequate intravascular volume and hemodynamic stability while localizing the bleeding site and providing adequate therapy is the mainstay of successful management.
- Clinical predictors of ↑ mortality include age more than 60 years, multiple serious underlying illnesses, recurrent bleeding, bleeding requiring more than 5 units of blood, and red-colored stool with NG aspirate at presentation.
- Initial evaluation aims to assess patient's intravascular volume and rate of bleeding, and tailor degree of resuscitating efforts.
- *Patient's appearance:* Decreased mental status, diaphoresis, pallor, or complaints of light headedness, thirst, and nausea are usually associated with significant blood loss (>500 mL), except in the elderly, where smaller volumes may lead to same signs and symptoms.
- *Initial exam:* Aimed at assessing volume status:
  - Orthostatic hypotension manifested by a drop in systolic blood pressure (BP) of more than 10 mm Hg or ↑ in HR of more than 20 beats/min is associated with moderate blood loss (10–20% of circulatory volume)
  - Supine hypotension indicates severe blood loss (>20% of circulatory volume)
  - *Hypovolemic shock*: Manifested by hypotension, tachycardia, and multiorgan failure, i.e. oliguria, confusion, and myocardial ischemia. Examination will reveal pallor, cool skin, and delayed capillary filling due to peripheral vasoconstriction. Type and cross for 3–6 U of packed red blood cells (RBCs) should be done as well as initial CBC, platelets, PT, partial thromboplastin time (PTT), and serum chemistries, as well as an electrocardiogram (ECG).

Resuscitation

- Two large-bore IV (14–16 gauge) should be placed for rapid volume infusion. This is usually quicker and with less morbidity than placing central vein catheters.

- Rate of fluid infusion will depend on patient's hemodynamic status. 0.9% saline or Ringer lactate is adequate starting solutions while blood is available from the blood bank.
- *Blood transfusion*: Aim to keep hematocrit around 30% or until patient is hemodynamically stable. In actively bleeding patients, where more than 5 U of packed RBCs have been transfused; fresh frozen plasma (FFP) should be given to correct for dilution of clotting factors.

Further Evaluation

Once patient is stable, attention is focused on determining the source of bleeding.
- A pertinent concise history together with a careful physical examination will usually suggest the source. Look for peptic symptoms and past history of pepsin will degrade.
- *Inspection of the stool*: Melena, described as black, sticky, or tarry stool, is present when bleeding source is proximal to the cecum. Approximately, 100 mL of blood is necessary to produce melenic stools. If bleeding ceases, melena can be present for less than or equal to 3 days and stool may present with occult blood for up to a week. *Maroon stool* is usually seen when bleeding site is located at the distal ileum or proximal colon. *Hematochezia*, or passage of bright red blood per rectum, usually indicates a distal colonic or anorectal pathology, but can also be seen in very rapid UGI bleeding.
- *Nasogastric aspirate*: When a UGI source of bleeding is suspected and no hematemesis is present, NG aspirate is mandatory. In patients with a history of hematemesis, the NG aspirate helps to assess the presence of continuous bleeding. There is a 16% false negative rate for NG aspiration in patients with endoscopically proven UGI bleeding. Therefore, a negative aspirate does not completely rule out an upper source. This may be due to coiling of the NG tube in the stomach or esophagus, or pylorospasm in patients with active duodenal ulcer bleeding. After the diagnostic aspirate is performed, the NG tube should be removed unless persistent vomiting or signs of gastric outlet obstruction are present, given that the continuous presence of an NG tube may lead to mucosal trauma and gastroesophageal reflux.
- It is important to recognize other manifestations of GI bleeding. Pulmonary complaints are not uncommon, especially in the patient with altered mental status, and protection of the airway by endotracheal intubation may be necessary to prevent recurrent aspiration. The hematocrit is not a good indicator of acute GI bleeding, given that it takes hours to equilibrate. The BUN is elevated more than 30 mg/dL in less than or equal to 75% of patients with UGI bleeding due to resorption of nitrogen products from the proximal small bowel.

UPPER GASTROINTESTINAL BLEEDING

The four most common causes of UGI hemorrhage are—(i) peptic ulcer, (ii) erosive gastritis, (iii) variceal bleeding, and (iv) Mallory-Weiss tear. These account for more than or equal to 90% of UGI bleeds.

Diagnosis

The diagnostic approach to the patient varies depending on clinical stability, rate of bleeding, and procedural expertise:
- Upper gastrointestinal endoscopy has largely supplanted barium studies of the GI tract in the evaluation of GI bleeding. Not only does it accurately identify the source of bleeding (90% accuracy), it also offers therapeutic options for hemostasis.
- Barium studies may identify the source of hemorrhage but suffer from the following drawbacks—they may not identify mucosal lesions (Mallory-Weiss tear and erosive gastritis); the identified lesion may not be the actual source of bleeding; and the presence of barium may hamper future endoscopic or angiographic examination.
- *Arteriography*: In the presence of continuous bleeding and a negative endoscopic examination, or with massive hemorrhage (blood loss of ≥0.5 mL/min), selective angiography may localize the site. In addition to identifying the site, it can also offer therapeutic options like intra-arterial, continuous vasopressin infusion in patients with Mallory-Weiss tear, or gastric ulcer. Additionally, embolization into the selective bleeding vessel may be undertaken.

Peptic Ulcers

They are the most common cause of UGI bleeding, but 85% will stop bleeding spontaneously.
- *Therapeutic endoscopy*: In large meta-analysis studies, has been shown to ↓ hospital stay, blood requirements, and emergency surgery. Modalities include injection therapy, bipolar electrocoagulation, laser therapy, and heater probe, all of which have similar success rates.
- *Surgery*: Mainly indicated for patients with intractable or recurrent bleeding. Surgical consultation should be obtained early in the patient's course.
- *Selective angiography*: Should be considered in patients who are not good surgical candidates and who have failed endoscopic therapy. Intra-arterial vasopressin infusion is successful in about 60-70% of peptic ulcers. Careful monitoring for evidence of ischemic organ damage (i.e. myocardial and mesenteric) should be done. Selective embolization is also an alternative.

Variceal Bleeding

Characteristically abrupt and massive. In the Western world, it is usually secondary to alcoholic cirrhosis via portal hypertension. Although a history of cirrhosis or chronic liver disease suggests the possibility of varices as the cause of bleeding, less than 50% of patients may have another source. Therefore, accurate identification of the source of bleeding is essential. After the patient is stabilized, early endoscopy should be performed to confirm the diagnosis. Admission to an intensive care unit (ICU) should be considered, and in patients with compromised mental status and active bleeding, endotracheal intubation for airway protection may be necessary.

Therapy

- Endoscopic sclerotherapy or rubber band ligation can achieve adequate hemostasis in less than 90% of patients. Sclerotherapy consists of injecting a sclerosing agent, such as sodium tetradecol into or around the varix, producing an inflammatory reaction that leads to thrombosis and eventually fibrosis of the vessel. Although significant rebleeding occurs, it usually responds to repeat treatment. Rubber band ligation is just as effective, and preliminary data suggest fewer complications.
- Intravenous vasopressin is effective in less than or equal to 60% of patients.
  - *Dosage:* Starting dose 0.4 U/min (100 U of vasopressin in 250 ccs of D5W). Increments should be started at a dose of 0.3 U/min for 30 min and, if ineffective, ↑ at approximately 30–60-min intervals to a max of 0.9 U/min. Once hemostasis is achieved, the infusion rate should be reduced. Because of its vasoconstrictive properties, common side effects include myocardial ischemia, arrhythmias, bowel ischemia, and even cardiac arrest. Patients should be monitored in an ICU setting and extreme caution should be taken in patients with known atherosclerotic disease or coronary artery disease. Concomitant nitroglycerin (NTG) infusion has been shown to ↓ side effects and may improve efficacy of vasopressin therapy. Infusion is started at 5 µ/min and ↑ by 5 µ /min q 3–5 min, titrated to a systolic BP of 100 mm/Hg. Sublingual NTG (0.6 mg q 30 min for 6 h) as well as nitropaste have also been used successfully.
- *Balloon tamponade*: The use of this method should be undertaken only with the aid of personnel experienced in this procedure. The reported success for controlling bleeding varies from 40% to 90%. Major complications of balloon tamponade include aspiration, esophageal necrosis and rupture, and airway obstruction. Because of the high risk of rebleeding and the serious nature of the complications, it should be viewed as a temporizing measure in patients who continue to bleed

in spite of routine therapy and IV vasopressin, while waiting for more definitive therapy either endoscopic or surgical.
- *Emergent shunt surgery*: Either with a portacaval shunt or a distal splenorenal shunt is very effective in controlling variceal bleeding but is associated with significant hospital mortality (12-50%) and postoperative hepatic encephalopathy. Elective shunt surgery should be considered in patients with good hepatic function (as measured by the child's classification) who fail sclerotherapy, are noncompliant, or cannot return for follow-up visits.
- Other therapies include the transjugular intrahepatic portosystemic shunt procedure, which involves creating a shunt via a transjugular approach between a hepatic and a portal vein. Preliminary results indicate that the technique is safe and effective. Orthoptic liver transplantation restores normal circulation and prevents further variceal bleeding, but few patients are candidates for this procedure.

Mallory–Weiss Tear

Vertical mucosal tear at the gastroesophageal junction. A history of repeated vomiting prior to hematemesis is a common symptom; its absence, however, does not exclude this diagnosis. Most bleeds are self-limited. In patients with persistent bleeding, endoscopic hemostasis or selective angiography is excellent therapeutic option. Surgery should be reserved for intractable bleeding, which is very rare.

LOWER GASTROINTESTINAL BLEEDING

- The most common etiologies for lower GI bleeding include anorectal pathology (hemorrhoids, fissures, and rectal trauma), angiodysplasia, diverticulosis, and neoplasms.
- Lower GI bleeding will stop spontaneously in less than or equal to 80% of cases
- Initially, patients should be stabilized as described earlier
- The patient's history is the most important diagnostic tool and can often lead to the source of bleeding. Blood mixed with stool, or coating or streaking of the stool, is usually from or distal to the sigmoid colon. Blood only seen in the toilet paper suggests anal canal pathology. A UGI source should always be suspected in the presence of massive hematochezia.

Diagnosis

- Digital examination, anoscopy and sigmoidoscopy should be performed in every patient with rectal bleeding. These will identify a bleeding source or will document bleeding coming from above the range of

the instrument detected, infusion of vasopressin, or embolization with a substance like gel foam, can be performed successfully to obtain hemostasis.
- Colonoscopy is indicated in patients who have ceased bleeding or who have a mild and hemodynamically stable GI bleed. In addition to localizing a specific colonic lesion, therapeutic interventions with electrocautery or laser therapy are possible.

BIBLIOGRAPHY

1. Acree M, Davis AM. Acute Diarrheal Infections in Adults. JAMA. 2017;318(10):957-8.
2. Chopra S, Waxman I. Gastrointestinal Diseases, Gastrointestinal Bleeding. In: KHAN MG, Bartlett JG, Chopra S, Topol EJ (Eds). Medical Diagnosis and Therapy. Pennsylvania: Lea and Febiger; 1994.
3. Ford AC, Lacy BE, Talley NJ. Irritable Bowel Syndrome. N Engl J Med. 2017;376:2566-78.
4. Shah SD, Cifu AS. Management of Acute Diverticulitis. JAMA. 2017;318(3):291-2.
5. Høivik ML, Moum B, Solberg IC, et al. Work disability in inflammatory bowel disease patients 10 years after disease onset: results from the IBSEN study. Gut. 2013;62:368-75.
6. Torres J, Mehandru S, Colombel JF. Crohn's disease. Lancet. 2017;389(10080): 1741-55.
7. Ungaro R, Mehandru S, Allen PB, et al. Ulcerative colitis. Seminar. 2017; 389(10080):1756-70.

CHAPTER 19

Liver Diseases

CIRRHOSIS

Major causes of cirrhosis include:
- Chronic hepatitis B virus (HBV) and hepatitis C virus (HCV) infection
- Alcoholism
- Nonalcoholic steatohepatitis
- Hepatitis C virus infection and nonalcoholic steatohepatitis are the causes that are primarily responsible for the growing burden of cirrhosis in healthcare.
- The increasing prevalence of nonalcoholic fatty liver disease, cirrhosis related to nonalcoholic steatohepatitis is predicted to surpass HCV-related cirrhosis as the most common indication for orthotopic liver transplantation in the United States.

The pathophysiological features of cirrhosis involve:
- Progressive liver injury and fibrosis resulting in portal hypertension and decompensation, including ascites, spontaneous bacterial peritonitis (SBP), hepatic encephalopathy, variceal hemorrhage, the hepatorenal syndrome, and hepatocellular carcinoma (Ge and Runyon).

Complications of severe liver disease can be dramatic and life-threatening. They are most frequently encountered in patients with cirrhosis of the liver. The complications are listed in Box 19.1.

Variceal Bleeding

Variceal bleeding is most often encountered in patients with cirrhosis of the liver and significant portal hypertension, defined as—elevation in the portal pressure more than 22 mm Hg when measured directly during surgery, a portal pressure more than that of the inferior vena cava (IVC) by more than 8 mm Hg when measured by the percutaneous transhepatic route, or a wedged hepatic venous pressure more than that of the IVC by more than 5 mm of mercury. This gradient, referred to as the portal vein pressure gradient, is more than 10 mm Hg in patients with clinically significant portal hypertension.

Box 19.1: Complications of liver disease.
- Variceal bleeding
- Hepatic encephalopathy
- Ascites
- Spontaneous bacterial peritonitis
- Hepatorenal syndrome
- Altered hemostasis
- Disorders of pulmonary function
- Abnormalities of the endocrine system
- Increased susceptibility to a variety of infections
- Primary hepatocellular carcinoma

- Esophageal varices are demonstrable in 50–75% of patients with cirrhosis of the liver. Rupture of varices is likely to occur in patients with large varices; with cirrhosis of the liver, grade child's B or C; and who at the time of endoscopy have cherry-red spots or red wale markings on the varices.

Portal hypertension is classified as:
- Presinusoidal
- Sinusoidal
- Postsinusoidal.

Presinusoidal causes of portal hypertension include portal vein thrombosis, splenic vein thrombosis, schistosomiasis, congenital hepatic fibrosis, sarcoidosis, and myeloid metaplasia.

Sinusoidal: Cirrhosis of the liver and severe chronic active hepatitis are example of sinusoidal portal hypertension.

Postsinusoidal portal hypertension include veno-occlusive disease, Budd–Chiari syndrome, congestive heart failure (CHF), and constrictive pericarditis.

The diagnosis of variceal bleeding is done by endoscopy.

The major aim is to stop the acute variceal bleeding. Steps to prevent recurrent variceal bleeding also need to be taken.
- Patients should receive appropriate blood and, if necessary, fresh frozen plasma replacement.
- If the bleeding is torrential, a bolus of 20 units of intravenous (IV) vasopressin in 100 mL of 5% dextrose should be given IV over a 10-minute period. Vasopressin infusion results in cessation of bleeding in a significant number of patients, but its utility is limited by a high rate of rebleeding and failure to show improvement in the rate of survival.
- Another agent that may be useful is somatostatin, 50–250 micrograms as a bolus and 250 μ/hours as an IV infusion.
- Balloon tamponade, endoscopic sclerotherapy, rubber-band ligation, and emergency shunts are employed.

Ascites

Causes of accumulation of serous fluid within the abdominal cavity (ascites) are listed in Box 19.2.

Box 19.2: Important causes of ascites.
- Cirrhosis of the liver
- Metastatic peritoneal carcinomatosis
- Congestive heart failure and constrictive pericarditis
- Tuberculosis peritonitis
- Fungal peritonitis
- Pancreatic ascites
- Budd–Chiari syndrome and veno-occlusive disease
- Nephrogenic ascites
- Myxedema ascites
- Bile ascites
- Peritoneal mesothelioma
- Pseudomyxoma peritonei
- Eosinophilic gastroenteritis
- Meigs syndrome

Ascites and edema in patients with liver disease occur as a result of avid Na^+ retention by the kidney, ↑ed splanchnic lymph flow, elevated hydrostatic pressure in the hepatic sinusoids or portal vein, and ↓ed plasma oncotic pressure. Major hypotheses for the formation of ascites include the following:
- In the underfill hypothesis, the primary event is portal hypertension. The ↑ed physical force drives fluid into the abdominal cavity, resulting in redistribution of the plasma volume. Although the total volume is ↑ed, the effective circulating volume—that is, the component of circulating plasma volume that stimulates volume receptors—decreases. As a result, "the kidneys believe their owner is underfilled," leading to avid Na^+ and water retention by the kidneys and further aggravation of the existing fluid derangement. Na^+ retention is mediated by the hormone aldosterone (the renin - angiotensin - aldosterone system is stimulated).
- In the overflow hypothesis, the primary event is believed to be inappropriately ↑ed Na^+ retention by the kidneys. Vasomotor derangements [arteriovenous (AV) shunting and ↓ed peripheral resistance] commonly occur in patients with cirrhosis, thus initiating this primary event. The result is ↓ in renal blood flow. Na^+ retention by the kidneys leads to expansion of the plasma volume, which is preferentially sequestered in the peritoneal cavity secondary to ↑ed hydrostatic pressure and ↓ed oncotic pressure within the portal venous bed and hepatic sinusoids.
- In the peripheral arterial vasodilation hypothesis, cirrhotics have peripheral arterial vasodilation because of the presence of AV fistulas in the dermal and pulmonary circulation and the splanchnic vascular bed.

This leads to a ↓ed "effective" plasma volume and activation of compensatory hormonal systems (renin – angiotensin – aldosterone, and vasopressin), with resultant Na⁺ retention by the kidneys.
- Nitric oxide (NO) acts as an endogenous vasodilator mediating the hyperdynamic circulation of cirrhosis. The trigger for NO release is bacterial endotoxin.

Systemic endotoxemia occurs because of portosystemic shunts and is commonly present in patients with cirrhosis.

Clinical Features

Ascites may be first noticed by the patient, a friend, or a physician. Its presence can be detected on physical examination by demonstrating shifting dullness and/or a positive fluid wave. Patients with tense ascites may have an everted umbilicus. In patients in whom it is not certain on clinical examination whether ascites is present, ultrasonic examination should be performed prior to a diagnostic paracentesis. Patients with ascites may, on occasion, have pleural effusions and striking penile, scrotal, and peripheral edema. Ascites is present in virtually all patients having SBP, hepatorenal syndrome, Budd–Chiari syndrome, and veno-occlusive disease.

Complications of ascites include abdominal discomfort, respiratory embarrassment, rupture of umbilical hernia, and SBP.

Analysis of Ascitic Fluid

Traditionally, the fluid is characterized as a transudate or exudate based on its protein content. Patients with a protein concentration more than 2.5 g/dL are considered to have exudative ascites. Common causes of exudative ascitic fluid include metastatic peritoneal carcinomatosis, tuberculous peritonitis, pancreatic ascites, Budd–Chiari syndrome, myxedema ascites, and peritoneal mesothelioma. About 10% of patients with uncomplicated cirrhosis of the liver may have ascitic fluids classifiable as exudative based on the above criteria. Additionally, patients with CHF may have exudative ascitic fluid (based on protein content). Causes of transudative ascites include cirrhosis of the liver, alcoholic hepatitis, chronic active hepatitis, and nephrotic syndrome. Hemorrhagic or bloody ascites occurs on patients with malignant disease (notably hepatoma), Budd–Chiari syndrome, tuberculous peritonitis, or trauma. Chylous ascites refers to the presence of grossly milky, creamy, or turbid peritoneal fluid and an elevated triglyceride more than 200 mg/dL. Causes of chylous ascites in children include malignancy and congenital abnormalities of the lymphatic system. Trauma and tuberculosis are other causes. The protein concentration of chylous ascites ranges from less than 2 g/dL to more than 6 g/dL. Pancreatic ascites refers to the accumulation of ascitic fluid in a patient with complicated pancreatitis such as a ruptured pancreatic duct or a leaking pseudocyst. The ascitic fluid amylase is always elevated. Recently, it has been proposed that ascitic fluid can be classified based on serum-ascites albumin concentration gradient (SAAG). SAAG = (A serum albumin) − (Ascitic fluid albumin). If the SAAG is more than 1.1 g/dL, the patient has portal hypertension with greater than 90% accuracy.

Management

- In rare instances, treatment aimed at correcting the underlying pathophysiologic abnormalities results in the cure of ascites. Examples include tuberculous peritonitis, pancreatitis ascites, and Budd–Chiari syndrome due to the presence of a web in the IVC.
- Bedrest and dietary—Na^+ restriction. Na^+ intake should be restricted to 500 mg–1 g of Na^+.
- Spironolactone, 200–400 mg per day and even higher doses were recommended but hyperkalemia can be dangerous.
- Caution, spironolactone is no longer recommended by the author (since 2000) and is not advised in the UK because the drug has hormonal effects including gynecomastia and genital secretions do occur in some women. Caution if renal dysfunction is present because hyperkalemia is dangerous.
- Amiloride 5–10 mg/day is now used but both drugs may cause hyperkalemia when furosemide is not given. Caution if renal dysfunction is present.
- Some claim that spironolactone is superior to furosemide in initiating diuresis in patients with cirrhosis and ascites, although furosemide or hydrochlorothiazide should be added, if high-dose spironolactone therapy is not effective.
- Large-volume paracentesis. Up to 5 L of fluid may be removed slowly while patients are clinically monitored. Paracentesis should be followed by IV infusion of 40 g of albumin, particularly if there is no peripheral edema or if renal function is marginal.
- Peritoneovenous shunts (LeVeen or Denver shunts) may be useful in 5% of patients with ascites refractory to all medical therapy. Complications include disseminated intravascular coagulation, shunt occlusion, fever, and a unique form of small bowel obstruction.
- Portosystemic shunts—side-to-side portocaval shunts decompress both the splanchnic and hepatic sinusoidal bed.

Spontaneous Bacterial Peritonitis

- Spontaneous bacterial peritonitis may be defined as bacterial peritonitis that occurs in patients with ascites in the absence of demonstrable causes of peritonitis such as intra-abdominal abscesses or bowel perforation. It occurs in 10–25% of hospitalized patients with ascites. The unifying feature of the type of ascites susceptible to SBP is a low protein

concentration of ascitic fluid (characteristically <1 g/dL). Patients are at risk for developing SBP because of defects in reticuloendothelial system function, defects in neutrophil function, complement deficiency, and opsonization impairment.
- All cirrhotic patients with ascites and evidence of any clinical deterioration (which may be subtle and include mild worsening of hepatic encephalopathy, low-grade fever, leukocytosis, hypotension, hypothermia, low back pain, or refractoriness to diuretics) should undergo a diagnostic paracentesis.
- The diagnosis can be made when the ascitic fluid contains more than 250 polymorphonuclear leukocytes. The highest yield on ascitic fluid cultures is derived by obtaining 10 mL of ascitic fluid and inoculating it at the bedside into blood culture bottles.
- The most common organisms include *Escherichia coli*, pneumococcus, and *Streptococcus*. Polymicrobial organisms and anaerobes are encountered very infrequently, and their presence should raise the suspicion that the patient has secondary bacterial peritonitis due to an intra-abdominal process.
- The distinguishing features of spontaneous bacterial peritonitis and secondary bacterial peritonitis include the initial ascitic fluid white count and protein concentrations. In patients who have an exudative fluid or an initial ascitic fluid WBC more than 10,000, the assumption can be made that they have bacterial peritonitis secondary to an intra-abdominal abscess or perforation. Computed tomography (CT) scans, barium contrast studies, and surgical consultation are required in such patients.

Treatment

Empiric antibiotic therapy with the third-generation cephalosporin (cefotaxime or ceftriaxone) should be instituted in suspected cases. Aminoglycosides should not be used, as they may result in precipitation of renal failure and confusion with hepatorenal syndrome. Cefotaxime, 2 g IV q 8 hours for a total of 7-10 days is frequently effective.

Mortality is 30-40%. Poor prognostic factors include a serum bilirubin more than 8 mg/dL, serum albumin less than 2.5 g/dL, serum creatinine more than 2.1 mg/dL, hepatic encephalopathy, and development of hepatorenal syndrome. Recurrence of SBP is common in patients surviving an episode. SBP is an expression of severe end-stage liver disease, and patients should be evaluated for liver transplantation.

Hepatorenal Syndrome

- This dreaded complication occurs in patients with end-stage liver disease. It is defined as unexplained renal failure occurring in patients with liver or biliary tract disease in the absence of clinical, pathologic,

or anatomic evidence of other known causes of renal failure. Its pathogenesis is unknown. Pathologic abnormalities in the kidneys are trivial and inconstant. Postmortem angiography shows striking reversal of the pronounced corticomedullary shunting of blood in the kidney.
- Recovery from hepatorenal syndrome can occur after successful orthotopic liver transplantation. Kidneys from patients with hepatorenal syndrome have functioned normally when transplanted into patients with end-stage kidney disease and normal hepatic function. All this points to the fact that the nature of renal failure is indeed functional.
- Hepatorenal syndrome is almost invariably encountered in patients who have already been admitted to a hospital with severe end-stage liver disease, are suffering from a number of complications, and are being subjected to a variety of treatments. Thus, in some patients it appears that hepatorenal syndrome is precipitated by gastrointestinal (GI) bleeding, paracentesis, excessive diuretic use, infection, or medication. Aminoglycosides and nonsteroidal anti-inflammatory drugs (NSAIDs) should be avoided in patients with severe liver disease.

Diagnosis

- Most patients with hepatorenal syndrome have severe hepatocellular disease with characteristic abnormalities in hepatic synthetic function such as prolongation of the prothrombin time and a low serum albumin. Hyperbilirubinemia is common. The serum aspartate aminotransferase (AST) and alanine aminotransferase (ALT) levels are variably elevated. Hyponatremia is common, and partially compensated respiratory alkalosis is frequently encountered. The blood urea nitrogen (BUN) and creatinine values are elevated in the mild-to-moderate range.
- The salient urinary analysis findings include a normal urine sediment, a urine osmolality that is more than or equal to 100 mOsm more than plasma osmolality, a urine to plasma creatinine more than 30:1, and a daily urine Na$^+$ excretion of less than 10 mEq (urine Na$^+$ is frequently <3 mEq/liter and often 0 mEq/liter). These findings are not specific for hepatorenal syndrome and can be identical to those seen in patients with prerenal azotemia.

Management

- Avoid making the diagnosis, which is a way of saying that the physician should look for causes of "pseudohepatorenal syndrome." Exclude hypovolemia, obstructive uropathy, urinary tract infection, and electrolyte imbalances.
- Discontinue any potentially offending drugs, such as aminoglycosides, NSAIDs, or lactulose.

- Trial of volume expansion. Ideally, salt-poor albumin should be infused under carefully monitored conditions with the use of a Swan–Ganz catheter with measurements of pulmonary capillary wedge pressure (PCWP) as a guide.
- Appropriate nutritional support
- There is no proven therapy for hepatorenal syndrome, with the exception of liver transplantation.

Hepatic Encephalopathy

Hepatic encephalopathy can be defined as a neuropsychiatric syndrome characterized by intellectual deterioration, altered state of consciousness, and personality changes in a patient with severe liver diseases and/or portosystemic shunting. It can occur in two major settings:
1. Acute fulminant hepatic failure, and
2. Portosystemic encephalopathy and variant syndromes.

Pathogenesis

The diffuse nature of the neurologic process and its potential for restoration to complete normality suggest that metabolic factors are operative. The diseased liver is unable to detoxify a toxin or a number of toxins, which then affects cerebral function, resulting in encephalopathy. The inability to detoxify is due to severe hepatocellular injury. Alternatively, although liver function is intact, the putative toxin (s) bypasses the liver because of shunting. The various putative toxins include ammonia, mercaptines, short-chain fatty acids, and gamma-aminobutyric acid.

The diagnosis of hepatic encephalopathy is based on a constellation of findings that include the following:
- The obligatory presence of liver disease and/or portosystemic shunting
- Abnormal mental state (confusion, restlessness, and reversal of sleep rhythm)
- Abnormal neuromuscular state (asterixis)
- Variably present clinical features (fetor hepaticus and hyperventilation)
- Characteristic pathologic findings [elevations in arterial ammonia and an abnormal electroencephalography (EEG)]
- A favorable response to appropriate therapy in most patients.

Hepatic encephalopathy should be a clinical diagnosis and can be easily made by the astute clinician. If the patient has evidence of liver disease by either physical examination or laboratory features and has any of the above-mentioned features, the diagnosis should be made and therapy instituted. Obtaining an EEG or arterial pneumonia is not usually necessary.

The precipitating causes of hepatic encephalopathy and their presumed mechanism are shown in Table 19.1. They are nitrogenous or non-nitrogenous. Examples of the former include dietary protein, constipation,

Table 19.1: Causes of hepatic encephalopathy and their mechanism.	
Cause	Presumed mechanism
Gastrointestinal bleeding	Substrate for increased production of ammonia and other nitrogenous toxins. 100 mL of blood = 15–20 g protein. Contribution of ammonia in stored blood. *Hypovolemia*—decreased hepatic, cerebral, and renal perfusion
Sedatives and tranquilizers	Hypoxia from depression of respiratory center. Direct depressant effect on brain.
Constipation	Increased production and absorption of toxins (e.g. ammonia) due to increased contact time between nitrogenous substances in gut and intestinal bacteria. Straining leads to increased portal pressure and may induce variceal rupture.
Uremia (spontaneous or diuretic)	Increased enterohepatic circulation of urea nitrogen with increased ammonia production. Direct depressant effect of uremia. Increased renal vein ammonia output if alkalosis present. Hypovolemia (overvigorous diuresis) leads to decreased vital organ perfusion.
Infection	Increased tissue metabolism, leading to increased endogenous nitrogenous load, and increased ammonia production, hypoxemia, and hyperthermia augment ammonia toxicity.
Excess dietary protein	Increased substrate for ammonia production

GI bleeding, uremia, and infection. Non-nitrogenous precipitants include sedative drugs, hepatocellular injury, and infection.

Treatment

- Identify and correct precipitating factors.
- Dietary protein restriction is instituted for patients with stage 1 and 2 encephalopathy. For patients with Stage 3 or 4 encephalopathy, protein intake is withheld and then reinstituted in slow increments (10–20 g/day) every 3-5 days as the patient's condition improves (Table 19.2). Some patients better tolerate vegetable proteins.
- Cleansing the bowel is important. Lactulose is administered in a daily dose of 60–120 mL in divided amounts to promote 2 or 3 soft stools daily. In patients with coma, lactulose may be given as an enema of 300 mL in 700 mL of water.
- *Caution:* Lactulose can precipitate or worsen hepatorenal syndrome. In refractory cases, neomycin 1 g per oral (po) may be given bid.
- Experimental agents that appear promising include benzodiazepine receptor antagonists such as flumazenil.

Table 19.2: Stages of hepatic encephalopathy.				
Stage	Mental state	Asterixis	EEG	% mortality*
I	Loss of affect, depression, and altered sleep pattern	(±)	Normal	20
II	Confusion, disorientation, and drowsiness	(+)	Abnormal	60
III	Stuporous, incoherent but arousable	(+)	Abnormal	60
IV	Not arousable, decerebrate or decorticate posturing	Not testable	Abnormal	80

(EEG: electroencephalography)
*Applicable to patients with massive hepatic necrosis. Age of patient is important prognostic indicator. Mortality rate higher in patients over 40 years of age.

HEPATOBILIARY MANIFESTATIONS OF AIDS

Hepatobiliary disorders are frequently encountered in patients with acquired immunodeficiency syndrome (AIDS). This phenomenon is undoubtedly a reflection of the profound immunosuppression present in these patients and leads to the ↑ed propensity for a multitude of opportunistic infections and neoplasms. In addition, the epidemiologic risks for AIDS, such as homosexuality and IV drug abuse, expose the patient to a variety of infectious processes that can occur prior to the onset of AIDS. Laboratory assessment of hepatic function discloses abnormalities in the vast majority of patients. At times, the hepatic or biliary disorder is asymptomatic or trivial in its significance, while in other instances, it is the cause of significant morbidity and even mortality.

Hepatitis B

Worldwide, the annual number of deaths attributable to viral hepatitis rose by 63% from 1990 to 2013—from 8,95,000 to 14,54,000—according to a Lancet study.
- Hepatitis B and C accounted for 96% of hepatitis mortality in 2013; most hepatitis deaths occurred in East Asia.
- Hepatitis was the seventh leading cause of death and disability in 2013—up from tenth in 1990 and ahead of AIDS, malaria, and tuberculosis.

The lead researcher said, "We have tools at our disposal to treat this disease, we have vaccines to hepatitis A and B, and we have new treatments to C. However, the price of new medicines is beyond the reach of any country—rich or poor".
- Markers of HBV infection are very common in patients with AIDS. Serologic evidence of past or current HBV infection is present in 80-95% of patients. Most of these markers reflect previous (80%) rather than active (10-20%) infection.
- Patients with established HIV infection who subsequently become infected with HBV have a substantially ↑ed risk of becoming chronic

HBV carriers compared with HIV seronegative controls. However, despite active HBV replication, patients have minimal biochemical and histologic signs of inflammation.
- The immunologic impairment secondary to HIV infection appears to be responsible for the attenuated clinical course of acute and chronic HBV infection seen in these patients.
- Fulminant viral hepatitis B in a patient with AIDS has been reported in the setting of hepatitis Delta virus coinfection.
- In a recent study, the prevalence of hepatitis B surface antigen (HBsAg) was more than twice as great (10.7% vs. 4.7%; $p < 0.02$) in patients with AIDS compared with human immunodeficiency virus (HIV) positive patients without AIDS. However, survival of HBsAg positive patients was similar to that of HBsAg negative patients. These findings support the notion that patients with the more advanced immunosuppression characteristic of AIDS are more likely to have reactivation of latent HBV infection, are less likely to clear HBV infection after exposure, or both. However, survival was not influenced in either group by the presence of HBsAg.

Hepatitis C

Voelker provides an excellent JAMA review article for Hepatitis C, an 8-week cure.
- Hepatitis C virus infection is common in patients who are HIV positive. In about 15% of HIV positive patients, the HCV antibody is positive. Of these patients, 50% have hepatitis C viremia.
- Recent studies suggest that there is a tendency for HIV positive patients to have higher levels of viremia.
- Severe liver disease with rapid progression to cirrhosis and liver failure has been noted in some patients with both HIV and HCV antibody positivity
- There is limited data on the efficacy of alpha-interferon in the treatment of such patients. In a recently published study, 4 of 12 patients had a complete response, while 3 of 12 had a near-complete response. However, a sustained response, that is, persistently normal liver function tests (LFTs) after cessation of interferon treatment, was only seen in a single patient.

New Drug

- The Food and Drug Administration (FDA) approved a second medication for HCV infection. The newer entry into the treatment arena is the first drug capable of suppressing viral load to undetectable levels in only 8 weeks (marketed as Mavyret).
- The recently approved medication is a combination of glecaprevir and pibrentasvir. Clinical trials involving about 2,300 adults with any of the six HCV genotypes showed that 92% or more who received the combination for 8, 12, or 16 weeks had no detectable virus in their blood 12 weeks after treatment ended, suggesting their infections were cured.

Other Infections

- Approximately, 30–50% of liver biopsies performed in patients with AIDS will yield evidence of an infectious organism. Infections may be multiple.
- *Mycobacterium avium-intracellulare* (MAI), *Cytomegalovirus* (CMV), *Mycobacterium tuberculosis*, *Pneumocystis carinii*, histoplasmosis, cryptococcosis, leishmaniasis, coccidioidomycosis and microsporidiosis, have all been reported.
- *Mycobacterium avium-intracellulare* is often associated with a substantial elevation of the serum alkaline phosphatase (mean 750 IU/L) and a normal serum bilirubin. Pathologically, there may be granulomas which are often poorly formed. Occasionally, the cultures will be positive with no tissue evidence of infection. This has been seen with MAI and tuberculosis.
- Hepatosplenomegaly is commonly present in patients with MAI infections. 80% of MAI-infected individuals have liver involvement at autopsy. Currently, recommended regimens for the treatment of MAI include a combination of amikacin, rifampin (or rifabutin), ethambutol, and ciprofloxacin.

Peliosis Hepatis

- Sinusoidal dilation, perisinusoidal fibrosis, and peliosis hepatis are frequently encountered in patients with AIDS.
- The lesion consists of multiple, small, and blood-filled cystic spaces in the liver without zonal predominance.
- Patients frequently have hepatomegaly and splenomegaly.
- On average, the serum ALT and AST are twice the upper limit of normal, and the serum alkaline phosphatase is five times the upper limit of normal. The serum bilirubin is normal or slightly elevated,
- Both peliosis hepatis and cutaneous bacillary angiomatosis have been reported in patients with HIV infection.
- Recent evidence suggests that peliosis hepatis is due to a *Rickettsia*-like organism closely related to *Rochalimaea quintana*. Patients may respond favorably to erythromycin.

Tumors

- Neoplastic lesions are present in 10–20% of liver biopsies.
- Kaposi's sarcoma (KS) is a frequent finding at autopsy but is rarely seen at liver biopsy lymphomas both of the Hodgkin's and non-Hodgkin's variety also frequently involve the liver.
- Patients with non-Hodgkin's lymphoma involving the liver have a marked elevation of the serum alkaline phosphatase (mean 900 IU/L) and a mild elevation of the serum bilirubin (4 mg/dL).
- Primary bile duct lymphoma has also been described.

Box 19.3: Biliary system in AIDS.
- Acalculous cholecystitis
- Sclerosing cholangitis
- Papillary stenosis
- Bile duct lymphoma

(AIDS, acquired immunodeficiency syndrome)

Biliary System in AIDS

Disorders of the biliary system noted in patients with AIDS are listed in Box 19.3.

Acalculous Cholecystitis

The triad of right upper quadrant (RUQ) abdominal pain, fever, and an elevated serum alkaline phosphatase is present in a number of syndromes which on occasion overlap.
- The range of symptoms includes mild RUQ pain, evaluation of which may reveal thickening of the gallbladder wall on sonographic examination, as well as fulminant gangrenous cholecystitis.
- Acalculous cholecystitis has been associated with CMV, *Cryptosporidiosis*, *Candida*, *Campylobacter*, and *Serratia*.
- Both acute and chronic changes may be present at the time of histologic examination. The gallbladder mucosa is often hemorrhagic, with focal punctuate ulcers and exudates. Severe necrotizing inflammation can be present in patients with acalculous cholecystitis secondary to CMV. The characteristic inclusions can be seen in epithelial and endothelial cells.

Sclerosing Cholangitis

- Patients may be asymptomatic or have mild symptoms. On occasion patients can have severe RUQ or epigastric pain with nausea and vomiting.
- It may be complicated by acute polymicrobial cholangitis and sepsis.
- Some patients have accompanying papillary stenosis.
- Sclerosing cholangitis has been reported in patients with CMV, *Cryptosporidiosis*, MAI, and microsporidia.
- Endoscopic retrograde cholangiopancreatography (ERCP) reveals the characteristic picture with strictures, dilation, and ulcerations of the biliary tree.
- Endoscopic sphincterotomy has resulted in symptomatic improvement in some patients. Rapid drainage of contrast material can be achieved with successful sphincterotomy. Although the serum alkaline phosphatase will decline in some patients, in others it will continue to rise and

may reflect intrahepatic disease that is not benefited by endoscopic sphincterotomy or coinfection with intrahepatic MAI.

Papillary Stenosis

- Patients with papillary stenosis have a similar clinical presentation to those with sclerosing cholangitis.
- The ERCP reveals stenosis of the distal common bile duct that may extend to the intraduodenal segment.
- Biopsies of the ampulla have revealed the characteristic CMV inclusions in some patients.
- Some patients have both sclerosing cholangitis and papillary stenosis.
- Patients may benefit by the endoscopic placement of a biliary stent or from a sphincterotomy. These procedures may need to be repeated.

Hepatobiliary abnormalities are common in patients with AIDS. Patients may be asymptomatic or have severe and disabling symptoms. The liver may be the site for a multitude of infections that are often part of a disseminated process. In addition, neoplastic lesions such as KS and lymphoma are frequently present. An intriguing lesion is peliosis hepatis, which was seen in the past with another chronic wasting disorder, namely, tuberculosis, as well as with the use of androgenic anabolic steroids. However, the peliosis hepatis noted in patients with AIDS appears to be uniquely associated with the presence of a Rickettsia-like organism. The spectrum of extrahepatic biliary involvement encountered in patients with AIDS includes acalculous cholecystitis, sclerosing cholangitis, and ampullary stenosis.

In approaching these patients, the differential diagnosis of abnormalities of LFTs should be noted. It is worth remembering that there is no specific pattern of biochemical abnormality that points to a particular disease process. However, marked elevations of the serum alkaline phosphatase with mild-to-modest hyperbilirubinemia or a markedly elevated serum lactate dehydrogenase (LDH) should suggest the possibility of lymphoma. Radiographic studies, such as hepatobiliary iminodiacetic acid (HIDA) scan, ultrasonography, and CT, may provide important clues favoring a diagnosis of acalculous cholecystitis or sclerosing cholangitis with or without ampullary stenosis. Fundoscopic examination (looking for CMV retinitis), blood cultures, and bone marrow examination may be helpful in suggesting a diagnosis. If these tests point to a specific diagnosis, treatment can then be initiated. Often the LFT abnormalities will improve or resolve and one can infer that the same process that was occurring elsewhere in the body was also affecting the liver. In patients with unexplained abnormal elevations of LFT and symptoms, a liver biopsy should be performed. The diagnosis may offer important prognostic insight. On occasions, therapy can result in substantial palliation of the patient's symptoms. Liver biopsy may be accompanied by an ↑ed bleeding risk in patients with AIDS; prior to performing this procedure, or an endoscopic sphincterotomy, it is prudent to check the routine coagulation parameters as well as a bleeding time.

LIVER ABSCESS

Diagnosis

Liver abscesses are classified by etiologic agent as pyogenic or amebic.
- Pyogenic abscesses may be extremely elusive with little more than fever, chills, leukocytosis, and modest changes in LFTs, especially the alkaline phosphatase. Some patients have positive blood cultures.
- The diagnosis is usually established with CT scans. The microbiology may be established with percutaneous aspiration. Detection of *E. histolytica* is generally based on serology (complement fixation, indirect hemagglutination, or gel-diffusion-precipitin test); stool examination for ova and parasite is occasionally positive.
- Many patients will have a history of presence in countries where amebiasis is prevalent. Thus, the diagnosis of liver abscess is suspected in the patient with high fever [often fever of unknown origin (FUO)], hepatomegaly and/or RUQ tenderness, and abnormal LFTs (especially alkaline phosphatase elevation and hypoalbuminemia).
- The diagnosis is generally confirmed with CT scans or ultrasound of the abdomen showing typical ring-enhancing lesions of the liver. The microbiologic diagnosis is established by blood cultures for pyogenic bacteria and serology for *E. histolytica*; needle aspiration of an abscess may be required.
- The distinction between pyogenic and amebic abscess is important because the role of surgery, the selection of antibiotics and the prognosis are very different.

Treatment of amebic abscesses—metronidazole (750 mg tid or 500 mg IV q 6 hours) for 5-10 days. Oral absorption is nearly 100%, so po preferred.
- The alternative is emetine (1 mg/kg/day to a maximum of 65 mg) for 10 days or chloroquine (250 mg qid for 7 days followed by 250 mg bid for 3-4 weeks).
- A luminal amebicide such as diiodohydroxyquin should be given concurrently to eliminate cysts. Needle aspiration is not indicated except to establish the diagnosis, for some large abscesses (greater than 10 cm in diameter), for impending rupture, or for failure to respond after 5 days of antibiotic treatment.
- Most patients respond rapidly and completely; surgery is rarely required. Treatment of pyogenic abscesses—drainage is often required although the frequency is debated.
- Some patients have multiple small abscesses which cannot be drained. The prognosis is variable, but most patients with a single abscess do well

and those with multiple small abscesses do poorly. Various authorities recommend three fundamentally different approaches:
- *Antibiotics alone*: Often advocated for patients who have multiple small abscesses which cannot be drained surgically or for patients who show an impressive clinical response to antibiotic treatment during diagnostic evaluation.
- *Antibiotics combined with needle aspiration:* This affords the opportunity to define bacterial pathogens and to decompress large abscesses.
- Antibiotics combined with surgical drainage or drainage with a tube placed by CT, ultrasound, or fluoroscopic guidance. This is traditional management.

Antibiotic selection: The dominant bacteria are coliforms (especially *E. coli* and *Klebsiella*), streptococci (especially *S. milleri* and anaerobic streptococci), *Enterococcus* and anaerobes (especially Fusobacteria and *Bacteroides* species).
- Empiric antibiotics are directed against these organisms. Regimens that include metronidazole have the advantage of including treatment against *E. histolytica* if suspended—metronidazole (500 mg po or IV q 6-8 hours) or clindamycin (600 mg IV q 8 hours) *plus* gentamicin or tobramycin (2.0 mg/kg IV; the 1.7 mg/kg q 8 hours) or 3rd-generation cephalosporins such as ceftazidime (1.5-2 g q 8-12 hours) or ceftriaxone (1-2 g q 24 hours) *plus* ampicillin (2 g IV q 6 hours) or aminoglycosides such as gentamicin or tobramycin (2.0 mg/kg IV then 1.7 mg/kg q 8 hours) *plus* antipseudomonad penicillin such as piperacillin (4-5 g IV q 6 hours).

CHOLECYSTITIS

Diagnosis

Typical symptoms are acute RUQ pain, anorexia, nausea, vomiting, and fever (about 38°C). Examination shows RUQ tenderness, guarding, and Murphy's sign (increased tenderness with palpation in subhepatic area during deep inspiration).
- Over 95% have stones that are most easily and reliably detected with ultrasonography.
- Radionuclide scan of the gallbladder with ^{99}Tc DISIDA or related compounds is the preferred method to confirm the diagnosis; filling of the gallbladder makes the diagnosis unlikely.

Treatment

Supportive measures: Nasogastric suction and IV hydration—antibiotics:
- Early in cholecystitis the gallbladder is sterile; within a week the gallbladder is infected in 30-50% of cases. The primary pathogens in

rank order are *E. coli,* other coliforms (*Klebsiella, Enterobacter,* etc.), *Streptococcus, Enterococcus* and *Clostridium* species.
- Anaerobic bacteria are infrequent except with ascending cholangitis. Although bile is sterile in about 50% of gallbladders resected for acute cholecystitis, infection is responsible for some of the major complications-empyema, gangrene, and perforation. Suggested antibiotics are—ampicillin (2 g IV q 6-8 hours) *plus* gentamicin or tobramycin (2.0 mg/kg IV, then 1.7 mg/kg q 8 hours), *or* cefoperazone (1-2 g IV q 12 hours) alone or in combination with gentamicin or tobramycin. Other second- or third-generation cephalosporins are probably equally effective.

Surgery

Surgeons continue to debate the relative merits of early or late surgical intervention. *Advantages of early intervention* (within 1-2 days of onset of symptoms) are—the procedure is as safe as with delayed procedures; resection is easier without fibrosis, the duration of hospitalization and recovery is reduced, delay may overlook serious complications such as empyema or perforation; and the disease may recur during the waiting period. *Advantages of delayed intervention* are—the patient will be in optimal condition, there is time to clearly establish the diagnosis, resection may be easier if acute inflammation has resolved and the frequency of postoperative complications is reduced.

Laparoscopic surgery is now the intervention of choice in most patients.

BIBLIOGRAPHY

1. Abul-Husn NS, Cheng X, Li AH, et al. A protein-truncating HSD17B13 variant and protection from chronic liver disease. N Engl J Med. 2018;378:1096-106.
2. Bartlett JG. Infectious Diseases. In: Khan MG, Bartlett JG, Chopra S, Topol EJ. Medical Diagnosis and Therapy. Philadelphia; Lea and Febiger; 1994.
3. Choi IJ, Kook MC, Kim YI, et al. *Helicobacter pylori* therapy for the prevention of metachronous gastric cancer. N Engl J Med. 2018;378:1085-95.
4. Chopra S. Liver Diseases. In: Khan MG, Bartlett JG, Chopra S, Topol EJ (Es). Medical Diagnosis and Therapy. Philadelphia: Lea and Febiger; 1994.
5. Ge PS, Runyon BA. Treatment of patients with cirrhosis. N Engl J Med. 2016;375:767-77.
6. Herman O, Sadoughi S. (2016) Global Burden of Viral Hepatitis Rose Sharply Over Past Two Decades. [online] available from http://response.jwatch.org/t?ctl=B61F:F82014DE957000380DBA18BD126FE472&. [Accessed August, 2018].
7. Petersen M, Balzer L, Kwarsiima D, et al. Association of implementation of a universal testing and treatment intervention with HIV diagnosis, receipt of antiretroviral therapy, and viral suppression in East Africa. JAMA. 2017;317(21):2196-206.
8. Voelker R. The 8-week cure for hepatitis C. JAMA. 2017;318(11):996.

CHAPTER 20

Neurologic Disorders

COMA

Altered consciousness or loss of consciousness is one of the most worrisome of neurologic problems. Therapy is dictated by the etiology, and rapidity of diagnosis is essential for a good prognosis. In many cases, the pattern of progression or resolution of the problem is highly informative (Lechtenberg)

To help monitor the severity of altered consciousness, several rating scales have been developed. The one most widely used is the Glasgow coma scale; on this scale a low score (0-7) correlates with profoundly impaired consciousness or severe psychiatric disturbance.

Glasgow coma scale: The unimpaired individual scores 15.
- *Verbal response:*
  - Orientated—5
  - Disorientated but in context—4
  - Inappropriate words—3
  - Incomprehensible sounds—2
  - Mute—2.
- *Motor response:*
  - Obeys verbal instruction—6
  - Localizes to stimulus—5
  - Withdraws from noxious stimulus—4
  - Postures with arm flexion—3
  - Postures with arm extension—2
  - No response to noxious stimulus—1.
- *Eye opening:*
  - Spontaneous—4
  - With verbal inducement—3
  - With pain—2
  - No voluntary eye opening—1.

If a history can be obtained, items of special interest include a history of substance abuse; prescription drug use; chronic diseases, such as diabetes mellitus and epilepsy; and head trauma. The examination must include a rigorous search for evidence of head trauma, substance abuse,

Table 20.1: Eye signs in comatose patients.

Clinical finding	Possible causes
• Pupils midposition (4–6 mm) and fixed	Midbrain damage
• Pupils dilated and fixed unilaterally	Third nerve damage
• Pupils dilated and fixed bilaterally	Uncal herniation
• Pupils small and reactive	Protracted anoxia
	Methyl alcohol
	Scopolamine
• Disconjugate gaze	Metabolic encephalopathy
	Opiates or opioids
	Pontine damage
	Diencephalic damage
• Absence of all eye movements	Cranial nerve damage
	Brainstem damage
	Pontine damage
	Metabolic encephalopathy
	Drug overdose

Source: Lechtenberg R. In: Khan. MDT. Philadelphia: Lea & Febiger; 1994.

and metabolic problems. The possibility of a psychiatric disturbance, such as catatonia, must be kept in mind, but no case of altered consciousness should be dismissed as a purely psychiatric problem even if the patient has a history of schizophrenia or severe depressive reactions (Lechtenberg).

Pay special attention to eye signs (Table 20.1).

- *Blood from the ears*—consider probable evidence of a basilar skull fracture until proven otherwise.
- *Fluid from the nose*—should be checked for glucose to determine whether or not it is cerebrospinal fluid (CSF) leaking through a meningeal tear.

Unless there is reason not to expect alcohol abuse, the patient should be given thiamine 100 mg intravenous (IV) prior to dextrose (see Wernicke's encephalopathy below). Hypoglycemia should be assessed as part of the examination with a bedside test.

- In addition to routine blood chemistries, arterial blood gases (ABGs) and hematologic studies, in case of unexplained coma, the patient's urine should be screened for amphetamines, barbiturates, cocaine, opiates, opioids, and any substances that are abuse problems in the region. A blood alcohol level may be informative, if the patient's breath smells of ethanol. An electrocardiogram (ECG) should be obtained routinely to look for arrhythmias. The stomach contents should be pumped out and examined.
- With coma or even transient loss of consciousness associated with head trauma, a computed tomography (CT) or magnetic resonance imaging (MRI) scan should be obtained. This is cost-effective because substantial head trauma or intracranial abnormalities is less likely to be missed.

Benign intracranial findings will support the decision to allow the patient to leave the hospital. Traditionally, X-rays and observation are used to screen patients with head trauma or other causes of transient loss of consciousness. During observation, other tests may be obtained, but the presumption is that significant intracranial problems, such as subdural hematomas, cerebral contusions, and meningeal tears, will be obvious after 24–48 hours of observations. With MRI and CT techniques, the likelihood of significant intracranial lesions can be much more directly assessed. The patient who has a brief (15 minutes) loss of consciousness after head trauma, but a normal CT or MRI scan may more confidently be sent home to be watched by a friend or relative than the individual assessed with little more than a skull X-ray and careful physical examination. Because a basilar skull fracture may be inapparent on a CT scan, many physicians recommend getting a skull X-ray with basilar views to further assess the victim of head trauma if the CT is negative.

Further studies and therapy should be performed as dictated by the probable cause of the coma. However, the physician must maintain adequate ventilation, circulation, and body.

EPILEPSY

Seizures are episodes of disorganized electrical activity in the brain. This disorganized electrical activity may produce loss of consciousness, alteration of consciousness, focal sensory disturbances, focal motor activity, inappropriate affective displays, or other neurologic or psychologic phenomena. These signs of disorganized electrical activity may occur individually or in combination.

A careful patient history and physical examination, electroencephalography, and brain imaging are necessary to separate patients with acute symptomatic seizures, single unprovoked seizures, and nonepileptic events from those with new-onset epilepsy.

Diagnosis

Seizures are considered generalized or partial according to whether or not the electrical disturbance in the cortex appears to arise diffusely or focally. Generalized seizures described as tonic-clonic involve loss of consciousness and transient tonic muscle contractions followed by transient clonic muscle contractions. With some generalized seizures, such as generalized absence seizures, the loss of consciousness may be so brief and so isolated that it goes unrecognized. Some types of partial seizures need not involve loss of consciousness, but those described as complex partial seizures invariably involve alteration or loss of consciousness.

Table 20.2: Antiepileptic dosage for adults.

Drug name	Brand name	Usual dose (mg/kg/day)	Therapeutic level (mg/mL)	Days to steady state	Serum half-life (hrs)
Carbamazepine	Tegretol	10-25	6-12	3-6	8-19
Valproate	Depakote	10-70	50-100	2-4	7-17
Valproic acid	Depakene	10-70	50-100	2-4	7-17
Phenytoin	Dilantin	4-10	10-20	5-10	22-40
Ethosuximide	Zarontin	20-40	40-100	6-12	50-60
Primidone	Mysoline	10-25	6-12	1-5	8-16
Phenobarbital	—	1-5	15-35	16-21	50-96
Clonazepam	Klonopin	0.03-0.10	.013-.072	6	16-60

Pathophysiology

Seizures are assumed to arise because of disorganized electrical activity in the cerebral cortex. The many forms that seizures assume suggest that more than 1 defect underlie this problem. This idea is supported by the vast differences in treatability exhibited by different types of seizures.

Therapy

Recurrent seizures often prompt visits to emergency rooms but are not usually true emergencies. The patient who has a seizure because of poor compliance with medication instructions often needs little more than a change in drug regimen to ensure better compliance (Table 20.2). Drug levels should be checked at the time of the seizure recurrence, and a routine reevaluation of the patient's overall health status is appropriate, but IV or intramuscular (IM) administration of antiepileptic medications is usually unnecessary and inappropriate (Lechtenberg).

DRUG-RELATED SEIZURES

Seizures may develop because of withdrawal from or intoxication with drugs, the most common of which is ethanol.

Diagnosis

Many patients exhibit signs of drug use when they present with drug-related seizures, but toxicologic screens may be needed to establish which drug was taken closest to the time of seizure. Signs of alcohol use do not ↓ the probability of concurrent cocaine or opiate use. If a consistent history of ethanol or cocaine use can be established, the seizure should be assumed to be related to use of the substance most implicated and treated accordingly.

Other causes or consequences of seizures, such as subarachnoid hemorrhage, meningitis, or post-traumatic epilepsy, should not be dismissed simply because circumstantial evidence points convincingly at substance abuse.

Pathophysiology

Seizures are presumed to occur with neuroexcitatory agents, such as amphetamines and cocaine, because of a direct effect of the substances on neurotransmitters in the brain. Inhibitory circuits responsible for coordinating neural activity may be disturbed by the stimulant drugs. A similar mechanism is also presumed for seizures that develop because of withdrawal from depressant drugs.

With barbiturate or benzodiazepine withdrawal, excess membrane channels created by neurons to deal with the burden of drug-related ion channel blockade may seriously impair maintenance of ion balances across the cell membranes. With ethanol abuse, changes in membrane channel populations are established, and seizures with ethanol withdrawal are assumed to develop because ion disequilibrium develops as channels blocked by ethanol becomes active.

Therapy (For Adults Only)

- *Ethanol withdrawal*: Administer 100 mg thiamin IV prior to dextrose infusion and for more than or equal to 2 days thereafter. Detoxify with chlordiazepoxide 25–100 mg po four to six times daily.
- *Barbiturate withdrawal*: Administer phenobarbital 200 mg IV acutely. Give phenobarbital 100 mg IV or po once daily for 2 days after the seizure. Taper by 35 mg qd over the subsequent 3 days.
- *Cocaine, amphetamines, and methaqualone:* Stabilize autonomic functions. Monitor cardiac function closely and intervene if arrhythmias develop. Hold antiepileptic medication unless more than 1 seizure occurs. Phenobarbital 100 mg IV for 2 days, if recurrent seizures develop. Taper phenobarbital with IV or po doses over the course of 3 days (Lechtenberg).

Cannabidiol for Refractory Epilepsy

A branded formulation of cannabidiol has now turned up positive results in three randomized controlled trials—one in Dravet syndrome and two in Lennox-Gastaut disease. Updated findings from two of those trials were reported at the 2016 American Epilepsy Society meeting.

"The bottom line is that cannabidiol works", Orrin Devinsky, MD, of NYU Langone Medical Center in New York City, who is a coauthor on the Dravet study, told *MedPage Today* during the meeting, "There are side effects, but the overall safety and tolerability are good, especially compared with other antiepileptic drugs."

Drug maker GW pharmaceuticals expect to file a new drug application with the Food and Drug Administration (FDA) for the drug in mid-2017, with hopes to be on the market the following year.

"So much has been written about medical marijuana with so little hard science behind it", said Gregory Barkley, MD, of Henry Ford Hospital in Detroit. "It is nice to see a company doing the testing the time-honored way".

FEBRILE SEIZURES

A seizure associated with high fever may be a sign of meningitis or encephalitis in adults but is more likely benign when it occurs in children. These childhood febrile seizures are considered simple if they are not likely to manifest debilitating central nervous system (CNS) disease or epilepsy.

Diagnosis

For the child less than 5 years old, simple febrile seizures are:
- Generalized, tonic-clonic movements may be observed in all limbs, and focal weakness is not evident during the postictal period.
- Seen between 1 year and 5 years of age. Seizures with fever before 6 months of age must be assumed to be a consequence of meningitis or encephalitis.
- No more than 15 minutes long. The postictal period may extend for several minutes or hours after the obvious seizure ictus, but the ictus itself should persist for less than 15 minutes.
- Associated with a normal neurologic examination
- Unassociated with a family history of epilepsy.

Complex febrile seizures are:
- Complex partial or simple (usually focal motor) seizures.
- Apparent before 1 year of age. Seizures in feverish children who are more than 5 years old must be viewed with as much suspicion as fever-associated seizures in adults.
- Longer than 15 minutes in duration.
- Associated with a persistent neurologic deficit.
- Associated with a family history of epilepsy.

Complex febrile seizures must be investigated aggressively with metabolic, electroencephalographic, bacteriologic, and neuroimaging studies. Simple febrile seizures are usually not investigated beyond metabolic and electroencephalographic studies (Lechtenberg).

Pathophysiology

The cause of simple febrile seizures is unknown. The susceptibility of the young child's brain to pyrexia is presumed to be related to its immaturity.

Therapy

- *Simple febrile seizures*: Antipyretics, such as acetaminophen orally or by suppository, alcohol rubs, and cooling baths.
- *Complex febrile seizures*: Antiepileptic medication (phenobarbital and valproate sodium); treat cause if established.

STATUS EPILEPTICUS

Diagnosis

Status epilepticus is seizure activity that is unremitting. The patient does not recover from the postictal state before the next seizure occurs. The most common, obvious, and lethal form of status epilepticus is tonic-clonic status. The most common settings for status epilepticus are after withdrawal of antiepileptic medications (patient compliance problems), with substance abuse (alcohol or barbiturate use especially), and with new onset seizure activity (previously undiagnosed epilepsy). Individuals with no prior history of seizures who develop status epilepticus should be investigated for intracranial lesions, such as neoplasms and arteriovenous (AV) malformations; metabolic disturbances, such as hyperglycemia and hyponatremia; acute infections, such as meningitis and encephalitis; and substance abuse.

Pathophysiology

The physiologic basis for status epilepticus is unknown. Presumably, inhibitory controls over some neural circuits are completely disabled, and disorganized neuronal activity continues unabated after the initial episode occurs.

Therapy

Status epilepticus is a potentially lethal condition, so the management of this problem must be aggressive and comprehensive (Box 20.1). Autonomic problems associated with status epilepticus include hyperthermia, blood pressure (BP) instability, and impaired respiratory control (Lechtenberg).
- Breathing disturbances are usually quite obvious, but not usually life-threatening. Many clinicians intubate patients as soon as status epilepticus is diagnosed, but most patients do not require ventilatory support. Intubation may provide some protection against aspiration, but the principal advantage of the maneuver is to simplify mechanical ventilation, if respiratory depression develops during drug treatment.
- Hyperthermia should be managed with a cooling blanket and antipyretics.

Box 20.1: Treating patients with status epilepticus.

- Stabilize autonomic function.
- Check blood gases, glucose, electrolytes, magnesium, and calcium.
- Administer thiamine 100 mg IV if alcohol abuse is probable.
- Administer glucose as $D_{50}W$ in a 50-mL bolus IV if hypoglycemia is probable.
- Start intravenous antiepileptic medications.
- Intubate if respiratory effort is depressed.
- Monitor vital signs and cardiac rhythm.
- MRI or CT if cause not apparent.
- EEG if diagnosis is in doubt.

(CT, computed tomography; EEG, electroencephalogram; MRI, magnetic resonance imaging)

- Hypotension may develop with the seizure activity, but it is more commonly seen as a consequence of antiepileptic therapy. In any case, BP must be monitored and managed.
- Renal problems may develop secondary to myoglobinuria. This is especially likely with violent seizure activity that produces considerable muscle injury. Dehydration and hypovolemia must be avoided to minimize the risk of myoglobin accumulation in the kidneys.
- If hypoglycemia is probable, a 50 mL bolus of $D_{50}W$ should be given IV.
- If alcohol abuse is probable, thiamine 100 mg IV prior to dextrose should be given as soon as possible and repeated po qd for 3 days.

Drug therapy should be administered IV. The doses of antiepileptic medications used for status epilepticus are higher than those conventionally applicable in seizure management (Box 20.2). The physician should wait for more than or equal to 10 minutes, but no more than 20 minutes, between successive treatments to determine whether or not seizures are persisting.

- *Phenytoin:* Most clinicians use phenytoin as their first-choice drug in the management of status epilepticus. It is given IV up to a total daily dose of 20 mg/kg. Individual doses are usually about 500 mg (5–12 mg/kg) and are infused at a rate not more than 50 mg/min. This drug should be pushed directly into the IV line (albeit very slowly) to avoid its precipitation into holding chambers or IV bottles and to avoid accidental delivery of a bolus more rapidly than is appropriate (dilute in 0.9% NaCl; avoid mixing with dextrose to prevent precipitation; flush the vein immediately with saline to avoid thrombosis). After the first dose of phenytoin (500 mg), lorazepam or diazepam may be given. If seizures have not stopped after two or three boluses of benzodiazepine, the second dose (500 mg) of phenytoin may be administered. Contraindications—complete heart block, CHF. Do not administer concomitantly with dopamine or lidocaine.
- *Lorazepam and diazepam* are favored as second-choice drugs because of their rapid onset of action. They are cleared from the body much more quickly than phenytoin, and so phenytoin should be given first to provide continuing antiepileptic drug levels. Diazepam is given IV (never

Box 20.2: Antiepileptic medication for status epilepticus in adults.

- Phenytoin (Dilantin) 500 mg at no more than 50 mg/min IV
  - Repeat phenytoin 500 mg every 30 minutes until seizures stop up to maximum of 20 mg/kg/day.
- Lorazepam 5 mg at no more than 2 mg/min IV
  - Repeat lorazepam 5 mg IV every 10 minutes until seizures stop up to maximum of 0.1 mg/kg/day.
- Phenobarbital 260 mg at no more than 100 mg/min IV
  - Repeat phenobarbital 260 mg IV every 20 minutes until seizures stop up to a maximum of 20 mg/kg/day.
- Diazepam 10 mg at no more than 5 mg/min IV
  - Repeat diazepam 10 mg IV every 10 minutes until seizures stop up to a maximum of 0.25 mg/kg/day.
- Consider general anesthesia if all else fails.

(IV, intravenous)

IM) at a maximum daily dose of 0.25 mg/kg at an infusion rate of no more than 5 mg/min. Lorazepam is given IV at a maximum daily dose of 0.10 mg/kg at an infusion rate of not more than 2 mg/min. Diazepam is usually given in individual boluses of 10 mg with doses repeated q 10–20 minutes until seizure activity stops, autonomic problems (i.e. hypotension) develop, or a maximum dose (usually not more than a total of 40 mg in 1 day) has been administered. Lorazepam is usually administered in boluses of 5–7 mg.

- *Phenobarbital*: If phenytoin and a short-acting benzodiazepine have not stopped seizure activity, phenobarbital may be tried. This barbiturate is usually given in 260–300-mg boluses administered at a rate of 100 mg/min. The maximum tolerated dose is usually less than 1,200 mg or a total daily dose of less than 20 mg/kg. Successive doses of phenobarbital should be more than or equal to 20 minutes apart. Hypotension or respiratory depression is likely, if more than 1,000 mg of phenobarbital is delivered over the course of 1 hour.

If all these measures fail, the patient may need general anesthesia. Most anesthetic agents have little or no antiepileptic activity, but the anesthetic agent will at least alter brain activity and simplify immobilization of the patient.

WERNICKE'S ENCEPHALOPATHY

Diagnosis

Features of Wernicke's encephalopathy include:
- Abnormal eye movements, such as ophthalmoplegia, ophthalmoparesis, or nystagmus
- Altered mentation, such as obtundation, disorientation, apathy, or confabulation
- Gait disorders, such as ataxia or disturbed tandem gait.

More worrisome, but less constant features include dysautonomia with hypothermia and hypotension. Individuals with autonomic abnormalities are at more immediate risk of dying.

The severity of the syndrome is quite variable, and individuals with relatively mild cases may appear to recover substantially with little or no treatment. The individual at risk is usually one with a nutritional disturbance, either as a result of dietary habits or concurrent illness.

Pathophysiology

The underlying disorder is thiamin deficiency. Symptomatic individuals are most often alcoholic. An acute deterioration often occurs when the individual at risk is given IV glucose or dextrose. CNS lesions evident in patients dying from Wernicke's encephalopathy include hemorrhagic necrosis in periventricular thalamic and hypothalamic gray matter (especially in the mammillary bodies), periaqueductal gray matter, and brainstem and cerebellar midline structures. Acute changes are evident in these structures on MRI scanning, but are not usually apparent on CT scanning until hemorrhage into necrotic tissue is substantial.

Therapy

Any reason to suspect this potentially lethal condition justifies parenteral thiamine administration. Thiamine 100 mg IV should be given as soon as the condition is suspected. It is preferable to give the thiamine prior to the patient's receiving dextrose because a glucose challenge will often precipitate an acute attack of Wernicke's encephalopathy. Supplements of 50–100 mg of thiamine should be given po or IV for 3 days.

Ocular and gait changes are sensitive to even low doses of thiamine. Improvement of an ophthalmoplegia to slight nystagmus and of severe ataxia to a disturbance of tandem gait should not be taken as an indication of adequate treatment. If treatment is delayed or inadequate, cognitive changes may be permanently disabling, with amnestic syndromes the most apparent.

NEUROLEPTIC MALIGNANT SYNDROME

Diagnosis

Core features of neuroleptic malignant syndrome (NMS) include:
- Encephalopathy (disorientation, agitation, catatonia, and altered consciousness)
- Hyperthermia (fever)
- Dysautonomia (labile BP, tachycardia, diaphoresis, and cutaneous vasoconstriction)
- Muscular rigidity (lead-pipe rigidity and bradykinesia).

Occasional features include tremor, dyskinetic movements, sustained postures (waxy rigidity), gaze abnormalities, dysphagia, elevated creatine phosphokinase (CPK) myoglobinuria, and acute renal failure.
- The evolution of signs and symptoms may be limited to hours or develop over days. Most cases occur within the first 2 weeks after the start of neuroleptics.
- Neuroleptic malignant syndrome may develop with first exposure to neuroleptics at relatively low doses. Alternatively, it may evolve when the neuroleptic dose is ↑ed or the type of neuroleptic changed.
- Men are more commonly affected than women. The incidence for patients on neuroleptics is less than 1%. Patients with psychotic disorders are more at risk for the syndrome. Lethal catatonia is often indistinguishable from NMS. Malignant hyperthermia may also seem similar to NMS, but it invariably develops after exposure to an anesthetic agent and is not associated with the early appearance of encephalopathy and dysautonomia.
- Syndromes difficult to distinguish from NMS may develop with exposure to amphetamines; tricyclic antidepressants in combination with monoamine oxidase inhibitors, tryptophan, or lithium; cocaine; reserpine; or tetrabenazine, and with withdrawal from antiparkinsonian medications.

Pathophysiology

Neuroleptic agents probably act primarily on the D_2 dopamine receptor because they produce postsynaptic blockade and interfere with the dopaminergic system.
- Responsible neuroleptic agents include phenothiazines (especially fluphenazine), butyrophenones (especially haloperidol), and substituted benzamides (such as metoclopramide and droperidol).
- Neuroleptic malignant syndrome is an idiosyncratic reaction—it is not dose related.

Therapy

Without treatment, mortality is usually more than 20%. Death usually results from cardiopulmonary failure, aspiration pneumonia, or renal failure. Complications of NMS include disseminated intravascular coagulation, renal tubular acidosis, inappropriate antidiuretic hormone, hyperglycemia, and pancreatic necrosis. Most important in treatment is the withdrawal of the neuroleptic agent. The patient must be observed in a critical care unit (CCU) to manage the dysautonomia. Cooling blankets, rehydration, antipyretics, and other supportive measures should be instituted as problems appear. Pharmacotherapy of NMS includes using dantrolene or dopaminergic drugs (bromocriptine, L-DOPA, lisuride, pergolide, and amantadine). The dose of drug necessary to ↓ the NMS symptoms is usually arrived at empirically. The useful range of bromocriptine doses is from less than 10 mg qd to more than 100 mg qd. One dopaminergic agent may be effective when others are not. If dantrolene is used it may be given as 0.25 mg/kg IV bid.

MIGRAINE

Diagnosis

- Pain over one side of the head usually develops after premonitory signs. These signs may be transient visual obscurations or more dramatic focal neurologic deficits (hemiplegia and ophthalmoplegia).
- Aura symptoms may include visual disturbances (e.g. wavy lines or bright or dark spots), other sensory changes (e.g. numbness or tingling), language dysfunction, and vertigo. Cutaneous allodynia (the experience of normal touch as uncomfortable) is also a common component of a migraine attack.
- Multiple medications can exacerbate migraine, including oral contraceptives, postmenopausal hormone therapy, nasal decongestants, selective serotonin-reuptake inhibitor antidepressants, and proton-pump inhibitors. In some patients, the frequency and severity of attacks can be dramatically reduced by adjusting or discontinuing these medications (Charles).
- Women are more likely to be affected than men, and there often is a family history of similar attacks. Attacks usually begin during adolescence and abate in the sixth or seventh decade of life.
- The most common premonitory sign is an evolving scotoma, often surrounded by a scintillating border. The scotoma may enlarge over the course of 10–60 minutes. The pulsatile pain characteristic of the migraine usually develops as the premonitory signs resolve. Nausea and vomiting in association with the attacks is common.
- Symptoms during migraine attacks include photophobia, phonophobia, and irritability as well as headache.
- Other types of hemicranial pain include the cluster headache. This typically occurs in men, develops late at night, awakens the sufferer from sleep, and is associated with personality changes during the attack. The episodes usually start with pain behind one eye that extends to much of the rest of the hemicranium.

Pathophysiology

- Migraines are called vascular headaches and are assumed to arise with disturbances in the autoregulation of intracranial (and to a lesser extent extracranial) vasculature. A variety of neurotransmitters have been

implicated as participants in the evolution of the headaches, but none has been convincingly established as the cause.
- Inflammation around sensory nerves and dilation of large intracranial blood vessels may produce much of the pain that is experienced.
- The long-standing concept of migraine as primarily a vascular disorder, in which headache is caused by dilation of blood vessels and is throbbing in quality due to the vascular pulse, has been refuted by substantial evidence during the past two decades. It is now clear that constriction of blood vessels is not a required mechanism of therapies for migraine. Although migraine is associated with an increased relative risk of stroke and cardiovascular disease, the mechanisms underlying this association remain uncertain, and it is exceedingly rare for cerebral ischemia or infarction to occur during a migraine attack.

Neck pain is another common symptom of migraine, but it is frequently misinterpreted as a manifestation of a disorder in the cervical spine, often leading to unnecessary scans of this region.

Caffeine intake, sleep, and exercise are a sensible approach to reducing migraine frequency. There are, however, no randomized trials of skipped meals, irregular caffeine intake, irregular sleep, and stress are commonly identified as migraine triggers. Migraine attacks are more common before and during the menstrual period in women. These observations reinforce the concepts that migraine attacks may be precipitated by environmental or hormonal change and that day-to-day consistency of diet-lifestyle modifications to support the efficacy of any specific approach, such as caffeine withdrawal or dietary restrictions.

Multiple medications can exacerbate migraine, including oral contraceptives, postmenopausal hormone therapy, nasal decongestants, selective serotonin-reuptake inhibitor antidepressants, and proton pump inhibitors. In some patients, the frequency and severity of attacks can be dramatically reduced by adjusting or discontinuing these medications.

Therapy

Selected therapies for acute migraine—triptans [selective activators of the 5-hydroxytryptamine (5-HT), or serotonin, receptors of type 1B, 1D, and 1F] are effective in aborting an attack in the majority of patients with migraine, but clinical trials indicate that a minority of patients are pain-free by 2 hours.

Preventive therapies (e.g. beta-blockers, candesartan, tricyclic antidepressants, and anticonvulsant agents for chronic migraine) should be considered on the basis of the frequency and severity of attacks, response to medications for acute migraine, and coexisting conditions (Charles).

In clinical practice, a substantial percentage of patients report dissatisfaction with triptans because of a slow or incomplete response. For some, the addition of a nonsteroidal anti-inflammatory drug (NSAID) (including nonprescription preparations), or taking one of these medications independently, can be effective. Multiple ergotamine preparations are available, and IV dihydroergotamine in particular is a mainstay of treatment for refractory migraine in urgent care or inpatient settings.

- Ergotamine in various forms is the traditional therapy for acute attacks of migraine. It is available in oral, sublingual, intranasal, IM, and rectal preparations. It is often used in fixed combination with caffeine. The tolerable dose of ergotamine varies with the type of preparation, route of administration, and individual sensitivity. It is usually taken in multiple small doses, starting at the first indication of a migraine attack. The dose is titrated up to a maximum daily and maximum weekly allowance. For example, oral ergotamine tartrate 1 mg tablets should be taken no more than four times qd and no more than 2 days consecutively in any week. Individual doses of 1 or 2 mg may be repeated at 1- or 2-hour intervals during a migraine attack.
- More conventional analgesics, such as acetaminophen, naproxen, propoxyphene, and aspirin, and NSAIDs are sometimes useful for mild attacks.
- For many individuals, prophylaxis is simpler and more effective than treatment of an acute attack. Beta-adrenergic blocking agents, such as propranolol, have been especially useful, but they are contraindicated in individuals with chronic obstructive pulmonary disease (COPD). Low doses (propranolol 40-120 mg qd) are usually effective in susceptible individuals. The ergot alkaloid methysergide is useful in prophylaxis, but has been associated with some reports of retroperitoneal fibrosis. Some physicians use NSAIDs and amitriptyline, but the effectiveness of these agents is quite variable from individual to individual.
- Sumatriptan is a serotonin-receptor agonist, the drug seems to abort migraine episodes by acting selectively at 5-SRT_1 (A and D subtypes) receptors in the carotid circulation. The presumption is that sumatriptan inhibits the development of perivascular inflammation that evolves with inappropriate stimulation of pain fibers.
Dosage SQ (6-12 mg): Repeat in 1 hour. If needed; orally—100 mg tablet, maximum 300 mg/d. It appears effective in many individuals with either migraine or cluster headaches. Contraindications—angina or CRD.
- Therapies for acute migraine (e.g. triptans, NSAID, and antiemetic agents individually or in combination) should be taken as early as possible after the onset of a migraine attack.
- Preventive therapies (e.g. beta-blockers, candesartan, tricyclic antidepressants, and anticonvulsant agents as well as botulinum toxin for chronic migraine) should be considered on the basis of the frequency and severity of attacks, response to medications for acute migraine, and coexisting conditions.

- Recent clinical trials support the efficacy of new therapies targeting calcitonin gene-related peptide (CGRP) for the treatment of acute migraine and for migraine prevention.

All currently available preventive medication therapies for migraine were initially developed for other indications and have been secondarily adopted as treatments for migraine. Antihypertensive agents (e.g. beta-adrenergic blockers and candesartan), anticonvulsant agents (e.g. topiramate and divalproex sodium), and tricyclic antidepressants (e.g. amitriptyline and nortriptyline) are standard preventive therapies for migraine.

Selected Preventive Therapies for Migraine

For some patients, these agents can be highly effective, although the average difference in headache days per month between preventive therapies and placebo has been small in clinical trials. Adverse effects are common for most of the preventive therapies, and patients often report an initial response that "wears off" despite increasing doses. Adherence to treatment is generally poor.

DIZZINESS VERTIGO

Diagnosis

- Acute or chronic positional instability develops with damage to or irritation of the inner ear, the VIII cranial nerve, the brainstem, or the brain. Feelings of instability are usually considered dizziness. The perception of environmental movement in association with the feeling of instability is usually considered vertigo. Nausea and vomiting routinely occur with severe vertigo.
- If the vertigo that develops is short-lived and evident only when the head assumes certain positions, it is often classified as benign paroxysmal positional vertigo. With this type of vertigo, nystagmus can be consistently elicited when the head is positioned appropriately.
- Meniere syndrome is the association of recurrent episodes of vertigo with episodes of tinnitus and progressive hearing loss.
- Persistent vertigo should be investigated with CT and MRI studies of the posterior fossa. If structural lesions are not evident, the vertigo is probably attributable to labyrinthine damage or dysfunction. In patients at risk for ischemia, digital subtraction angiography or MRI angiography of the vertebrobasilar circulation may point to a vascular basis for the complaint.

Pathophysiology

- Most cases of dizziness or vertigo remain unexplained after routine evaluations. If the symptom remains independent of other more

localizing signs and symptoms, the patient should be periodically reassessed to be sure that a slowly evolving but treatable lesion, such as an acoustic schwannoma, is not responsible for the symptom.
- In any case of labyrinthine dysfunction, exposure to ototoxic drugs or other substances must be considered.
- An acute inflammatory lesion of the labyrinth (acute labyrinthitis) may produce a vertigo that is substantially exacerbated by abrupt changes in head position.
- Meniere's is often ascribed to an endolymphatic hydrops, but the underlying problem may be a disturbance of ion balance in the endolymph.
- Brainstem and cerebellar lesions routinely produce vertigo or dysequilibrium. With structural damage to these structures, instability may persist for years. Transient episodes may occur with ischemia.

Therapy

- Because the cause of dizziness or vertigo is often unknown, much of the treatment must be symptomatic. Antiemetic agents are helpful with vertigo severe enough to elicit vomiting. These medications include droperidol 2.5–5.0 mg IM, prochlorperazine 10 mg IM, and promethazine 25 mg PO or PR. Problems associated with these antiemetic agents include sedation, dystonia, and extrapyramidal reactions. Consequently, they should be used at the lowest feasible doses. Sublingual and rectal preparations are available for some of them.
- Drugs believed to act more directly on the labyrinth to suppress vertigo include diazepam 5–10 mg po, IM, or IV; meclizine 25 mg po, and dimenhydrinate 50 mg po. Scopolamine is also believed to suppress vertigo and is available as a patch.
- Meniere's syndrome may respond to diuretic [hydrochlorothiazide (HCTZ)] treatment, but many physicians will attempt an endolymphatic shunt to ↓ symptoms in long-suffering patients.
- Destruction of part of the vestibular nerve is sometimes attempted with intractable vertigo, but the risk of damaging the cochlear division of the auditory nerve is high, and the likelihood of permanently eliminating the vertigo is low. The vertigo may have started at the end organ and evolved as central (brainstem) mechanisms became disabled by the persistence of misleading sensory input.

TRANSIENT ISCHEMIC ATTACKS

Diagnosis

A transient ischemic attack (TIA) is an episode of focal neurologic deficit that lasts less than 24 hours and is caused by vascular insufficiency. Identifying a

TIA early is important because individuals suffering from them are at high risk of developing stroke. The intracranial problem may be secondary to acute myocardial infarction (MI), valvular heart disease, or arrhythmia. Diagnostic measures appropriate on an emergency basis include:

- Neuroimaging studies to establish that infarction has not occurred. A good MRI scan may detect ischemic damage as small as 5 mm across. This should be done as an emergency procedure the first time the patient presents with what appears to be a TIA, because cerebral, cerebellar, or brainstem infarction will require a different approach from that appropriate for a TIA.
- Screening blood and urine tests to establish that the focal deficits are not a result of a metabolic or hematologic disorder. Elderly individuals with severe anemia may develop focal neurologic deficits. Hyperglycemia, hyponatremia, and hypercalcemia may all produce neurologic changes easily confused with a TIA. Coagulopathies, vasculitides (systemic lupus), and hemoglobinopathies (sickle cell disease) must also be investigated
- Electrocardiogram to exclude MI or a cardiac arrhythmia; echocardiography and Holter monitoring are selectively requested.

Pathophysiology

The prevailing assumption is that TIA produces no structural damage, but improvements in neuroimaging have weakened this assumption. What can be said of structural CNS damage is that it is relatively occult and may only be evident in a redundant system, if the brain or spinal cord deteriorates.

Therapy

Attempts to arrive at a consensus on the management of TIAs have only emphasized the diversity of opinions in this area. Many physicians believe that TIAs suggestive of the carotid system should be managed with carotid endarterectomy. Most advocate some type of anticoagulation in the management. Typical approaches include:

- Reducing postural stress by keeping the patient recumbent. With focal ischemia, local autoregulation of blood flow is disturbed and postural changes may stress the ischemic tissue to the point that infarction occurs.
- Limiting serum glucose levels. Many investigators believe that abnormally high glucose levels may worsen the stress imposed upon neurons by ischemia. This means that glucose infusions are ill advised.
- Clopidogrel 75 mg or soft chew aspirin 80–81 mg daily is advisable (not enteric coated aspirin as it is less effective because of poor absorption).
- Hospitalizing the patient and monitoring the course of the TIA. In many cases, the patient presents after the episode has completely resolved, but observation is still warranted. How long the patient should be watched is controversial. After the first episode of TIA, recommendations range

from days to more than 1 week. If the patient has had several prior episodes of TIA, protracted observation is less warranted (and less likely to be acceptable to the patient), especially if the TIA is much the same each time it occurs. A change in the pattern of the TIA or a shortening of the interval between TIAs is more worrisome and should prompt closer observation of the patient.
- Carotid endarterectomy has been in and out of favor for several decades, but it is currently favored in cases of TIA or even nondisabling stroke in which a high-grade carotid stenosis is found on the same side as the neurologic deficits.
- Whether or not endarterectomy is being contemplated, the patient with TIAs should have an evaluation of the aortic arch and the vasculature supplying the head. Improvements in transcranial Doppler studies and MRI angiography have made this an increasingly atraumatic investigation. Problems with resolution of the blood vessels may ultimately require angiography, but vascular anomalies and large lesions should indicate considerably less invasive studies.
- Patients at risk for stroke and not on warfarin or heparin are usually given aspirin daily, in doses ranging from 80 qd to 325 mg tid. The addition of dipyridamole appears to have no clinical value in individuals with occlusive vascular disease. Ticlopidine 250 mg bid is advisable for patients who cannot tolerate aspirin; rare neutropenia is a problem with ticlopidine, and fatalities have been reported.
- After endarterectomy, many physicians prescribe aspirin and dipyridamole. They are ineffective in reducing the frequency or extent of restenosis. Restenosis of carotid vessels managed with endarterectomy occurs in as many as one out of four patients within 1 year of the surgery.

STROKE

Diagnosis

The individual who acutely develops focal neurologic deficits, such as hemiparesis, aphasia, ataxia, dysarthria, hemisensory deficits, or cranial nerve disturbances, may have suffered a stroke—an acute vascular injury to the CNS.

Alternative explanations for the neurologic findings include:
- *Transient ischemia*: If the deficits clear within 24 hours, there may prove to be no structural damage to the CNS.
- *Seizure*: The deficits rarely persist for more than 1 hour, but some individuals may exhibit a Todd's paralysis that persists for more than 1 day.
- Acute decompensation from a chronic lesion, such as a tumor
- Profound metabolic disturbances, such as hypoglycemia.

Seizures may be the first sign of a stroke and may delay diagnosis. Focal deficits are difficult to assess during the ictal and postictal periods associated with seizure activity. Individuals with hemorrhagic stroke, especially if the hemorrhage extends into the subarachnoid space, may give severe headache as the first complaint.

Risk factors for stroke include hypertension, diabetes mellitus, hypercholesterolemia, cigarette smoking, atrial fibrillation (AF), valvular heart disease, and left ventricular (LV) hypertrophy. Hemorrhagic strokes must be considered likely in any individuals on anticoagulant therapy who acutely develop focal neurologic deficits.

In many cases, stroke is suggested by the combination of signs and symptoms reported or exhibited by the patient. Concurrent face and ipsilateral hand numbness or weakness suggest damage to the cerebral cortex about the central sulcus in the distribution of the middle cerebral artery. Hemiparesis, affecting the dominant hand, associated with aphasia suggests damage to the dominant frontal lobe. A hemisensory deficit that extends onto the face from the affected side of the body suggests a thalamic injury, such as that seen with hypertension and lacunar infarction.

Pathophysiology

Stroke is irreversible brain damage secondary to occlusive or hemorrhagic vascular disease. Occlusive lesions may develop with arterial thrombosis, spasm, dissection, atherosclerosis, or inflammation. Even an adjacent neoplasm may produce stroke by compressing the arterial lumen. With hemorrhage into the parenchyma of the brain or spinal cord, damage to CNS tissue may be very direct and immediate. Hemorrhage into the subarachnoid space may produce focal or nonfocal disturbances which are often complicated by ischemic damage as vascular spasm develops in association with the subarachnoid blood.

Intracranial hemorrhage is most commonly seen with chronic hypertension or with rupture of an intracranial aneurysm. The latter is more likely to produce subarachnoid accumulation of blood (subarachnoid hemorrhage) than an intraparenchymal blood clot. Rupture of a vessel damaged by chronic hypertension is more likely to produce an intraparenchymal clot than a subarachnoid hemorrhage.

Ischemic injuries to the brain are especially likely with—systemic hypoperfusion, such as that associated with cardiac arrest; intracranial vasculitis, such as that developing with systemic lupus erythematosus (SLE); emboli, arising in the heart, emissary vessels to the head, or intracranially as reflux from occluded vessels; or thrombosis, such as that commonly occurring in association with atherosclerosis.

Focal neurologic deficits developing after trauma suggest a subdural, epidural, or subarachnoid hemorrhage. Deficits noted on awakening in the morning are likely to be ischemic injuries associated with intracranial thrombosis. A preexisting infection, such as a pneumonia or otitis media, which evolved shortly before the appearance of the neurologic deficits, may point to a meningoencephalitis or vasculitis as the cause of the stroke syndrome.

Investigations

These are similar to those required for TIAs:
- Patients believed to have suffered a stroke should have emergency neuroimaging studies. CT scanning is especially useful in revealing hemorrhagic lesions. MRI scanning reveals ischemic injuries early in their evolution. With evidence of intracranial hemorrhage, an angiogram should be performed to determine the site of bleeding and to assess the likelihood of subsequent hemorrhage. The patient with multiple aneurysms should have surgical intervention to ↓ the risk of recurrent bleeding. Complete blood count (CBC), urinalysis, and ECG are routine; echocardiography is required, if embolic stroke is suspected.
- There are some situations in which a lumbar puncture (LP) is clearly appropriate or inappropriate, but in many cases the clinician must decide whether or not to do an LP on the basis of how comfortable he or she is with the diagnosis. Ischemic stroke developing in the setting of an acute infection should be investigated with an LP so that CSF can be collected for culture. A hemorrhagic stroke with substantial distortion of the brain, especially if posterior fossa structures are involved, should make the clinician forgo an LP.

Therapy

- Much of acute stroke therapy is supportive. IV hydration must be started as soon as possible so that the patient can be made nil per os (NPO) and intravascular volume readily adjusted. Because of concern over the deleterious effects of IV dextrose, as already discussed for TIA, many clinicians start with a saline infusion at 30 mL/h.
- If a seizure occurs at the time of the stroke, antiepileptic medications are usually administered, unless there is an associated metabolic disturbance to which the seizure activity may be attributed. The antiepileptic of choice is phenytoin; the preferred route is IV. A loading dose of 10–15 mg/kg infused at a rate of no more than 50 mg/min is usually sufficient to control seizures during the first day after the stroke appears. If seizures recur, phenytoin 300 mg qd should be administered as a single dose (see earlier discussion).
- A respiratory arrest may occur, especially if aspiration has complicated the stroke.

The high risk of aspiration makes oral intake of nutrition or drugs inadvisable. The patient should be kept NPO for at least the first day or 2 if there is any evidence of speech, swallowing, or alertness problems.
- Autonomic disturbances may cause substantial damage. Falling BP associated with changes in position may exacerbate the ischemia that caused the dysautonomia. Patients with even minor strokes should be kept recumbent or nearly so until their deficits have stabilized for at least a few days. Hypertension may develop acutely with the stroke, but must be managed cautiously (see Chapter 1). An expanding intracranial hematoma may produce the Cushing effect (rising BP and slowing pulse), but aggressive lowering of the systemic BP may impair cerebral perfusion and ↑ the area of ischemic injury surrounding the area of initial infarction or hemorrhage.
- Antihypertensives given to the stroke patient with hypertensive emergency should be titrated to produce a slow and only moderate ↓ in BP—not more than 20% ↓ in the baseline systolic and never to less than 140 mm Hg. Many clinicians use sodium nitroprusside (see Chapter 1). If volume status is normal, gentle diuresis will suffice.
- Thrombolytic agents are not yet approved for use outside research protocols, and experience with those currently available suggests that they may be of value only in highly selected patients, under well-controlled conditions, and if treatment can be initiated within the first 2 hours after deficits appear.
- Surgery is not considered a viable option for acute stroke, but opinions are changing as surgical and anesthetic techniques produce less morbidity and mortality in these extremely unstable patients, and as neuroimaging techniques help to select patients most likely to profit from invasive strategies. The carotid system, rather than the vertebrobasilar system, is the most amenable to surgical intervention. The patients most likely to profit from acute surgical intervention are those with acute occlusive disease of the internal carotid artery who do not have profound neurologic deficits—such as impaired consciousness, aphasia, or hemiplegia—or intracerebral hemorrhage, and who do evidence contrast medium reflux in the petrous portion of the internal carotid artery.
- Successful surgical procedures on appropriate patients include internal carotid thromboendarterectomies, proximal remnant angioplasties (stumpectomies) with concurrent external carotid endarterectomies, and superficial temporal-to-middle cerebral artery bypass procedures.

Managing Catastrophic Deterioration

Strokes occasionally produce a catastrophic deterioration, such as brain herniation, status epilepticus, massive intracranial hemorrhage after infarction, or vasospasm after intracranial hemorrhage (see previous discussion).

Herniation may be transfacial (across the falx cerebri), transtentorial (across the tentorium cerebelli), or transforaminal (through the foramen magnum). It should be suspected in any stroke victim, whether that stroke is ischemic or hemorrhagic, who exhibits rapid deterioration, especially if that deterioration involves clouding of consciousness and autonomic dysfunction.

A variety of measures ↓ the risk of herniation. These include minimizing agitation, restricting fluids, and inducing hyperventilation.

- Acutely, the patient may be given a rapid (5–20-min) infusion of 20% mannitol solution at a dose of 0.5 g/kg. With this infusion, the patient must be watched closely for hypervolemia.
- Many clinicians use megadoses (10–100 mg) of dexamethasone or other corticosteroids as a single injection at the first sign of herniation.
- Centers with aggressive neurosurgical teams may opt for surgical decompression if an extensive area of necrotic tissue is evident. The surgical evacuation of intracerebral hemorrhages has generally produced poor results. Removal of intracerebellar hemorrhages and infarction has had much better outcomes.

Ischemia Associated with Vasospasm

The patient with subarachnoid bleeding or extension of intracerebral or intracerebellar hemorrhage into the subarachnoid space is at high risk for vasospasm. Consequently, the individual with few symptoms of subarachnoid blood may acutely develop evidence of extensive cerebral ischemia. Ca channel blockers, such as nimodipine, seem to ↓ the risk of vasospasm associated with subarachnoid hemorrhage and improve the outcome in patients with signs of cerebral vasospasm. *Dosage*—nimodipine 60 mg po q 4 hours for 3 weeks, commenced within 4 days of symptoms.

PARKINSON'S DISEASE

Diagnosis

- There are four characteristic features of Parkinson's disease—(1) rigidity, (2) tremor, (3) bradykinesia, and (4) dementia. If any or all of these signs occur with conditions that are not Parkinson's disease but imitate it, the situation is referred to as parkinsonism.
- The tremor associated with Parkinson disease and parkinsonism is a resting tremor. It is less evident or remits completely when a movement is initiated in the affected limb.
- The rigidity is usually lead pipe or cogwheel in character. Lead-pipe rigidity is a fairly constant resistance to movement while the affected

limb is passively moved. With cogwheel rigidity, the examiner can feel abrupt, but very brief, changes in the degree of resistance to movement. The cogwheel character of the tremor is especially likely to be evident if the affected limb is moved passively while the patient tries to perform mental calculations.
- Causes of parkinsonism include drugs (phenothiazines and butyrophenones), hereditary basal ganglia disease (Wilson's hepatolenticular degeneration and progressive supranuclear palsy), and metabolic encephalopathy [carbon monoxide poisoning and 1-methyl-4-phenyl-1,2,3,6-tetrahydropyridine (MPTP poisoning)].

Pathophysiology

Parkinson's disease develops with disease of the brain stem and diencephalon; the substantia nigra is severely damaged early in the course of the disease. Dopamine-dependent pathways in the basal ganglia are disturbed and eventually degenerate. Neuronal loss is obvious and extensive.

Therapy

Okun et al. give an excellent review in JAM, 2017. Levodopa is currently the most effective and safest agent and should be administered as soon as possible.

Dopamine agonists (ropinirole and pramipexole) can be useful but may cause impulse control disorders. But combination therapy is often needed with addition of dopamine agonists (pramipexole or ropinirole).

Bromocriptine and pergolide are not used as they may cause valvular disease and pulmonary fibrosis (Okun).

Amantadine is effective for suppression of Parkinson disease dyskinesia that develops after a few years of levodopa therapy.
- Dopamine does not cross the blood–brain barrier, and so L-DOPA, which is converted to dopamine in the CNS, is used to ↑ the overall level of dopamine in the CNS. Dopamine produces gastrointestinal (GI) disturbances when it reaches appreciable levels in the systemic circulation, and so a DOPA decarboxylase inhibitor (e.g. carbidopa) is usually combined with L-DOPA to ↓ the total dose of L-DOPA needed to achieve therapeutic levels in the CNS. DOPA decarboxylase inhibitors like carbidopa cross the blood–brain barrier poorly. Most physicians delay the introduction of L-DOPA or carbidopa treatment until other treatments fail to control the patient's symptoms. When treatment is started, a tablet with 25 mg carbidopa and 100 mg L-DOPA is given bid or tid. The dose is ↑ to maximize the benefit unless akathisia, GI distress, hallucinations, or other serious adverse effects develop.
- Alternative dopaminergic drugs include bromocriptine, lisuride, and pergolide mesylate. These drugs are usually introduced when L-DOPA

preparations fail to produce substantial improvement. Bromocriptine is usually started at a dose of 1.25 mg qd and gradually ↑ed to as much as 7.5 mg per day. Pergolide mesylate is given 0.05 mg each day initially and gradually ↑ed to less than or equal to 1 mg tid. Hallucinations and agitation are common problems with these dopaminergic drugs and are often dose limiting.
- Attempts to restore dopaminergic function in the brain have included the transplantation of adrenal or fetal tissues into the basal ganglia. The experience with this approach has been very inconsistent, but some groups have demonstrated convincing improvement in patients receiving transplants of fetal tissue.

MYASTHENIA GRAVIS

Diagnosis

- Myasthenia gravis is a disease of the neuromuscular junction that produces muscle weakness. It is characterized by antibodies to and consequent degeneration of the postsynaptic elements of the junction. The muscles most often symptomatic early in the disease are the ocular motor muscles and the levator palpebrae. Women are more commonly affected than men. Changes in the thymus, ranging from hyperplasia to malignancies, often appear in association with the disease. Hyperthyroidism may occur with myasthenia or as an independent cause of muscle weakness.
- The affected individual typically weakens as an activity is continued or the day passes. Strength usually peaks shortly after awakening.
- An IV injection of less than or equal to 1 mg edrophonium chloride (Tensilon), a short-acting, cholinesterase inhibitor, will produce a transient improvement in strength in affected individuals. An alternative, but much more hazardous, screening test involves the injection of a minuscule (1/70th of a curarizing dose) amount of curare. The individual with myasthenia is excessively sensitive to this neuromuscular blocking agent.
- The diagnosis is usually confirmed with electromyography (EMG) and nerve conduction studies. The affected individual will exhibit decreasing amplitudes of muscle action potentials with repeated (several times per second) stimulation of the nerve innervating the muscle. Muscles not obviously symptomatic will exhibit this decrementing pattern of action potentials, as will those which are symptomatic.
- Antiacetylcholine receptor antibodies are usually detectable in the serum. CT studies of the mediastinum may reveal thymic enlargement.
- Several conditions produce myasthenic syndromes, that is, disorders symptomatically similar to myasthenia gravis but arising from distinctly different causes. These include the Eaton–Lambert syndrome, in which

disease of the presynaptic elements of the neuromuscular junction develops in the setting of a malignancy. The most common malignancy to produce the Eaton–Lambert syndrome is bronchogenic carcinoma.

Pathophysiology

Myasthenia is presumed to arise because of damage to the acetylcholine receptor on the postsynaptic membrane of skeletal and ocular motor muscles. Cardiac muscle is not affected, but the diaphragm is often involved. Prior to the development of successful therapies, death usually occurred because of respiratory insufficiency. The affected individual would have a respiratory arrest or develop pneumonia because of inadvertent aspiration or recurrent hypoventilation.

Therapy

- Anticholinesterase inhibitors have been used successfully for several decades. By interfering with the breakdown of the neurotransmitter acetylcholine at the synapse, these drugs ↑ the exposure of the defective postsynaptic receptor to acetylcholine and potentiate the effect of acetylcholine. Pyridostigmine bromide 60 mg po q 4 hours during the day is a common regimen. The major disadvantage of these drugs is their cholinergic activity independent of the skeletal muscles. GI motility is ↑ed and may be especially disabling. Attempts to modulate this nonmuscular effect of cholinesterase inhibitors with atropine and similar anticholinergic drugs have been problematic because of the risks of overdose.
- Mediastinal exploration and resection of thymic tissue have been associated with substantially improved long-term prognoses in individuals with myasthenia gravis. Complete thymectomy is now generally recommended for all young (40 years old) individuals who become symptomatic. Some physicians recommend the procedure at any age, once the diagnosis has been firmly established.
- Because this is presumed to be an autoimmune disorder, a variety of immunosuppressant approaches have been tried. The most successful has been treatment with corticosteroids. After initiating treatment with relatively high doses (prednisone 60–100 mg each morning for days or a few weeks), maintenance therapy may require little more than a few mgs every other day. Strength may deteriorate when the steroids are started; some physicians start at low doses of prednisone and gradually ↑ the daily dose to avoid this deterioration.
- Many physicians use azathioprine as adjunctive immunosuppressant therapy for a few months at the start of treatment. The dose is 2.5–4 mg/kg/day, tapered over the course of weeks, unless the patient exhibits leukopenia or other serious reactions to the drug.

ACUTE POLYNEUROPATHY

Diagnosis

- Guillain-Barré syndrome is one of the most common and most lethal forms of acute polyneuropathy. It is an inflammatory, pure motor neuropathy, or nearly so (Lechtenberg).
- A Lancet Seminar is provided by Willison et al. Guillain-Barré syndrome is the most common and most severe acute paralytic neuropathy, with about 100,000 people developing the disorder every year worldwide (Willison et al.).
- The syndrome is usually preceded by infection or other immune stimulation that induces an aberrant autoimmune response targeting peripheral nerves and their spinal roots.
- The severe, generalized manifestation of Guillain-Barré syndrome with respiratory failure affects 20-30% of cases. Treatment with IV immunoglobulin (IVIg) or plasma exchange is the optimal management approach, alongside supportive care.
- All patients with Guillain-Barré syndrome need meticulous monitoring and supportive care. Early initiation of IVIg or plasma exchange is of proven benefit and crucial, especially in patients with rapidly progressive weakness. Because a quarter of patients need artificial ventilation and many develop autonomic disturbances, many patients need admission in the high or intensive care setting. Symptoms peak within 4 weeks, followed by a recovery period that can last months or years, as the immune response decays and the peripheral nerve undergoes an endogenous repair process.
- The acute progression of limb weakness, often with sensory and cranial nerve involvement 1-2 weeks after immune stimulation, proceeds to its peak clinical deficit in 2-4 weeks. When patients present with rapidly progressive paralysis, the diagnosis of Guillain-Barré syndrome needs to be made as soon as possible.
- The affected individual usually develops progressive weakness, starting in the legs and progressing cephalad over the course of 2 weeks. The deficits usually appear within weeks of an upper respiratory infection (URI). Bladder and bowel control are retained, but diaphragmatic paralysis may develop. Sensation is usually preserved throughout the limbs, but many patients note paresthesias about the feet or ankles and occasionally in the hands. Areflexia or hyporeflexia are invariably present at some time during the course of the illness.
- Transient autonomic disturbances, such as hypertension, tachycardia, mydriasis, and disturbances of sweating, commonly develop during the course of the illness and usually do not require treatment
- Ocular motor control is usually unaffected. In the rare Miller-Fisher variant, strength may be relatively little affected, but ataxia, areflexia, and ophthalmoplegia prominent

- At the time the weakness (or ophthalmoplegia) evolves, the patient is afebrile. The CSF exhibits a high protein content (usually >100 mg/dL), with little or no associated ↑ in the white cell content. This is usually referred to as cytoalbuminemic dissociation and was originally used to differentiate acute polyneuropathy from poliomyelitis.
- Electromyography and nerve conduction studies will establish that a neuropathy is present, but this test may give deceptively normal results early in the evolution of symptoms. Within days or weeks of the first signs of weakness, the patient will have a conduction block.

Pathophysiology

Guillain-Barré syndrome is idiopathic, but there are forms of acute polyneuropathy that are attributable to specific infectious agents, such as diphtheritic polyneuropathy. The underlying defect in acute inflammatory polyneuropathy is demyelination of peripheral nerves.

Guillain-Barré syndrome is a typical postinfectious disorder, as shown by the rapidly progressive, monophasic disease course (<1 month) shortly after infection, usually without relapse. Two-thirds of adult patients report preceding symptoms of a respiratory or gastrointestinal tract infection within 4 weeks of onset of weakness. Many different preceding infections have been identified in patients with the disorder, but only for a few microorganisms has an association been shown in case-control studies. *Campylobacter jejuni* is the predominant infection, found in 25-50% of the adult patients, with a higher frequency in Asian countries. Other infections associated with Guillain-Barré syndrome are *Cytomegalovirus* (CMV), *Epstein-Barr virus*, *Influenza A virus*, *Mycoplasma pneumoniae*, and *Haemophilus influenzae*. An association of Guillain-Barré syndrome with hepatitis E has been identified in patients from both the Netherlands and Bangladesh. An emerging relation between Guillain-Barré syndrome and acute arbovirus infection including Zika and chikungunya is being closely monitored and is the subject of major interest as the global epidemic spreads in the UK and the Netherlands at least 25% of Guillain-Barré syndrome cases are preceded by *C. jejuni* infection (Willerson et al.)

Therapy

- The most important measure is supportive treatment. At the first sign of respiratory embarrassment, the patient must be intubated. Individuals with respiratory insufficiency must be maintained on ventilators, and care must be taken to manage any pulmonary problems, such as atelectasis or pneumonia that develop.
- Repeated trials with corticosteroids have demonstrated no efficacy for this traditional therapy.
- Plasmapheresis has been attempted in several trials. There is a growing consensus that this is efficacious in acute inflammatory polyneuropathy. Routinely, five exchanges are completed over the course of 7-14 days.

- Intravenous gamma-globulin infusions appear to be as effective, if not more effective, than plasmapheresis. If IVIg or plasma exchange is be started, they should, in principle, be started as soon as possible, before irreversible nerve damage has taken place (Willison et al.). Immunosuppressive therapy does not improve the outcome.
- None of the treatments currently available influence the severity of the deficits that evolve, but plasmapheresis and gamma globulin do ↓ the duration of hospitalization. Only 15% of patients will recover with no residua. About 3-8% die from complications, such as infection.

ACUTE SPINAL CORD COMPRESSION

Diagnosis

- Cord compression usually produces sensory and motor deficits at or below the level of the compression. The sensory level is 3-4 dermatomal levels lower than the motor level and is most apparent contralateral to the motor deficits. Both of these features of the sensory level are related to the crossing of the spinothalamic tracts after ascending in Lissauer's tract (substantia gelatinosa). With massive compression, deficits will be evident bilaterally, and quadriplegia or hemiplegia associated with hypesthesia or anesthesia below the level of the motor deficit will develop.
- Bladder and bowel control may be lost relatively early in the course of spinal cord compression. With involvement of the cauda equina alone, bladder and bowel dysfunctions are likely to be prominent elements of the symptomatology.

Pathophysiology

- Common causes of spinal cord compression include malignancies, benign neoplasms, trauma, and infection. Malignancies impinging upon or arising in the spinal cord are usually metastatic lesions. The most common benign neoplasms impinging upon the cord are meningiomas and neurofibromas. Trauma sufficient to cause cord compression is usually in the cervical region. Trauma to the lumbar region may produce spinal root compression, but is unlikely to involve the cord because the conus medullaris in the adult rarely extends much below the L1 vertebral body. Infections involving the vertebral bodies or the intervertebral discs may impinge directly on the cord or produce cord compression as tissues around the cord are damaged and vertebrae sublux.
- Subluxation of the atlas and the axis (C1 and C2) may develop in juvenile rheumatoid arthritis and produce cervical spinal cord compression that is insidiously progressive.
- Cord compression develops in some instances secondary to enlargement of a cyst (syrinx) within the cord. Syringomyelia is most commonly seen

in the cervical or lumbar cord regions. Pain and temperature sensory deficits may be substantial early in the course of the cyst enlargement, presumably because the anterior decussation of the spinothalamic tract is compressed by the syrinx.
- Patients from regions in which the parasite *Schistosoma mansoni* is endemic, such as Puerto Rico, may develop a rapidly enlarging granulomatous reaction to the ova of this worm as they accumulate in the lumbar spinal cord. The affected individual will have paraparesis; sensory deficits in the legs; and bladder, bowel, and sexual dysfunction evolving over the course of days.

Therapy

- What is causing the cord compression must be ascertained as soon as cord compression is suspected. This is often evident on MRI of the spinal cord. The histologic character of the lesion may be suggested by the image, but in many cases an ambiguous mass must be biopsied.
- With acute deterioration, high-dose corticosteroids usually help ↓ symptoms and provide additional time for more definitive treatment. Dexamethasone 40–100 mg IV is administered as soon as the cord injury can be ascribed to compression. Subsequent treatment with 4–10 mg IV q 6 hours may be useful on a short-term basis.
- If a circumscribed, extraparenchymal mass is evident, surgical resection is usually appropriate. Surgery should be performed as soon as feasible— protracted cord compression will produce irreparable dam-age. If functional transection of the cord persists for much more than 24 hours, the probability of recovering much function is remote.
- Patients with metastatic disease impinging on the cord should have radiation therapy on an emergency basis. Decompressive surgery along with radiation provides little if any additional benefit, but it is often performed when the diagnosis is uncertain. Radiation therapy of the tumor may produce a transient ↑ in the local mass effect of the lesion; steroids are usually continued for several days or weeks to counter this phenomenon. The dose of radiation and character of the ports are determined by the probable nature of the tumor. Surgery is curative for some infectious lesions such as epidural abscesses.

INFECTIONS OF THE CENTRAL NERVOUS SYSTEM

Infections of the CNS produce clinical expression by three processes—each may cause headaches:
1. Inflammation
2. Increased intracranial pressure
3. Tissue necrosis.

Meningeal Inflammation

Causes

- *Meningismus*: Inability to straighten a leg when the hips are flexed (Kernig's sign) and leg flexion occurs when the head is flexed (Brudzinski's sign). Primarily with chronic meningeal inflammation, cranial nerve palsy is possible.
- Inflammation within the brain parenchyma (encephalitis) or necrosis (cerebral abscess) may alter consciousness, and cause focal neurologic deficits or seizures. Any of the three may result in increased intracranial pressure with altered consciousness and fever.

Diagnostic Studies

Cerebrospinal fluid (CSF): Guidelines for interpretation for CSF analysis are provided in Table 20.3 for normal findings, abnormal CSF with noninfectious causes, and the differential diagnosis for major infectious conditions. CT and MRI.

- Patients with focal neurologic defects or evidence of increased intracranial pressure (vomiting or papilledema) should have brain imaging prior to LP. Hypodense area in scans suggests encephalitis or meningoencephalitis; ring-enhancing lesions suggest cerebral abscess (Bartlett).
    - *Traumatic tap*: ↑ed protein; red blood cells (RBCs); white blood cell (WBC) count, and differential proportionate to RBCs. In peripheral blood, clear and colorless supernatant of centrifuged CSF. Usually 1 WBC/700 RBC.
    - Chemical meningitis (injection of anesthetics, chemotherapeutic agents, air, and radiographic dyes) ↑ed protein, and lymphocytes [occasionally polymorphonucleocyte (PMNs)].
    - Cerebral contusion, subarachnoid hemorrhage, and intracerebral bleed RBCs. ↑ed protein (1 mg/1,000 RBCs), disproportionately. Increased PMNs (peak at 72–96 hours); ↓ed glucose in 15–20%).
    - Vasculitis (SLE, etc.), ↑ed protein (50–100 mg/dL), ↑ed WBCs (usually mononuclear cells and occasionally PMNs), and normal glucose.
    - *Postictal (repeated generalized seizures)*: RBCs (0–500/mm^3), WBCs (10–100/mm^3 with variable % PMNs with peak at 1 day) and protein normal or slightly ↑ed.
    - Tumors (esp. glioblastomas, leukemia, lymphoma, breast cancer, and pancreatic cancer)—low glucose, ↑ed protein, and moderate PMNs.
    - *Neurosurgery*: Blood; ↑ed protein; and WBCs (disproportionate to RBCs with predominance of mononuclear cells) up to 2 weeks postoperative.
    - *Sarcoidosis*: ↑ed protein; WBCs (up to 100/mm^3 predominantly mononuclear cells); and low glucose in 10% (Bartlett).

Table 20.3: Cerebrospinal fluid analysis.

	Cell count/dL and predominant type	Protein (mg/dL)	Glucose (mg/dL)	Microscopic examination	Culture
Normal	0–5, mononuclear cells	15–45	40–80 (>6 × serum level)	Negative	Negative
Meningitis Viral	10–2,000, early-PMNs; late-mononuclear cells	Normal 100	Normal	Negative	Usually negative
Bacterial Untreated	100–100,000 PMNs 100–10,000 PMNs	Normal 600 Usually ↑	Low in 50–80% Normal or low	Positive: 60–80%* Variable*	Positive: 90% Variable
Partially treated					
Tuberculosis	10–1,000 mononuclear cells	100–500	Normal or low	Rarely positive	Usually positive
Fungal	5–1,000 mononuclear cells	50–500	Low	Antibody and antigen detection*	Usually positive
Syphilitic	5–100 mononuclear cells	50–100	Normal or low	VDRL positive in 75%*	Negative
Encephalitis	0–2,000, early-PMNs, late-mononuclear cells	50–120	Normal	Negative	Negative
Brain abscess Noninfectious diseases**	5–500, variable	50–500	Normal	Negative	Negative

*Serum serology for syphilis, HIV, fungal (coccidioidomycosis and histoplasmosis). CSF serology (coccidioidomycosis—syphilis nontreponemal tests) and antigen detection (cryptococcosis meningitidis, S. pneumoniae, and H. influenzae type B)
**Abnormal CSF with non-infectious causes.
(PMN: polymorphonucleocyte)

Neurologic Disorders 477

Table 20.4: Pathogens causing pyogenic meningitis.		
	Commonly acquired (253 cases)	Nosocomial acquired (151 cases)
Streptococcus pneumoniae	97 (38%)	8 (5%)
Gram negative bacilli	9 (4%)	57 (38%)
M. meningitidis	35 (14%)	1 (1%)
Streptococci	17 (7%)	13 (9%)
Enterococcus	0	4 (3%)
Staphylococcus aureus	13 (5%)	13 (9%)
Listeria monocytogenes	29 (11%)	5 (3%)
Haemophilus influenzae	9 (4%)	6 (4%)
Mixed	6 (2%)	10 (7%)
Staphylococcus (coagulase-negative)	0	13 (9%)
Other	4 (2%)	5 (3%)
Negative culture	34 (13%)	16 (11%)

(Bartlett)

Pyogenic Meningitis

Diagnosis

- The CSF generally shows a total WBC exceeding 100/mm^3 with a predominance of neutrophils, increased protein, and decreased glucose.
- Blood cultures are often positive. Most cases show typical bacteria on Gram stain, positive antigen assays *(Streptococcus pneumoniae, H. influenzae type B, and N. meningitidis)*, and positive cultures. Major pathogens in community-acquired and nosocomial infections are listed in Table 20.4.

Treatment

Therapeutic decisions are dictated by etiologic agent. The guidelines below are provided for initial empiric treatment assuming no specific clues with the initial evaluation pending culture results according to host status (Table 20.5). After the putative agent is identified, antibiotic treatment is simplified according to the agent recovered and, in some cases, in vitro susceptibility tests and pharmacologic properties for penetration across the blood–brain barrier (Tables 20.6 and 20.7).

Tuberculous Meningitis (Table 20.8)

This represents hematogenous spread during miliary disease or reactivation and rupture of a latent tubercle.

Table 20.5: Empiric treatment of pyogenic meningitis.

Setting	Likely agents	Treatment
Adult, community acquired, immunocompetent	Streptococcus pneumoniae Neisseria meningitidis	Cefotaxime—2 g IV q 4 hours Ceftriaxone—2–3 g IV q 12 hours Ceftizoxime—3 g IV q 8 hours Penicillin allergy: Chloramphenicol—1 g IV q 6 hours
Immunosuppressed Defective humoral antibody, asplenia, and complement defect Defective cell-mediated immunity	Streptococcus pneumoniae Neisseria meningitidis Listeria Cryptococcosis	As above

Ampicillin. 3 g IV q 6 hours ± gentamicin. 1.7–2.0 mg/kg IV q 8 hours Penicillin allergy: Trimethoprim sulfamethoxazole, 3–4 mg/kg (trimethoprim) IV q 6 hours |
| Post-neurosurgical procedure or cranial trauma | Enterobacteriaceae Pseudomonas species Staphylococcus aureus | Tobramycin—1.7–2.0 mg/kg IV q 8 hours + piperacillin, mezlocillin, or ticarcillin. 40 mg/kg IV q 4 hours + vancomycin. 1 g IV q 12 hours Alternative to penicillins is ceftazidime, 2–3 g IV q 8 hours |
| Ventricular shunt | Staphylococcus epidermidis | Vancomycin, 1 g IV q 12 hours + rifampin, 300 mg po or IV q 12 hours |

* Assumes negative CSF Gram stain and negative tests for bacterial antigens.
(IV, intravenous)

Diagnosis

- With miliary disease, there is often false-negative purified protein derivative (PPD).
- With reactivated CSF disease, there may be no other organ involved, but the skin test is usually positive. CSF may be similar to viral meningitis in early stages; in late-stage disease, there may be cranial nerve palsies and obstructive hydrocephalus, with CSF glucose often low.
- Positive acute febrile encephalopathy (AFE) stains and positive cultures establish the diagnosis, but long delays in culture results and the organism may prove difficult to recover making empiric treatment necessary.

Treatment (Initial)

- Isoniazid, 5 mg/kg/day (usually 300 mg) po or IM plus

Table 20.6: Treatment of pyogenic meningitis by organism.

Organism	Preferred drug	Alternative	Comment
Streptococcus pneumoniae	Penicillin G or ampicillin Cefotaxime Ceftriaxone	Chloramphenicol Cefuroxime Ceftizoxime	Test susceptibility to penicillin Resistant strains chloramphenicol or vancomycin + rifampin Treat ≥10 days
Neisseria meningitidis	Penicillin G or ampicillin	(As above)	Intimate contacts should receive rifampin Treat ≥ 7 days
Haemophilus influenzae	Ampicillin (Ampici 11 insensitive strains)	Chloramphenicol Cefotaxime Ceftizoxime Ceftriaxone Ceftazidime	If children <4 years in household, contacts should receive rifampin prophylaxis (type B only) Treat ≥10 days
Listeria monocytogenes	Ampicillin ± gentamicin	Trimethoprim sulfamethoxazole	Cephalosporins are not effective Treat 14-21 days
E. coli and other coliforms	Cefotaxime Ceftizoxime Ceftriaxone Ceftazidime	Aminoglycoside ± anti-pseudomonad— penicillin or ampicillin sulfatrimethoprim	In vitro sensitivity tests required MBC data preferred Chloramphenicol lacks bactericidal activity vs GNB—not recommended Aminoglycoside is given systemically ± intrathecally Treat ≥21 days Ceftazidime should be reserved for suspected or established Pseudomonas aeruginosa
Pseudomonas aeruginosa	Aminoglycoside + ceftazidime	Aminoglycoside + antipseudomonad penicillin (ticarcillin, mezlocillin, and piperacillin)	Sulfa-trimethoprim- Acinetobacter, P. cepacia and Flavobacterium Aminoglycoside is given systemically ± intrathecally
Staphylococcus aureus	Antistaphylococcal penicillin ± rifampin	Vancomycin + rifampin Trimethoprim-sulfa + rifampin or ciprofloxacin	Vancomycin + rifampin for methicillin resistant Staphylococcus aureus
Staphylococcus epidermidis	Vancomycin + rifampin	Teicoplanin	

(MBC, minimum bactericidal concentration; GNB, gram-negative bacteria)

Table 20.7: Doses of drugs for CNS infections.

Aminoglycosides and vancomycin

Agent	Systemic	Intrathecal or intraventricular
Gentamicin	1.7–2.0 mg/kg q 8 hours	4–8 mg q 24 hours
Tobramycin	1.7–2.0 mg/kg q 8 hours	4–8 mg q 24 hours
Amikacin	5.0–7.5 mg/kg q 8 hours	10–20 mg q 24 hours
Vancomycin	1 g q 12 hours	5–20 mg q 24 hours

Cephalosporins
   Cefuroxime—9 g/day in 3 doses
   Cefotaxime–12 g/day in 6 doses*
   Ceftizoxime–9 g/day in 3 doses*
   Ceftriaxone–4–6 g/day in 2 doses*
   Ceftazidime–6–12 g/day in 3 doses*
Chloramphenicol: 4–6 g/day in 4 doses*
Penicillins
   Ampicillin—12 g/day in 6 doses*
Antipseudomonad penicillins
   Ticarcillin—18–24 g/day in 6 doses (40–60 mg/kg q 4 hours)
   Mezlocillin—18–24 g/day in 6 doses (40–60 mg/kg q 4 hours)
   Azlocillin—18–24 g/day in 6 doses (40–60 mg/kg q 4 hours)
   Piperacillin—18–24 g/day in 6 doses (40–60 mg/kg q 4 hours)
Antistaphylococcal penicillins
   Nafcillin—9–12 g/day in 6 doses
   Oxacillin—9–12 g/day in 6 doses
   Penicillin G—20–24 million units/day in 6 doses*
Trimethoprim-sulfamethoxazole: 15–20 mg/kg/day (trimethoprim) in 4 doses
   Metronidazole—2 g/day in 2–4 doses
   Vancomycin—2 g/day in 2 doses*

*Assume adult patient with normal renal function
(Bartlett)
(CNS: central nervous system)

- Rifampin, 10–20 mg/kg/day (usually 600 mg) po or IV plus
- Pyrazinamide, 15–30 mg/kg/day (usually 2 g) plus
- Ethambutol, 15–25 mg/kg/day (usually 2.5 g) *or*
- Streptomycin, 15 mg/kg/day 1M (usually 1 g).

Cryptococcal Meningitis

The major fungal pathogen is *Cryptococcus neoformans,* which is the most common pathogen in patients with meningitis plus defective cell-mediated immunity including organ transplantation, acquired immunodeficiency syndrome (AIDS), lymphoma, corticosteroid therapy, and cancer chemotherapy.

Table 20.8: Some causes of chronic meningitis: the differential diagnosis includes the following causes of chronic meningitis.*

Infectious		Neoplastic	Miscellaneous
Bacteria	Fungi	Leukemia	SLE*
M. tuberculosis	Cryptococcosis	Lymphoma	Wegener's
Atypical	Coccidioides**	Metastatic	granulomatosis
mycobacteria	Histoplasma**	Breast	CNS vasculitis
Treponema	Blastomyces	Lung	Granulomatous
pallidum**	Sporotrichum	Thyroid	vasculitis
Borrelia	Pseudallescheria	Renal	Sarcoidosis
burgdorferi**'	Alternaria	Melanoma	Behcet's disease
Leptospira	Fusaria	Primary CNS	Vogt–Koyanagi
Brucetia	Aspergillus	Astrocytoma	and Harada's
Listeria	Zygomycetes	Ependymoma	syndromes
Actinomyces	Cladosporium	Pinealoma	Benign
Arachma	Viruses	Medulloblastoma	lymphocytic
Nocardia	HIV		meningitis
Parasites	Echovirus		
Toxoplasma gondii			
Cysticercus			
Angiostrongylus			
Spinigerum			
Schistosoma			

*Defined as illness present for more than or equal to 4 weeks with or without therapy CSF analysis usually shows lymphocytic pleocytosis. Analysis of 83 previously healthy persons in New Zealand showed 40% had tuberculosis, 7% had cryptococcosis, 8% had malignancy, and 34% were enigmatic.
**Evaluation culture, serum serology. CT scan or MRI (brain abscess cysticercosis, toxoplasmosis) cytology CSF (lymphoma, metastatic cal. eosinophilic (parasitic coccidioidomycosis), CSF serology or antigen (cryptococcosis, coccidioidomycosis, and syphilis histoplasmosis), blind meningeal biopsy (rarely positive), empiric treatment (TB then penicillin, then amphotericin B, and then corticosteroids) (Bartlett)
(CNS: central nervous system)

Diagnosis

- The *serum* cryptococcal antigen is positive in over 95% of patients with AIDS and cryptococcal meningitis.
- Cryptococcal antigen is virtually always positive and false-negative antigen assays are extremely rare when properly done.
- An India ink stain will usually show the agent and may be used as a substitute for the antigen assay for patients with AIDS.

Treatment

- Amphotericin B (0.5–0.7 mg/kg/day) IV ± flucytosine (75–100 mg/kg/day) po until total dose of amphotericin B is 15 mg/kg *and* negative CSF culture, then fluconazole (200 mg/day) indefinitely. Alternative for patients with favorable prognosis (normal mental status, high CSF leukocyte count, and relatively low number of organisms)—amphotericin B (0.5-0.7 mg/kg/day) IV ± flucytosine (75-100 mg/kg/day) po × 10-14 days, then fluconazole (400 mg/day) po × 8 weeks, then fluconazole (200 mg/day) po indefinitely.

Treatment for Patients without AIDS
- Amphotericin B (0.3 mg/kg/day) IV + flucytosine (150 mg/kg/day) po × 6 weeks. Alternative for immunocompetent host without neurologic complications—above regimen x 4 weeks.

Viral Encephalitis

Diagnosis

The clinical picture provides minimal help with etiology, although travel and contact histories may be important. Findings include confusion, delirium, ataxia, seizures, and cranial nerve palsies. The most important to recognize because of its devastating consequences and susceptibility to effective therapy is *Herpes simplex* encephalitis which often shows evidence of a temporal lobe lesion by MRI, CT scan, or EEG. A definite diagnosis is made with brain biopsy with histopathology, culture, or fluorescent antibody staining. There is generally no evidence of *H. simplex* lesions on mucocutaneous surfaces.

Treatment

Acyclovir, 10 mg/kg IV q 8 hours for 10-14 days.

Cerebral Pyogenic Abscess (Table 20.9)

Diagnosis

Cerebral abscess should be suspected in patients with focal neurologic signs accompanied by systemic evidence of infection (fever or leukocytosis) and/or associated conditions most often found with this complication. Fever is found in only about one-half of cases so that the absence of fever fails to help in excluding this diagnosis. Common associated conditions include sinusitis, otitis or mastoiditis, head trauma, prior neurosurgery, endocarditis, and congenital cyanotic heart disease. An MRI or CT scan with contrast shows a ring-enhancing lesion adjacent to the site of entry where the pathophysiologic mechanism is direct extension as with sinusitis, otitis, head trauma, or prior neurosurgery. Cerebral spinal fluid shows nonspecific findings with an increased protein and modest pleocytosis with a dominance of mononuclear cells. The diagnosis is established with an aspirate of the lesion or at neurosurgery with Gram stain of purulent exudate

Table 20.9: Some causes of brain abscess.

Associated condition	Likely pathogen	Drugs to be used based on bacteriology
Sinusitis	Anaerobic, microaerophilic, and aerobic streptococci Bacteroides species	Metronidazole, 500 mg IV or po every 6 hours plus Penicillin G 5–6 million units IV q 6 hours
Otitis	Bacteroides fragilis	Chloramphenicol, 1 g IV q 6 hours plus Penicillin G, 6 million units IV q 6 hours
Trauma, post neurosurgery	Bacteroides species, streptococci, Enterobacteriaceae	As above
	Staphylococcus aureus Enterobacteriaceae Pseudomonas aeruginosa	Oxacillin or nafcillin, 2–3 g IV q 4 hours or Vancomycin, 1 g IV every 12 hours Cefotaxime, 2 g q 4 hours Ceftazidime, 2–4 g q 8 hours ± aminoglycoside
Endocarditis		Tobramycin, 2 mg/kg, then 1.7 mg/kg q 8 hours plus
	Staphylococcus aureus Streptococcus species	Ceftazidime, 2–4 g q 8 hours or Piperacillin, 4 g q 6 hours Methicillin sensitive: Oxacillin or nafcillin
Cyanotic heart disease	Streptococcus species	methicillin resistant— vancomycin penicillin G, 5–6 million units IV q 6 hours or ampicillin, 2 g IV q 4 hours ± aminoglycoside As above

(IV, intravenous)

showing typical bacteria. Cultures should be obtained for both aerobic and anaerobic bacteria; cultures should also be submitted for mycobacteria and fungi. Putrid discharge indicates anaerobic bacteria; a polymicrobial flora on Gram stain also suggests anaerobic bacteria.

Treatment

Antibiotic selection is based on bacteriology using care to correlate clinical symptoms, Gram stains and culture results. Most pyogenic cerebral abscesses involve anaerobic bacteria or mixtures of anaerobes or coliforms and/or streptococci. Empiric therapy for pending cultures and in the event that surgery is not performed is based on anticipated bacteriologic patterns according to associated conditions using the guidelines shown in Table 20.9.

Liver Abscess

Diagnosis

Liver abscesses are classified by etiologic agent as pyogenic or amebic. Pyogenic abscesses may be extremely elusive with little more than fever, chills, leukocytosis, and modest changes in liver function tests, especially the alkaline phosphatase. Some patients have positive blood cultures. The diagnosis is usually established with CT scans. The microbiology may be established with percutaneous aspiration. Detection of *E. histolytica* is generally based on serology (complement fixation, indirect hemagglutination, or gel-diffusion-precipitin test); stool examination for ova and parasite is occasionally positive. Many patients will have a history of presence in countries where amebiasis is prevalent. Thus, the diagnosis of liver abscess is suspected in the patient with high fever [often fever of unknown origin (FUO)], hepatomegaly and/or right upper quadrant (RUQ) tenderness, and abnormal liver function tests (especially alkaline phosphatase elevation and hypoalbuminemia). The diagnosis is generally confirmed with CT scans or ultrasound of the abdomen showing typical ring enhancing lesions of the liver. The microbiologic diagnosis is established by blood cultures for pyogenic bacteria and serology for *E. histolytica;* needle aspiration of an abscess may be required. The distinction between pyogenic and amebic abscess is important because the role of surgery, the selection of antibiotics and the prognosis are very different.

Treatment of Amebic Abscesses

Metronidazole (750 mg tid or 500 mg IV q 6 hours) for 5-10 days. Oral absorption is nearly 100% so po preferred. The alternative is emetine (1 mg/kg/day to a maximum of 65 mg) for 10 days or chloroquine (250 mg qid for 7 days followed by 250 mg bid for 3-4 weeks). A luminal amebicide such as diiodohydroxyquin should be given concurrently to eliminate cysts. Needle aspiration is not indicated except to establish the diagnosis, for some large abscesses (greater than 10 cm in diameter) for impending rupture or for failure to respond after 5 days of antibiotic treatment. Most patients respond rapidly and completely; surgery is rarely required.

Treatment of Pyogenic Abscesses

Drainage is often required although the frequency is debated. Some patients have multiple small abscesses, which cannot be drained. The prognosis is

variable, but most patients with a single abscess do well and those with multiple small abscesses do poorly. Various authorities recommend three fundamentally different approaches:
1. *Antibiotics alone*: Often advocated for patients who have multiple small abscesses, which cannot be drained surgically or for patients who show an impressive clinical response to antibiotic treatment during diagnostic evaluation.
2. *Antibiotics combined with needle aspiration*: This affords the opportunity to define bacterial pathogens and to decompress large abscesses.
3. Antibiotics combined with surgical drainage or drainage with a tube placed by CT, ultrasound, or fluoroscopic guidance. This is traditional management.

Antibiotic selection—the dominant bacteria are coliforms (especially *E. coli* and *Klebsiella*), streptococci (especially *S. milleri* and anaerobic streptococci), *Enterococcus* and anaerobes (especially fusobacteria and Bacteroides species). Empiric antibiotics are directed against these organisms. Regimens that include metronidazole have the advantage of including treatment against *E. histolytica* if suspended: Metronidazole (500 mg po or IV q 6-8 hours) or clindamycin (600 mg IV q 8 hours) *plus* gentamicin or tobramycin (2.0 mg/kg IV; the 1.7 mg/kg q 8 hours) or third-generation cephalosporins such as ceftazidime (1.5-2 g q 8-12 hours) or ceftriaxone (1-2 g q 24 hours) *plus* ampicillin (2 g IV q 6 hours) or aminoglycosides such as gentamicin or tobramycin (2.0 mg/kg IV then 1.7 mg/kg q 8 hours) *plus* antipseudomonad penicillin such as piperacillin (4-5 g IV q 6 hours).

Cholecystitis

Diagnosis

Typical symptoms are acute right upper quadrant pain, anorexia, nausea, vomiting, and fever (about 38°C). Examination shows RUQ tenderness, guarding, and Murphy's sign (increased tenderness with palpation in subhepatic area during deep inspiration). Over 95% have stones that are most easily and reliably detected with ultrasonography. Radionucleoside scan of the gallbladder with ^{99}Tc DISIDA or related compounds is the preferred method to confirm the diagnosis; filling of the gallbladder makes the diagnosis unlikely.

Treatment

Supportive measures: Nasogastric suction and IV hydration—antibiotics: early in cholecystitis the gallbladder is sterile; within a week the gallbladder is infected in 30-50% of cases. The primary pathogens in rank order are *E. coli*, other coliforms (*Klebsiella, Enterobacter*, etc.), *Streptococcus, Enterococcus* and *Clostridium* species. Anaerobic bacteria are infrequent except with ascending cholangitis. Although bile is sterile in about 50% of gallbladders resected for acute cholecystitis, infection is responsible for some of the major complications—empyema, gangrene, and perforation. Suggested antibiotics are—ampicillin (2 g IV q 6-8 hours) *plus* gentamicin or tobramycin (2.0 mg/kg IV, then 1.7 mg/kg q 8 hours) *or* cefoperazone (1-2 g IV q 12 hours) alone or in combination with gentamicin or tobramycin. Other second- or third- generation cephalosporins are probably equally effective.

Surgery

Surgeons continue to debate the relative merits of early or late surgical intervention. *Advantages of early intervention* (within 1-2 days of onset of symptoms) are—the procedure is as safe as with delayed procedures; resection is easier without fibrosis, the duration of hospitalization and recovery is reduced, delay may overlook serious complications such as empyema or perforation, and the disease may recur during the waiting period. *Advantages of delayed intervention* are—the patient will be in optimal condition, there is time to clearly establish the diagnosis, resection may be easier if acute inflammation has resolved and the frequency of postoperative complications is reduced.

REVIEW ARTICLE

Brown et al provide a New England Journal of Medicine review article. "Amyotrophic lateral sclerosis (ALS) is a progressive and paralytic disorder characterized by degeneration of motor neurons in the brain and spinal cord. It begins insidiously with focal weakness but spreads relentlessly to involve most muscles, including the diaphragm. Typically, death due to respiratory paralysis occurs in 3-5 years".

"The drugs riluzole and edaravone, which have been approved by the FDA for the treatment of ALS, provide a limited improvement in survival. Riluzole acts by suppressing excessive motor neuron firing and edaravone by suppressing oxidative stress. Numerous other compounds that have been investigated have not been shown to be effective".

BIBLIOGRAPHY

1. Berkovic SF. Cannabinoids for Epilepsy—Real Data, at Last. N Engl J Med. 2017;376:2075-6.
2. Brown RH, Al-Chalabi A. Amyotrophic Lateral Sclerosis. N Engl J Med. 2017;377(2):162-72.
3. Charles A. Migraine. N Eng J Med. 2017;377:553-61.
4. Gittler M, Davis AM. Guidelines for Adult Stroke Rehabilitation and Recovery. JAMA. 2018;319(8):820-1.

5. Gavvala JR, Schuele SU. New-Onset Seizure in Adults and Adolescents: A Review. JAMA. 2016;316(24):2657-68.
6. Gladstone DJ, Spring M, Dorian P, et al. Atrial Fibrillation in Patients with Cryptogenic Stroke. N Engl J Med. 2014;370:2467-77.
7. Okun MS. Management of Parkinson Disease in 2017: Personalized Approaches for Patient-Specific Needs. JAMA. 2017;318(9):791-2.
8. Lechtenberg R. In: Khan. MDT. Philadelphia: Lea & Febiger; 1994.
9. Willison HJ, Jacobs BC, van Doorn PA. Guillain-Barré syndrome. Lancet. 2016; 388(10045):717-27.

CHAPTER 21

Renal Diseases

INTRODUCTION

Because the kidneys are required for many homeostatic functions, renal diseases can manifest in a wide variety of ways, including: fluid, electrolyte, and acid-base disorders; renal failure with accumulation of nitrogenous wastes in the blood; hypertension; and abnormal urinary excretion of blood cells, leukocytes, and protein. This chapter focuses primarily on the diagnosis and management of the causes of acute and chronic renal failure (CRF) and glomerular diseases.

ACUTE RENAL FAILURE

Renal failure is categorized as acute or chronic, either of which will result in end-stage kidney disease (ESRD) if not reversed (Box 21.1). Acute renal failure (ARF) is defined as rapid or abrupt onset of renal failure in a few hours or days of this illness characterized usually but not always by oliguria (urine volume <400 mL/day) with severe decrease in glomerular filtration rate (GFR), increase in blood urea nitrogen (BUN) and creatinine, and abnormality of other renal functions.

The major causes of ARF are classified anatomically into prerenal, renal, and postrenal.

Box 21.1: Major causes of acute renal failure.
Prerenal
- Low cardiac output
- Acute renal artery disease

Renal
- Acute glomerular disease
- Acute vascular disease
- Acute tubular and interstitial disease

Postrenal
- Acute urinary tract obstruction
  - Chronic renal failure
  - End-stage renal disease (ESRD)

Box 21.2: Causes of prerenal acute renal failure.
- Intravascular volume depletion
  - Actual losses
    - Hemorrhage
    - Gastrointestinal: diarrhea, vomiting
    - Renal: salt wasting, diuretics
    - Skin: burns, exudative dermatitis
  - Reduced effective circulating volume
  - Redistribution of fluid
    - Ascites
    - Peritonitis
    - Pancreatitis
    - Abdominal surgery
  - Peripheral vasodilation
    - Sepsis
    - Anaphylaxis
- Cardiac dysfunction with low cardiac output
  - Myocardial infarction
  - Cardiac tamponade
  - Other causes of cardiogenic shock
- Acute renal artery disease
  - Acute stenosis
  - Acute thrombosis
  - Acute embolism

Prerenal Acute Renal Failure

The causes of prerenal ARF are listed in Box 21.2. Structurally, the kidneys are normal and respond appropriately to the various prerenal causes, in particular, sudden marked decrease in vascular volume and/or cardiac output, which leads to hemodynamic changes, such as low blood pressure (BP) and decreased renal perfusion, and hormonal changes. The end result is:
- Decreased renal blood flow, decreased GFR.
- Increased tubular absorption of Na^+, H_2O, and urea (not creatinine).

The final outcome is:
- Oliguria
- More concentrated urine
- Low-urine Na^+ concentration.

Diagnosis

A relevant history and physical examination will often reveal the correct diagnosis. Urinalysis is normal (Table 21.1). Urinary indices in the diagnosis of ARF are given in Table 21.1. Renal ultrasound is normal.

Management

Early recognition and treatment of the underlying cause before the more severe form of acute tubular necrosis (ATN) sets in is crucial.

Table 21.1: Urinary indices in the diagnosis of acute renal failure.

Parameters	Prerenal	Renal ATN
Urine volume	Low	Low
Urinalysis	Normal	Active, i.e. protein, RBC, epithelial cells, epithelial cell casts, pigmented granular casts
Urine (Na$^+$) mEq/L	<20	>40
Urine (Osm) mOsm/L	>500	<300
U/P creatinine	>40	<20
RFI (UNa)/(U/P Cr)	<1%	>3%
Fractional excretion of Na$^+$	<1%	>3%
(U/P Na$^+$)/(U/P Cr) x 100		

(ATN, acute tubular necrosis; Cr, creatinine; Na, sodium; RBC, red blood cell; RFI, renal failure index; UNa, urine sodium concentration; U/P, urine:plasma ratio)

- Conditions with contracted intravascular volume often require central venous pressure (CVP) line to monitor volume replacement with 0.9% saline, blood, or albumin, depending on the type of loss. Typically, 110.9% saline is infused over 30-60 minutes then titrated to achieve adequate urine output and BP.
- Third-space losses can be reversed by using colloids (albumin or blood) and fewer crystalloids (isotonic saline).
- Cardiogenic shock requires the insertion of a Swan-Ganz catheter to monitor pulmonary capillary wedge pressure (PCWP).
- Low-dose dopamine and dobutamine are titrated to maintain BP.

The following cautions should be taken:
- Avoid furosemide if the patient is volume depleted.
- Avoid nonsteroidal anti-inflammatory drugs (NSAIDs) which may further aggravate ARF.
- Urinary indices are of no value if the patient is already given furosemide or has underlying CRF.

Postrenal Acute Renal Failure

Obstruction to the flow of urine leads to oliguria or complete anuria. Oliguria or anuria interspersed with polyuria is indicator of urinary tract obstruction. Sites and common conditions causing urinary tract obstruction include the following:
- Urethra and bladder neck: prostatic hypertrophy, urethral stricture or valves, meatal stenosis, phimosis.
- Bladder: neurogenic, calculus, carcinoma, blood clot.
- Ureter: intrinsic obstruction (calculus, sloughed necrotic renal papilla, clots, carcinoma), extrinsic obstruction (uterine prolapse, ureterocele, strictures, pelvic or retroperitoneal tumors), retroperitoneal fibrosis.

- Ureteropelvic junction: intrinsic (calculus, clots, sloughed necrotic renal papilla), extrinsic (stricture, fibrous bands, aberrant arteries).
- Renal pelvis: calculus, clots, papilla, carcinoma, tuberculosis (TB).

Look for suprapubic fullness indicating distended urinary bladder usually caused by bladder neck obstruction (e.g. enlarged prostate), if trauma, consider bladder rupture. Obstruction higher up (e.g. bilateral calculi) leads to hydronephrosis. Ultrasound may show dilation of the collecting system; however, retrograde pyelogram may be necessary to rule out postrenal obstruction. Obstruction leads to:
- Increased intratubular pressure.
- Decreased glomerular transcapillary pressure and GFR.
- Afferent arteriolar vasoconstriction.
- Further decrease in GFR.

Management comprises removal of obstruction surgically or by percutaneous nephrostomy.

Renal Acute Renal Failure

Causes include:
- Most commonly: ATN.
- Glomerulonephritis (GN): rapidly progressive GN and acute diffuse proliferative GN (e.g. poststreptococcal).
- Tubulointerstitial disorders such as acute hypersensitivity tubulointerstitial nephritis (HTIN) and intratubular obstruction (abnormal proteins or drugs).
- Vascular disorders, such as thrombotic microangiopathies [e.g. malignant hypertension, thrombotic thrombocytopenic purpura (TTP), hemolytic uremic syndrome (HUS)], thromboembolic disorders [e.g. disseminated intravascular coagulation (DIC), cholesterol embolization], vasculitis.

Acute Tubular Necrosis

Various terms describe this condition at different stages, e.g. ARF (clinical), ATN (pathologic), and vasomotor nephropathy (pathophysiologic).

The two basic pathogenic mechanisms for ATN are ischemia and nephrotoxicity (Box 21.3):
- Ischemia is caused by the mechanisms listed in Box 21.2. If the hypoperfusion that causes prerenal failure continues, a second mechanism sets in that maintains oliguria. This involves tubular epithelial injury resulting in tubular permeability causing leak and reabsorption of fluid back into the circulation (backleak theory) and tubular obstruction due to debris (cells, casts, etc.; obstructive theory). There is also vasoconstriction of the afferent arteriole leading to decrease in GFR (tubuloglomerular feedback).
- Drug nephrotoxicity is a major cause of nosocomial nephrotoxic ARF. Aminoglycosides remain the most common cause of drug-induced ATN.

Box 21.3: Causes of ischemic and nephrotoxic acute tubular necrosis (ATN).
- Ischemic ATN
  Same as Box 21.2
- Nephrotoxic ATN
  - Endogenous toxins
    - Hemoglobin
    - Myoglobin
  - Exogenous toxins
    - Drugs (e.g. aminoglycosides and other antibiotics, chemotherapeutics)
    - Radiocontrast dyes
    - Heavy metals (e.g. mercury, arsenic)
    - Organic solvents (e.g. carbon tetrachloride, ethylene glycol)
    - Anesthetics (e.g. methoxyflurane, enflurane)

Box 21.4: Causes of hemoglobinuria and myoglobinuria.
- Hemoglobinuria
  - Transfusion reactions
  - Snake and arthropod venoms
  - Hemolytic anemia
  - Amniotic fluid leak
- Rhabdomyolysis
  - Crushing trauma
  - Muscular ischemia
  - Muscular overexertion (e.g. seizures)
  - Hyperthermia
  - Hypothermia
  - Infection (e.g. influenza)
  - Snake and arthropod venoms
  - Drugs and toxins (e.g. alcohol)
  - Inflammation (e.g. dermatomyositis)
  - Hereditary enzyme defects

Although, some aminoglycosides (e.g. gentamicin) are more nephrotoxic than others (e.g. tobramycin), all have nephrotoxic potential.
- Patients with preexisting renal disease, multiple myeloma, or dehydration are at greatest risk for developing radiocontrast-induced ATN.
- In patients with ATN associated with hemoglobinuria and myoglobinuria, poorly understood factors in addition to urine excretion of hemoglobin (Hb) and myoglobin contribute to the nephrotoxicity. Box 21.4 lists causes for hemoglobinuria and myoglobinuria.

Diagnosis: It is clarified by:
- The clinical identification of the causes listed in Boxes 21.3 and 21.4
- Urinalysis and urinary indices (Table 21.1)
- Urinalysis for myoglobin and Hb.

Prevention: It involves the following:
- Maintenance of intravascular volume, cardiac output, BP, and thereby adequate renal perfusion is crucial to prevention of ischemic ATN; it also reduces the toxicity of most nephrotoxins. Adequacy of intravascular volume can be achieved by giving crystalloids (0.9% saline), albumin, or blood and mannitol. These measures are particularly important in cardiac or cardiovascular surgery, in patients at high risk for hemoglobinuria or myoglobinuria, and when radiocontrast dyes are used.
- Alkaline diuresis (urine pH > 7.0) is recommended to prevent ARF in conditions with high uric acid load, myoglobinuria, or salicylate overdose.
- Allopurinol 600 mg prior to and 300 mg qd after chemotherapy in various myeloproliferative disorders.
- Avoid NSAIDs in high-risk cases, such as the elderly, in patients with volume-depleted status with high-renin activity, and in those with compromised renal function. Avoid concomitant use of triamterene-containing diuretics.
- Avoid using multiple nephrotoxic drugs, e.g. aminoglycoside antibiotic and methoxyflurane anesthesia.

Management: Management of ATN focuses on its two phases: (i) oliguric and (ii) diuretic.

Oliguric phase:
Most ischemic ATN is oliguric. Nonoliguric ATN is more often nephrotoxic; thus, the recognition of renal failure may be delayed, resulting in hyperkalemia and fluid overload. Morbidity and mortality is reported to be less if patients are nonoliguric to start with or are converted to a nonoliguric state with high-dose furosemide (≤1,000 mg).
- Do not exceed 4 mg/min infusion since ototoxicity may occur with high-dose bolus.
- Maintain meticulous fluid and electrolyte control: Dialysis can be delayed if the fluid and electrolyte balance is maintained tightly and intake and output are carefully monitored. Intake is calculated based on the daily losses. Good guidelines are the daily weight (usually 0.5 lb weight loss daily), presence or absence of edema, and BP status. Protein is restricted to 0.6–0.8 g/kg body weight, Na^+ to 2 g qd, K^+ to 40–60 mEq qd.

Hyperkalemia can be controlled by a combination of the following measures:
- Strict reduction of K^+ in the diet; eliminate oral K^+ supplements and drugs containing K^+.
- Correct acidosis with sodium bicarbonate ($NaHCO_3$) PO; 600 mg bid, up to 1.2 g tid; goal carbon dioxide (CO_2) 16–20 mEq/L, with care not to cause volume overload and/or congestive heart failure (CHF).
- Glucose-insulin infusion, e.g. 2 g glucose with 1 U of regular insulin (50 cc 50% D/W with 10 U of regular insulin over 15–20 min).
- Resins. Kayexalate PO or as a rectal enema, or Ca resonium PO.

- Cardioprotection with IV CaCL or Ca gluconate.

Hemodialysis or peritoneal dialysis may be required. Indications for dialysis are:
- Clinical signs of uremia [encephalopathy, nausea and vomiting, gastrointestinal (GI) hemorrhage, pericarditis] and fluid overload causing intractable CHF and pulmonary congestion.
- Biochemical BUN (>120 mg/dL), uncontrollable hyperkalemia, acidosis.

Diuretic phase:
Carefully monitor fluid and electrolyte balance to prevent severe volume depletion that can result in significant morbidity and mortality.

Prognosis: Despite modern technology, morbidity and mortality remain high, mostly because of the underlying conditions that caused the ATN, e.g. postcardiac or vascular surgery, sepsis, cardiogenic shock. Death is usually caused by these underlying conditions, hyperkalemia, fluid overload, or GI hemorrhage.

Acute Hypersensitivity Tubulointerstitial Nephritis

Hypersensitivity tubulointerstitial nephritis accounts for 15-20% of ARF. Acute infectious tubulointerstitial nephritis (TIN) (acute pyelonephritis) rarely causes ARF but may lead to chronic pyelonephritis and CRF. The most common causes of acute HTIN are drugs, e.g. penicillins, sulfonamides, NSAIDs, cephalosporins, furosemide, rifampin, and phenytoin.

Diagnosis: The classic signs and symptoms begin 1-2 weeks after initiation of drug administration: fever, rash, and eosinophilia. However, all three features occur only in 113 of patients. Eosinophilia is most frequent (80% of patients). Typical urinalysis findings are sterile pyuria, eosinophiluria, white blood cell (WBC) casts, proteinuria (<2 g/24 h) and slight hematuria.

Management: Identify and remove potential inciting agent (renal function should begin to improve within several days). If no response to discontinuation of drugs or no inciting agent identified, steroid therapy may facilitate recovery (prednisone 1 mg/kg/day PO for 4-6 weeks). If ARF is severe, dialysis and management of fluid and electrolytes as described previously for ATN is required.

Prognosis: If an inciting agent is identified and removed, full recovery usually ensues within 1-2 weeks. However, recovery may take less than or equal to 2 months. Persistence of ARF for more than 2 weeks and absence of an apparent inciting agent are signs of poorer prognosis.

CHRONIC RENAL FAILURE

International guidelines define chronic kidney disease (CKD) as decreased kidney function, GFR of less than 60 mL/min/1.73 m^2 (an adjustment is made in Blacks) or markers of kidney damage, or both, of at least 3 months duration, regardless of the underlying cause (Nagler et al., 2017).

Most individuals with CKD are asymptomatic or complain of weakness, lethargy, itch, and anorexia with added symptoms caused by the underlying disease:
- Hypertension
- Diabetes
- Lethargy, and
- Chronic nephritis.

Loss of appetite and presence of proteinuria [albumin:creatinine ratio (ACR) ≥30 mg/g] is associated with increased risk of progression of CKD and death (Nagler et al., 2017).

Normal function includes less than 150 mg of protein and less than 30 mg of albumin in urine daily. Complications include anemia due to reduced production of erythropoietin (EPO) by the kidney. Death from cardiovascular disease often occurs prior to end-stage CKD.

For those with an estimated GFR of 60 mL/min/1.73 m^2, up to a quarter will have a measured GFR less than 42 or more than 78 mL/min/1.73 m^2.

Many people are asymptomatic or have nonspecific symptoms such as lethargy, itch, or loss of appetite and presence of proteinuria [albumin:creatinine ratio (ACR) ≥30 mg/g] is associated with increased risk of progression of CKD and death (Nagler et al., 2017).

Complications include anemia due to reduced production of EPO by the kidney.

The presence of cells, casts, and crystals in the urinary sediment might give clues to the causes of underlying kidney disease. Glomerular disease can result in urinary red blood cells (RBCs), whether visible or invisible to the naked eye, whereas WBC might be seen in TIN or, along with hematuria, in various forms of GN.

Chronic renal failure occurs slowly over many years. It is irreversible. As the nephron population decreases, the remaining nephrons adapt (intact nephron hypothesis), ultimately leading to additional nephron loss through sclerosis. There is also extrarenal adaptation and trade-off. Therefore, these patients enjoy a symptom-free life until the GFR drops to less than 25% of normal. Life support with dialysis and/or renal transplant is necessary when the nephron population is less than 5%.

Causes in Adults

Causes in adults include diabetic glomerulosclerosis, chronic GN, hypertensive arterionephrosclerosis, renovascular disease, adult polycystic kidney disease, chronic pyelonephritis, analgesic abuse, hereditary disorders.

Natural History

Hemodynamic, hormonal, structural, and adaptive events occur during the progression of CRF.
- *Hemodynamic*: Initially there is increase in renal blood flow (hyperperfusion), leading to increase in intraglomerular pressure and increase GFR per remaining nephron and therefore increase in filtered load of nonprotein nitrogen (urea, creatinine, uric acid), electrolytes, and other solutes.
- Hormonal changes predominantly regulate the tubular functions of absorption and secretion [e.g. aldosterone, atrial natriuretic hormone, antidiuretic hormone (ADH), and parathyroid hormone (PTH), which control Na^+, K^+, H_2O, Ca^{++}, and phosphate (PO_4), respectively]. A steady state is maintained for a long time and the patient is asymptomatic until progressive glomerulosclerosis leads to azotemia and uremia.
- *Structural*: Progressive glomerulosclerosis may develop as a result of glomerular hyperfiltration.
- Extrarenal adaptations and trade-offs. As the Hb concentration decreases, there is a shift to the right of the O_2-Hb dissociation curve, unloading O_2 at the tissue level (favorable). Therefore, blood transfusion is usually not needed until the Hb drops to less than 7–8 g/dL (70–80 g/L), at which time the patient becomes symptomatic.
- As the serum PO_4 level rises, serum Ca^{++} falls. This in turn stimulates PTH, causing phosphaturia and mobilization of Ca^{++} from bones. With the progression of renal failure, metabolic bone disease can appear in the form of renal rickets/osteomalacia (deficiency of vitamin D), osteitis fibrosa (↑ PTH), and metastatic calcification (increased PO_4 x Ca^{++} product).
- Chronic acidosis is associated with mobilization of calcium carbonate ($CaCO_3$) from bones (which are rich reserves of $CaCO_3$), which may ultimately contribute to metabolic bone disease.

Signs and Symptoms

Almost any system can be affected during the course of CRF. The earliest symptoms are related to:
- Gastrointestinal system: morning nausea, anorexia, intermittent vomiting, and weight loss.
- Central nervous system: leg cramps (especially at night), fatigue, asterixis, and lack of concentration.

Late and usually severe and alarming features are:
- Cardiovascular system: uremic pericarditis, cardiac tamponade.
- Central nervous system: encephalopathy, neuropathy.
- Musculoskeletal: metabolic bone disease, intractable itching.

Table 21.2: Guidelines to differentiate between acute and chronic renal failure.

Features	Acute	Chronic
Etiology	Prerenal Renal Postrenal	Diabetes mellitus Chronic glomerulonephritis Hypertensive arterionephrosclerosis Adult polycystic kidney disease Chronic pyelonephritis Hereditary disorders Analgesic abuse
Urine volume	Usually oliguric	Usually polyuric until late stages
Endocrine function Hb Ca PO_4	Usually normal Normal Normal Normal	Abnormal Anemia Abnormalities of vitamin D metabolism and 2° ↑ PTH (e.g. ↓ Ca, ↑ $CaPO_4$) ↑ PO_4
Blood pressure	Normal or low	High with hypertensive changes: fundi and ECG/LVH pattern
Kidney size	Normal	Small in chronic glomerulonephritis, nephrosclerosis and chronic pyelonephritis. Large in polycystic kidneys, amyloidosis, hydronephrosis, and diabetes
Course	Usually reversible	Irreversible with slow deterioration

(Ca, calcium; $CaPO_4$, calcium phosphate; ECG, electrocardiogram; Hb, hemoglobin; LVH, left ventricular hypertrophy)

Diagnosis

Table 21.2 differentiates between ARF and CRF.

Management

The goals are to slow the progression of renal failure, control the manifestations of uremia, and maintain proper nutritional status. In order to slow the progression of CRF:
- Control hemodynamic factors, i.e. hyperperfusion, increase in intraglomerular pressure, and hyperfiltration in remaining nephrons. Dietary restriction of protein is very important. Research data indicate that diets low in protein and phosphorus slow the progression of CRF, whereas diets high in lipids may accelerate it. There is increasing evidence that angiotensin-converting enzyme (ACE) inhibitors may retard the progression of CRF by reducing intraglomerular pressure in residual hyperfunctioning glomeruli, which is thought to cause progressive glomerulosclerosis.
- Control both systolic and diastolic hypertension.

- Control factors known to aggravate renal failure: prerenal factors such as volume depletion and hypotension; CHF; infection; and drug toxicity due to aminoglycosides, radiocontrast dyes, NSAIDs, and postrenal obstruction.
- Control the underlying disease process that is causing CRF, e.g. diabetes mellitus.

General treatment of CRF requires management of protein intake, fluid balance, K^+, Ca, phosphorus, acidosis, hypertension, and anemia.

- Fluid and Na^+ balance: CRF impairs the ability to handle a Na^+ load and to conserve Na^+. Because of reduced glomerular filtration and tubular reabsorption, Na^+ intake more than the limited renal capacity for excretion results in Na^+ and H_2O retention, which can cause hypertension, edema, and CHF. Conversely, because of impaired renal conservation of Na^+, inadequate Na^+ intake causes Na^+ depletion and reduced extracellular fluid volume, which can cause reduced renal blood flow and worse renal failure. Na^+ intake of 2-3 g qd is appropriate in most circumstances in nondialyzed CRF patients, depending upon BP and presence of edema. Na^+ intake of 1-2 g/day is usually more appropriate for dialysis patients. Some CRF patients with salt-losing nephropathy may require more Na^+ intake to prevent volume depletion and further decrease in GFR. If Na^+ balance is maintained, thirst will usually maintain normal H_2O balance until the GFR is less than 5 mL/min. Thereafter, careful control of fluid intake may be required.
- Protein and calorie control: Experimental and clinical studies suggest that protein restriction slows the progression of CRF. Protein should be restricted to 0.6-1.0 g/kg body weight, one-third of which should be of high biological value (i.e. rich in essential amino acids), e.g. milk, eggs, fish, meat. To prevent malnutrition and catabolism, the diet should contain 35-40 kcal/kg/day. In patients with proteinuria, the protein intake must be increased by approximately 1 g/day for every 1 g/day proteinuria.
- Potassium: Usually not a problem unless the patient is oliguric or has a sudden overload of K^+. Contributing factors that may cause hyperkalemia include the use of nonselective β-blockers, ACE inhibitors, K^+-sparing diuretics, salt substitute, NSAIDs, and severe metabolic acidosis and hyporeninemic hypoaldosteronism, especially in noninsulin-dependent diabetes mellitus (NIDDM).
- Calcium and PO_4: CRF can cause vitamin D deficiency and resistance to vitamin D. Ca supplement and an active form of vitamin D are usually given to prevent metabolic bone disease. Phosphorus should be restricted to minimize hyperparathyroidism and possibly to retard progression of CRF. Besides dietary restriction of PO_4 to 300-700 mg/day, $CaCO_3$ 0.5-1 g tid, which binds PO_4 in the gut, may be administered to keep serum levels of PO_4 at a lower concentration; $CaCO_3$ avoids aluminum overload, which may occur with aluminum compounds.

- Acidosis: Because of impaired excretion of acidic metabolites and renal loss of bicarbonate, metabolic acidosis is common in patients with CRF who are not on dialysis. Keep serum HCO_3 level close to 20 mEq/L and arterial pH less than 7.35. Mild acidosis can be controlled with $NaHCO_3$ 600 mg bid or tid or $CaCO_3$ 500–1,000 mg bid or tid. More severe acidosis may require intravenous (IV) alkali or dialysis.
- Hypertension: CRF alters the metabolism and excretion of some antihypertensive drugs. Antihypertensive drugs can beneficially influence problems in CRF patients in addition to hypertension, e.g. fluid overload (diuretics) and glomerular hyperfiltration (ACE inhibitors). ACE inhibitors may have special significance because they not only reduce systemic BP but also intraglomerular pressure. Volume overload often requires diuretics, especially furosemide, because thiazides are not effective in patients with severe CRF. The action of antihypertensive drugs, as well as other drugs, may be altered in CRF because of decreased renal excretion, altered metabolism, altered volume of distribution, and, in patients on dialysis, removal by dialysis. This requires appropriate dose adjustment.
- Anemia: Avoid transfusions unless the patient is symptomatic because of low Hb. Patients with CRF usually tolerate a Hb of 7 g/dL without symptoms except those with concomitant angina or CHF, who require judicious infusion of packed RBCs with added furosemide. Recombinant human EPO should be used in order to decrease the need for blood transfusion. The usual dose of EPO is 40–100 IU/kg SC three times per week. The dose of EPO can be adjusted depending on the response (Hb should be kept ≤12 g/dL).
- Dialysis: A point will be reached in the course of the disease when conservative management with diet and drugs fails to control signs and symptoms of uremia and hyperkalemia. At this point dialysis and/or renal transplant is indicated. Consider dialysis at the early manifestation of uremia, which can appear when urea is approaching 30–40 mEq/L (BUN 80–100 mg/dL, 28.5–35 mmol/L) and creatinine 8–10 mg/dL (800–1,000 μmol/L).
- Types of dialysis: Hemodialysis can be done in hospital, or the patient can be trained to do the same at home or in a self-care unit. Arteriovenous (AV) fistula or a graft provide vascular access. Sometimes a subclavian catheter can be inserted for urgent or short-term dialysis. The most common form of peritoneal dialysis is continuous ambulatory peritoneal dialysis (CAPD). This type is preferable for elderly people with difficult vascular access, individuals with cardiovascular instability and diabetics. CAPD is easier than hemodialysis and can be done without much extra assistance. Some of the common problems with CAPD are peritonitis, protein loss, hyperglycemia, and respiratory embarrassment.

- Transplantation is the preferred replacement therapy for end stage renal disease. It may restore the quality-of-life to normal and is more economical than chronic dialysis in the long run.

GLOMERULAR DISEASE

The steps in the assessment and management of a patient with glomerular disease are:
- Clinical recognition of glomerular disease
- Determination of the type of glomerular disease
- Identification of the cause or pathogenic category
- Determination of the prognosis and selection of treatment.

Clinical Recognition

Glomerular injury manifests as:
- Evidence of *structural* damage to the glomerulus: abnormal urinalysis demonstrating proteinuria, casts, hematuria, and other cells
- Evidence of *functional* damage to the glomerulus: azotemia, salt and H_2O retention, hypertension, oliguria.

With structural and functional damage to the glomerulus, certain clinical syndromes result that indicate the presence of glomerular disease.
- Nephritic syndrome: Hematuria, proteinuria (3 g/day), cells in the urine (RBC, WBC), urine casts (all types, with RBC casts most specific), azotemia (↑ BUN, creatinine), hypertension, edema.
- Nephrotic syndrome: Proteinuria more than 3 g/day, lipiduria (free fat droplets and oval fat bodies with Maltese crosses under polarized light), hypoalbuminemia, hypercholesterolemia, and edema.
- Combined nephritic and nephrotic syndrome.
- Asymptomatic proteinuria or hematuria: Proteinuria or hematuria without the other features of nephritis or nephrotic syndrome.
- Rapidly progressive GN: More than or equal to 50% loss of renal function within 3 months, often with oliguria or anuria.
- Chronic GN: Nephritis or nephrotic with gradual progression of renal failure over many years.

Determination of Type of Glomerular Disease

Once the clinical diagnosis is made, the second step is to determine the type of glomerular injury responsible for the clinical syndrome (Tables 21.3 to 21.5). Accurate diagnosis, therapeutic decisions, and prognostication may require renal biopsy. Pathologic evaluation usually requires three procedures: (i) light microscopy, (ii) immunofluorescence microscopy (IM), and (iii) electron microscopy (EM).

Table 21.3: Characteristics of some of the common types of proliferative and mixed glomerulonephritis (GN).

Types of GN	Light microscopy	Immunofluorescence microscopy	Electron microscopy	Cause, therapy and prognosis
1. Mesangial GN	(a) Mesangial proliferation (focal segmental)	IgA-dominant C3 granular, mesangial	Mesangial deposits	IgA nephropathy (Berger's disease) Rx: Supportive Prognosis: Variable (features of poor prognosis: nephrotic syndrome, hypertension) Differential diagnosis: Henoch–Schönlein purpura, liver cirrhosis
	(b) Same as 1(a)	IgG-dominant C3, C1q, IgM, IgA	Same as 1(a)	SLE (type II) Rx: None Prognosis: Generally good
2. Diffuse proliferative GN	(a) Hypercellularity: endothelial, mesangial ± epithelial (± crescents) proliferation and leukocyte influx	IgG C3 granular capillary wall	Subepithelial humps	Postinfectious GN Rx: Supportive Prognosis: Good, especially in children
	(b) Same as 2(a) plus wire loop lesions	IgG, IgA, IgM C3, C1q (full house)	Mesangial, subendothelial and subepithelial deposits Microtubular arrays	SLE (type IV) Rx: Steroids, imuran, cyclophosphamide Prognosis: Variable, guarded

Contd...

Contd...

Types of GN	Light microscopy	Immunofluorescence microscopy	Electron microscopy	Cause, therapy and prognosis
3. Crescentic GN/ Rapidly progressive GN (RPGN)	(a) Crescents (cellular, fibrous, mixed)	IgG C3 linear GBM	No dense deposits	Anti-GBM GN, (Goodpasture disease) Rx: Steroids, Imuran, plasmapheresis Prognosis: Variable, guarded
	(b) Same as 3(a)	IgG C3 granular	Subendothelial Subepithelial humps	SLE, postinfectious GN, other immune complex GN Rx: Steroids, Imuran, cyclophosphamide for SLE Prognosis: Fair
	(c) Same as 3(a)	No deposits	No dense deposits	Pauci-immune GN, Wegener's granulomatosis, microscopic polyarteritis Rx: Steroids, cyclophosphamide Prognosis: Variable
4. MPGN type I	Mesangial proliferation, thick capillary walls, lobular pattern, double contour of BM	C3-dominance IgG, IgM	Subendothelial and mesangial deposits	(a) Idiopathic (most common in children) Rx: No therapy Prognosis: Poor (b) Secondary to infection, neoplasm, cryoglobulinemia Rx: Treat primary cause Prognosis: Variable
5. MPGN type II (dense deposit disease)	Lobular, pattern, ribbon-like thickening of capillary walls	C3 capillary, mesangial	Intramembranous dense deposits	(a) Idiopathic (b) Secondary to partial lipodystrophy Rx: No therapy Prognosis: Poor

(MPGN, membranoproliferative glomerulonephritis; BM, basal membrane; GBM, glomerular basement membrane; SLE, systemic lupus erythematosus)

Table 21.4: Characteristics of nonproliferative glomerular disorders.

Characteristics	Light microscopy	Immunofluorescence microscopy	Electron microscopy	Cause, therapy and prognosis
Minimal change glomerulopathy	Normal	Negative	Nonspecific fusion of foot processes. No dense deposits	(a) Idiopathic (most common in children) Rx: Usually steroids alone or with cyclophosphamides for poor responders Prognosis: Excellent. Relapse is common but responds to retreatment (b) Secondary to lymphoid malignancy Rx: Treat neoplasm
Focal segmental glomerulosclerosis	Sclerosis of part of glomerular tuft	IgM and C3 in sclerosis	Nonspecific fusion of foot processes. No dense deposits	(a) Idiopathic (most common in children) Rx: No therapy Prognosis: Slow progression to renal failure (b) Secondary to obesity, reduced renal mass Reflux nephropathy
Membranous glomerulopathy	Thickening of capillary walls, no proliferation of cells Spike formation	IgG-dominant C3 granular capillary	Subepithelial dense deposits (staging I–IV)	(a) Idiopathic (most common in adults) Rx: Steroids, chlorambucil, cyclophosphamide; varying reports of benefits Prognosis: Spontaneous remission in 20–25%; slow progression to renal failure (b) Secondary to malignancy lymphoma, SLE, drugs, hepatitis
Diabetic glomerulosclerosis	Nodular sclerosis and thickened GBM	IgG linear GBM	Thick GBM	Diabetes mellitus Rx: Control diabetes, ACE inhibitor Prognosis: Poor

Contd...

Contd...

Characteristics	Light microscopy	Immunofluorescence microscopy	Electron microscopy	Cause, therapy and prognosis
Amyloidosis AL	Acidophilic effacement of tufts	Immunoglobulin light chains (λ > κ)	10 nm fibrils	May be secondary to B cell neoplasm Rx: Treat neoplasm
AA	Same as AL	Amyloid A protein	10 nm fibrils	May be secondary to chronic inflammatory disease (e.g. TB, rheumatoid arthritis) Rx: Treat inflammatory disease

(ACE, angiotensin-converting enzyme; GBM, glomerular basement membrane; SLE, systemic lupus erythematosus)

Table 21.5: Characteristics of glomerular injury in systemic diseases.

Characteristics	Light microscopy	Immunofluorescence microscopy	Electron microscopy	Therapy and prognosis
SLE (WHO classification types I–V)				
Type I	Normal	Negative	Negative	No therapy
Type II (Mesangial) IIa	Normal	IgG, IgM, IgA C3, C1q granular mesangial	Mesangial dense deposits	No therapy
IIb	Mesangial proliferation	Same as IIa	Same as IIa	No therapy
Type III [focal (<50%) glomeruli involved]	Proliferation of endothelial mesangial and ± epithelial cells, leukocyte influx, necrosis	IgG, IgM, IgA C3, C1q	Subendothelial and mesangial dense deposits	No therapy unless severe

Contd...

Contd...

Characteristics	Light microscopy	Immunofluorescence microscopy	Electron microscopy	Therapy and prognosis
Type IV [diffuse (>50%) glomeruli involved]	Proliferation of endothelial mesangial and epithelial cells, vessel necrosis	IgG, IgM, IgA C3, C1q	Subendothelial and mesangial dense deposits	Rx: Steroids, Imuran, cyclophosphamide Variable response Prognosis: Guarded
Type V (membranous GN)	Thickening of capillary walls	IgG, IgM, IgA C3, C1q	Subepithelial dense deposits most numerous	No therapy
Microscopic polyarteritis	Necrotizing glomerulonephritis and vasculitis, usually crescents	Negative	No dense deposits	Rx: Steroids, cyclophosphamide Prognosis: Fair
Wegener's granulomatosis	Necrotizing glomerulonephritis and vasculitis, usually crescents	Negative	No dense deposits	Rx: Steroids, cyclophosphamide Prognosis: Fair
Thrombotic microangiopathies (HUS, TTP, pSS, malignant hypertension)	Glomerular consolidation, arteriolar necrosis, arterial intimal expansion, thrombi	Negative or fibrin	Lucent subendothelial expansion	Rx: Plasmapheresis, control hypertension Prognosis: Guarded
Mixed cryoglobulinemia	Same as MPGN type I	IgG, IgM C3	Subendothelial and mesangial dense deposits	Rx: Steroids, cyclophosphamide, plasmapheresis
Henoch–Schönlein purpura	Same as IgA nephropathy	IgA-dominant C3	Mesangial dense deposits	No therapy unless very severe Prognosis: Good

(HUS, hemolytic uremic syndrome; MPGN, membranoproliferative glomerulonephritis; pSS, primary Sjögren's syndrome; TTP, thrombotic thrombocytopenic purpura; WHO, World Health Organization)

Light Microscopy

Morphologic changes involve glomeruli primarily. However, tubules, interstitium, and blood vessels often are involved secondarily. Glomerular injury can be diffuse (most or all glomeruli involved), focal (only some glomeruli involved), segmental (segments of glomeruli involved), or global (whole glomeruli involved). Blood vessels may be involved by the same inflammatory process that is in the glomeruli in some forms of systemic vasculitis, e.g. microscopic polyarteritis and Wegener's granulomatosis.

Glomerular morphologic changes can be classified into:
- Proliferative disorders involving proliferation of various cells located in the glomerulus, e.g. mesangial cells (mesangial proliferative GN), endothelial cells, and epithelial cells (crescentic GN); and sometimes accompanied by influx of leukocytes.
- Nonproliferative disorders in which glomeruli may have no histologic abnormalities (minimal change glomerulopathy), thickening of capillary walls (membranous GN), segmental scarring (focal segmental glomerulosclerosis), nodular sclerosis (diabetic glomerulosclerosis), or infiltration by proteinaceous material (amyloidosis).
- Mixed disorders with both proliferative and nonproliferative changes [types I and II membranoproliferative GN (MPGN)].

Immunofluorescence Microscopy

This is of great value in defining specific categories of disease based on:
- Patterns of immune deposits: Granular (lumpy-bumpy), signifying injury due to immune complex localization, as seen in postinfectious GN or lupus nephritis. Linear deposition of immunoglobulin signifying injury due to antiglomerular basement membrane antibodies (anti-GBM Ab), as seen in Goodpasture syndrome.
- Composition of immune deposits, e.g. IgA-dominance of immunoglobulin in IgA nephropathy, Henoch–Schönlein purpura and cirrhotic liver disease; IgG and conspicuous C1q in lupus nephritis; C3-dominance in MPGN.
- Absence of immune deposits, e.g. idiopathic (pauci-immune) crescentic GN, microscopic polyarteritis GN, and Wegener's granulomatosis GN.

Electron Microscopy

This defines:
- Epithelial foot process effacement (fusion), which is a nonspecific finding seen in any condition with significant proteinuria.
- Electron-dense deposits and their locations, e.g. mesangial (IgA nephritis, lupus nephritis), subendothelial (lupus and MPGN type I), subepithelial

(membranous GN, poststreptococcal GN), and intramembranous (MPGN type II).
- Abnormal material, e.g. amyloid deposits.

Identification of Cause or Pathogenic Category

The third step in defining glomerular injury is to determine the cause or pathogenesis.
- Granular immune deposits by IM and dense deposits by EM indicate immune complex disease. The composition of the immune deposits, other laboratory data (serology, complement levels), and additional clinical data [associated diseases: systemic lupus erythematosus (SLE), cryoglobulinemia, endocarditis, streptococcal infection, hepatitis, malaria] may indicate specific forms of immune complex GN, such as IgA nephropathy, lupus nephritis, or poststreptococcal GN.
- Linear immunoglobulin binding to GBM by IM and detection of anti-GBM antibodies by serology indicate anti-GBM GN. Concurrent pulmonary hemorrhage indicates Goodpasture syndrome.
- No immune deposition is characteristic of idiopathic (pauci-immune) crescentic GN and the GN in patients with microscopic polyarteritis and Wegener's granulomatosis. Antineutrophil cytoplasmic autoantibodies are a serologic marker for these diseases.
- A concurrent systemic disease may be the cause of glomerular diseases: diabetes, amyloidosis, systemic sclerosis, and SLE.

Prognosis and Treatment

The final step is to determine the prognosis and to select the treatment for glomerular injury (Tables 21.3 to 21.5). The treatment of GN generally consists of:
- Supportive measures in keeping with the functional changes in the glomerulus, e.g. fluid and electrolyte balance, and control of BP. If ARF or CRF ensue, treat as detailed earlier in this chapter.
- Treatment of the primary cause, if possible, e.g. diabetes, infection, neoplasm, drug exposure.
- Steroid and immunosuppressive treatment of inflammatory diseases and immune-mediated diseases.

RENAL STONES

Crystallization of new stone and an increase in present stone would occur. Only three things would help: 1 and 2 are definite.
1. Lowering calcium filtered. Your calcium is 2.55, normal is 2.2–2.6; you are high although not abnormal, but filtering a higher amount increases concentration and favors crystal deposit.

2. More water to dilute the filtered urine so lowering calcium concentration (need to collect 24 hours urine to see if passing >2 L/d) only then you know it is dilute. Increasing fluid intake to facilitate at least 2.5-3 L of urine volume on a daily basis (do this test once per week or fortnight).
3. Diet: Low calcium foods help only 10-20% as if we try to lower blood calcium some comes out of bone to normalize the slightly lowered blood calcium.

Hydrochlorothiazide (HCTZ) 50 mg/day (too big a dose but may be the only hope) or indapamide 2.5 mg/day is advised.

It is advised 12.5 mg HCTZ twice daily plus amiloride 5 mg/day. Add amiloride 5 mg/day to conserve potassium.

12.5 mg twice daily as although no clinical trial proof; it likely does lower filtered calcium (as even 12.5 often used for BP and less often 25 mg/day does increase bone calcium and prevent fractures). Thus, it is believed it must lower urinary calcium at 25 mg (12.5 twice daily) but no trial proof.

The value of increasing urine volume was demonstrated in a randomized clinical trial lasting 5 years. In that study, stones recurred in only 12 (12%) of the 99 patients who maintained a urine volume of about 2.6 L/day over 5 years, whereas stones recurred in 27 (27%) of the 100 patients in the control group, whose urine volume was about 1.2 L/day ($p = 0.008$). In addition, the time to recurrence was longer in the experimental group than in the control group [38.7 (standard deviation 13.2) months vs 25.1 (standard deviation 16.4) months; $p = 0.016$]. The relative risk reduction ratio for subjects with higher fluid intake (and hence greater urine volume) was about 0.45.

A recently published meta-analysis of randomized trials on preventing the recurrence of calcium oxalate stones suggested that the greatest benefit from pharmacologic intervention is associated with thiazide diuretics.

Five trials involving thiazide diuretics and a single trial with the closely related drug indapamide suggested a risk reduction for developing new stones of 21.3% (95% confidence interval: 29.2-13.4%) in the patients receiving medication.

The combination of HCTZ, 25-50 mg, with amiloride, 5 mg, to prevent potassium wasting was appropriate. Benefits were seen only after 3 years of treatment, so therapy should not be abandoned if stones recur early.

SCLERODERMA (SYSTEMIC SCLEROSIS)

This is an immune-mediated uncommon rheumatic disease that is characterized by fibrosis of the skin and internal organs, vasculopathy, with high morbidity. Some patients present with musculoskeletal pain that might mimic inflammatory joint disease. Mortality is particularly high with renal involvement. The disease may be limited:
- Variable skin thickening of the fingers of both hands, extending proximal to the metacarpophalangeal joints.

- Raynaud's phenomenon.
- Pulmonary arterial hypertension.
- Interstitial lung disease or fibrosis in about 80% but less than half develop progressive interstitial lung disease.
- Pulmonary arterial hypertension affects about 15% of patients with systemic sclerosis particularly in those with minimal skin manifestations.
- Currently, death is caused by lung disease—pulmonary fibrosis and pulmonary hypertension.
- The upper GI tract is commonly affected causing reflux, bloating, distension, constipation, diarrhea, and anorectal incontinence.
- Renal crisis with thrombotic microangiopathy, accelerated-phase hypertension and progressive acute kidney injury carry a high mortality. Treatment with ACE inhibitor should be urgently commenced.

BIBLIOGRAPHY

1. Denton CP, Khanna D. Systemic sclerosis. Lancet. 2017;390(10103):1685-99.
2. Jindal SL, Jennete FC. Medical Diagnosis and Therapy. In: Khan MG, Bartlett JG, Chopra S, Topol EJ (Eds). Pennsylvania: Lea and Febiger; 1994.
3. The Lancet. Systemic sclerosis: advances and prospects. Lancet. 2017;390(10103):1624.
4. Webster AC, Nagler EV, Morton RL, et al. Chronic kidney disease. Lancet. 2017;389(10075):1238-52.

CHAPTER 22

Hematologic Disorders

ANEMIA

The history and physical examination should reveal the likely cause of anemia. Classification of anemia (morphological) is given in Box 22.1. The mean corpuscular volume (MCV) taken in context with the peripheral blood smear should yield a presumptive diagnosis (Table 22.1) (*NB*: Reticulocytes have a large diameter and will ↑ MCV). Corrected reticulocyte count = Measured reticulocyte count × hematocrit ÷ by 40. Further tests requested and interpreted in logical steps should confirm the diagnosis. Table 22.2 gives appropriate laboratory tests and results that may be helpful in evaluating the cause of microcytic anemia (Roath and Gross).

MICROCYTIC HYPOCHROMIC ANEMIA

Iron Deficiency

- The classic example of a microcytic hypochromic anemia is iron deficiency. In the newborn infant, iron deficiency may be a consequence of premature delivery, or from nutrition inadequate to the task of supplying the growing hematopoietic mass.
- Total body iron in a term infant is about 220 mg and in a 70-kg adult is 3.5 g (range 2–5 g). In the newborn, 85% of the iron is in the red cell; in the adult, it is 65%. Smaller amounts are present in the tissues as

Box 22.1: Classification of anemia (morphological).
- *Normocytic normochromic*:
  - Membrane defects
  - Metabolic disorders
  - Aplastic anemia
  - Pure red blood cell aplasia
  - Secondary anemia (simple chronic anemia)
  - Anemia with marrow disruption
  - Defects in globin chain synthesis
  - Hemolytic anemia.
- *Microcytic hypochromic*:
  - Iron deficiency
  - Thalassemias
  - Erythropoietic porphyria.
- *Macrocytic (megaloblastic)*:
  - Folic deficiency
  - B_{12} deficiency
  - Orotic aciduria
  - Refractory
  - Drug induced.

Table 22.1: Peripheral blood morphology—diagnostic aids.

MCV (fl)	RBCs	Suggest
<78	Microcytic hypochromic	• Iron deficiency • Thalassemias • Sideroblastic • Chronic disease.
78–98	Normocytic	• Acute blood loss, hemolytic anemia • Neoplasm, renal failure • Hypothyroidism, aplasia • Chronic disease.
>100	• Macrocytic • Oval macrocytes • Normal macrocytes.	• B_{12} or folate deficiency • Liver disease • *Rarely*: Aplasia, myelodysplasia.
	Dimorphic	• Sideroblastic • Treated iron deficiency • Megaloblastic and iron deficiency • Hemolytic anemia.
	Reticulocytes ↑	• Blood loss • Hemolysis • Response to therapy.
	Fragmented cells: • Helmet, schistocytes • Irregular contracted cells.	• Fragmentation • Hemolysis • DIC.
	Basophilic stippling	• Sideroblastic • Thalassemias, lead poisoning.
	Target cells	• Thalassemias • Sickle cell disease • Liver disease • Postsplenectomy states.
	Spherocytes	• Hereditary spherocytosis • Warm immune hemolysis • Burns • Gas gangrene • Rarely G6PD.
	Sickle forms	Sickle cell anemia
	Spiculated (Burr cells)	• Liver • Splenectomy, uremia • Severe malnutrition.
	Blister cells	G6PD
	Rouleaux formation	Myeloma, macroglobulinemia
	Howell–Jolly bodies (nuclear fragments)	• Megaloblastic, splenectomy • Hemolytic anemia.
	Nucleated red cells	Leukoerythroblastic

Contd...

Contd...

MCV (fl)	RBCs	Suggest
	Myelocytes metamyelocytes	• Infiltration • Severe hypoxemia • Blood loss (severe) • Severe hemolysis • Neonates.
	Hypersegmented neutrophils	• Megaloblastic (characteristic) • Inflammatory processes • Renal failure • Rarely hereditary.

(DIC, disseminated intravascular coagulation; G6PD, glucose-6-phosphate dehydrogenase; MCV, mean corpuscular volume; RBCs, red blood cells)

Table 22.2: Laboratory aids to microcytic anemia.

Normal	Iron deficiency	Thalassemia*	Chronic disease	Sideroblastic
MCV 78–98 fl	<78	<70	N or <78	<78–110
Ferritin M 20–250 ng/mL (2–250 µg/L) F 12–250 ng/mL (12–250 µg/L)	<12**	N or ↑	20–1,000 (usually ↑)	>250
Serum iron 65–175 µg/dL (12–32 µmol/L)	<30 µg/dL <5 µmol/L	N or ↑	<30 µg/dL <5 µmol/L	>200
TIBC 250–410 µg/dL 45–73 µmol/L Transferrin saturation 25–50% Basophilic stippling Marrow iron stores sideroblasts RDW 12–15	>360 µg/dL >64 µmol/L >16 No Absent 16–24	N N or ↑ Yes/No N or ↑ <15	<300 µg/dL <54 µmol/L <16 No N or ↑ Variable usually >15	N >80 Yes/No ↑Abnormal sideroblasts >18

*In minor or intermediate cases.
**Diagnostic only if low: May be normal with infections, malignancies, and severe liver disease.
(F, female; M, male; N, normal; RDW, red cell distribution width; TIBC, total iron binding capacity)

storage iron, with significantly lesser amounts as enzyme and transport iron. With the exception of the actively menstruating female, iron requirements for a normal adult are very email—usually no more than 0.5 mg/kg/day. Iron-rich foods contain more than adequate amounts of iron, and save for the premature infant and/or the childbearing or menstruating female, iron supplementation is unnecessary.

- Iron absorption is governed by demand and occurs in the duodenum and jejunum following a complex uncoupling process of apoferritin to ferritin. It is then transported in the plasma on a β1-globulin (transferrin) to nursing cells in the marrow, where it is injected by pinocytosis into developing red cell precursors, at which point it is stored in the mitochondria for subsequent attachment to protoporphyrin to form heme.
- Iron deficiency is not expressed clinically until iron stores are used up and demands for further utilization of iron go unmet. The net effect is an ↑ in the free transferrin and the appearance of hypochromic microcytic anemia.
- In the older patient, lassitude, stomatitis, esophageal webbing, koilonychia, and achlorhydria are progressive entities. In the term infant, the most common cause is inadequate dietary iron. In the adult, the most likely causes are gastrointestinal (GI) bleeding and excessive menstrual losses. In the tropics, hookworm infestation plays a role.
- Adult treatment consists of ferrous sulfate ($FeSO_4$) or equivalent (1-3 × 325 mg) by mouth (PO) once daily (qd) between meals. Orange juice (citric acid) enhances iron absorption by hastening its valence change. Milk or milk products and cereals, impair iron absorption because of the high phosphate load characteristic of these and similar foodstuffs and which render the iron insoluble. Therapy is usually continued for about 3 months, by which time the anemia is corrected and the stores are replaced. Of all the iron preparations, $FeSO_4$ tablets are the most effective and least expensive. Red cell transfusions are rarely, if ever, indicated. Parenteral iron is often prescribed when oral iron is intolerable. Intramuscular (IM) iron is never indicated.
- Normal bound iron: 60-90 μg/dL; total iron binding capacity: 180-270 μg/dL. Normal ferritin: 30-120 mg/dL (20-250 μg/mL) (Table 22.2).

NORMOCYTIC NORMOCHROMIC ANEMIAS

Membrane Disorders

The red cell membrane is composed of a highly mobile bilayer of intercalated phospholipids, glycolipids, and nonesterified cholesterol penetrated by a protein structure that includes antigens, receptors, and transport proteins on a supporting submembrane lattice of spectrin and actin, which in turn control H_2O content in combination with an adenosine triphosphate (ATP) energy-derived cation pump.

Hereditary spherocytosis (HS) is the single most common membrane defect. It is inherited as an autosomal dominant.
- Classical findings often include neonatal jaundice, pallor, modest splenomegaly, abdominal pain (with gallstones), and after the neonatal period, intermittent nonobstructive jaundice. Patients may go for years with minimal symptoms or may experience waxing and waning periods of heightened hemolysis on aplasia following either viral or bacterial infections.
- Hematologic findings include anemia, reticulocytosis, ↑ indirect reacting bilirubin, spherocytes, and increased osmotic fragility in hypotonic saline. The defect, which resides in the spectrin fraction of the membrane, impairs membrane flexibility and results in splenic trapping. The red blood cell (RBC) membrane in HS is also highly permeable to sodium (Na).
- Treatment of choice is splenectomy, preferably after the patient reaches less than 3 years of age or at a time when the patient is responsive to active immunization with polyvalent pneumococcal and *Haemophilus influenzae*. Postsplenectomy penicillin is administered for more than or equal to 5 years. This approach applies to any splenectomized individual, irrespective of the underlying disorder (Roath and Gross).

Hereditary elliptocytosis (HE) is twice as common but much less severe than HS.
- It is inherited as a single dominant and codominant inheritance may be fatal. A peripheral blood film reveals prominent elliptocytosis.
- The defect resides in the spectrin-actin interface of the red cell membrane. It often presents in the newborn with prominent jaundice. The osmotic fragilities mimic that of HS.

Splenectomy is rarely if ever required, and HE is less pronounced in the older patient.

Cation permeability disorders induce minimal hemolysis, the result of either Na^+ or K^+ losses. In the former, the picture is that of stomatocytosis, the result of ↑ H_2O absorption. In the K^+-loss group, the cells tend to desiccate (desiccocytosis).

Inheritance is unclear, and splenectomy is effective in the occasional serious case.

Disorders of physical or thermal injury include the so-called "Waring blender syndrome" defects, which result from vascular damage and are known as microangiopathic hemolytic anemia. Mechanical factors, as in eddy currents initiated by prosthetic material (e.g. heart valves), may also affect similar findings which, on occasion, may be so severe as to initiate consumption of clotting factors, leading to disseminated intravascular coagulation (DIC). Thermal injury produces a cell bubble effect, not unlike yeast, which has all the clinical and laboratory features of HS.

Metabolic Disorders

Hexose monophosphate pathway: Glucose-6-phosphate dehydrogenase (G6PD) deficiency is the classic example of the hexose monophosphate shunt disorder, with millions of people affected by a sex-linked inheritance of an abnormality that includes more than 100 variants. The two most common variants are the type that occurs predominantly in American Blacks and the type that is most common in the Mediterranean basin, or the more unstable "African" type.

The gene for G6PD is inherited as an X-linked recessive and is characterized by inability to summon electrons (e.g. hydrogen atoms) to respond to oxidant-induced membrane stress. Common inducers of oxidant stress are drugs and infections. With infections, hydrogen peroxide generated during phagocytosis is very likely the initiating agent. Drug-induced stress is produced by agents that impair the electron transfer system (the list is extensive). Fava bean-induced hemolysis occurs mainly in the Mediterranean population, is usually severe-even lethal—and may occur merely by inhalation of the pollen. Dopaquinone, a metabolite of L-3,4-dihydroxyphenylalanine (L-DOPA), is a powerful oxidant, and is probably responsible for the severe hemolysis in a limited number of fava bean-sensitive populations. The reason for the dopaquinone effect is probably a distinctly separate, gene-related inability to metabolize L-DOPA.

- Treatment consists of separation from the offending agent (when possible), aggressive hydration to minimize heme-induced renal damage, red cell transfusions for symptomatic anemia, and iron to replace hemoglobinuric losses. Counseling is a necessary prophylactic course (Roath and Gross).

Apart from the (often massive) hemoglobinuria, and the anemia and reactive reticulocytosis (which contain sufficient G6PD to limit further oxidant attack at the same dose level, e.g. tachyphylaxis), the peripheral smear reveals occasional red cells with retracted areas of hemoglobinization (blister cells) (Table 22.1).

Embden–Meyerhof pathway: Pyruvate kinase (PK) deficiency is the most common example of a glycolytic enzymopathy. Because the defect occurs subsequent to 2,3-diphosphoglycerate (2,3-DPG) formation, patients with PK deficiency tend to be more symptomatic than those with G6PD deficiency. In addition, the abnormality is constant and not triggered by an external source. Although inherited as an autosomal recessive, the disease varies in severity, very likely due to subsets. Infection-induced marrow hypoplasia also adds to the severity.

Hematologic findings include chronic anemia of variable severity, reactive reticulocytosis, and nonspecific anisocytosis. All patients have degrees of splenomegaly. The hemolysis is entirely within the reticuloendothelial (RE) system.

- Treatment may include red cell transfusion for symptomatic anemia. Splenectomy helps only in patients who develop hypersplenic events. Folate supplementation probably helps those individuals whose dietary folate is inadequate to replace red cell synthesis demands. Iron administration is contraindicated.

Aplastic Disorders

Anemia characterized by normal mean corpuscular hemoglobin concentration (MCHC) and reticulocytopenia are hypoproliferative (anemia of marrow failure or ineffective erythropoiesis).
- Aplastic anemia is a classic example of such a disorder, although only rarely if ever is the marrow totally acellular. Scattered areas of trilineage activity are usually present in such individuals.

Acquired disorders: Factors known to induce marrow aplasia include: ionizing radiation, aromatic hydrocarbons (e.g. benzene and toluene), virtually all anticancer agents, a variety of inorganic poisons (e.g. arsenicals), certain antimicrobials (e.g. chloramphenicol), anticonvulsants (e.g. phenylhydantoin), antithyroid agents (e.g. tapazole, hypoglycemics, and mood elevators), insecticides [e.g. dichlorodiphenyltrichloroethane (DDT)], solvents (e.g. carbon tetrachloride), viruses, such as those that cause hepatitis, bacterial agents (e.g. tubercle bacillus), and certain immune-mediated hemolytic anemia (e.g. PNH) that often terminate in either aplastic anemia or malignancy. In more than 112 of the affected population, the etiologic agent is unknown (Roath and Gross).

Inherited disorders: Inherited, or constitutional aplastic anemia, also referred to as Fanconi anemia and often accompanied by various combinations of abnormalities involving the skin, bones, and kidneys, has an associated high risk of late-occurring leukemia, usually of the monocytic type.
- Aplastic anemia is usually slow in onset and characterized by petechiae, frequent infections, and signs and symptoms specifically related to low levels of circulating hemoglobin (Hb). Hematologic findings, as noted, include reticulocytopenia with a normocytic normochromic anemia, thrombopenia, and granulocytopenia. Marrow biopsy usually reveals skip areas of hematopoietic activity, most commonly lymphocytes and plasma cells, as well as reticulin, fat, and supporting tissue.

  Severe aplastic anemia by definition is characterized by a reticulocyte count less than or equal to 0.1%, an absolute granulocyte count less than or equal to 500% mm^3, and a platelet count less than or equal to 20,000/mm^3. Iron turnover is marginal; the iron-binding protein (β1-globulin, transferrin) is highly saturated with much of the iron present in the RE system. Organomegaly is an uncommon finding, and when present, suggests an underlying malignancy, infectious disorder, or autoimmune process.

- Treatment of choice for all severe aplastic anemias, including the Fanconi type, is bone marrow transplantation (BMT) preferably with a matched-related donor, with therapy designed to minimize graft-versus-host disease (GVHD). Match-unrelated donors (MUDs) are acceptable, although they carry a high risk for severe GVHD and its associated ↑ in morbidity. The response to matched sibling donor BMT is a 75% disease-free survival leading to cure in the absence of an appropriate donor. Leukocyte-poor, carefully screened, and temporally sequenced red cell and platelet transfusions are needed in order to maintain adequate function and minimize the occurrence of alloimmunization and platelet refractoriness, respectively. Rigid infection surveillance is also warranted in order to minimize the chances of overwhelming sepsis. Red cell and platelet transfusions should be performed at levels of 6 g/L and 10,000/mm^3 or less, respectively. Human leukocyte antigen (HLA)-matched platelets are the preferred donor source.

The use of such cytokines as erythropoietin (Epo), granulocyte colony-stimulating factor (G-CSF), or granulocyte-macrophage colony-stimulating factor (GM-CSF) has provided modest, albeit unsustained success, but only in the less severely affected patients. Combination of interleukin-3 (IL-3) and Epo may prove to be somewhat more successful in effecting trilineage responses, but responses, when they occur, are sustained only as long as the cytokines are administered. In patients with evidence of T-cell-mediated suppression, the use of antithymocyte globulin, cyclosporine A (CSA), or even cyclophosphamide has achieved limited success. Spontaneous remissions occur in approximately 15% of cases and are essentially unpredictable. Combinations of corticosteroids and androgens offer only marginal responses.

SECONDARY ANEMIA

Red cell hypoplasia or aplasia has been identified in patients with renal failure whose severity is roughly proportional to the degree of uremia. Both red cell mass and plasma volume are depressed in these patients, who are further compromised by a shortened red cell survival and bleeding secondary to impaired platelet function. Although platelet and white cell levels are usually normal, 10% of end-stage renal disease (ESRD) patients have granulopenia, apparently the result of high-density lipoprotein (HDL)-induced suppression of granulopoiesis. Red cell deformation with helmet cells is a common feature of this disease.
- *Treatment*: For anemic, uremic patients unresponsive to Epo (25 mg/kg twice weekly), carefully monitored red cell transfusion is the only efficacious therapy.

Deficiencies in pituitary, thyroid, adrenocortical, or gonadal hormonal function can produce a normochromic normocytic anemia, although the anemia of thyroid deficiency may be microcytic and hypochromic, the result of inadequate foodstuff iron absorption in association with hypometabolic states; or macrocytic if the major inadequacy is folate.

ANEMIA WITH MARROW DISRUPTION

Primary or marrow metastatic disorders, or marrow encumbered by increased numbers of metabolically inert cells (as in the lipid storage disease) may also lead to severe pancytopenia. Agnogenic myeloid metaplasia, a rare disease of unknown etiology, resulting in marrow fibrosis accompanied by extramedullary myeloproliferation, ultimately results in pancytopenia with massive splenomegaly.
- The peripheral blood film is characterized by distorted and fragmented cells (ordinarily captured and removed from the circulation by the spleen), schistocytes, tear drops, giant platelets, and immature forms. Proper diagnosis mandates proper evaluation of biopsy material. There is no known effective therapy.
- Fibrosis is relentless but usually slow (upward of 5–7 years), and the disease terminates either in hematopoietic failure or refractory myeloid leukemia. Splenectomy does not affect cures and may actually be counterproductive if the spleen is both RE tissue and a major hematopoietic organ.

Sickle Cell Disease

Of the 200 known hemoglobinopathies, sickle cell disease is the most common and the most destructive.
- "Every year approximately 300,000 infants are born with sickle cell anemia, which is defined as homozygosity for the sickle hemoglobin S (HbS) gene [i.e. for a missense mutation (Glu6Val, rs334) in the β-globin (*HBB*) gene] and that this number could rise to 400,000 by 2050" (Piel et al.).
- In most of these disorders, the physical defect is a single amino acid substitution in either the α, β, γ, or δ subunits. Virtually, all the diseases are inherited as an autosomal codominant, and in the vast majority of cases, detection is readily apparent by gel electrophoresis at variously adjusted pH.

Molecular features of human Hb variants fall into five major groups of single or double amino acid substitution.
  - Examples of single substitution include Hb S, C, D, E, and G on the β chain, HbI on the α chain, HbF on the γ chain, and HbA2 on the δ chain.
  - Of the amino acid deletions identified to date, all are found on the β chain. None produces serious clinical findings, the classic sample being Hb Freiberg.
  - A third category is the fusion Hbs, which result in nonhomologous crossing over, e.g. Hb Lepore, a γ-β fusion with clinical findings consistent with the thalassemias.

- A fourth group includes the elongated subunits, which have either a base substitution or a frameshift. An example of the former is Hb Constant Spring, and of the latter, Hb Wayne, both occurring on the α chain. There are no known β-chain frameshifts. Symptomatology is minimal.
- A fifth classification includes the unstable Hbs: those producing the Heinz bodies and hemolysis, those with high O_2 affinity without cyanosis (e.g. familiar erythrocytosis), and those that result in cyanosis (e.g. M-Hbs). The unstable variants as well as the high O_2-affinity group, including the M-Hbs, appear only as heterozygotes. The homozygous state is felt to be lethal.

- Of all African Americans, 1.5% are homozygous and 8% heterozygous for sickle cell disease.
- The disease is not uncommon in Nigeria, the Democratic Republic of the Congo, and India.
- It appears that heterozygosity for the sickle cell mutation in *HBB* provides against severe malaria.
  Of all homozygous sickle cell disease patients, 30% have approximately 80% of all the major symptomatology, and it is postulated, although unproven, that a haploid subtype of the disease accounts for the severity of findings. Sickle cell disease is the only hemolytic disorder marked by serious intravascular clotting. Major untoward events include strokes, relentless priapism, and infarction of any system, including the renal medulla or segments of the GI tract. Early in life, splenic sequestration presents a hazard and may result in more than 50% of the total blood volume being acutely trapped in the splenic circulation at a given time.
- Treatment of sequestration includes cautious transfusion and monitoring for autoreinfusion of entrapped cells. Because of the propensity for repeated episodes, splenectomy following a second event is appropriate.
- "Early diagnosis, penicillin prophylaxis, blood transfusion, transcranial Doppler imaging, hydroxyurea, and hematopoietic stem cell transplantation can dramatically improve survival and quality of life for patients with sickle cell disease" (Piel et al.).
  By 5–7 years of age, the spleen tends to shrink in size following repetitive infarctions, but it may be enlarged and become nonfunctional before it involutes.
  It is likely that minor repetitive central nervous system (CNS) infarctions account for changes in mental function. There are data to support the likelihood that CNS vascular reserve is impaired as a result of these episodes. Infarction-induced changes in the renal medulla impair concentrating ability; most SS patients consequently develop hyposthenuria by age 10 years, necessitating frequent trips to the drinking fountain and toilet.
- The single most effective diagnostic test of hemoglobinopathy is electrophoresis of peripheral blood. Abnormal Hb can also be identified

in utero via analysis of amniocentesis fluid. The solubility test, which depends on differences in the solubility of deoxyhemoglobin-S when compared to other Hbs, is far less reliable.

Pathophysiology of sickle disease results from β-chain substitution of valine for glutamine. It occurs in the deoxy form wherein Hb elongates into bundles of fibers which ultimately gel into "permanent" sickle forms. The extent of this phenomenon is controlled by the initiating insult and the nature of the associated β chain. A normal associated β chain (e.g. HbA), as in sickle cell trait, ↓ the degree of gelation, whereas HbC on the paired chain enhances this phenomenon. For example, homozygous (100%) deoxyhemoglobin-S requires 24 g HbS/100 mL red cells to induce gelation. Equal concentrations of deoxyhemoglobin-S and deoxyhemoglobin-C require 30 g/100 mL for gelation to occur, and equal concentrations of HbS and F require 36.9 g/100 mL. The obvious combination for maintenance of a symptom-free disorder is the SF or the β-d combination. The net effect of the elongated and rigid red cells is obstruction of blood flow, initially at the capillary level and subsequently, as the clot propagates, to larger vessels. Reoxygenation may effect a reversal of sickle cells to a normal shape only prior to gelation, i.e. only prior to their assumption of the permanent sickled form. Prolonged minimal deoxygenation, abrupt severe deoxygenation, or an environment, will induce the appearance of irreversible, sickled forms, the most prominent symptom of which is pain and the worst finding of which is stroke (Roath and Gross).

Treatment

Pain crises require analgesia and hydration.

Piel et al. indicated that "hydroxyurea treatment is the sole approved pharmacologic therapy for sickle cell disease and is increasingly used in both adults and children; hematopoietic stem cell transplantation is potentially curative, although its use is restricted by the high cost, toxicity, and limited availability of suitable donors" (Piel et al.).

- The patient with a serious vascular event should receive exchange transfusion in order to maintain HbS less than 30% in the presence of a hematocrit less than or equal to 33% in order to minimize the risk of viscosity-induced stroke.
- With impaired splenic function, there is an associated immunologic deficit, including diminution in immunoglobulin M (IgM) production and opsonization, the latter resulting in ↓ ability to recognize encapsulated organisms.

As a consequence, patients with HbS disease or sickle cell Hb in combination with another abnormal Hb should receive pneumococcus, *Haemophilus influenzae*, and meningococcus vaccines. Because of the uncertainty of the efficacy of vaccination less than 2 years of age, all patients should also receive 5 years of penicillin, commencing in the first 4 months of life.

Sickle cell Hb electrophoretic patterns in older patients are the inverse of those of the newborn, i.e. 5% F and 95% S. By the time, the patient presents to the doctor with local or diffuse pain, it is usually hard to distinguish between infarction and infection. Radionuclide scanning is helpful at times, but infections may include an infarction component, and many infarctions result in secondary infections. It is best to treat any suspected infarction as both infarction and infection, irrespective of the presence or absence of fever. Another area of major concern is the abdominal pain crisis. The distinction between sickle cell-induced abdominal pain crises and so-called "surgical" abdomens is the absence of bowel sounds, or the hypodynamic bowel, in sickle pain crisis. Bowel sounds in inflammatory bowel disease are hyperactive, save for the onset of typhlitis or septic shock.

Genetic counseling is a major therapeutic endeavor and is designed to enable parents to make decisions about risks and consequences. Male sickle cell disease patients produce variably viable sperm, and sickle cell disease females are generally able to conceive and bear children but only with careful Hb control and prolonged obstetrical monitoring. For severe sickle cell disease, i.e. those with stroke or repeated infections/infarction, BMT is the treatment of choice.

Sickle cell disease can occur, as noted, with other hemoglobinopathies, including thalassemia and HbC. Heterozygous HbS–HbC disease is less symptomatic than the former and occurs about 25% as commonly as HbS disease, but it is almost as common among adults because of the diminished life expectancy of Hb SS disease. Hb CC anemia is mild to moderate, and includes target cells and occasional precipitated Hb clumps. Splenomegaly is common.

Red cell transfusion for sickle cell disease is rarely indicted. Its value is essentially limited to patients with prolonged symptomatic aplastic crises or who acquire "adult" Hb prior to surgery (reduction of HbS to <30%) or who develop massive pneumonias with ineffective oxygenation. The advantage of supplemental folate (1 mg/day) as a means of addressing ↑ utilization needs remains controversial.

- There are around 55 unstable Hbs, all of which cause varying degrees of hemolysis in the heterozygous state. The homozygous disorder is apparently lethal. The amino acid substitution occurs in the heme pocket of the β chain, which enhance oxidization to methemoglobin, following which the heme forms precipitate out (Heinz bodies). Symptomatology is minimal and does not require therapy (Roath and Gross).

IMMUNOHEMOLYTIC ANEMIA

Immunohemolytic diseases are characterized by a group of disorders in which hemolysis is mediated by autoantibodies of the immunoglobulin G (IgG) or IgM type and more than or equal to one components of complement—usually activated C3 and occasionally C4-coating the red cell. Antibody identification is carried out by the direct Coombs', also known as antiglobulin test. Antibodies of the IgG type coat, but do not agglutinate, red cells in vitro in the absence of antiglobulin, and are accordingly termed "incomplete antibodies". A direct positive test is the sine qua non of the immunohemolytic process. The indirect test detects serum antibodies. Any serum with suspected antibody is incubated for 30 minutes at 37°C with red cells, following which the serum is washed away and the red cells are treated with reagent to determine both presence and antibody specificity. Classification of immunohemolytic anemia includes chemical and structural relationships: (i) warm activation (primarily at body temperature), (ii) cold activation (room temperature or lower), (iii) whether it is an IgG [molecular weight (MW) 160,000] or an IgM (MW 1,000,000), and (iv) ability to activate complement. Warm antibodies do not injure the red cell membrane per se, although they bring about spheroid changes in shape and corresponding ↑ in osmotic fragility. In summary, the IgG antibodies have a MW in the 160,000 range, an optimal temperature of 37°C, little or no activation of complement, a positive direct Coombs' test, a frequently positive indirect Coombs' test, and only rare specificity but strong avidity for red cell antigens. Most of the cases of IgG autohemolytic anemia are of unknown etiology; approximately 20% are the result of drug-induced phenomena, and 10–15% is the result of malignancies. Because of the "incomplete" nature of these antibodies and the fact that they rarely activate complement, phagocytosis occurs within the RE system, the net effect of the anemia being ↑ bilirubin production (Roath and Gross).

Antibodies that activate complement usually cause abrupt and extensive hemolysis, usually in the intravascular space, resulting in rapid utilization of haptoglobin and resultant levels of less than or equal to 5 mg. Unlike 7S warm (IgG) antibodies, the 19S cold (IgM) antibodies are optimally reactive at 2–4°C. Above 10°C, affinity ↓, and at about 30°C, antibodies dissociate from the cell itself. In effect, IgM antibodies remain bound to red cell antigens only at low temperatures. Agglutination is, therefore, often limited to the peripheral circulation of the extremities. Warming an extremity may cause the disappearance of the cold antibody effect. In any suspected cases of cold antibody disease, studies ideally should be carried out at bedside using serially diluted anticoagulated blood drawn from a cold extremity in order to determine the lowest concentration at which hemagglutination is observed. Factors determining the potency of hemolysis include:
- Mechanical destruction when cold exposure is accompanied by muscular exertion.
- Complement activation inducing profound intravascular hemolysis.
- Temperature controlling the distribution and reactivity of the antigen on the red cell membrane.
- Antigen.

Complement-mediated hemolysis is an orderly sequence of interactions that usually creates perforations in the red cell membrane. Activation begins with the C1q subunit. Conversion of C4 and C2 into activated components leads to an unstable complex activating C3, which in turn, causes segments of C5–C9 to alter lipids and bind proteins, thereby creating membrane depressions. The properdin system is an alternate activation pathway that bypasses the first three components. Why one or the other of the pathways occurs is unclear, but either should be looked for in any patient with massive intravascular hemolysis leading to hemoglobinuria.

Immunoglobulin G disorders are usually self-limited but on occasion, progress to a chronic and unremitting state. Icterus, as opposed to hemoglobinuria, is its common pathologic expression. Splenomegaly is a rare occurrence. Reticulocytosis and leukocytosis usually accompany hemolysis. In some patients, there is an associated thrombocytopenia, also known as Evans syndrome. Drugs known to induce warm autoimmune hemolytic disease—such as quinine, quinidine, and sulfonamides—form an antigenic protein complex. Penicillin may also induce an autoimmune process that differs from other drug complexes in that the cell–drug complex is antigenic, which elicits IgG antibodies directed against penicillinized red cells.

Therapy for warm autoantibody disease depends on the underlying situation. Most patients respond to the administration of glucocorticosteroids, which poison monocyte function and impair lymphocyte (antibody) production. Patients refractory to corticosteroids usually respond to a high-dose of gamma globulin or splenectomy.

Ten percent of patients are refractory to all forms of therapy. For any identifiable etiologic mechanism, effective treatment must eliminate the autoimmune process. Immunohemolytic anemia secondary to cold antibodies may occur in patients with mycoplasma, pneumonia, and similar infectious disorders or be associated with certain myeloproliferative diseases. Symptoms are due to a vas occlusion in portions of the circulation exposed to cooling. Hemolysis may range from mild to severe, with impressive amounts of intravascular lysis leading to free Hb, followed by conversion to methemoglobin, and following consumption of haptoglobin to methemalbumin, which is then released in the kidneys as methemoglobinuria. Splenomegaly is uncommon.

Because the IgM is largely confined to the circulation, corticosteroids and/or hyperimmune globulin are not effective, and the single most effective approach is the intense use of plasmapheresis, usually every 3–4 weeks, until the process subsides. When transfusions are needed to raise the Hb levels in the severe cases, we must recognize the likelihood of an impaired cross-match, followed by an attempt to identify a basis for intravascular lysis and hemoglobinuria. In these situations, a large volume of intravenous (IV) fluids is required to "wash out" excess free Hb and avoid renal damage (Roath and Gross).

THALASSEMIA

Unlike sickle cell disease and related disorders where defective globin production results in a shortened red cell life span, the thalassemias are characterized by impaired production of otherwise normally structured globin chains. The net result is ineffective erythropoiesis.

- α-chain development begins early in fetal life; β-chain development begins shortly before parturition, with a typical distribution at birth as follows: 100% α chains, 75% γ chains, and 25% β chains. By 6 months, there is a 50% decline in γ chain, and a corresponding ↑ in β-chain production. The significance of the embryonic chains, epsilon, zeta, etc. the production of which ceases at around the 12th week of gestation, is unknown.
- Whereas β-thalassemia is characterized by ↓ synthesis, β-thalassemia has essentially no β-chain synthesis. Save for β-thalassemia, incorporation of radioactive material in β-thalassemia is less than or equal to 30% of that incorporated into the α chains.
- *Both α- and β-thalassemias are inherited as autosomal dominants*: 50% chance for heterozygous offspring (25% chance for homozygous disease and 25%, for normal offspring) from two heterozygous parents. β-thalassemia is common to the Mediterranean subbasin of southern Italy and Greece. In the Orient, α-thalassemia is the common form. In Africa, both α- and β-thalassemia occur with almost equal frequency rate and gross
  In the heterozygous form, the anemia varies from nil to mild. In the homozygous form, anemia is severe and characterized by marked microcytosis, targeting fragmentation, tear drops, and stippling. In heterozygotes, there is a corresponding elevation in δ-chain synthesis (HbA2) to 4–6% (normal, <3%) and in γ-chain synthesis (HbF) to as much as 20%. Neither HbA2 nor HbF is ↑ in heterozygous α-thalassemia. Although the reason for the differences in HbF synthesis among the various β-thalassemia patients is unknown, those with ↑ HbF synthesis tend to have milder symptoms than those who do not.
- δ-β-thalassemia, an uncommon type, occurs as the result of deficient δ-β-chain synthesis and is accompanied by a corresponding ↑ in fetal δ-chain production to 2:5%. Hb Lepore is another uncommon disorder that consists of two α chains and the fusion products of one β and one δ chain. Both δ-β and Lepore disorders are essentially asymptomatic. However, the combination of Hb Lepore and β-thalassemia minor will produce a double heterozygote of Hb Lepore-β thalassemia minor, which is clinically indistinguishable from homozygous β-thalassemia. Although the thalassemias morphologically appear to be iron deficient, these patients have ↑ iron stores. Treatment would add further oxidant stress and ↑ the risks of already existing iron overload, progressing to irreversible hemosiderosis.

- Clinically, homozygous thalassemia is classified as thalassemia major, a classification particularly germane to the β-thalassemias and which is expressed as severe (major) or moderate (intermedial). With the ↓ in β chains, there are ↑ numbers of residual, or unattached, α chains, which in the free form, are unstable and tend to precipitate out as inclusion bodies. These bodies damage the cell membrane and effect a corresponding ↑ in permeability, with concomitant loss of ATP and premature uptake by the RE system, leading to ↓ survival.

Treatment

Untreated β-thalassemia major results in severe debilitation. Blood transfusions and folate supplementation (the latter designed to address ↑ demands), in association with aggressive chelation therapy, will enhance life span and quality of life. However, transfusion carries a high risk of alloimmunization and hemosiderosis (even with aggressive chelation).

Overall, growth and development are poor. The typical habitus is one characterized by hepatosplenomegaly, massive medullary and extramedullary hematopoiesis, multiple exocrine disorders, and as noted, transfusion-induced hemosiderosis.

Patients with HbH diseases have 20–30% β chains in tetrads (B4). Typical findings include hypochromia, poikilocytosis, and mild anemia.

Treatment with the exception of the occasional aplastic crisis, patients with HbH disease uncommonly requires blood transfusions. In the rare extreme case, splenectomy is moderately effective in combating the severity of the anemia.

Patients with α-thalassemia major have only tetrads of δ chains, e.g. Hb Bart—which, as the sole Hb, is ineffective in providing O_2 delivery. α-thalassemia homozygotes are virtually hypoxic, and if not still born, die within minutes of birth with classic hydropic features, including macerated placentae.

Genetic counseling of heterozygotes is an important part of overall medical care. Prenatal diagnosis can be made by amniocentesis during the 1st trimester using either two-dimensional chromatography or by polymerase chain expansion of deoxyribonucleic acid (DNA) molecules.

Treatment of choice for thalassemia major is BMT. In the absence of an appropriately matched related or unrelated donor, blood transfusion, folate supplementation, and in many cases, splenectomy (with immunization) represents the only life-sustaining alternatives.

PORPHYRIA

Porphyria is a unique group of multisystem disorders with microcytic hypochromic anemia, characterized by ↑ production of uroporphyrins and their precursors, viz. aminolevulinic acid (ALA) and porphobilinogen (PBG)— as a result of blocks along various steps in the heme biosynthetic pathway.

Glycine and succinyl CoA combine to form ALA in the presence of ALA synthetase and pyridoxal phosphate. Condensation of two ALAs catalyzed by ALA dehydrase forms PBG, a red, H_2O-soluble compound which is a diagnostic end-product of acute intermittent porphyria.

Increased production of porphyrin or porphyrin precursors results in erythopoietic porphyria or hepatic porphyria. Erythropoietic porphyria is characterized by dermatitis with bullous lesions, stained teeth, ineffective production as well as ↑ destruction of red cells, and splenomegaly. As in hepatic porphyria, a less severe disorder of little hematologic significance, large amounts of uro- and coproporphyrin-1 are present in bone marrow cells as well as in urine, stool, and tissues. The light sensitivity of the fluorescent porphyrins causes the skin and teeth changes. PBG imparts a red color to the urine, which also fluoresces in the presence of ultraviolet (UV) light as the result of the concomitant presence of porphyrins. Tests that identify PBG also identify UBG, which is distinguished from the former compound by solubility, e.g. the addition of a fat solvent, such as chloroform to a red solution suspected of being either PBG or UBG will entrap the UBG if it is present.

Treatment

Erythropoietic porphyria and erythropoietic protoporphyria require red cell transfusion support for maintenance of life. The only curative therapy is marrow transplantation, without which patients rarely live beyond 20–25 years of life.

MACROCYTIC (MEGALOBLASTIC) ANEMIA

The classic example of megaloblastic anemia is that secondary to vitamin B_{12} or folic acid deficiency. Megaloblastic anemia is a disorder resulting from impairment of DNA synthesis and involving changes in any or all hematopoietic cell lines. As a consequence, megaloblastic erythroid cells are larger (macro-ovalocytes), have a higher cytoplasmic-to-nuclear ratio, and possess more granular chromatin than do normal erythroid forms. The white cell series are also larger than their normal components and have strangely shaped nuclei with ragged chromatin, which in the mature form, become hypersegmented. Granulation tends to be deficient. Megakaryocytes are sometimes bizarrely shaped but may be normal in appearance.

Mean corpuscular volumes usually exceed 100 μ^3 (Table 22.1); the reticulocyte count is low and sometimes absent. With progressive disease, erythroid precursors with obvious megaloblastic features may be found in the circulation. Neutrophil nuclei usually exhibit 5–6 segments, sometimes as many as 18 (Table 22.1). The marrow is usually cellular and characterized by megaloblastic transformation and frequent mitotic figures. Pancytopenia may ensue.

Clinically, the anemia is slow in onset and characterized by fatigue, shortness of breath. Patients appear both pale and lemony yellow.

Serum bilirubin, serum iron, lactate dehydrogenase (LDH), and muramidase levels are invariably increased.

FOLIC ACID DEFICIENCY

The role of the pterins in human nutrition assumed major importance following the discovery of pteroylmonoglutamic acid (folic acid), which consists of three components: (i) a pteridine, (ii) an aminobenzoic acid, and (iii) a glutamic acid. Its nomenclature is N-(2-amino-4-hydroxypteridine-6-ethyl)-p-aminobenzoic acid, an acyl radical with the generic term "pteroylglutamate". The catalytic reduction of folic acid by dihydrofolate reductase to 5, 6, 7, 8-tetrahydrofolic acid ensures its role in enzyme reactions. Dihydrofolate reductase is sensitive to folic acid analogs, which contain the 4-amino group, which is the fundamental reason for its anticancer activity.

In humans, the major form of folate is N5-methyltetrahydrofolic acid. The N5 methyl group is a *Leuconostoc citrovorum* growth factor, which accounts for one of its earlier names: Citrovorum factor. It is also commonly referred to as folinic acid. Functionally, this family of folate compounds, or one-carbon constituents, serves as the source for DNA synthesis.

Although widely distributed in nature, the richest sources are vegetables, such as asparagus, spinach, and lettuce. The minimum daily requirements for adults are 40–60 µg, and approximately twice that amount for the premature newborn.

Folates are absorbed primarily in the proximal jejunum. Most of what is ingested is absorbed, following which it is protein bound for transportation.

With both bioassay (*Lactobacillus casei* systems) and chemical assay, the normal range of bound serum folate is 4–20 ng/mL.

Folate deficiency leads to a megaloblastic anemia associated with glossitis, ↑ levels of LDH, and weight loss. Neurologic changes do not occur as a consequence of folic acid deficiency.

Typical laboratory findings include ↓ serum and red cell folate and ↑ excretion of folic acid intermediates (e.g. formiminoglutamic acid following a loading dose of histidine).

Infants fed solely goat's milk, which is essentially folate free, develop folic acid deficiency. Ascorbic acid participates in the reduction of folic acid to tetrahydrofolic acid. As a consequence, dietary deficiency of vitamin C may induce folic deficiency in an individual whose folate intake is marginal.

The most common cause of folate deficiency is inadequate intake or aggressive cooking of foodstuffs. With poor intake, folate deficiency may become manifest in less than 3 months.

Malabsorptive disorders, so-called celiac diseases, and parasitic infestations induce folate deficiency because of changes in the GI mucosa.

Oral administration of folic acid, even in the presence of celiac syndrome, will result in improvement in serum folate levels.

Certain pharmacologic agents (dilantin) may also impair folate absorption.

Additionally, oral contraceptives have been shown to block absorption. Increased requirements are imposed by pregnancy or in patients with various chronic hemolytic anemias. Patients with severe anorexia secondary to neoplastic diseases profit from the additional administration of folic acid.

Folic acid antagonists used in the treatment of leukemia and related diseases·interfere with the conversion of folic acid to tetrahydrofolate by blocking dihydrofolate reductase. This is corrected only via tetrahydrofolate (Citrovorum factor) administration.

Treatment of folic acid deficiency with as little as 1 mg/day for 7-10 days is sufficient to correct the disorder, but 5 mg is usually given to adults. Folinic acid is rarely needed in deficiency states.

VITAMIN B_{12} DEFICIENCY

Both ineffective production and ↑ hemolysis contribute to vitamin B_{12} deficiency anemia. Normal red cells transfused into B_{12}-deficient patients have ↓ survival.

The source of vitamin B_{12} in human nutrition is essentially tissues of animal origin as well as fish, eggs, and milk. The total daily dietary requirement is 2-5 µg.

Because vitamin B_{12} is stored and reused, deficiency states take 2-3 years to develop after cessation of B_{12} ingestion. Functionally, vitamin B_{12} is a cyanocobalamin molecule.

Systems impaired by vitamin B_{12} deficiency include those involved with methionine-methyl synthesis (which relates ultimately to tetrahydrofolic acid regeneration) and methylmalonyl-CoA isomerization (which relates to metabolism of propionic acid). The impairment in DNA synthesis accounts for the megaloblastic transformation and all related features. More specifically, defective methylmalonyl-CoA metabolism impairs the neurologic processes, a feature prominent in such patients. Absorption occurs in the ileum following its conjugation with parietal cell secreted intrinsic factor, which is enhanced by histamine, methacholine, and gastrin production and eliminated by gastrectomy.

Plasma B_{12} levels are 150-500 pg/mL, all of which is transcobalamin bound.

Transcobalamins prevents loss of body secretions and provides transport through cell membranes. Transcobalamin-2 is the initial transport mechanism. Transcobalamin-1 carries most of the vitamin B_{12} in plasma, and the role of transcobalamin-3 is uncertain, although much of it appears to rise from granulocytes. Neurologic abnormalities consist of combined system disease of the spinal cord. Vitamin B_{12} levels are determined by bioassay or isotope dilutions. In the absence of a coexisting folate deficiency, folate levels are increased in the presence of vitamin B_{12} deficiency.

Vitamin B_{12} deficiency is rarely the result of inadequate diet except in vegans. It is most often due to:
- Diminished intestinal absorption, secondary to either intrinsic factor deficiency (defective synthesis or antibody blocked)
- Gastric resection
- Overgrowth of intestinal bacteria, as in the blind loop syndrome
- Intestinal stasis
- Infestation by the vitamin B_{12}-utilizing fish tapeworm
- Organic disease of the bowel wall itself, or
- Increased requirements during pregnancy and in premature infants
- Occasionally, low folate levels may give a falsely low B_{12} result.

The term pernicious anemia is reserved for deficiencies of intrinsic factor irrespective of the basic underlying pathology.

The Schilling test measures absorption of vitamin B_{12} and is an effective means of identifying the various etiologic factors. Variations of this test with and without intrinsic factors clarify diagnosis.

Treatment

Response to therapy is dramatic. As little as 100 µg of cyanocobalamin will induce a marked reticulocyte rise, and maintenance with 100–1,000 µg every 4-6 weeks will maintain adequate levels. Most patients are given 4 × 1,000 µg over 2-3 weeks as a loading dose and then maintained on 1,000 µg 1 M monthly for the rest of their lives.

It is inappropriate to treat vitamin B_{12}-deficient patients with folic acid unless there is an associated folic acid deficiency, in which case both folate and B_{12} are used simultaneously. In the solely B_{12}-deficient patient, folate administration will produce a modest hematologic response and a marked impairment in the neurologic abnormalities.

Sublingual B_{12} is used for B_{12} deficiencies in nonpernicious anemia patients.

DISORDERS OF HEMOSTASIS

Patient may bleed inappropriately, clot excessively and undesirably, or have disorders where combinations of these occur. The individual patient's problem must be accurately diagnosed, often in a stepwise fashion, as appropriate management must be precisely directed. A brief understanding of the systems involved in hemostasis and of the tests that may be applied to localize defects within the system is essential before proceeding to list clinical problems and their management.

Table 22.3: Characteristics of blood coagulation factors.

Factor numbers	Common synonyms	Approximately molecular weight	Approximately plasma half-life (years)
I	Fibrinogen	340,000	120
II	Prothrombin	68,000	85
III	Tissue factor		
IV	Calcium ions		
V	Labile factor	350,000	15
VII	Stable factor	60,000	5
VIII	Antihemophilic factor	1,200,000	14
IX	Christmas factor	55,000	20
X	Stuart–Prower factor	63,000	60
XI	Plasma thromboplastin antecedent (PTA)	160,000	60
XII	Hageman factor	82,000	60
XIII	Fibrin stabilizing factor	350,000	100
	High-molecular-weight kininogen (HMWK)	110,000	
	Prekallikrein	80,000	

Note: Italicized synonyms indicate that the synonym is used more commonly than the factor number.

Hemostasis is complex and by no means fully understood. Its major components are:
- *The vessel wall:* Musculature, endothelial lining, and products
- *Blood platelets:* Contractile mechanisms, products, and surface characteristics
- *Blood leukocytes:* Relationships with platelets and vessel walls; production or surface siting of coagulation proteins
- *Hemostatic factors:* Classical coagulation factor pathways, natural coagulation inhibitors, fibrinolytic factors, and inflammatory cascade factors influencing coagulation.

Table 22.3 illustrates the characteristics of blood coagulation factors. Flowcharts 22.1A to D demonstrate some of the characteristics of these systems; tests that are relevant to various components of these systems are listed in Table 22.4.

Diagnosis

Unexpected bleeding in the newborn (e.g. from the umbilical cord or from needle stick punctures) and major bleeding events (such as intracranial hemorrhage or scalp hematoma) arising within the first few days of life should raise the possibility of a quantitative or qualitative deficiency of a

Flowcharts 22.1A to D: Characteristics of blood coagulation systems.

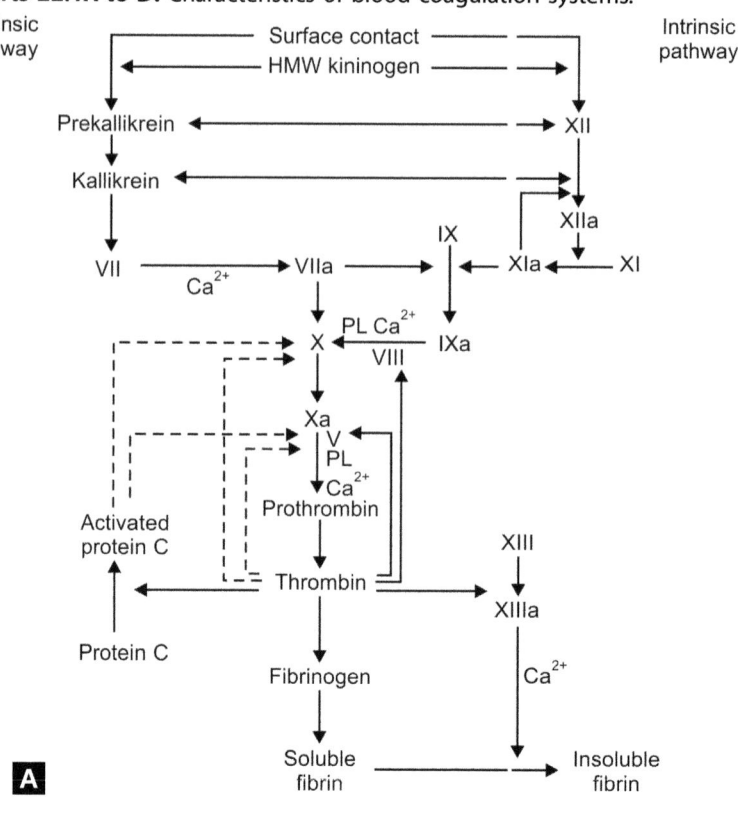

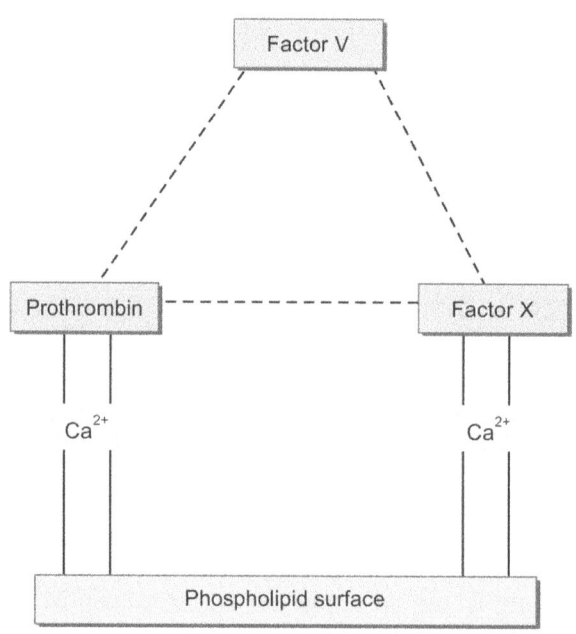

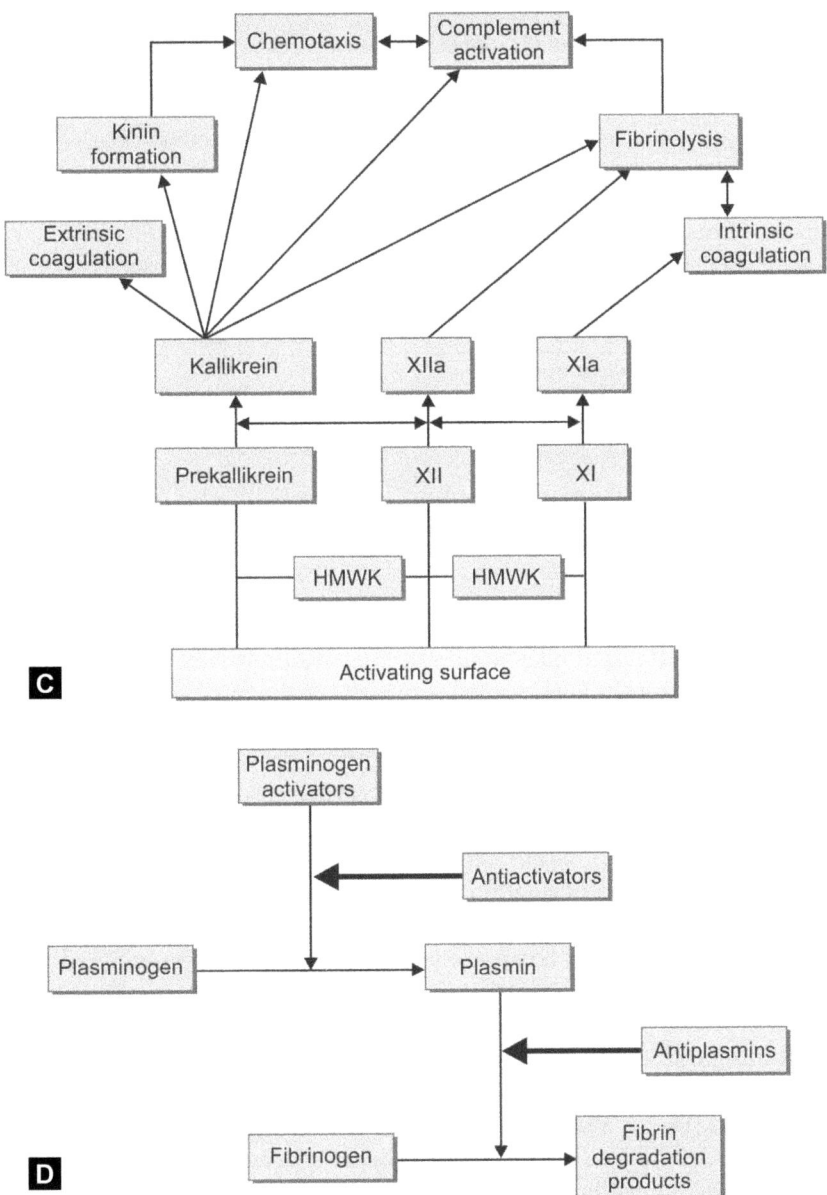

(HMWK, high-molecular-weight kininogen)

clotting factor. In those societies where circumcision is performed at this time, undue bleeding following this procedure is also especially significant.

Assuming that vitamin K has been given, assessment should take place as follows:
- If not already available, a thorough family history for bleeding disorders must be undertaken. Even if this is negative, if there is a strong suspicion

Table 22.4: Clotting problems and relevant tests.

Parameters	Tests
Platelet defects	• Bleeding time (template) • Aggregation (aggregometer) • Adhesion (glass beads).
Platelet numbers (thrombocytopenia or thrombocythemia)	Platelet count
K-dependent factor defects (qualitative and quantitative) (V, VII, and X)	Prothrombin time (PT) (INR)
VIII, IX, V, XI, and XII deficits	Partial thromboplastin time (APTT or =)
Anticoagulants (natural or added)	PT ± APTT
Fibrinogen defects	Thrombin time (--T)
	Direct fibrinogen assay
Fibrinolysis	Fibrin degradation products (FDPs, XDPs, and D-dimer)

(APTT, activated partial thromboplastin time; INR, international normalized ratio)

that a factor deficiency is involved, the neonatal period is often an excellent occasion in which to take blood samples from relatives. With a definitive family history, it should be possible to institute therapy as soon as screening or assessment blood tests have been done, without waiting for results.
- In the absence of a positive family history, a drug history must be taken. Anticonvulsants may have an effect on K vitamin-dependent coagulation-factor production, and rarely, other maternal medications may be significant.
- If no "leading" information is available, then the routine screening tests for the more common coagulation defects should be carried out [prothrombin time, international normalized ratio (INR), partial thromboplastin time (PTT), and fibrinogen level]. A plasma sample should be retained frozen for a more precise factor assay. Bleeding time determinations: The bleeding time is of little value in the newborn as a screening test, but the observation of protracted or recurrent bleeding (e.g. from heel prick) is important.
- The most common factor deficiencies are the hemophilias and related disorders. Factor VIII, IX, and von Willebrand disease (vWD), and less likely, factor XIII, V, VII, and dysfibrinogenemias (fibrinogen is factor I, but name rather than factor number tends to be used clinically).

Hemophilia (see also Hemophilia A under Inherited Coagulation Defects)

- *Factor VIII deficiency*—The role of molecule in factor X activation and thereby thrombin formation is well recognized. The carrier mother may be unaware of her status, new mutations occur in hemophilia (at a rate of as high as 25%), and bleeding due to factor VIII (C) deficiency may occur in females.

- The lyonization hypothesis for activation of the X chromosome would account for a small percentage of carrier females who have very low factor VIIIC levels, and of course, individuals with a single X chromosome (Turner's syndrome) might also be unfortunate enough to have the hemophilia gene on this chromosome. The diagnosis is usually made in newborn males who are severely affected. Ten percent of hemophiliac infants may be expected to show bleeding in the newborn period. Circumcision bleeding, intracranial hemorrhage and cephalohematomas, and bleeding from the umbilical cord stump are probably the most common sites of bleeding in these newborn.
- *Diagnosis*: A PTT more than 50 seconds in the presence of a normal prothrombin time (not >2 seconds prolonged over the top of the normal range for your laboratory) would make one suspect hemophilia A. The test is repeated adding a normal pooled plasma sample that will correct it if due to a factor deficiency (but in the presence of an anticoagulant mimicking factor VIII deficiency, normalization of the APTT will not take place). A specific coagulation factor assay should then be carried out using correction tests and antigenic determination against a precipitable antibody. The approach for hemophilia B is very much the same as that for hemophilia A, and vWD rarely presents and is quite difficult to diagnose in the newborn. Although the type 3 might show itself by bleeding from the umbilical stump or following heel prick, only in this form the bleeding time is markedly prolonged.

Most individuals with congenital acquired defects of coagulation (both bleeding and clotting tendencies) develop symptoms in childhood or adult life. Some will come to light as a result of family studies, some will bleed on provocation (dental extraction, minor surgery, and trauma), and others will be investigated, e.g. epistaxis or unexpected menstrual spotting. Another group will come to light because of apparently unprovoked thrombosis. Some will have mixed thrombotic and hemostatic problems, and sometimes the state of the vessel wall itself will contribute toward bleeding. Conditions include:
- Thrombocytopenias and thrombopathies
- Factor deficiencies
- Thrombotic states
- Mixed thrombotic/bleeding states [DIC and thrombotic thrombocytopenic purpura (TTP)]
- Acquired inhibitors of clotting factors.

FUNCTIONAL PLATELET DISORDERS

Most are discovered during the investigation of the patient with a bleeding problem. They are characterized by a bleeding time (>10 minutes). Aspirin, nonsteroidal anti-inflammatory drugs (NSAIDs), penicillins, and cephalosporins can cause platelet dysfunction. A few rare hereditary thrombopathies are difficult to distinguish from each other: Glanzmann's thrombopathy, Bernard-Soulier syndrome, vWD variants, glycoprotein 1a deficiency, the gray platelet syndrome, and storage pool deficiency. In these disorders, membrane defects and platelets associated with poor adhesion or aggregation can be found. There is usually a positive family history. Management, if indicated, is by platelet transfusion or BMT.

INHERITED COAGULATION DEFECTS

Hemophilia A

Hemophiliacs are graded for severity according to the percentage of factor VIII coagulant present (VIIIC). The most severe have less than 29% moderate 2-10%, and mild more than 10% normal levels. Severe hemophiliacs will have persistent abnormal bleeding at any site, although characteristically into the joints, muscles, and soft tissues. This is an enormous problem, especially during early childhood, and if untreated will result in considerable morbidity and crippling deformations. Bleeding from cuts is often unimpressive, and epistaxis, e.g. tends only to follow injury. Occasionally, intrarenal or GI hemorrhage, or hematuria occur. Individuals tend to follow the same disease bleeding pattern throughout their childhood. Those with moderate or mild hemophilia tend to bleed only after significant trauma, dental extraction, surgery, etc. These divisions are guidelines only and should not influence management in an individual patient.

The individual should regularly attend a hemophilia clinic and wear an identity bracelet or hemophilia card. The parents should be aware of the problem.

Treatment of the Acute Bleeding Episode

The principle of treatment is to raise the factor VIII C level to 2-4 times its basal level and hopefully bring it into the lower end of the hemostatic functional range. Many mildly affected hemophiliacs benefit from Desmopressin (DDAVP) 0.3 µg/kg in saline by IV infusion, but this can only be used for a few days as patients may be refractory to a second dose. When a major bleeding episode has occurred, most hemophiliacs, and certainly severely affected ones as well as many mildly affected one will need factor VIII concentrates. Enough needs to be given to raise the factor level to about 50% of the normal value and to keep it there for 3-4 days. Many older hemophiliacs will present early on during the bleeding episode, as they are aware that this is taking place and that rapid induction of treatment can often prevent a more severe episode. As little as 15 U/kg of factor VIII may abort a major hemarthrosis. Brief periods of bed rest only are usually recommended, and rapid mobilization in the case of muscle and joint problems is currently recommended with physiotherapy under cover with factor VIII concentrate. Adequate analgesia is necessary during the acute event; drugs, such as acetaminophen (paracetamol) and codeine are recommended. Aspirin is contraindicated.

Patients with head injuries should receive a CT or equivalent scan. All hemophiliacs with head injuries should be hospitalized and given prophylactic factor VIII treatment. If there is documented evidence of intracranial hemorrhage, therapy should normalize their factor levels initially and they should be so treated for 10-14 days thereafter. Neurosurgery is not contraindicated in these patients.

Dental treatment is a problem in hemophiliacs. First dentition gives surprisingly little trouble, and fillings under local anesthetic could be covered without factor replacement treatment (use DDAVP). Extractions certainly need to be covered as well as being given tranexamic acid 25 mg/kg tid for 5 days. Surgery, such as synovectomy should be covered in much the same way as intracranial hemorrhage; levels should be maximized initially to approaching 100% and kept around 50% for the next 10 days.

Prophylactic Treatment

Depending on the programs available, severely affected boys with frequent hemorrhages may need prophylactic treatment with factor VIII concentrate. 20 U/kg twice a week IV is effective, and parents can be trained to give such treatment, as indeed can older hemophiliacs themselves. DDAVP before scheduled minor surgery reduces the need for blood products.

Treatment of Hemophiliacs with an Inhibitor

About 5-10% of patients with hemophilia will develop antibodies to factor VIII. This makes their bleeding much more difficult to control because of their inability to have their factor VIII levels ↑ by concentrates. The factors influencing both the development and the aggressiveness of antibody production are poorly understood and may be genetic. They present a considerable management problem, and if low levels of inhibitors are present (<10 plasma U), they may respond to increasing the dose of factor VIII concentrate. The clinical response is clearly critical rather than the measurement of the rise in plasma units. The use of recombinant factor VIII, prothrombin complexes, and activated factor VIII may be of value, and porcine factor VIII has been lifesaving in covering severe serious bleeds. However, this is highly antigenic, and its use in anyone individual is bound to be very limited. Exchange plasmapheresis to reduce the inhibitor has been used. DDAVP appears to retain its effectiveness, presumably because native factor VIII may be less affected by antibody. Certainly any hemophiliac who has received numerous factor VIII concentrates should have his antibody status checked, especially before planned surgery. Differing administrative schedules for factor VIII use and even immunosuppressive treatment have been promoted to minimize this problem. Success seems to be variable at best.

von Willebrand's Disease

- von Willebrand's disease is an inherited bleeding disorder characterized by defective platelet adhesion and aggregation; it is the most common inherited bleeding disorder and has an autosomal inheritance pattern (Leebeek and Eikenboom).

von Willebrand factor (vWF), genetically controlled form chromosome 12, is nonvitamin K-dependent and produced by the endothelium. It acts as a cofactor with VIIIC, and because of its action in facilitating platelet adhesion to the endothelium, its manifestations are largely those of a bleeding tendency rather than a hemostatic defect. However, because it "carries" VIIIC, there is often a functional ↓ in this factor that may be enough to give a coagulation defect as well.

Diagnosis

Findings:
- Bruising and epistaxis, hematomas, menorrhagia, and bleeding from minor wounds. The majority of patients (60–80%) have bleeding after surgery or dental extractions (Leebeek and Eikenboom).
- The diagnosis of vWD is based on a personal history of bleeding, a family history of bleeding, or both, in combination with laboratory tests showing abnormalities in vWF, factor VIII, or both (Leebeek and Eikenboom).

If there is a bleeding diathesis associated with a prolonged bleeding time, in the presence of a normal platelet count and in the absence of drugs, such as aspirin, some form of vWD may be present (excluding acutely ill patients who may have acquired severe disorders of hemostasis). The activated partial thromboplastin time (APTT), always prolonged in hemophilia A, is not diagnostic of vWD although it is often prolonged. Similarly, the factor VIIIC level is often but not always below the normal range. The vWF antigen may be quantitated immunologically. Most patients with vWF deficiency will have absent or reduced ristocetin-induced platelet aggregation. However, one type (2B) behaves aberrantly in this fashion. A direct assay for the ristocetin cofactor is probably the best assay for the diagnosis.

Table 22.5 shows the main subtypes of vWD; this is an incomplete description and new subtypes continue to be described. The types are based on the quantity and quality of polymer (multimer) circulating or found on platelets. The largest multimers appear to be most effective in attaching to platelets. In type 1 vWD, these forms are still detectable; type 2 shows loss of these large multimers and generally speaking the disease is worse than type 1. Type 3 shows minimal levels of all components of the VIII vWF

Table 22.5: Classification and characteristics of von Willebrand's disease.

Types	Bleeding time	von Willebrand factor (vWF) plasma	VIIIC level	Multimer	Platelet aggregates (ristocetin)	Ristocetin cofactor
I	Increase	Reduced	Normal	Normal	Normal or ↓	Reduced
IIa	–	Normal or ↓	Normal or ↓	Large, absent	Reduced	Reduced
IIb	–	–	–	–	Enhanced	Normal or ↓
IIc	–	–	–	Small and abnormal	Reduced	Reduced
III	–	–	–	Variable and abnormal	Very reduced	Reduced

complex and tends to resemble hemophilia with the addition of vWD, and often presents in infancy.

Management

- This depends largely on the type and severity of the vWD. DDAVP seems to be the treatment of choice for type 1 and certainly transiently corrects the bleeding time. It is less effective in type 2, but subtype 2a may respond relatively well.
- Treatment of vWD is based on normalizing vWF and factor VIII levels in case of bleeding or before an intervention. This can be achieved by increasing the endogenous factor levels with the use of DDVAP or by infusing exogenous coagulation factors in the form of a high-purity vWF concentrate or a low-purity factor VIII—von Willebrand.
- Tranexamic acid is sometimes recommended with DDAVP for its effect on inhibiting plasminogen activation. Factor VIII concentrates need to be used in the remainder of vWFs but do have a variability of vWD multimer content. Cryoprecipitate, however, contains everything needed to correct the defects in vWD but, of course, like any biological product, carries the risk of disease transmission, however well the donor is screened. Single-donor rather than pooled units should always be used if possible.

Individuals with vWD bruise easily and bleed from cuts and from the gums and nose. Menorrhagia is also common, and some of the most severe type-3 vWDs have tissue and joint hemorrhages characteristic of classic hemophilia. Most cases, however, are very mild and are diagnosed in family studies or because of bleeding, e.g. following dental extraction. It is thought that the incidence may be as high as 1% of the population at large.

Factor IX Deficiency (Hemophilia B; Christmas Disease)

Most of what has been said about classic hemophilia (hemophilia A) is true for hemophilia B. It is about five times less common than hemophilia A, the frequency being one per 10,000 of the population. Factor IX is produced by the liver and is vitamin K dependent. The APTT is still the best screening test to indicate that this form of hemophilia is present, and direct estimation of the factor IX level would confirm the diagnosis. Unlike classic hemophilia, where a dysfunctional form of the clotting factor appears to be present, factor IX-deficient individuals may also have failure to synthesize the molecule in any form. Carriers are often highly symptomatic in this disorder as well. Other variations from classic hemophilia include a lesser tendency to form antibodies, and the relatively long half-life of factor IX means that less frequent doses need to be given.

Management is as for hemophilia A, but factor IX concentrate rather than factor VIII is used.

ACQUIRED COAGULATION FACTOR DEFICIENCIES

Hepatic Failure

Most patients with established hepatocellular failure will have some abnormality in their coagulation tests (*see* prothrombin time and APTT) but are often asymptomatic insofar as their coagulation is concerned. It has to be remembered that some of both procoagulant- and anticoagulant-produced (actors depend on hepatocytes and vitamin K for their synthesis). If there is a coagulopathy associated with liver disease, it is always worth giving vitamin K in adequate amounts (1 mg IM as a test dose) initially. If, however, factor replacement is necessary (e.g. for an investigative or surgical procedure), then covering with fresh frozen plasma (FFP) to bring the prothrombin time to within about 3 seconds of normal and the APTT to within about 5 seconds of normal should be adequate. Fibrinogen levels tend not to be markedly diminished in stable liver disease, and fibrinogen itself or cryoprecipitate rarely needs to be given.

Chronic Malabsorption Syndromes

These present with a functional vitamin K deficiency and a hemostatic defect that is correctable by IM vitamin K.

Disseminated Intravascular Coagulation

This condition invariably presents with bleeding. However, thrombosis in small vessels can be the main feature [e.g. in hemolytic uremic syndrome (HUS) or TTP]. DIC has been reported in several clinical situations:

Infections, malignancies, obstetric emergencies, following major surgery, and a host of other conditions. Patients with clinically significant DIC show a consumptive coagulopathy associated with heightened fibrinolysis: Low levels of those factors which are consumed in the coagulation process, particularly factors V, VIII, and X, and fibrinogen and prothrombin themselves. Thus, both the prothrombin time and APTT or equivalent will be prolonged. In addition, platelets will be consumed; sometimes markedly so, especially in states where bone marrow function is impaired (e.g. leukemias, severe infections). The procoagulant side of DIC that results in thrombin formation also triggers protein C activity and plasmin formation. This degrades the increased amount of fibrin produced, resulting in an excessive level of fibrin split products: Fragments X, Y, D, and E. Most laboratories are capable of measuring more than or equal to one of these.

About 5–10% of patients who develop acute myeloid leukemias (AMLs) have a partially differentiated promyelocytic form and its characteristic cytogenetic karyotype (15;17 T). Many patients have died of hemorrhage either prior to or during induction treatment. The role of the leukemic cells in activating DIC is still not completely certain, but the syndrome, if unrecognized, carries a considerable mortality.

The principal treatment of DIC is the removal of the underlying insult. However, while this is being managed, the patient will need to be supported through the period of risk from DIC. Replacement of clotting factors, usually with FFP, and if necessary, cryoprecipitate or even factor VIII concentrates, should be undertaken. Assuming that thrombocytopenia is present, platelet concentrates should also be given. The use of these products should be monitored by INR, APTT, and platelet counts. There is no merit in giving fresh blood that cannot be obtained by specific correction of factors as described earlier. Hb levels, however, should be maintained, as should adequate BP; shock itself may contribute to DIC. Prednisolone and heparin have been recommended for the treatment of DIC, but their firm role has never been established. Generally, defibrinolytic treatment is said to be contraindicated, but newer antiproteases, such as aprotinin may well be strikingly valuable in this situation, especially for short-term use.

Hemolytic Uremic Syndrome and Thrombotic Thrombocytopenic Purpura

These syndromes represent microangiopathies with clotting and are predominantly those of intravascular coagulation. The former is associated in childhood with a febrile illness and is characterized by renal failure. TTP affects adults where many of the manifestations are neurologic, variable, and difficult to assemble diagnostically. It has been suggested that abnormally high levels of vWF may be related to the onset of both these diseases. HUS tends to be self-limiting, and with supportive care, and if necessary, renal dialysis, recovery can be expected.

Treatment of TTP is uncertain, but plasmapheresis is of proven value.

Acquired Inhibitors of Coagulation

Apart from inhibitors acquired in hemophilia itself, by far the most common is the lupus anticoagulant. This is so-called because of its association with systemic lupus erythematosus (SLE) or other autoimmune disorders, but can certainly be diagnosed in the absence of these underlying problems. The anticoagulant itself is an immunoglobulin that reacts with platelet membranes, particularly activating prothrombin production. Patients with the lupus anticoagulant, therefore, are at risk from clotting as well as bleeding, and principally show thromboses, pulmonary embolism, and in pregnant women, a high incidence of abortion. Patients with the lupus anticoagulant will not often need treatment as they will not have a bleeding problem. Corticosteroids diminish or abolish the clotting abnormalities, as will immunosuppressive drugs.

Other Conditions Associated with Coagulation Failure

Patients receiving massive blood transfusions may develop dilution of clotting factors and platelet deficiencies. Patients receiving plasmapheresis or an extracorporeal circulation may also show the same phenomena and citrate intoxication may complicate this. Such patients may need replacement clotting factors and platelets.

THROMBOTIC DISORDERS

The natural hemostatic balance is maintained by inhibitors of the procoagulation system, and fibrinolytic mechanisms. The level of natural coagulation inhibitors is normally genetically regulated, and they include protein C, S, and antithrombin III (ATIII).
- Protein C deficiency can present at any age from the neonatal period onward; presentation neonatally is usually of DIC-like syndrome characterized by a widespread thrombosis and purpura; most such patients often die during this period. Most, however, present later, and the heterozygotes of the autosomal variety will have characteristically recurrent venous thromboses. Protein C is vitamin K-dependent and is produced by the liver, as are many other coagulation factors. Its level is also affected by warfarin treatment, so its assay, which is usually immunologic, cannot be carried out in patients who are on this anticoagulant. Family studies in individuals with protein C deficiency are essential, especially in the recessive type, and antenatal diagnosis

is now possible. Management is generally with warfarin, but human protein C concentrates may become available. Factor IX concentrates are also rich in protein C. Although warfarin is the treatment of choice in adults, in children, of course, with indefinite administration of the drug, there may be long-term problems with bone growth and development.
- Protein S acts as a cofactor for protein C. Two types of patients have been described: (1) One with protein S complexed to C4B binding protein and less available functionally, and (2) Another where manufacture of the protein seems to be severely affected. Few cases have been reported, but the management would appear to be similar to that for protein C deficiency.
- Antithrombin III deficiency is probably incompatible with life in the homozygous form, and heterozygotes are variably affected, but rarely in the neonatal period (one or two cases have been reported, but they have been homozygous cases). Children and adults have a tendency to both venous and arterial thromboses, and as ATIII provides most of the plasma antithrombin activity, the chance of being affected by recurrent venous thrombus or embolism is almost 100%. Treatment with heparin is effective in the short term, and long-term anticoagulation with warfarin is usually recommended.
- *Problems of the vessel wall*: Vasculitides include mainly the so-called allergic purpuras (Henoch–Schönlein type), some drug-induced purpuras that are nonthrombocytopenic, and those associated with a variety of infections. Rarely such purpuras may also be seen because of defects in connective tissue or paraproteinemias.
- Allergic purpuras occur most often in children or adolescents but can be seen at any age, usually as an acute illness with systemic symptoms, such as headache, fever, or abdominal or joint pain. The purpura, which is often over the joints, fingers, or ear tips, may be accompanied by urticaria or erythema. Frank hemorrhage may often occur, and renal involvement resembling acute nephritis may be found. There are no characteristic blood findings, but the vascular injury has been demonstrated to be a result of immunoglobulin A (IgA)-based immune complexes, and IgA levels may be in some cases of the disease. Drug-induced vascular purpuras may have a similar skin lesion, but patients are usually less ill. Treatment is supportive (Roath and Gross).

PLATELET DISORDERS: THROMBOCYTOPENIA AND THROMBOPATHY

In the adult, the normal platelet count is 150–400 × 10^9/L. Platelet counts of 450–1,000 may be seen in patients with chronic hemolytic disease, severe iron deficiency and malignancy, and following splenectomy.

Thrombocytopenia is due to either failure of platelet production or increased platelet loss. Some causes of impaired platelet production include:
- Aplastic and hypoplastic anemias
- Vitamin B_{12} or folate deficiency
- Occupation of the marrow by, e.g. tumor, leukemia, or fibrosis
- Antitumor chemotherapy.

Disorders causing increased platelet loss include:
- Immune [iso- and auto-l thrombocytopenic purpuras (iso-, e.g. associated with previous platelet transfusions or pregnancy; autoimmune, e.g. immune thrombocytopenic purpura (ITP); other immune purpuras associated, e.g. with SLE or hemolytic anemia—Evans syndrome)].
- Hypersplenism with platelet sequestration
- Consumptive coagulopathies (DIC, TTP, and some vascular purpuras)
- Drugs can cause both immune and occasionally nonimmune thrombocytopenias.

Immune Thrombocytopenic Purpura

Immune thrombocytopenic purpura occurs in about four per 100,000 children per year and a lesser incidence in adults. Most cases present acutely, often after viral illnesses, and a number may be associated with infectious mononucleosis. A few present in the chronic phase. The acute disease manifests with the sudden onset of spectacular bruising with widespread petechiae and purpuric lesions. There is often epistaxis and occasionally conjunctival or retinal hemorrhages. Hematuria, intrajoint bleeding, or widespread ecchymoses often point to coagulation defects rather than ITP. Physical examination is otherwise unremarkable, and it is said that splenomegaly does not occur in this condition. Frequent splenic palpation may cause subcapsular hemorrhages or rupture, so they should be limited and gentle. The pathologic findings include platelet counts of levels, such as $10 \times 10^9/L$, and recent studies have shown the presence of platelet-associated immunoglobulins, including IgM and IgG antibodies and to glycoproteins 1V, 2V, or 3A. It is assumed that these are virally induced but also recognize a platelet-based antigen. The rest of the blood count should be normal, but if there is any doubt, bone marrow aspirate should be undertaken, especially if steroids are to be given, as the steroids might mask, e.g. an underlying leukemia. The marrow shows plentiful megakaryocytes and is otherwise normal.

Management of Acute Form

The disease is often self-limiting, but the impressive clinical findings and the occasional risk of cerebral hemorrhage indicate positive management. Although there are no good data regarding survival of patients given different treatment, conventionally, prednisolone in doses of 1 mg/kg/day until the platelet count rises to normal levels and then reduced over the next 6 weeks would be orthodox treatment. Intravenous immunoglobulin (IVIG) may be equally effective, but individuals given prednisolone can often be quickly discharged from hospital and monitored easily on an outpatient basis. Most individuals will remit and spontaneously be cured on this regimen, but a few, often identifiable by suboptimal responses, will become cases of chronic ITP.

Chronic ITP may well have a somewhat different etiology from the acute form, and the platelet-associated immunoglobulin is often IgG rather than IgM and should be found in most cases. Some cases of chronic ITP will be subclinical, with platelet counts of 225–50 × 10^9/L. They need no management but should be observed, and a careful search for associated autoimmune states should be made. Those that need treatment can be offered a course of IVIG. This is often again of temporary benefit, as is pulsed steroid therapy. Vinca alkaloids and cytotoxic immunosuppression probably have little place in the treatment of chronic ITP. Newer treatments include, interferon, and more successfully, danazol. In some reports, half of patients with chronic ITP make an excellent and sustained response, but this drug would need to be given for 2:6 months. The initial dose should be 800 mg/day, but it may be tapered to 200 mg/day after about 2 months.

Splenectomy is the established treatment for chronic ITP, and in children, the success rate is about two-thirds; many adults will at least have higher platelet counts following a splenectomy, which makes their management easier. The operation, however, is not without morbidity, and in children especially, there is always a risk of sepsis, especially from encapsulated organisms. Vaccination against pneumococcal and *Haemophilus* should be undertaken preferably prior to splenectomy. Children should be given penicillin V PO bid for many years following splenectomy, and adults for more than or equal to 1 year.

Other Immune Purpuras

- That associated with infectious mononucleosis may be indistinguishable from ITP but is usually of less than or equal to 6 weeks duration and may not be as severe. Splenic rupture is a possible complication in this combination of disorders.
- Human immunodeficiency virus (HIV)-associated immune thrombocytopenia is a complication of acquired immunodeficiency syndrome (AIDS) and can be an early finding. The disease mimics chronic ITP and can be managed in much the same way.
- Drug-induced immune thrombocytopenia behaves like chronic ITP, but the offending antibody seems to be addressed against a drug, so the mechanism of platelet involvement is not well understood. The platelet

count normalizes when the drug is removed. Drugs implicated include: Cimetidine, heparin, phenytoin, sodium valproate, rifampicin, sulfa compounds, and NSAIDs.

PROBLEMS WITH LEUKOCYTES AND THEIR MANAGEMENT

Clinical problems due to, or associated with, leukocytes fall into natural categories: Too few, too many, or poorly functioning leukocytes.

Leukopenia

Most problems associated with leukopenias are due to inadequate numbers of neutrophils/neutropenias. In children less than 12 years, neutrophil counts as low as 1.5×10^9/L probably represent the lower limits of the normal range, except in the first few months of life after the immediate neonatal period when they may drop as low as 1×10^9/L. In adults, anything less than 1.8 should be regarded as significantly low.

It is essential to establish that neutropenia actually exists. A cause or association should be detected for the neutropenia. Assuming morbidity to be associated with a neutropenia, steps need to be taken to eliminate the cause of the neutropenia or ameliorate its effects.

- Serial full blood counts need to be carried out to make sure this is not one of the cyclic phenomena occasionally described and associated with cyclic changes in other blood cells, platelets, and oral ulcers.
- Assuming the neutropenia is persistent, if long standing and relatively asymptomatic, it is worth carrying out a neutrophil mobilization test, preferably using both hydrocortisone and adrenalin as stressor agents [5 mL/kg of hydrocortisone hemisuccinate IV and 0.03 mL/kg of 1-10,000 adrenalin subcutaneous (SC)]. Monitor neutrophil counts at 15-minute intervals for 1 hour and hourly thereafter, up to 6 hours. Functionally, neutropenic patients fail to show a normal neutrophil count during either part of this procedure, whereas those who have adequate reserves but slightly low circulating numbers of neutrophils show responses well within the normal range.

True persistent neutropenia can be due to:
- Congenital (extremely rare) conditions, e.g. Kostmann's syndrome.
- *Immune neutropenias*: The isoimmune neutropenia of the neonatal period and autoimmune neutropenias, occasionally detected later (disorders analogs to idiopathic autoimmune thrombocytopenic purpura).
- *Generalized disorders of bone marrow*: Bone marrow failure, e.g. aplastic anemia.
- Drug-induced neutropenias.
- Miscellaneous causes, such as Felty's syndrome.
- Some infections.

Antibiotic Policy in Severe Neutropenia

"Neutropenic fever" should be assessed through cultures of blood or other materials, but therapy should be initiated as soon as these are taken, not awaiting the results. There is no fixed protocol for such treatment, but combinations of, e.g. aminoglycosides, such as gentamicin or amikacin with a synthetic penicillin, such as azlocillin, are often used. Many such protocols for children, however, use cephalosporins, such as cephtrioxasole, which appear to be equally effective and avoid the renal and ototoxicity and the necessary monitoring of aminoglycoside blood levels. Frequently no organism will be found, and hopefully the symptoms will resolve within 48 hours. Antibiotics should be administered for more than or equal to 5 days and for 24 hours following the dehiscence of fever. If pyrexia persists, further microbial culture should be attempted, including fungal and viral studies. A switch to "second-line" antimicrobial therapy, including a potent antifungal agent, should be considered.

Prevention of neutropenic fever: Prophylaxis of infection in neutropenic and other immunocompromised patients should be considered, especially when the host defensive mechanisms are temporarily defective. The use of "barrier" procedures or protective isolation accompanied by careful personal hygiene on the part of the patient and all visitors and attendants is more important than prophylactic antibiotics or other measures. Laminar air flow and aggressive decontamination of patient cubicles are also effective, but expensive. Oral antibiotics should not be necessary under ideal isolated conditions. All blood products should be carefully screened, as described earlier, and there may be a case for a simple oral antifungal agent, such as fluconazole. Acyclovir 215 mg/m tid is effective in reducing the incidence of recrudescent herpetic infection and may have some value against cytomegalovirus (CMV). Trimethoprim-sulfamethoxazole (TMP-SMX), as described, is also known to prevent Pneumocystis infection—certainly in some groups of patients. It may also be effective against toxoplasmosis. Long-term prophylactic antibiotics are rarely used except in splenectomized patients or those with recurrent single-site infection.

Leukocytosis

All blood counts reporting leukocytosis are not necessarily due to leukemia. It is also true that many patients with leukemia do not have leukocytosis or may indeed be leukopenic as far as the peripheral blood is concerned. Generally, leukocytosis shows an increase in mature or near-mature, forms of white cells, with essentially normal bone marrow processes, and unless there are separate causes for them, no involvement of the nonleukocytic elements of the bone marrow (red cells, platelets).

Leukocyte counts of less than or equal to $100 \times 10^9/L$ have been observed in severe infections. Reactive leukocytosis can present a diagnostic problem, especially in children and with some of the less common infections. Lymphocytes or monocytes may be raised (e.g. in mycoplasma pneumonia or pertussis), and modest raises may be seen in, e.g. pregnancy or Hodgkin's disease and some patients with progressive cancer. In the latter, especially the myelophthisic, appearance in the blood of immature forms may initially give rise to diagnostic difficulties, especially in relation to some of the more indolent myeloproliferative disorders.

Leukemia

Leukemias can be conveniently divided into the acute and chronic myeloid and lymphatic types. The diagnosis can only be safely made through examination of bone marrow material when the number of immature cells can be assessed, cytochemistry, cell markers and cytogenetics carried out, and gene rearrangement noted, where appropriate.

Acute Myeloid Leukemia

Elihu Estey, in the N Engl J Med, editorial quoting the findings of investigators emphasized the following:
- Patients with AML generally receive stereotypical treatment.
- Young patients receive cytarabine for 7 days and an anthracycline for 3 days (known as "7 + 3 induction").
- Thus, treated some groups, predictably, have an approximately 50% chance of "cure" (favorable risk) whereas others, also predictably, have a survival of 6–18 months (unfavorable risk). This nonrandom heterogeneity after homogeneous treatment suggests that, like pneumonia, AML is several diseases (Elihu Estey).
  "Acute myeloid leukemia is primarily defined according to leukemia-cell karyotype and an increasing number of molecular aberrations". It follows that different types of AML should ideally be treated differently.
- This concept is best exemplified by acute promyelocytic leukemia, in which arsenic trioxide plus all-*trans* retinoic acid (ATRA) eliminates the causative molecular abnormality and results in routine cure without the need for cytotoxic chemotherapy (Elihu Estey).
- "Patients with AML and *TP53* mutations, which are readily detectable with the use of validated commercial platforms, should receive decitabine for 10 days, as might as the far larger group of patients with unfavorable-risk cytogenetic profiles. Unlike cytarabine and anthracycline induction, decitabine is routinely administered on an outpatient basis" (Elihu Estey).

Table 22.6: AML and ALL FAB classifications.		
AML FAB classification		
M0	Undifferentiated (positive myeloid markers)	
M1	Poorly differentiated	
M2	Differentiated	
M3	Promyelocytic	
M4	Myelomonocytic	
M5	Monocytic	
M6	Erythroid	
M7	Megakaryocytic	
ALL FAB classification		
	Cells	*Cytoplasm*	*Nucleoli*
L1	Small	Scanty	Indistinct
L2	Large (or mixed)	Abundant	Prominent
L3	Large	Abundant (often vacuolated)	Prominent

(ALL, acute lymphoblastic leukemia; AML, acute myeloid leukemia; FAB, French–American–British)

Patients may present with:
- Anemia, bleeding, and/or fever; skin lesions (infiltrates and/or bleeding); gum infiltrates (especially in M4 and M5 varieties), and,
- Less often, testicular, ophthalmic, or CNS manifestations.
- The bone marrow should contain more than or equal to 30% blasts, most of which should type antigenically as myeloid cells, and in the more differentiated forms, should show at least the cytochemical characteristics of development with, e.g. myeloperoxidase or nonspecific esterase. TDT is occasionally positive (10–15%). Seven subtypes of AML are known (Table 22.6).
- The M1, M2, and M3 leukemias represent different degrees of myeloid differentiation, but the M3 variety has special features that include very prominent granules and bundles of Auer rods. This seems to be a rather precisely defined group of patients with a specific karyotypic abnormality (TI5:T17) and a clinical course initially accentuated by severe bleeding associated with a DIC-like syndrome. The morbidity and mortality in the presentation and early treatment induction phase of this disease is high, but if patients survive this period, their prognosis is said to be better than with other myeloid acute leukemias.
- The M1 and M2 leukemias have no special features and are associated with a number of different cytogenetic abnormalities. The M4 and M5 types involve monocytes and myeloblasts in different proportions, and the M6 is an erythroleukemia known earlier as the Di Guglielmo type; many patients have multinucleated marrow erythroblasts that may

be periodic acid-Schiff (PAS) positive. Some of these leukemias may terminate in what appear to be myeloblastic forms. The M7 variety involves megakaryocytes and may be associated with considerable marrow fibrosis.

Management of acute myeloid leukemias: This is similar for all types, with the exception of M3. Treatment consists of a regimen designed to induce remission:
- Usually chemotherapy with an anthracycline, and cytarabine. Usually two courses are given, followed by consolidation treatment using similar drugs, with the addition of, e.g. etoposide and µ-amsacrine.
- Thioguanine is often used somewhere in the scheme. There are a number of programs available, and there is little evidence that anyone is superior to any other at present. The response of the different leukemic subtypes is also similar, although it is said that the M5 variety does more poorly in childhood. Overall, survivals at 5 years vary with age, being about 50% in childhood and 20% overall in adults less than 55 years. M3 leukemias deserve special attention during the induction phase, where ATRA has recently been shown to have an excellent effect in inducing differentiation and giving a form of remission with good platelet counts and Hbs. The white count may rise considerably, however, and such remissions are not durable, so in practice such patients should be admitted to "orthodox" induction programs as soon as is practical.
- Allogenic BMT with a matched sibling donor gives the best survival in acute myelogenous leukemia in children and young adults. Such allogenic transplantation is carried out early in first remission. All patients should be tissue typed early in their disease, when peripheral blood leukocytes are available and their family members matched. Matched, unrelated donor transplants can also be successful, assuming there is access to a donor registry and a successful search is made. The problems associated with GVH disease are greater in this latter group of patients and the morbidity and mortality due to this phenomenon is increased.

Autologous BMT is now a part of many AML treatment programs. This is usually carried out by marrow harvesting following completion of remission induction and consolidation treatment and the bone marrow either given back directly following further chemotherapy or held in reserve in case relapse should occur.

Acute Lymphatic Leukemia (Acute Lymphoblastic Leukemia)

This is the most common form of childhood cancer that, although more frequent in children, occurs in adults at all ages. The etiology is unknown although, like AML, there is a relationship between sizable doses of radiation, either accidental or related to treatment of other disorders, and the incidence of disease. A virus has been implicated in one rare form of acute lymphoblastic leukemia (ALL)—the human T-lymphotropic virus type 1 (HTLV1)—which appears to be passed on in maternal milk.

Classification of ALL is by a French–American–British (FAB) classification into L1, L2, and L3. L1 consists mostly of smaller lymphocytes, L2 larger, and L3 more Burkitt cell-like. Phenotypically, most belong to a common "pre-β" ALL type and are CD10 [common acute lymphoblastic leukemia antigen (CALLA)] positive. A few, especially very young children, are null cell ALLs, where immunophenotyping is not helpful; about 10% are T cells and about 3% are B cells. Most ALLs will be TDT positive.

Prognostic features in ALL are related to the height of the white blood cell (WBC) (poor if $50 \times 10^9/L$), age, and sex (males do worse than females). Cytogenetic abnormalities are common, and those with most hyperdiploidy do worse, as do those with the Philadelphia chromosome. Other cytogenetic abnormalities involve a number of chromosomes, and although related to B- or T-cell lineage, may not be related to prognosis in aggressively treated patients.

Treatment: Long, complex, and usually consists of an induction program with vincristine, prednisolone (prednisone), and L-asparaginase. Intensification programs typically use cyclophosphamide, methotrexate, L-asparaginase, and an anthracycline and corticosteroids, specifically-directed CNS treatment with radiotherapy, and/or intrathecal methotrexate followed by continuing maintenance treatment, usually with oral drugs on an outpatient basis. Typically, vincristine and methotrexate are used in such regimens. About 2 years' continuing therapy is the minimum requirement for relapse prevention. This complicated treatment regimen, with many side effects and problems with growth and mental development in children, needs a considerable amount of support. Also, in older patients, since the chances of cure ↓ with age, this prolonged treatment is often abbreviated (i.e. no maintenance). About one-half of all children may expect to be cured by current treatment; some may relapse with new clonal leukemias. The incidence of cure is probably about 25% in young adults, and is minimal over age 50 years.

Bone marrow transplantation: Because of the high cure rate in childhood, most centers reserve BMT for high-risk cases (males with high counts, Philadelphia chromosome, or hyperdiploidy) where matched donors are available. Even if a suitable donor presents, many centers will not treat "average" ALL cases in this manner unless they relapse. Since the chances of obtaining a second remission are good, this is usually found to be an acceptable philosophy. Autologous bone marrow, usually with purging of the appropriate lymphoid population, has been used, but it is not yet clear whether this is an established treatment for either primary or relapsed ALL.

Although relapse most commonly occurs in the bone marrow, as does AML, about 10% of patients with this disease will relapse in the CNS despite the preventive treatment that is part of the induction program.

This is meningeal leukemia and presents very much as meningitis. Blasts can usually be found in the CNS fluid, although the numbers may be quite low. Quite often such patients are not in overt hematologic relapse. The treatment is by methotrexate and craniospinal irradiation. Cytosine arabinoside is probably equally effective. Patients treated in this way have historically been neurologically or intellectually limited in follow-up. It is probably also best to treat as if there were a systemic (bone marrow) relapse as well, with the same kind of treatment as was used for initial induction and consolidation. Occasionally, AML will relapse similarly and should be treated in the same way.

Testicular relapse is a relatively common relapse in boys and may occur in less than or equal to 10% of treated individuals (it is much less common in AML, although it certainly occurs). Testicular irradiation is not recommended, but treatment as for a systemic relapse is effective.

Rarely, relapse occurs at other sites, such as the ovary or eye. Ocular radiotherapy is recommended for the rare cases with eye disease, and again, systemic treatment as for bone marrow relapse should be carried out.

Chronic Myelogenous Leukemia

This disease occurs at all ages, although its peak frequency is in mature adults is 40–60 years of age. Many patients present without impressive clinical or laboratory findings, except for an ↑ WBC. The WBC differential invariably shows immature WBCs and frequently a mild basophilia or eosinophilia. More florid cases have the full-blown disorder with splenomegaly and very high WBCs up to 500×10^9/L, with all types of bone marrow cells, including normoblasts and sometimes precursor megakaryocyte fragments in the peripheral blood. Presentation may be with anemia, splenic pain, sudden visual failure, gout, and rarely bleeding. Some of these symptoms are due to leukostasis.

The biology of chronic myelogenous leukemia (CML) is well worked out, and 90% of cases have the Philadelphia chromosome (9/21 translocation). Most that do not have this exchange of chromative material in an overt manner will still have the presence of the *BCR-ABL* oncogene arrangement.

Management: Drug treatment of CML is palliative. The mean survival is around 4 years, a figure that has not changed since the introduction of busulfan about 30 years ago. This drug and hydroxyurea are the main standbys. Allopurinol should be given (300 mg once daily) to all patients with CML when treatment is proposed. Rarely, the Philadelphia chromosome disappears or is found in a smaller percentage of cells under such treatment, but latterly α-interferon has been introduced and in about one-half of the cases of CML seems to be able to suppress leukocyte production after initial cytoreduction with conventional chemotherapy. About one-third of these patients will achieve some kind of lessening of the percentage of Philadelphia positive cells prefect. The only other long-standing management for this disorder is radiotherapy, which is effective in reducing the spleen size where this is a particular problem, and when bony pain occurs, presumably due to infiltration, it is also effective. AML-type treatment has been tried and is still being evaluated in some centers. At present, its value is unproven.

Allogenic BMT is the only hope for cure in CML at present, and all individuals who have a matched sibling donor should be offered allogenic BMT. This has been carried out in patients up the age of 60 years with success. About 50% of patients overall may be cured by this technique. There are, of course, the usual problems with GVH disorders, and if MUDs are used, these are enhanced.

Chronic Lymphocytic Leukemia

Peak incidence is over the age of 65 years. Most patients run an indolent course. Presentation is often incidental: The patient is observed to have an increased lymphocyte count. Patients may present with anemia, adenopathy, and/or splenomegaly, infections, or rarely, thrombocytopenic bleeding. The pathology of the disorder involves proliferation of mature B lymphocytes in more than or equal to 95% of cases. T-lymphocyte chronic lymphocytic leukemia (CLL) is also described, and there are a number of CLL variants with special features. Attempts have been made to stage CLL so that prognosis, and more importantly perhaps, management can be appropriately recommended. Two systems have been used, one described by Rai and Binet. Table 22.7 describes these categories. Unfortunately, although these are of some value in a nosologic sense, their use in assessing individual patients at a single point in time is not always satisfactory.

Management: Many patients need no specific therapy. If the patient is not anemic and does not have troublesome adenopathy or splenomegaly, despite a high peripheral blood lymphocyte count and the presence

Table 22.7: CLL classifications.

Rai:
- Blood lymphocytes
- One blood lymphocytes + enlarged nodes
- Two blood lymphocytes + splenomegaly
- Three blood lymphocytes + anemia
- Four blood lymphocytes + thrombocytopenia.

Hb (g/L)	Pl × 10^9/L	Clinical involvement
Binet:		
A ≥100	≥100	<Three areas
B ≥100	≥100	≥Three areas
C <100+/or	<100	Any

(CLL, chronic lymphocytic leukemia; Hb, hemoglobin)

of considerable bone marrow disease, there is no urgency in initiating treatment. Treatment is indicated for symptomatic anemia, falling Hb, progressive thrombocytopenia, uncomfortably enlarging lymph nodes, or rarely, spleen.

Immune dysfunction is a complication of CLL. It may present as autoimmune disease, particularly hemolytic anemia, and less often thrombocytopenia. Deficient immunoglobulin production may be associated with recurrent infections of the upper respiratory tract, lung, and urinary tract.

Treatment: Many will respond, although will not be cured, by chlorambucil in doses 20 mg/week. Patients with CLL are usually elderly and frail, and if it is possible to treat in a simple manner and they are kept well, this is probably the treatment of choice. Patients who fail this regimen, or who are younger and have bulky disease, may be considered for a more aggressive combination of chemotherapy, e.g. monthly cyclophosphamide and an anthracycline, oncovin, and prednisone (CHOP) for 6 months. There seems to be little vogue for single-agent anthracyclines, but fludarabine at monthly intervals for 6 months has shown considerable success in patients who have failed on other therapy; new agents, such as chlorodeoxyadenosine also look promising. Prednisolone may be useful in the treatment of complications, such as acquired hemolytic anemia or immune thrombocytopenia, but is not recommended in the usual management of CLL, although it certainly is lympholytic.

Radiotherapy to bulky disease areas or enlarged spleen is effective in reducing tumor mass. In patients with immune suppression and history of recurrent infections, a program of IVIG at monthly intervals is of value.

A very small number of "young" patients have received allogenic matched BMTs with success rates comparable to CML. Such younger patients are in a considerable minority and may represent a fundamentally more aggressive form of CLL, so the usual palliative approach may certainly be amended for this group of patients.

Although a disorder, such as a B-cell CLL would seem a tempting target for immunotherapy, trials with interferons have been disappointing, and monoclonal antibodies, either against CLL-associated antigens or linked with cytotoxins, have not fulfilled some animal work-based promise.

Chronic Lymphocytic Leukemia Variants

A "splenic" form of CLL has been described where the major problem is splenomegaly accompanied by anemia and/or thrombocytopenia. Frequently these latter become accentuated when drug treatment is given, while the spleen size stays persistently large. This group of patients seems to benefit from splenectomy, which reduces the tumor bulk and may restore good quality survival and freedom from transfusion. X-irradiation of the spleen is also effective but may be of less permanent benefit. The borderline between CLL and small-cell lymphocytic leukemia is poorly defined, and when in doubt, especially in younger patients, if therapy is needed, the more aggressive protocols are probably indicated.

Prolymphocytic leukemia: This is usually a B- but occasionally a T-cell variant. It may be a transformed chronic leukemia, although it certainly presents de novo from time to time. The morphologic features of this disease are an increased number of prolymphocytes with their characteristic large single nucleoli and an increased cytoplasmic content compared with "adult" small lymphocytes. The disorder has a high mortality.

Hairy cell leukemia is a proliferation of what are hybrid lymphocytes with many B-cell features, some T-cell features, and some conforming to those of histiocytes. The presence of both heavy- and light-chain gene rearrangements suggests its B-cell origin. There are probably a number of hairy cell leukemia-like disorders.

The syndrome usually presents with nonspecific symptoms, such as malaise, fever, and weight loss. Patients present with abdominal discomfort, splenomegaly, adenopathy, anemia, and associated asymptomatic thrombocytopenia. Most patients show hairy cells in the peripheral blood on close examination. The bone marrow shows a characteristic morphologic picture where the cells' oval or indented nuclei are separated widely from each other. The cells show the typical hairy features and are defined by their tartrate-resistant acid phosphatase activity. Several karyotypic abnormalities have been reported: 14q plus or abnormalities of chromosome 12 are most common, but there is no specific abnormality. Treatment of hairy cell leukemia is usually splenectomy, which should not be done until the patient is symptomatic, as many will have a very indolent course. The use of corticosteroids and lymphoma-type chemotherapy has not been helpful in the past, but successful results have been obtained with α-interferon, deoxycoformycin, and chlorodeoxyadenosine. All these agents appear to be effective in inducing remission; hopefully, some kind of intermittent/maintenance regimen can be established that will allow long-term survival, but at the moment even these regimens do not appear to be curative.

MYELOPROLIFERATIVE DISORDERS

Polycythemia is either "true" [polycythemia vera (PV)] or secondary. PV is a panmyelopathy where, sooner or later, all three of the major bone marrow products are increased in the peripheral blood: Red cells, neutrophils, and platelets. In secondary polycythemias, sometimes called erythemias, only the red cell component is increased. There are also pseudopolycythemias. If all the classic features are present, PV is clearly distinguishable from the others, but in some cases, the distinction may be blurred, at least initially.

Polycythemia Vera

Polycythemia vera is a disorder affecting mature adults with a peak incidence in the mid 50s. The presentation may be with plethora, headaches, vertigo, stroke, or myocardial infarction (MI). Peripheral vascular disease (PVD) with endangered digits or limbs may occur, the incidence of gout is increased, and paradoxically, a number of patients may present with bleeding from the GI tract. On examination, if the full-blown syndrome is present, splenomegaly will undoubtedly be found or detected on abdominal ultrasound. Hepatomegaly is usually not prominent, and adenopathy is unusual.

The peripheral blood contains ↑ RBCs. This may be matched by a high Hb and hematocrit; but, if the patient has bleed, these may be normal or low. The neutrophil count should be raised but with no immature cells circulating. The platelet count should be raised with variations in platelet size but not all of these features may be present.

All patients suspected of being polycythemic should have a RBC mass. This should be accompanied by a plasma volume. Males living at sea level or thereabouts should have less than or equal to 30 mL/kg RBCs, and females about 25 mL/kg. The total blood volume of males should be around 60 mL/kg and slightly less for females (exact values should be those obtained in your own laboratory). Increase in red cell mass beyond the normal levels plus your accepted standard deviation should indicate a diagnosis of "polycythemia". This does not help distinguish true from secondary polycythemias but will eliminate some pseudopolycythemias, such as stress polycythemia, where the problem seems to be one of a reduced plasma volume only. Tests that help distinguish between true and secondary polycythemias include:

- *Erythropoietin levels*: Patients with PV have normal Epo levels (again these should be your own reference laboratories values); 90% of patients with secondary polycythemias for whatever reason will have ↑ Epo.
- *Bone marrow biopsy*: Bone marrow aspirate is often unhelpful in the diagnosis of PV, but a biopsy should show increased cellularity and especially increased numbers of megakaryocytes. There will also be some increase in reticulin fibers. Secondary polycythemias at best show some erythroid hyperplasia.
- *Bone marrow colony growth*: Bone marrow cells from patients with PV will form spontaneous erythroid colonies in vitro. Normal individuals and those with the secondary polycythemias will not.
- *Uric acid levels*: Uric acid levels are usually normal or ↑ in PV. They are rarely ↑ in secondary polycythemias.
- Leukocyte alkaline phosphatase level, if reliably available, will be ↑ in PV and may be normal in other polycythemias.

Management is palliative. Good management can lead to the achievement of a normal life span with good quality of life in most patients. The form of management depends on the symptoms, findings, and age of the patient.

- Patients with principally an erythremic component of their polycythemia can be managed by venesection, which should be sufficient to achieve a hematocrit of less than or equal to 45.
- This usually requires energetic venesection initially until iron stores are depleted, but the frequency can then be reduced. The red cell numbers may be ↑ at 7 or 8 × 10^{12}/L, but it is the PCV that has the major effect on blood viscosity rather than red cell numbers, so symptomatically patients treated in this manner may avoid the complications of the disease.
- Some patients need cytoreductive treatment initially, and most eventually because of pruritus, perisplenitis, or evidence of hyperviscosity [transient ischemic attacks (TIAs), PVD] or gout. Cytoreduction can be accomplished by oral medications, such as hydroxyurea or busulfan in a dose-dependent fashion.
- Monitoring of WBC and platelets is necessary during the maintenance period of treatment, which may last for many years.
- This is probably the preferential treatment for young individuals (<55 years of age); thereafter, radiophosphorus (P32) is equally effective and more convenient. A dose of 200 mbeq initially repeated as necessary causes of "remissions" (treatment-free periods) for many years. It is not recommended for younger patients because of the suspicion that it may be leukemogenic. However, the incidence of leukemia is still very low in patients treated with P32.

Individuals with PV often survive 10–20 years, but about 5% develop acute leukemia; some develop myelofibrosis.

Secondary Polycythemia

There is a pure red cell mass elevation without any evidence of myeloproliferation.

- *Respiratory*: The relationship between the red cell mass and O_2 saturation is well established, and if Hb is relatively desaturated due, e.g. to respiratory disorders or living at high altitudes, then compensation through elevation of the red cell mass will take place. Smokers traditionally have a hematocrit which may be 5–10% higher than nonsmokers. Patients with suspected respiratory polycythemia should have their arterial blood gases (ABGs) estimated; arterial saturation of less than 92% is abnormal.
- The cyanotic Hb variants, including methemoglobinemia, usually produce mild Hb elevations only, but erythrocytosis in both these and many of the high-affinity Hbs is relatively asymptomatic.
- However, O_2 dissociation curves will show the abnormality, and in most cases, the Hb variant is identifiable with structural abnormalities in both the α and β chains of the globin-suspected variant.
- Cardiac erythrocytosis may occur with congenital cyanotic heart disease.

- *Renal erythrocytosis*: Renal carcinoma, adenomas, Wilms' tumors, cysts, hydronephrosis, and polycystic kidneys have been reportedly associated with secondary polycythemia.
- *Other tumors*: Hepatocellular cancer, hepatic tumors, cerebellar hemangioblastomas, and uterine leiomyosarcoma have been associated with erythrocytosis.

OTHER MYELOPROLIFERATIVE SYNDROMES

Essential thrombocythemia occurs in middle adult life. Patients present with thrombotic complications, but bleeding may also occur. Splenomegaly should be found, but the spleen may be atrophied due to infarction.

The differential diagnosis is from reactive thrombocytosis. In each, the platelet count may be abnormally high (>700 × 10^9/L), but patients with counts of, e.g. 2,000 × 10^9/L are almost invariably myeloproliferative, and clusters of megakaryocytes in the bone marrow confirm the diagnosis.

Management of the disease is based on cytoreduction. Anticoagulants or aspirin should not be regarded as adequate. Alkylating agents, such as busulfan, antimetabolites, such as hydroxyurea, or radiophosphorus are all effective. The latter is somewhat slower than, e.g. hydroxyurea or cyclophosphamide. If there are no treatment complications, many years' survival can be achieved, although, like PV, some patients die of associated acute leukemia or bone marrow failure due to myelofibrosis.

Myelofibrosis

In elderly patients, malignant fibrosis of the bone marrow accompanied by myeloid metaplasia (myelofibrosis) may be found. In this form, the marrow stroma is taken over by reticulin and then collagen fibers, and hematopoiesis is found in the spleen and liver, both of which become enlarged. The disease is accompanied by severe wasting, anemia, thrombocytopenia, perisplenitis, and cachexia.

Management is difficult: Splenectomy is useful in prolonging good quality of life if carried out early in the disease, but often is of little value in later stages. Blood transfusion and supportive therapy are probably as effective. α-interferon may be of value in some instances, but its use has not yet been established. Epo may help with the anemia (androgen therapy had traditionally been used but response was poor). A more aggressive form of this disease may be seen in young women, where it behaves like AML.

PARAPROTEINEMIA

Myeloma

- Myeloma is a disorder characterized by overgrowth of monoclonal plasma cells in the bone marrow and the presence of an abnormal M

protein in the plasma of 80–90% of myeloma patients and the urine in 50–80% (techniques for identifying abnormal urinary proteins continue to improve).
- More than 5% of myeloma patients have no detectable paraproteins in the plasma or urine.

Clinical Presentation

Myeloma may present with bone pain with (or without) associated fractures, anemia, infection, neurologic problems (either associated with cord compression or polyneuropathy), renal failure, hypercalcemia, or hyperviscosity.
- The diagnosis is confirmed by bone marrow aspirate showing increased numbers of plasma cells that must show monoclonality by their surface light chain typing.
- The peripheral blood findings are variable but a normocytic normochromic anemia with rouleaux formation is commonly observed and there may be leukopenia and thrombocytopenia in advanced cases. Only in the rare plasma cell, leukemia are the characteristic cells actually seen in the peripheral blood.
- There may be signs of bone destruction in the blood chemistry assessment (hypercalcemia), but the alkaline phosphatase is often normal or marginally increased.
- A monoclonal immunoglobulin of any class may be found sometimes in very high concentrations in the plasma, and there may be a reduction in the normal immunoglobulin levels.
- The urine shows Bence Jones protein in more than one-half of cases, representing synthesis of excess light chains. The urine may also contain excess albumin due to tubular damage by these same light chains. IgG "spikes" are the most common in one-half to two-thirds of patients, with IgA in about 20%, and IgM, which is often separately classified, probably forming 10–15%. About 15% may have urine protein abnormalities only.
- There is a certain degree of correlation between the paraprotein type and clinical attribute. IgM, IgA, and IgG3 myelomas are more likely to be associated with hyperviscosity syndromes, the rarer IgD myeloma (1%), is rather like a generalized lymphoma with hepatosplenomegaly and extramedullary disease.
- Light-chain disease is associated with a poorer-than-average prognosis, as may be nonsecretory myelomas. A few patients will have double paraproteins: the so-called biclonal gammopathies.

The differential diagnosis is between myelomatosis and other monoclonal gammopathies, such as monoclonal gammopathy of undetermined significance (MGUS) (see later); polyclonal elevations of immunoglobulins are frequently seen in collagen vascular disorders or chronic infections and an increase in plasma cells in the bone marrow may also be seen in these conditions. Occasionally, myeloma presents with generalized osteopenia, especially in elderly females, and this is difficult to distinguish from the osteoporosis commonly seen in such individuals.

Assessment and Prognosis

Assessment and treatment may need to be undertaken on an emergency basis but, if not, a clinical staging system based on clinical and laboratory parameters is worth considering. The several systems available tend to reflect the total tumor burden. Older prognostic features, such as the Hb level and blood urea nitrogen (BUN) now appear to be of less value.

Management Strategy

Despite the success of novel targeted agents in newly diagnosed multiple myeloma, an upfront stem cell transplant remains the best treatment choice.

Immediate management includes hydration, especially in patients with renal failure, correction of anemia (but take care in patients with hyperviscosity), reduction of hypercalcemia, if symptomatic, with doses of prednisolone, e.g. 16 mg/L^2/day, and the use of bisphosphonates, such as etidronate 7.5 mg/kg qd. Mithramycin has also been used in patients resistant to all these maneuvers (25 µg/kg once or twice). The other emergency needing immediate treatment is pathologic fracture, and in the case of vertebral collapse with or without paravertebral disease, neurosurgical intervention may be indicated. Orthopedic repair of, e.g. fractured neck of femur is not contraindicated in myeloma.

Unlike many leukemias, myeloma treatment has traditionally been palliative. Recently, only allogenic BMT has been used in a small number of patients, but it may be the only way of curing the disease, especially in younger patients. For most, the expected best result is the induction of a "remission", i.e. a period when the disease is apparently controlled, the level of paraprotein reduced, and the patient symptom free with an improved quality of life until relapse.

In younger patients previously untreated, a typical treatment program would consist of six courses of adriamycin, BCNU, cyclophosphamide, and prednisone (ABCM) at approximately monthly intervals. The alternative is probably single-agent treatment with an alkylating agent, such as melphalan or cyclophosphamide. Typically, with the former, a dose of 0.25 mg/kg/day is given for 4 days (there is some doubt as to whether adding prednisone is helpful at this time). The treatment can be repeated every month until plateau has occurred, as measured by no further fall in the serum paraprotein. Cyclophosphamide can be used in a similar way, either IV or PO, at doses of 2–250 mg/L^2 qd for 4 days.

MESNA and extra fluids need to be given at this time to reduce the risk of hemorrhagic cystitis.

For relapsed patients, if they have not received combination chemotherapy, it is worth trying programs of high-dose melphalan; hemibody radiation is also worth considering. The role of interferons in the treatment of myeloma, especially in maintenance regimens, is currently uncertain. Interferons do have some suppressive effect on myeloma cells. Palliative radiotherapy to painful bone lesions is also useful. Elderly patients are probably best treated with oral melphalan as described. Plasmapheresis is temporarily effective in reducing the paraprotein level, but should be reserved for patients with acute hyperviscosity syndromes.

Other Paraproteinemia

Monoclonal Gammopathy of Undetermined Significance

A relatively benign condition of monoclonal gammopathy of unknown significance has been described, especially in elderly patients where it may reach an incidence of 3–4% in patients of 80 years of age. This must be distinguished from malignant paraproteinemia through a period of observation, and needs no treatment. A few patients with apparently benign disease develop frank myeloma after many years.

Solitary Plasmacytoma

This condition is self-explanatory and should be treated like a local tumor, usually with radiotherapy. Most such patients will develop myeloma eventually, but there is no proof that treating them systemically following the appearance and management of the solitary lesion prevents the onset of frank myeloma.

Waldenström's Disease (Macroglobulinemia)

Characterized by an elevation of monoclonal IgM, Waldenström's disease behaves differently to myeloma. It is almost exclusively a disease of the elderly, and again, may be often relatively benign. Presentation is most commonly that of anemia or bleeding or bruising. Bony fractures or renal disease are relatively uncommon, but occasionally neurologic symptoms can be found. Physical findings show hepatosplenomegaly in about one-half of the patients, and adenopathy may also occur. Diagnosis is made through detecting the abnormal paraprotein and by the presence of the Waldenström cells (lymphoplasmacytoid cells) in the bone marrow. They are also found in lymph nodes and spleen. Bone marrow biopsy is essential to confirm the nature of the disease.

Management and Treatment
When treatment is necessary because of anemia or increasing organ size, oral alkylating agents are the treatment of choice, and chlorambucil or melphalan are of value. Typically, melphalan 6 mg/L^2/day for 7 days at monthly intervals should suffice. Occasional patients can benefit from plasmapheresis, as hyperviscosity syndromes are sometimes life-threatening. A few younger patients with more aggressive disease can be treated in the same way as myeloma.

Heavy Chain Disease

Resembles the other paraproteinemias in that there is an abnormal serum protein that reacts to one of the heavy chains (α, γ, μ, or δ) but not with the κ and λ light chains. It is seen in younger patients, mostly 10–35 years old, and presents with lymphadenopathy, and GI and bone marrow involvement. A few circulating lymphoplasmacytoid cells may be seen in many cases. Prognosis is poor, and often, especially in tropical cases, there are associated diseases.

Treatment with alkylating agents, as in myeloma, may help in the short term, but this disorder is rare, and therapeutic trials of combination chemotherapy have not been conclusively carried out.

BIBLIOGRAPHY

1. Estey E. Sickle cell disease. N Engl J Med. 2018.??
2. Piel FB, Steinberg MH, Rees DC. Sickle cell disease. N Engl J Med. 2017;376:1561-73.
3. Roath S, Gross S. ?? In: Khan MG, Bartlett JG, Chopra S, Topol EJ (Eds). Medical Diagnosis and Therapy. Pennsylvania: Lea and Febiger; 1994.
4. Seymour JF, Kipps TJ, Eichhorst B, et al. Venetoclax-rituximab in relapsed or refractory chronic lymphocytic leukemia. N Engl J Med. 2018;378:1107-20.

CHAPTER 23

Rheumatic Disorders

DIAGNOSIS

Differential diagnosis of a musculoskeletal problem can be developed in two ways. First, however, decide whether the problem is regional and noninflammatory, such as osteoarthritis (OA); or localized, as a bursitis.

- Is it part of a systemic disorder? Table 23.1 provides the differential diagnosis in this manner. Tables 23.2, 23.3 and Box 23.1 provide a differential diagnosis based upon the number of joints involved. These tables present the major diagnostic considerations if the presentation is a single swollen joint (at times, the most difficult task for a rheumatologist); when the presentation consists of less than or equal to four swollen joints, often in an asymmetric pattern; or when onset presents with a symmetrical polyarthritis affecting more than five joints (hands and feet are considered as one joint for counting purposes, respectively) (Sheon).
- Inflammation is suspected when joints are either visibly inflamed or accompanied by morning stiffness or gelling of more than or equal to 30 minutes duration; fever, weight loss, and fatigue may occur.
- Nonarticular rheumatic pain disorders include myofascial pain, bursitis and tendinitis, structural disorders, nerve entrapment disorders, and fibromyalgia. It provides features that distinguish these from the inflammatory or systemic rheumatic diseases.
- Often, OA is a silent accompaniment to a nonarticular rheumatic pain disorder. Whereas OA would cause pain during use or weight bearing, a superimposed nonarticular disorder such as bursitis would cause pain at night. Night pain that is worse than daytime pain is unlikely due to an arthritis (Sheon).

Features of Rheumatic Pain Disorders

Inflammatory Rheumatic Diseases

- Pain during movement
- Palpable joint swelling

Table 23.1: Six major disease groups.

Connective tissue diseases				
B-cell mediated	*T-cell mediated*	*Hematologic*	*Metabolic*	*Neoplastic*
• Rheumatoid arthritis	• Dermatomyositis	• Hemophilia	• Gout	• Hypertrophic pulmonary osteoarthropathy
• Juvenile arthritis	• Polymyositis	• Sickle cell anemia	• Pseudogout	• Cancer arthropathy
• Acute rheumatic fever	• Giant cell arteritis	• Thalassemia	• Hyperparathyroidism	• Metastasis to joint
• Lupus erythematosus	• Wegener's granulomatosis	• Hemochromatosis	• Hyperthyroidism	• Osteochondroma
• Mixed connective tissue	• Churg–Strauss vascular syndrome	• Gaucher's disease	• Pancreatitis	• Villonodular synovitis.
• Felty's syndrome	• Kawasaki's disease	• Weber–Christian disease	• Acromegaly	
• Sjögren's syndrome	• Takayasu's arteritis	• Amyloidosis	• Ochronosis	
• Systemic sclerosis	• Ankylosing spondylitis	• Myeloma	• Hyperlipidemia	
• Mixed cryoglobulinemia	• Reiter's syndrome	• Leukemia	• Diabetes	
	• Psoriatic arthritis	• Lymphoma	*Allergic*	
	• Chronic ulcerative colitis	*Infectious*	• Henoch–Schönlein purpura	
	• Crohn's disease	• Gonococcal arthritis	• Stevens–Johnson syndrome	
	• Granulomatous colitis	• Tuberculous arthritis	• Drug lupus	
	• Whipple's disease	• Bacterial endocarditis	• Serum sickness	
	• Behçet's disease	• Hepatitis arthritis	• Hypersensitivity vasculitis	
		• Lyme arthritis	• Sarcoidosis	
		• Rickettsial infection		
		• Sporotrichosis		
		• Fungal arthritis		
		• Bacterial arthritis		
		• Viral arthritis		
		• Reactive arthritis.		

Table 23.2: Differential diagnosis of monoarticular arthritis.

Noninflammatory	Inflammatory	Septic
• Trauma/osteoarthritis • Internal derangements • Osteonecrosis • Reflex dystrophy • Hemarthrosis • Neuropathic/Charcot • Paget's disease • Joint tumors	• Rheumatoid monoarthritis • Gout/pseudogout • Juvenile monoarthritis • Spondyloarthropathy • Pigmented villonodular synovitis	*Bacterial* • Tuberculous • Gonococcus *Fungal* • Sporotrichosis *Viral* • Acquired immunodeficiency syndrome (AIDS) *Rickettsia*

Table 23.3: Differential diagnosis of polyarticular arthritis (approximately six joints).

Rheumatoid diseases	Hematologic	Infectious
• Seronegative rheumatoid arthritis (RA) • Seropositive RA • Sjögren's syndrome • Felty's syndrome. *Other connective tissue diseases* • Systemic lupus erythematosus • Mixed connective tissue disease • Dermatomyositis • Mixed cryoglobulinemia • Adult Still's disease *Reactive arthritis* • Acute rheumatic fever • Reiter's syndrome • Psoriatic arthritis • Spondyloarthritis	• Leukemia • Hemochromatosis. *Metabolic* • Polyarticular gout • Pseudogout • Dialysis arthropathy *Vasculitis* • Giant cell arteritis • Wegener's granulomatosis	• Endocarditis • Lyme disease • Parvovirus B19 • Rocky mountain spotted fever *Miscellaneous* • Serum sickness • Henoch–Schönlein purpura • Enteric arthropathy • Paraneoplastic syndrome • Sarcoidosis

Box 23.1: Differential diagnosis of pauciarticular polyarthritis (≤four joints).
- Spondyloarthropathies (HLA-B27 positive)
- *Reactive arthritis*:
  ○ Reiter's syndrome
  ○ Psoriatic arthritis
  ○ Acute rheumatic fever
  ○ Enteric arthropathies
- Metabolic and crystal-induced arthropathies
- Paraneoplastic syndromes
- *Septic arthritis*:
  ○ Acquired immunodeficiency syndrome (AIDS)-related arthritis
  ○ Parvovirus
  ○ Lyme arthritis
- Seronegative rheumatoid arthritis

- Abnormal tests
- Aggravating factors possible
- Diagnosis based on clinical examination and test results.

Nonarticular Disorders

- Pain after rest
- Swelling is only a sensation
- All laboratory tests normal
- Aggravating factors likely
- Diagnosis based on physical examination maneuvers and outcome.

Diagnosis Based on Features of Various Syndromes

Connective tissue diseases often lack pathognomonic feature. It is advisable to learn the elements of each disease syndrome and then elicit those features during the examination.

Table 23.4 provides a checklist for features important in a rheumatic history and physical examination.
- Is swelling visible or only a sensation? Morning stiffness/gelling duration and location will differentiate inflammatory disease from noninflammatory disease or gout. Gout seldom causes stiffness. Make certain stiffness is in true joint areas, not "all over", and not episodic, but present daily. Fibromyalgia and Parkinson's disease can cause "all-over" stiffness.
- Constitutional features of fever, chills, sweats, and weight loss indicate urgent diagnosis and treatment. Chills are rarely present in connective tissue diseases. Chills indicate infection.
- Weakness is a common complaint but must be objectively quantified. Can patient arise unassisted from a chair, lift head from bed, raise arms above head, etc.?
- If the onset followed trauma, elicit information regarding the extent of trauma (e.g. amount of damage to car); presence of abrasion, laceration, or fracture at the time of injury; and availability of X-rays. Is litigation pending? Has patient been able to perform usual daily routine at work or at home? Specify the disabilities (e.g. cannot dress, grasp, and climb).
- If an ominous feature or objective signs are not evident, include a misery index: "If you were so bad that you could not get out of bed, and if that was like being in the bottom of a pit, and being restored to perfect is like being out of the pit, and there are 100 steps down into the bottom of the pit, with step #1 being terrible, where is your level of misery this week?" This version of a pain scale can discriminate irrational pain concern or alert you to search more closely for evidence of ominous disease.
- The history taking will vary with the mode of presentation and age of the patient, but should quickly eliminate ominous features. Look early

Table 23.4: History and physical checklist (Sheon).

	History		Physical
Current illness	• Onset, pattern of spread • Was swelling visible? • Duration of swelling • Chills, fever, and rash • Weight loss/gain • Stiffness duration/location • Results of medications tried	General Skin HEENT	• Appearance, movement • Body symmetry, limb length • Flexibility, strength • Hair loss, rashes, and psoriasis • Nail fold infarctions, leg ulcer • Temporal arteries palpable • Conjunctiva, mucous membranes • Dentition, fundoscopy
Family history	• Inflammatory bowel diseases • Other rheumatic diseases • Migraine headaches • Joint laxity	Neck Cardiac/pulmonary	Thyroid abnormalities, pulses • Rubs, murmurs, and wheezes • Chest expanse
Social	• Stairs at home, location of bathrooms • Tic exposure • Smoking/drinking	Abdomen Lymph nodes Extremities	Organs, masses, and bruit Cervical, groin • Deformity, color, and temperature • Pulses, range of motion, and active • Passive, muscle symmetry
Past history	• Allergies/operations • Current medical diseases • Past medical diseases.	Joints	• Crepitus, tenderness • *Synovitis:* Boggy or not • Effusions • Periarticular tenderness • Inflammation

Contd...

Contd...

	History		Physical	
Current Rx	Prescription and nonprescription drugs	Spine		• Appearance of bending and extending • Effect on pain
Review of systems	• Skin rashes, psoriasis • Raynaud's phenomenon • Sun sensitivity and rash • *Alopecia • Jaw/fist clenching • Headache, convulsions • *Jaw claudication • Depression, stressful event • Dryness in eyes and mouth • Stomatitis • *Pleuropericarditis • Dyspnea, cough, and wheeze • *Edema, discoloration of limbs • Dysphagia, acid reflux • Liver diseases, peptic ulcers • Change in bowel habit • Kidney stones, hematuria • Dysuria, frequency • Nocturia, balanitis • Genital discharge • Cervicitis • Paresthesias, weakness	Neurologic		• Appearance, reflexes • Pathologic reflexes • Gait, ability to arise unassisted

*May be ominous sign.

and quickly for ominous features (Table 23.4) that should be assessed at the outset of the patient encounter.
- It is not rare for patients to have overlapping features, such as sicca complex, with another disease, or the pain of a nonarticular rheumatic disorder laid upon another rheumatic disease.
- Facial asymmetry can suggest temporomandibular joint pain and dysfunction with resulting neck pain and headache; or it may be associated with other skeletal deformities such as a short leg and scoliosis.
- Observe patient arising from a chair. Then, with legs bare, have patient walk away, and then toward you. Note gait, leg alignment or torsion, and balance.
- Swelling can be determined by palpating small joints with the examiner's two index fingers at the sides of the joint. Is the synovium normal, palpable, or boggy (like soft dough) thick? Always examine the feet; often they are deformed by a previous unrecognized attack of rheumatoid arthritis.
- Trigger points should be located when pain and symptoms occur beyond the joint boundary. Palpation should approximate 4 lb pressure. You can use the stylomastoid process as a control point. Palpation of the trigger point should reproduce the distant pain and paresthesia (Sheon).

INVESTIGATIONS

Order tests individually with thoughtful consideration of the disease presentation. For example, do not order a rheumatoid factor in young children: The various types of juvenile arthritis are usually seronegative; if more than or equal to three features of lupus are not present, the antinuclear antibody (ANA) is more likely to confuse than to help.

Complement determination and anti-DNA testing should be reserved for patients with active and diagnosed systemic lupus erythematosus (SLE).

Measurement of the complement component, C1q, is an inexpensive way to detect circulating immune complexes in patients suspected of having vasculitis, lupus, or systemic rheumatoid vasculitis.

The Westergren method for sedimentation rate discriminates better between normal and abnormal than other methods.
- Roentgenographic findings must be correlated to the age of the patient. Degenerative changes may be normal at advanced age and unrelated to the presenting problem.
- Imaging procedures of the cervical and lumbar spine have high sensitivity but low specificity: Findings in control groups reveal significant abnormality in 20% of normal 20-year-old, in 40% of normal 40–50-year-old, and in more than one-half of those normal persons more than

60 years of age. Do not order these scans if you have no evidence for an ominous disease process or if you lack criteria for surgical intervention, and be certain the patient would be willing to undergo surgery if findings indicated the need for a surgical procedure. Too often the physician presents the MRI finding of disk herniation only to be told by the patient, "Oh no, I am not that bad". Do not waste this resource (Sheon).

PHARMACOLOGY AND THE RHEUMATIC DISEASES

Nonsteroidal Anti-inflammatory Drugs

- *A large study indicated that* Celebrex 200 mg causes less gastrointestinal (GI) problems and is no worse than Naprosyn or ibuprofen and with no increase in cardiovascular disease (CVD). But the large population studied was not high CVD risk.

Patients at ↑ed risk for major nonsteroidal anti-inflammatory drug (NSAID) complications include those with hypertension, diabetes, poor renal function, liver disease, asthma or nasal polyps, peptic ulcer history, aspirin sensitivity, or advanced age.

Before initiating an NSAID, screen patient with appropriate history, complete blood count (CBC), and chemistry panel.

Once selection of NSAID proves satisfactory, follow-up with repeat laboratory tests at 2 months and then less frequently (annually or semiannually).

Adults with risks can be given nonacetylated salicylates such as choline salicylate, magnesium salicylate or salsalate, or combination.

Steroids

Oral steroids are not indicated unless systemic inflammation is evident and less hazardous treatment has failed, or life- and limb-threatening features are evident. Why add to the patient's problems? Do not use a short-term benefit when it carries a long-term catastrophic side effect. Steroid side effects include osteoporosis, diabetes, cataracts, glaucoma, and atherosclerosis. High doses may cause avascular necrosis of the shoulders or hips.

Calcium supplements, vitamin D, avoidance of simple carbohydrates, and excess salt are helpful when long-term steroid treatment is prescribed.

Intra-articular corticosteroid injection after joint aspiration is safer, provides more symptomatic benefit, and may retard loss of cartilage. Do not repeat injection in same joint more than 4-6 times a year. Boxes 23.2 and 23.3 provide principles for joint and soft-tissue injection.

Synovial fluid analysis is essential if acute inflammation is evident (Box 23.4).

Box 23.2: Principles for soft-tissue injection.
- Mark site of injection with circular end of ballpoint pen.
- Prepare a sterile field; use gloves or sterile technique.
- Use the shortest needle that will reach the lesion.
- For injecting tender points, use the needle as a probe.
- For injecting tendon sheaths, insert the needle parallel to the tendon.
- At site of nerve entrapment, wait a moment after needle is inserted; be certain the needle has not penetrated a nerve or vessel.
- Use 1% or 2% local anesthetic *without epinephrine.*
- Universal precautions apply.

Box 23.3: Principles for joint aspiration and injection.
- Prepare a sterile field. Use gloves.
- Use local anesthetic without epinephrine. Make skin wheal with #25 needle tip bevel flat to skin.
- Inject local anesthetic into synovium; withdraw needle.
- Use #16 needle for joint aspiration. Any smaller needle may get plugged by synovium or rice bodies.
- Use 30-cc syringe to aspirate larger joints. Aspirate slowly to avoid sucking synovium into needle tip and getting a dry tap.
- Transfer aliquot or synovial fluid to heparinized tube for synovianalysis.
- If crystalline steroid (methylprednisolone or triamcinolone hexacetonide) are mixed with xylocaine or procaine, a flocculant will occur with a likely prolongation of local effect.
- Use 20–40 mg of corticosteroid and 1 cc of 1% lidocaine for larger joints, and as little as 5–10 mg for smaller joints.
- Have patient apply ice locally to prevent a painful crystal reaction.
- Have patient avoid strenuous activity to the involved joint for 2 weeks.
- Universal precautions apply.

Box 23.4: Synovianalysis.
Basic information:
Volume, color, turbidity grade*, string sign for mucin content (one drop fluid on gloved finger, touch with thumb, and separate: A 3-inch or longer string IS normal: length varies inversely with inflammation).
Suspected problem:
- *Infection:*
  - White blood cell (WBC), differential: Gram stain: culture
  - Sugar (and concomitant serum glucose)
- *Gout*:
  - WBC, differential
  - Crystal study with polarizing microscopy and red compensator
- *Rheumatoid arthritis (RA), lupus, rheumatic fever, etc.:*
  - WBC, differential
  - *Latex RA titer.* Crystals

*Infected synovial fluid is a dirty or muddy brown (*Staphylococcus*), green (gonococcus), and all color grades in between. If in doubt, do Gram stain: sugar: culture

Get help early rather than too late. If disease is complex, or if treatment involves costly and potentially hazardous medication, consult rheumatologist.

If pain is persistent or if the disease is potentially deforming, consult occupational and physical therapy (Box 23.5). Box 23.6 presents some helpful hints for providing care to patients with rheumatic complaints.

Box 23.5: Joint protection guide.

Head and neck:
- *Principle:* Keep head aligned with trunk.
- Avoid jutting head forward ("Birdwatcher's neck", as if looking through field glasses); hold head up when reading; use large lap pillow for holding handwork. Higher, lower adjustable chair if worktable or desk is too low for long-waisted person. Avoid propping head forward when resting (use proper chair for support).

Shoulder:
- *Principle:* Avoid repetitive movements or prolonged overhead use.
- Vacuuming, performing push-ups, or sports in which the arm moves like a piston can lead to overuse injury. Such activities should be moderated. Women with heavy breasts may benefit from use of a support brassiere. When writing, keep the involved shoulder held backward and upward.

Elbow:
- *Principle:* Repetitive and rotating motions should be moderated.
- Fist clenching, using tools with a tight grip and using the hands to push off of chairs may lead to tennis elbow. Reduce grip pressure by using pipe insulation on tool handles.

Wrist and hand:
- *Principle:* Use larger muscles when possible, moderate repetitive activities.
- Grasp with flat open palms when possible. Repetitive movements and handwork should be interrupted with other activities. Never say "I am going to finish this even if it kills me". Use a plastic pencil holder during prolonged writing. Use foamy pipe insulation on tool handles.
- Avoid clenched fists at night (a tension state). Using nylon stretch gloves during sleep may help.

Low back:
- *Principle:* Avoid prolonged standing, prolonged sitting, and improper lifting.
- Bend at the knee not at the waist. Lift with the thighs. Avoid bending over with straight knees. When prolonged standing is necessary, use a 2 × 4 × 8 inch wood block and step up on it with one foot for a few minutes, then change it to the other foot (while working in the kitchen, or if working at a machine, or as a cashier). When carrying heavy objects, carry the object out in front, turn with the feet, not by twisting the trunk. Use cushion-soled shoes when standing or working on concrete.

Knee:
- *Principle:* Maintain good alignment and quadriceps (thigh muscle) strength.
- When arising from a chair, avoid using hands to push off of chair, use thigh muscles to push off. Avoid prolonged sitting. Avoid twisting the trunk; turn with the feet. Avoid stair climbing. If the home lacks a first floor toilet facility, place a portable toilet on the first floor.
- Avoid kneeling on hard floors; use a pad.

Contd...

Foot:
- *Principle:* Shoes were meant to cover and protect the feet, not to compress them. Aging feet sometimes enlarge or toes spread. Have shoe size measured while standing. Prolonged standing or squatting may result in foot strain. If you have flat feet, leg cramp may result from wearing flat shoes or slippers.

Source: Shean RP. Nonarticular rheumatism and nerve entrapment disorders. Res Staff Phys. 1989;35(12):65-70.

Box 23.6: Helpful hints.
- Laying on of the examiner's hands often provides more useful information than do roentgenograms.
- Osteoarthritis seen on roentgenograms is often unrelated to the pain syndrome
- Localized musculoskeletal pain disorders may be layered over another established disease process.
- When morning stiffness does not *mainly* involve the hands and second feet, rheumatoid arthritis is an unlikely diagnosis.
- Pain so severe that the limbs cannot be touched (the touch-me-not syndrome), and with no discernible spasm, is usually of psychogenic origin.
- Pain localized to a body quadrant seldom is due to a psychogenic cause.
- Observing the patient while seated, while rising from a chair, while standing, and while bending forward can lead to recognition of basic *structural* alterations. "Misuse" of the musculoskeletal system may also be observed.
- Drugs may be the least important part of treatment. Stretching exercises and avoiding aggravating factors often provide more sustained benefit than pills.

Source: Sheon RP, Moskowitz RW, Goldberg VM. Soft Tissue Rheumatic Pain: Recognition, Management, and Prevention, 2nd edition. Philadelphia: Lea & Febiger; 1987.

OSTEOARTHRITIS

Osteoarthritis should be considered as either compensated or decompensated. When accompanied by ligamentous instability or adjacent muscle weakness, decompensation occurs and a vicious cycle of pain, weakness, disuse, and finally, swelling occurs. Roentgenographic findings do not correlate with outcome.

When decompensated, treatment should be directed not only to pain relief, but more importantly, to restoration of muscle strength, joint protection, and elimination of bad habits and obesity.
Types include:
- *Primary OA*: Nodal, generalized, inflammatory (erosive), or spinal
- *Secondary OA*: Following trauma, inflammation, metabolic, endocrine, or neuropathic diseases.

Nodal Osteoarthritis

Features include bulbous enlargement of the terminal finger joints (Heberden nodes) or proximal interphalangeal (PIP) joints (Bouchard nodes); enlargement (bossing) of the great toe of metatarsophalangeal joint, often with bunion formation; and enlargement and limitation of movement of the first carpometacarpal joint.

Pathogenesis

Often genetically transmitted, pathology includes fibrillation, fragmentation, thinning, and eventual loss of cartilage; formation of osteophytes; and sclerosis of subchondral bone.

Differential Diagnosis

Distal finger nodes might be similar to psoriatic arthritis, tophaceous gout, or a benign tumor of bone.
- *Cost-effective workup*: Order X-ray only when trauma has occurred, if asymmetric, or if accompanied by warmth or redness.

Initial Treatment

Pain management is done with oral analgesics, salicylates, and NSAIDs in that order. Joints with effusions: Aspiration and injection. If synovial fluid is turbid, do synovianalysis (Boxes 23.3 and 23.4).

Teach patient long-term behavior modification by applying joint protection for each affected area (Box 23.5). Refer to an occupational therapist for joint protection and finger exercises; splinting ad-lib. Long-term behavior modification is more important than medication.

For patient education, call the Arthritis Foundation for pamphlets on osteoarthritis and joint protection.

Osteoarthritis of the Hip, Knee, and Spine

Often is asymptomatic; if pain awakens the patient, or is worse at rest, suspect other causes for pain, particularly bursitis, tendinitis, myofascial pain disorder, gout, and rheumatoid arthritis.

Features

Weight-bearing or use-related pain accompanied by ↓ed or painful passive range of joint motion. Knee buckling, locking, or giving way suggests an internal derangement such as a meniscus tear.

Initial Treatment

Pain management is done with either salicylates or NSAIDs. Joints with effusions of more than 10 days' duration, when pain limits essential activity, or if persistent despite quadriceps strengthening: Aspiration and corticosteroid injection. If synovial fluid is turbid, do synovianalysis (Boxes 23.3 and 23.4).

Chondroitin sulfate: High-quality chondroitin sulfate is as effective as celecoxib in treating knee OA, according to an international trial in the Annals of the Rheumatic Diseases.

Roughly 600 adults older than 50 years with primary knee OA were randomized to receive pharmaceutical-grade chondroitin sulfate (800 mg) plus placebo, celecoxib (200 mg) plus placebo, or double placebo daily for 6 months.

At the end of treatment, the chondroitin and celecoxib groups had significantly greater reductions in pain relative to the placebo group, with no difference between the two active treatments. Similarly, at 3 months and 6 months, chondroitin sulfate and celecoxib conferred significant improvements in function relative to placebo, again with no difference between the two active groups.

The authors, noting the risks associated with long-term use of NSAIDs and acetaminophen, say chondroitin sulfate "should be considered a first-line treatment in the medical management of knee OA".

(Link(s): Annals of the Rheumatic Diseases article (Free) http://response.jwatch.org/t?ctl=17012:F82014DE957000380F7CEDA6A1BC6AC4&.)

Background: NEJM Journal Watch General Medicine coverage of recent trial showing no benefit of glucosamine/chondroitin over placebo (Your NEJM Journal Watch subscription required) (http://response.jwatch.org/t?ctl=17013:F82014DE957000380F7CEDA6A1BC6AC4&.)

Referral to physical therapist for exercises and home program, dietitian for weight reduction, and occupational therapist for joint protection advice. This is as important as oral medication (Box 23.5).

Surgical referral for OA of the hip or knee should be restricted to patients with avascular necrosis; or patients who, after a trial of physical therapy and directed home exercises, cannot perform an essential function such as dressing, getting through a grocery store, having sex, or getting to the bathroom.

The symptomatic osteoarthritic joint will often improve with rest and modified behavior. Use NSAIDs cautiously.

- Strengthening exercises reduce pain, particularly at the wrist, hand, and knee. Elderly patients should be encouraged to use exercise therapy, rub-on medications, and acetaminophen.

Unless patient has features suggesting need for surgery and agrees to surgery, X-rays are not necessary.

NONARTICULAR RHEUMATIC DISORDERS

These very common symptom disorders include bursitis, tendinitis, myofascial pain syndromes, structural disorders such as joint laxity (hypermobility syndrome) or body asymmetry, and fibromyalgia. They lack objective measurement and may overlay other rheumatic disorders, creating significant disability. Reserve expensive imaging for patients who have objective abnormality or who fail conservative treatment.

Diagnosis is often based on subjective features and physical examination techniques that reproduce symptoms (Table 23.4).

Nonarticular rheumatic disorders are common and easily treated without invasive procedures and with a minimum of diagnostic study.

A six-step management plan should be followed:
1. Exclude other diseases through careful history, physical examination, and appropriate tests.
2. Identify habits and aggravations that will cause persistence or recurrence.
3. Provide an explanation for the pain and disability.
4. Provide pain relief, so that exercise will be performed.
5. Provide exercises to restore muscle flexibility and tone.
6. Provide an expected outcome.

Regional Soft Tissue Disorders

Features include local pain and tenderness; swelling is variable; and ominous findings are not present (Table 23.4). Pain at rest often is more severe than pain during movement. Numbness and tingling may occur if the local process is adjacent to a major nerve.

Passive movement and palpation, tests, and maneuvers (e.g. the Finkelstein maneuver, trigger point palpation) can reproduce the pain. Symptom relief should follow treatment, and this corroborates diagnosis.

Etiology is usually traumatic and often subtle, such as inappropriate body position, or habits (Box 23.5). Some common but often vague entities are:
- *Carotidynia*: Throbbing pain may occur over the side of the face, head, or neck. Marked tenderness, and sometimes swelling at the carotid bifurcation, may be palpated. The condition is probably related to migraine. No diagnostic studies are available. Treatment includes drugs useful in migraine.
- *Temporomandibular myofascial pain*: Pain is often referred to the neck and face, and often without jaw complaint. Palpation of the internal pterygoid muscles within the anterior pillars (with gloved finger) will elicit severe pain or tenderness. Malocclusion should be excluded with dental examination. Treatment includes use of a bite splint, behavior modification, and muscle relaxants such as cyclobenzaprine, or tricyclics, prescribed particularly at bedtime. Some patients have caffeine and theophylline sensitivity; a trial of abstaining from dark beverages may be helpful.
- *Scapulothoracic syndromes*: Aching discomfort throughout the shoulder girdle, usually unilateral, with nighttime aggravation and often with diffuse arm paresthesia, may result from a trigger point in the infraspinatus

muscle, located midway between the spine of the scapula and the lower scapular pole. Palpation of the indurated firm muscle bundle reproduces the pain. An important clue is painless passive arm rotation in any plane. Injecting the trigger point is helpful and diagnostic. Other parascapular muscles may be involved (Box 23.2 for injection technique and Box 23.5 for joint protection for the shoulder region). A common cause is repetitively reaching backward: For a seatbelt, into the back seat of the car, or when in the kitchen or at work.

- *Shoulder impingement syndrome*: Pain during arm abduction, elevation, often with paresthesias, may result from shoulder cuff impingement under the acromion. Tenderness occurs in the vicinity of the subcoracoid bursa, below the acromioclavicular joint and medial to the insertion of the biceps tendon. Impingement is reproduced by grasping the patient's elbow while the arm is abducted and externally rotated, then pressing arm into acromion and rotating slightly to reproduce symptoms. The best test is instillation of xylocaine (1 cc 1%) mixed with methylprednisolone (20–40 mg) into the subcoracoid space and adjacent tissues, after careful preparation. Then, active movement should be pain free. Treatment includes avoiding repetitive arm motion with elbow abducted. When necessary to perform repetitious movement, the patient should position the body so the arm can perform task out in front of the ipsilateral breast. In this manner, the biceps and supraspinatus muscles avoid impingement. Physical therapy consultation is appropriate before undertaking further evaluation or orthopedic consultation.

- *Carpal tunnel syndrome*: Pain, weakness, and paresthesias in median nerve distribution are suggestive. Physical examination findings include positive Tinel test, wrist compression test, or wrist tourniquet test. Electrodiagnostic study is recommended only if conservative treatment fails. If swelling is evident, or features include prolonged symmetrical morning stiffness, tests for rheumatoid arthritis should be obtained.

  Patients with suggestive symptoms but without weakness or atrophy should have such conservative measures as resting wrist splints, ↓ in repetitious motion, occupational and physical therapy consultation, and avoidance of excessive gripping of the steering wheel, tools, or nocturnal hand clenching (can be treated with nylon stretch gloves worn at night with the seams to the outside). NSAIDs or injection of the volar wrist area with methylprednisolone-xylocaine mixture (Box 23.2) can be helpful. If conservative measures fail, then surgery is indicated.

- *Trigger finger, trigger thumb*: Complaints include snapping or locking sensation of one or several digits, particularly upon arising. Usually follows unusual or repetitive hand tasks. Treatment is highly satisfactory with injection of the flexor tendon sheath with steroid-xylocaine mixture (Box 23.2). Splinting the digit is helpful. Provide joint protection advice (Box 23.5).

- *Myofascial chest wall pain syndrome (costochondritis)*: Inflammatory disease of the costochondral joints can occur in rheumatoid arthritis and ankylosing spondylitis (costochondritis). Much more commonly, the disorder is not inflammatory, and the term myofascial chest wall pain syndrome is preferred. What distinguishes this syndrome from other causes of chest pain is pain at rest relative to effort and exquisite costochondral tenderness. Causes include such repetitive effort as coughing, or transferring heavy objects such as moving log pile. Treatment includes behavior modification and chest wall stretching exercises. One simple exercise is for the patient to stand 2 feet out from the corner of a room and perform a push up slowly into the corner for 1 minute or 2 minutes several times a day.
- *Myofascial low back pain*: Perhaps as many as 90% of patients with persistent back pain lack objective causality determinants. If ominous features are not present, avoid labels suggestive of skeletal origin. Radiographic changes of disk degeneration or narrowing, spurs, unusual angulation, or congenital lumbosacral changes often have no relation to symptoms or outcome.

Much of the history and examination methods of the past have been proven unreliable.

Ominous features include a history of progressive pain that is worse with walking; paresthesia felt below the knee; leg pain that has become worse than back pain; weakness with giving way of leg; and/or physical findings of listing, flattening of the spine when patient bends forward, limitation of hip movement, diminished reflexes on one side, and weakness consistent with nerve root involvement.

If buttock claudication has occurred, spinal stenosis should be considered. Roentgenographic examination should be limited to those patients whose symptoms followed significant trauma, are older, have important objective features, or have a past history suggesting possible ominous disease (e.g. osteomyelitis, tumor, family history of ankylosing spondylitis, iritis, or other systemic features, including weight loss, fever, prolonged morning stiffness, or use of corticosteroids for extended periods of time). When ordering roentgenography, be sure to order a pelvis examination along with lumbar spine roentgenographs.

Imaging studies should likewise be reserved for the patient who has ominous features and would be willing to have surgery if the findings warrant it. Severity of pain alone is not an indication for imaging.

Conservative care includes assessment of trunk strength with corrective exercise prescription, proper shoes, and job and hobby activity modification, if necessary. Smoking and diet should be addressed. Smoking reduces O_2 content of disk and soft tissues, thus impairing natural healing. Physical therapy should be ordered early. Bedrest is of value only if an acute herniation is suspected, and then not for more than a few days.

Use of NSAIDs, muscle relaxants, and trigger point injections with steroid-xylocaine mixture are a means to provide pain relief and compliance with physical therapy.

Patients improve in direct proportion to the number of treatment modalities tried. In one study, 91% of patients with proved herniated nucleus pulposis improved without surgery if cord impingement was not severe and if the patient failing one therapy was provided several alternatives in sequence.

- *Bursitis of the hip or knee*: Pain in the hip or knee that is more disturbing during rest than when walking should suggest a regional bursitis, even when significant OA is evident. Night pain may be severe, is uncommon in OA, and suggestive of bursitis.

  Trochanteric bursitis with either superficial or deep tenderness at or posterior to the greater trochanter can be treated with either an NSAID, or if persistent, a corticosteroid-xylocaine injection. Relief is usual within a few days. Patient should be instructed in proper bending (with knees bent and back straight).

  Anserine bursitis along the inner aspect of the knee joint commonly occurs in elderly women with thick knee panniculi. Have the knees separated with a cushion between the thighs during sleep. Night pain is common and relieved by local steroid-xylocaine injection.

  Prepatellar bursitis may result from repeated kneeling or from foreign body penetration; septic bursitis can occur. If the bursa is swollen, do aspiration and synovial fluid examination for sugar, white blood cell (WBC), Gram stain, and culture. Leukocyte count may not be impressive; even as low as 1,000 cells/mL may be found in septic bursitis. Many rheumatologists prefer to use oral NSAIDs and not inject this bursa after aspiration. Many would similarly treat olecranon bursitis. Surgical excision may be necessary for persistent swelling.

- *Tarsal tunnel syndrome*: Foot pain that awakens the patient from sleep is characteristic. Nerve entrapment is common following ankle trauma, but may also occur from an adjacent tenosynovitis brought on by stretching the posterior tibial tendon by walking barefoot or in flat slippers. The Tinel test is best performed by rolling the examiner's thumb across the tarsal tunnel inferior to the medial malleolus. Pain reproduction is suggestive. Use of a local steroid-xylocaine injection (and proper footgear) should provide relief.

Generalized Soft Tissue Rheumatic Pain

When patients complain of diffuse stiffness and aching, or widespread arthralgia, and the sensation of joint swelling (My rings feel tight) but without evidence of illness or synovitis, two entities deserve consideration: (1) Fibromyalgia and (2) the hypermobility syndrome. A tender point count and examination for joint laxity should be performed. Only in the absence of other diseases can these entities be considered a primary disorder.

A lengthy workup is not needed. A chemistry panel, including creatine phosphokinase (CPK), thyroid-stimulating hormone (TSH), CBC, and Westergren sedimentation rate, may suffice. Unless objective features of connective tissue disease are in evidence, it is not necessary to order ANAs or rheumatoid factor: Since 5% of normal persons may have low titers of these tests, and only 6% of patients with the tender point count have underlying connective tissue disease, these tests are not cost-effective.

Fibromyalgia

Features include widespread aching and stiffness (aggravated following rest), nonrestful sleep, weather sensitivity, and fatigue. Other common features include migraine headache, Raynaud's phenomenon, irritable bowel syndrome, paresthesia, and weakness. Diagnosis requires 11 of 18 points and few control points. Use the mid-thigh region as a control for tenderness: The sensation that occurs when the examiner presses with about 4 lb pressure is called tenderness, whereas more than that is pain, particularly when the patient grimaces or withdraws. Other control points include the forehead, mid-dorsal forearm, thumbnail compression, and midway down the third metatarsal bone. The test points should be palpated and interspersed with the control points, and they should elicit a pain response rather than a tender-only response.

Laboratory features are normal unless fibromyalgia coexists with another disease. Most patients blame a stressful event for the symptoms. Many believe alteration in substance P and endorphins are involved.

Treatment begins by eliminating serious underlying disease with a comprehensive history and physical examination and judicious testing. When the control points are normal, the patient will be relieved to know that the examination demonstrates a nonpsychological disorder; the pain is not imagined.

Medication that improves mood and sleep is helpful, including tricyclics, trazodone, meprobamate, cyclobenzaprine, or carisoprodol. These agents also boost endorphins. Most important is a gradual and progressive fitness exercise program. Aquatic exercises, very light aerobic exercises, walking, and cycling can result in more prolonged pain relief than that which occurs with medication.

Severe incapacitation from fibromyalgia is rare; additional measures may include tender point injections or an ice rub and stretch routine. Behavior modification, biofeedback, and psychosocial counseling can be helpful.

Hypermobility Syndrome

Symmetrical joint pain and back or neck pain, stiffness, and a sensation of joint swelling that is of so short duration (hours) that inflammation is unlikely, may result from loss of muscle tone in persons with diffuse joint laxity. Such patients may not be aware of joint laxity, yet they can do the following: Bend over and touch palms to floor with knees straight, extend elbows and knees more than 10°, draw thumb into apposition with ipsilateral forearm, draw finger back and parallel to forearm, and/or invert or evert ankle excessively.

Patients with hypermobility syndrome show joint laxity in more than or equal to three locations. Since 5% of the population has joint laxity, another factor is needed before symptoms occur. Most patients have onset after a period of inactivity, such as following pregnancy, illness, study, or a career change to a sedentary state. Then, upon attempting a physically taxing chore or sport, symptoms occur. Treatment consists of exercises that emphasize extensor muscle strengthening for the involved joints. Symptoms usually improve after several months of exercise. For patients with spinal complaints, pool aerobics may be helpful.

MONOARTICULAR ARTHRITIS

Age at onset, personal and family history, lifestyle and personal habits history, palpation for synovial thickness, and synovial fluid analysis are essential elements for diagnosis. Reaching the diagnosis in monoarticular arthritis is often a taxing rheumatologic exercise.

Noninflammatory Monoarthritis

- *Osteoarthritis*: Discussed earlier.
- *Internal derangement* occurs in the knee, wrist, and temporomandibular joint, often without a history of trauma. The term implies a mechanical derangement that interferes with normal joint motion. Cartilage defects, ligamentous disruption, and intra-articular loose bodies are the more common disorders. Locking or buckling of the joint is usual symptoms. When the knee is affected to the point, the patient is unable to bear weight on it, refer to orthopedist. If less severe, prescribe a trial of conservative treatment. Most patients do not need surgery. Initiate use of crutches until swelling has subsided. Aspirate synovial fluid fully; do synovial fluid analysis if fluid has turbidity. Pain can be alleviated with instillation of corticosteroid and local anesthetic (Boxes 23.3 and 23.4). *Treatment* for all noninflammatory degenerative monoarthropathies should include physical therapy and extensor muscle strengthening exercises. Pain relief often follows return of strength, irrespective of cause. Most patients with features of a meniscus tear or internal derangement improve with conservative measures. At this writing, an MRI of the knee costs $1,500; conservative treatment costs much less. Treat first, test later.
- *Osteonecrosis, reflex dystrophy, Charcot joint, and hemarthrosis* have specific features of pain quality and severity and weight-bearing

aggravation or buckling, and require management by those experts in their care.
- *Paget's disease* of the spine, knee, or hip often presents with articular pain that results from secondary OA of the involved joints. Pain often responds to joint aspiration, corticosteroid injection, ASA, and physical therapy. Serum alkaline phosphatase and urine hydroxyproline reflect disease activity. Drug treatment is usually reserved for those with elevated test results and with bone pain or in preparation for joint replacement. Treatment: Salicylates are often helpful. Active Paget's disease can be treated with etidronate 5–10 mg/kg daily for 56 months. If joint destruction is severe, arthroplasty should be considered. Calcitonin and mithramycin are used in special circumstances.
- *Intra-articular tumors* are rare. Benign tumors present with swelling and moderate pain, and often cause locking. Malignant tumors generally cause much more pain both during movement and at rest; joint fluid is bloody and thin. MRI is helpful to diagnosis. Orthopedic consultation should be obtained for management.

Inflammatory Monoarthritis

Inflammatory features of local or systemic fever, redness, and visible swelling require efficient and prompt diagnosis. Synovial fluid examination should be performed at the first visit (Boxes 23.3 and 23.4). Simply noting the mucin string sign and degree of turbidity (cloudiness) is of more value than roentgenography or scans.

Rheumatoid Arthritis

If synovium is thick and boggy, rheumatoid arthritis is most likely. The joint fluid turbidity signifies the erosiveness of the inflammatory process. Joint fluid tests for rheumatoid factor would likely be positive in high titer in adults and negative in children less than 16 years. Treatment should be aggressive.

Treatment: Installation of a corticosteroid after aspiration can be performed if features of infection are not present. The injected joint should be protected from overuse for 2 weeks. NSAID in doses that parallel the degree of turbidity are prescribed, see next section's coverage of rheumatoid for comprehensive treatment.

Gout and Pseudogout

These conditions must be given top consideration if onset was abrupt and joint tenderness was severe. Primary gout, of genetic origin, occurs in the absence of any causative factor (diuretics, alcohol, renal disease, occult hematologic or other malignancy, lead poisoning, etc.).

Synovial fluid should be examined by experienced staff; red compensation and polarized microscopy are usually necessary for crystal identification. Gout should be worked up, including tests for renal function, liver function, CBC, and uric acid determination in serum and in a 24-hour urine specimen. A 24-hour urine uric acid should be obtained before institution of specific therapy but after the acute attack has subsided and nonsteroidals can be replaced with colchicine.

- A study published in the N Engl J Med indicated that in patients with gout and major cardiovascular coexisting conditions, Febuxostat was noninferior to allopurinol with respect to rates of adverse cardiovascular events (White et al.).
- All-cause mortality and cardiovascular mortality were higher with Febuxostat than with allopurinol (White et al.).

Colchicine does not affect urate metabolism and can be used while waiting for urine uric acid test results. In primary gout, urine uric acid is usually normal (500–900 mg/24 h). When urine uric acid is greatly elevated, consider tumor or Lesch–Nyhan syndrome.

Serum uric acid or joint fluid uric acid content, although usually elevated, may not always be so. Use of NSAIDs or aspirin may reduce the uric acid level to normal levels even though the patient is in the middle of an attack.

Treatment: Treatment of the acute attack includes NSAID treatment (indomethacin, if not contraindicated, 50 mg q 8 hours) until attack subsides, usually not more than 48 hours, or adrenocorticotropic hormone (ACTH) 40 U/24 h. If a diuretic is used for hypertension, try to change to other forms of antihypertensive treatment. If the diuretic is necessary, then, after the acute attack is over, and under cover of an NSAID or colchicine (0.5 mg bid or 0.6 mg bid), begin allopurinol 300 mg qd.

If renal function is good and several attacks have occurred, long-term treatment with probenecid is preferred. Again, this agent also requires cover of an NSAID or colchicine. Allopurinol is used if urine uric acid is high or if patient requires continued diuretic use or has hematologic or renal diseases.

The goal in using drugs that lower uric acid is to keep the serum uric acid level less than 6 mg/dL. Patients taking probenecid should not take ASA; rather, an NSAID or acetaminophen is preferred. Use maintenance NSAID or colchicine until patient is symptom free for several months and serum uric acid is normalized.

Examine all gouty patients for tophi. When present, the patient should be on life-long treatment with either allopurinol or probenecid as described earlier. 85% of patients with primary gout can be treated successfully with probenecid long term; it is preferred because of less severe side effects.

Allopurinol should be used with caution in patients on coumadin, antineoplastic agents, ampicillin, amoxicillin, or angiotensin-converting enzyme (ACE) inhibitors, and in low dose if patient is azotemic.

- Hyperuricemia in the absence of gout is not an indication for long-term treatment with agents that lower the uric acid.

Psoriatic Arthritis

- Usually begins with an acute dactylitis: A sausage-like swelling of a single digit. The digit is painful, red, cool to touch, and diffusely swollen. Or, it may present as a symmetrical polyarthritis, however, rheumatoid factor would be negative.
- Bulbous terminal finger joint with onycholysis or nail pitting is a characteristic finding. Search carefully for psoriatic involvement of the scalp, umbilicus, and gluteal cleft.
- Hyperuricemia is common in patients with psoriasis, but gout is not a consideration. Gout is much more abrupt in onset and much more painful; joint fluid urate crystals are not present in psoriatic arthritis.

Psoriatic arthritis occurs in about 30% of Caucasian patients with psoriasis and is uncommon in Asians and Blacks (Ritchlin et al.).

Rheumatoid arthritis is characterized by proximal, symmetric involvement of the joints of the hands and feet, with sparing of the distal interphalangeal joints, whereas in more than 50% of patients with psoriatic arthritis, the distal joints are affected (Ritchlin et al.).

Psoriatic monoarthritis, particularly involving the toes, or dactylitis may be misdiagnosed as gout or pseudogout. The uric acid level may be elevated in patients with psoriatic arthritis, as well as in those with gout, making the differential diagnosis difficult, particularly if crystal analysis of joint fluid is negative or cannot be performed. The distal-joint involvement that is characteristic of psoriatic arthritis is also observed in OA. In psoriatic arthritis, palpation of distal joints reveals soft swelling due to inflammation, whereas in OA, swelling arises from a bony osteophyte and is solid. Moreover, involvement of distal interphalangeal joints and nail disease (pitting or onycholysis) occur frequently in psoriatic arthritis but not in OA (Ritchlin et al.).

Ixekizumab, another interleukin-17 blocker, showed efficacy in phase three trials involving patients with psoriatic arthritis and was recently approved for the treatment of psoriasis (Ritchlin et al.).

Pseudogout

It may be monoarticular or polyarticular in onset. Fever can occur. Most common joints affected are the knee, ankle, and foot; rarely the great toe. The joint fluid is turbid but not "dirty"; synovial fluid microscopy with red compensator lens is important for identifying the weakly birefringent calcium pyrophosphate dihydrate crystals.

Treatment: Management of the attack is identical to treatment described for gouty arthritis attacks. Colchicine (0.5-0.6 mg bid) should be tried for intercritical treatment (Sheon).

Milwaukee Shoulder and Knee

A highly destructive basic calcium phosphate (hydroxyapatite, octacalcium phosphate, or tricalcium phosphate) arthropathy due to massive synovitis of a shoulder or knee in the elderly should be recognized early. Joint calcification and a creamy joint fluid or bloody effusions of large quantity are clues. Treat with frequent aspiration and NSAIDs.

Juvenile Monoarthritis

Without other diagnostic features, this condition may be extremely difficult to categorize. If family history is suggestive (arthritis, iritis, spondylitis, and IBO), an HLA-B27 test determination is appropriate. Teenagers should have rheumatoid factor test determination, but this is not necessary for younger children.

All children with monoarticular arthritis should have ophthalmologic study with slit lamp for iritis, and ANA test determination (if positive, anterior uveitis will be more likely to occur).

Young adults should be screened carefully for sexually transmitted disease. Females may require cervical smear for gonococcus if sexually active. Joint fluid analysis is imperative on the initial visit (Boxes 23.3 and 23.4).

Complete examination is essential for signs of related diseases (Table 23.4). Particularly examine the skin and genitalia for psoriasis and Reiter's syndrome, erythema nodosum, and erythema migrans. Perform the ear, nose, and throat (ENT) examination for signs of mucous membrane changes and streptococcal infection, and of course, a systematic examination as determined by the presentation.

Treatment: If joint fluid is turbid but not purulent, begin with NSAID and joint injection with corticosteroid. Lower-limb joints should be protected from weight bearing with use of crutches until joint swelling and tenderness have subsided. Defer roentgenographic examination except in patients with sepsis or trauma.

Oral anti-inflammatory treatment for children can be instituted if signs of inflammation are present: Fever, turbid joint fluid, abnormal Westergren sedimentation rate, or C-reactive protein. Preschoolers can be given nonacetylated salicylate either liquid (Arthropan; Trilisate liquid) or tablets; begin with 70-80 mg/kg in divided dosage.

Periodic determination of serum salicylate level taken 2 hours after first morning dose is important in proper dosing of young children. Try to maintain salicylate level within 20-25 mg%. Reye's syndrome is rare, but during influenza or chicken pox outbreaks, salicylate therapy should be replaced with an NSAID. Naproxen (15 mg/kg/day) or tolmetin sodium (25-30 mg/kg/day) may be used.

Physical therapy, home instruction is important and should begin as soon as the acute inflammation subsides.

Juvenile Spondyloarthropathies

Often affect the lower extremity joints and only occasionally begin as a monoarthritis. Look for signs of sacroiliac tenderness, limited chest expanse with tape measure, family history, genital lesions of Reiter's syndrome, and nail changes.

Treatment: See under Pauciarticular Polyarthritis here.

Pigmented Villonodular Synovitis

Usually involves the hip or knee. Synovial fluid is sanguineous. Consult an orthopedist.

Septic Arthritis

Bacterial infections often attack a single joint abruptly. The organism is usually spread hematologically. Older patients may not have systemic manifestations; often they suffer other debilitating diseases that lower their resistance to infection. Steroids and chemotherapy provide ↑ed risk for infection.

- In younger individuals, septic arthritis is common among drug abusers, alcoholics, or those who are sexually promiscuous. The organism varies with the patient's risk factors. When the inflamed joint is associated with a tenosynovitis, look for gonococcus and tuberculosis. When the onset began with a migratory arthritis, consider bacterial endocarditis and hepatitis. If the patient works in soil (gardeners, tree surgeons), consider sporotrichosis and fungal pathogens.
- The most important treatment is early recognition. Septic arthritis can be classified as late or too late. If treatment is delayed more than 72 hours, consider open drainage. Joint fluid should be removed daily in any event. Parenteral antibiotics are necessary in debilitated patients and those with compromised immune systems.

Acquired immunodeficiency syndrome (AIDS) presents most commonly with a secondarily infected joint; the organism varies with risk factors. Those who are drug abusers tend to get staphylococcal or *Pseudomonas* infections whereas prostitutes are more likely to have gonococcus, syphilis, or chlamydia organisms. Other organisms associated with AIDS include *Mycobacterium avium-intracellulare* and *Candida albicans*. Other AIDS patients may present with features of Reiter's syndrome (see next section).

Viral arthritis and Lyme arthritis rarely present as a monoarthritis and will be discussed later.

PAUCIARTICULAR ARTHRITIS

Arthritis presentation with less than or equal to four swollen joints usually signifies a diagnosis other than rheumatoid arthritis and is often called a rheumatoid-variant arthritis. When the spine is affected, the term spondyloarthropathy is often used, and the HLA-B27 gene is usually present. Other rheumatic diseases without spinal involvement and in the absence of HLA-B27, and with onset following infection, are known as reactive arthritis (Box 23.1). Treatment for the group is similar.

Diagnosis is based on extra-articular features combined with the joint findings. Extra-articular features may include involvement of the eye, heart, intestine, skin, and nails. Often the sites of tendon attachment become inflamed (enthesitis).

Spondyloarthropathies: Ankylosing Spondylitis

Onset varies with sex. Males most often start with low back stiffness and pain; the disease then slowly ascends; the neck is usually involved later. Lower extremity joints may be affected in adolescent males. Females more often present with lower limb symmetrical arthritis without spinal complaint. Chest expanse is restricted in most patients at first visit. Iritis is common.

Diagnosis should be based on the presence of more than or equal to three features: Back pain and stiffness not relieved by rest, sacroiliitis on X-ray or bone scan, limited chest expanse (<3 inches male, 2 inches female), history of iritis (anterior uveitis), positive HLA-B27, or symmetrical inflammatory arthritis of lower limb joints. In practice, it is not necessary to test both roentgenography and HLA-B27 positivity.

Exclusions include roentgenographic findings of diffuse idiopathic skeletal hyperostosis; inflammatory bowel disease (IBD); features of Reiter's syndrome; or psoriasis. Juvenile onset can occur, but rarely with simultaneous onset of rheumatoid arthritis; these patients then have spondylitis features and small upper limb joint involvement.

Differential diagnosis of sacroiliitis includes tuberculous spondylitis and other bacterial infections, amyloidosis, Whipple's disease, intestinal shunt-related arthritis, gout, hyperparathyroidism, Paget's disease, and neoplasia. Treatment is discussed here.

Reactive Arthritis

Inflammatory nonseptic arthritis in response to bacterial cell wall antigens has come to be known as reactive arthritis. Beginning with such well-established diseases as rheumatic fever and Reiter's syndrome, the group includes the arthritis associated with enteric pathogens and psoriatic arthritis, and the arthritis associated with IBDs.

Diagnosis is based on: Lower limb inflammatory arthritis, often involving articular and periarticular tissues; mucocutaneous lesions; urogenital lesions; and rarely, aortitis and other cardiac lesions.

Reiter's Syndrome

Classical features are conjunctivitis and painless stomatitis; nonseptic urethritis; lower limb arthritis (knee, ankle, and feet) of 21-month duration; nail changes; and a papular hyperkeratotic skin rash (keratoderma blennorrhagica). Circinate balanitis of the glans penis is common. Cervicitis is common in female patients. Unilateral sacroiliitis is also common.

The history must include sexual activity, risk factors for AIDS, and previous ocular, urogenital, or cutaneous involvement. Patients rarely volunteer the information.

If a joint effusion is present, synovial fluid analysis should be undertaken at the first visit to exclude infection. Joint fluid findings include moderate turbidity, ↓ mucin content, and WBC range 5,000–30,000/mm^3, often with inclusion cells. If very turbid, the joint fluid should be submitted for Gram stain, culture, and comparison of sugar content to simultaneous blood sugar result.

Sedimentation rate usually reflects the level of systemic disease. Leukocytosis may occur. HLA-1327 is not necessary for diagnosis and is often negative if the spine is not symptomatic.

Roentgenography of symptomatic joints may reveal sacroiliitis or a "fluffy" periostitis along the area of the plantar fascia attachment.

Pathogenesis: Prodromal sexually acquired or enteric infections are thought to be important in setting off the syndrome. Bacterial cell wall antigens can be found in some joint fluids. Presumably the host immune system is defective, allowing persistence of these antigens; these in turn lead to local immune-related tissue injury. Organisms that have been involved include *Chlamydia*, ureaplasmas, and *Neisseria gonorrhoeae*, *Shigella flexneri* and *Shigella sonnei*, *Campylobacter jejuni*, many salmonella and *Yersinia* strains; *Brucella*, *Blastocystis hominis*, *Clostridium difficile*, and *Borrelia burgdorferi*.

Differential diagnosis from rheumatoid arthritis usually is not difficult, but if onset includes symmetrical arthritis, the history is important. Urogenital or mucocutaneous lesions are required for the diagnosis of Reiter's syndrome. Erythema nodosum, arthritis, and sarcoidosis lack the stomatitis and urogenital feature. Sexually acquired infection, septicemias, and AIDS must be excluded.

The inflammatory process rarely may destroy ocular tissue, cause aortic insufficiency, and may rarely lead to articular bony erosions. The usual course of inflammation lasts several months to several years.

Treatment: For general management, see below. Patients with severe and prolonged disease may benefit from long-term antibiotic treatment as well as the measures described here.

Acute Rheumatic Fever

In recent years, young adults have been seen with rheumatic fever presenting as an acute migratory polyarthritis or sometimes a rheumatoid-like symmetrical polyarthritis. The more classical involvement of children ages 5–9 years is less common. Each joint swelling is painful, often red and warm, and classically completely resolves within 1 week.

A preceding sore throat may have been so inconsequential that it is not recalled. Because ↑ of streptococcal antibodies is common in carriers without disease, the diagnosis should be based on evidence of multisystem involvement and the presence of a very rapid Westergren erythrocyte sedimentation rate (ESR).

Jones criteria for diagnosis include two major criteria (carditis-valvulitis or heart block; polyarthritis; chorea; erythema marginatum; and subcutaneous nodules). A throat culture should be obtained for definitive evidence of a streptococcal infection, but a positive culture need not be present. Streptococcal antibodies should be elevated to several times to normal levels.

Treatment in young children: Aspirin is still preferred. Begin with 75 mg/kg in divided dose. Arthropan (brand) or Trilisate (brand) liquid, a liquid choline and choline-magnesium salicylate, respectively, is easy to give to small children. A salicylate level can be obtained 2 hours after a first morning dose. Try to keep the level within 20–25 mg%. The response to aspirin treatment is rapid and complete compared to that in other forms of juvenile arthritis.

If Reye's syndrome is a concern, or in teenagers and young adults, NSAIDs may be preferred. If serious carditis is present with features of pericarditis, tachycardia, heart block, or congestive heart failure (CHF), begin steroids at once, 1 mg/kg/day in divided dose.

Be certain to test all family members for occult streptococcal infection, and treat those infected. Patients should be followed closely for signs of carditis with weekly electrocardiogram (ECG) and auscultation.

Prevention: Penicillin or similar antistreptococcal agent should be administered in order to prevent recurrences. Most reliable prophylaxis is benzathine penicillin, 1.2 million U intramuscular (IM) monthly. Most experts recommend continued prophylaxis until age 40 years.

Enteropathic Arthritis

These include IBDs such as ulcerative colitis, Crohn's disease, granulomatous colitis, and collagenous colitis. Perhaps related are the arthritis associated with intestinal bypass procedures, and with diverticulitis.

Features include lower extremity joint synovitis, skin lesions of erythema nodosum, pyoderma gangrenosum, erythema multiforme, and a painful stomatitis. Iritis is common when sacroiliitis has developed.

The arthritis may precede bowel disease, but most commonly arthritis onset coincides with the bowel disease. Small hand joints are more commonly involved with regional enteritis.

Laboratory tests are nondiagnostic. Anemia, rapid sedimentation rate, and synovial fluid findings of nonspecific inflammation are usual findings. HLA-B27 is positive if sacroiliitis occurs. Endoscopy and small bowel biopsy may be necessary for diagnosis. Synovial biopsy is usually nonspecific, but granulomas characteristic of Crohn's disease can be found.

Treatment of Ankylosing Spondylitis and Reactive Arthritis

Large joint aspiration and corticosteroid injection should be performed on the first visit. NSAIDs are helpful. The pyrrole-acetic acid derivatives, particularly tolmetin, are preferable first. Indomethacin should be considered only when milder NSAIDs fail. Gastric cytoprotection with misoprostol is indicated in patients with a past history of ulcer or if using concomitant steroids.

Antibiotic therapy is controversial, but in patients with Reiter's syndrome, a 2-week course of a broad-spectrum tetracycline (doxycycline or minocycline 100 mg bid) has little downside risk. Patients with onset following sexually transmitted infection should be treated with an antibiotic (doxycycline 100 mg bid for 2 weeks, or azithromycin 250 mg/day for 5 days). Sex partners should also be treated.

Persistent disease or very severe onset is indication for use of sulfasalazine. The mechanism of action is unknown, but the sulfa moiety appears to be the active ingredient. It is contraindicated in patients known to be allergic to sulfa. Begin with 500 mg enteric coated tablets bid by mouth (PO) and followed with a full glass of water. Every few days ↑ dose until 1,000 mg tid PO is achieved. Headache may occur at higher doses; lower doses may be used. Rash, hepatitis, diarrhea, leukopenia, rarely pancytopenia, and hematuria demand termination of this treatment (Table 23.5).

Table 23.5: Disease-modifying antirheumatic drugs (DMARDs).

Drug brands	Dosage	Monitor requirements	Side effects
Methotrexate Rheumatrex	2–5 mg tablets; 5–20 mg single	CBC, SGPT q 2–4 weeks Chemistry panel q 3–6 months	Cytopenias, hepatic fibrosis, and CNS disturbances
Use with caution in patients with azotemia; avoid using with trimethoprim-sulfamethoxazole, phenylbutazone, retinoids, NSAIDs, probenecid, ethanol, cephalothin, and penicillin			
Gold salts Myochrysine reaction Solganol Ridaura	First dose 10 mg Second dose 25 mg then 50 mg/week to 1,200 mg, then every 2–4 weeks 3–9 mg	CBC, platelet count Urinalysis with each dose Chemical panel semiannually Monthly CBC/UA	Rash, stomatitis Nitritoid Nephritis marrow toxicity As earlier.
(Less effective than injectable salts; useful for patients unable to travel, or for those who develop allergic reactions to injectables)			
D-penicillamine Depen Cupramine	250 mg/day 1st month 500 mg bid 2nd months	CBC/UA weekly at first, then	Rash, headache, GI upset, and nephritis
Then may increase q 2–4 weeks, protein pneumonitis slowly to 3,000 mg/d dipstick weekly			
Sulfasalazine Azulfidine	500 mg/day 1st month 500 mg/day 2nd month then if need up to 3,000 mg/day	CBC/UA weekly at first than q 2–4 weeks Albustix weekly	Rash, headache, GI upset, nephritis Pneumonitis

Contd...

Contd...

Drug brands	Dosage	Monitor requirements	Side effects
Avoid in patients with positive ANA, past sulfa sensitivity, azotemia, and hepatitis			
Antimalarials			
Chloroquine	250 mg/day	Eye examination with slit lamp central fields, fundoscopy	Phototoxicity
Plaquenil	200 mg/bid		Ocular, neuro-, and cardiac toxicity
Immunosuppressors			
Azathioprine (Imuran)	1 mg/kg/day up to 200 mg/day	CBC q 2–4 weeks chemical panel q 6–12 months	Cytopenias, nausea, and hepatitis
Cyclophosphamide	1–2 mg/kg/day or 750–1,000 mg bolus	CBC, urinalysis chemical panel q 3–6 weeks	Cytopenias, hemorrhagic cystitis
Chlorambucil	2–8 mg/day	CBC q 1–4 weeks chemical panel q 6–12 months	Cytopenias, late-onset leukemias
>Cyclophosphamide and chlorambucil should be administered by those with experience. They are reserved for only life-threatening disease because of their association with late-onset malignancies.			

(ANA, antinuclear antibody; CBC, complete blood count; CNS, central nervous system; GI, gastrointestinal; NSAIDs, nonsteroidal anti-inflammatory drugs)

Benefit should be noticeable within 8 weeks. CBCs, including platelet count, and urinalysis should be done at 3-week intervals. Periodic chemistry analysis is recommended.

The course of psoriatic arthritis and IBD is often chronic and prolonged, with unpredictable remissions. Methotrexate is useful for severe or prolonged arthritis but should be left to those experts in its use. Gold salt therapy can be used in patients with persistent ankylosing spondylitis or psoriatic arthritis.

When spondylitis is present, physical therapy and home exercise instruction help breathing and prevent a stooped posture.

Metabolic and Crystal-induced Arthropathies

Gout and pseudogout can occur in multiple joints all at the same time. When this occurs and gout is the disease, look for underlying causes, including use of diuretics, severe calorie restriction, alcohol, renal disease, and occult neoplasm.

Pseudogout occurring in multiple joints may result from hemochromatosis or hyperparathyroidism. Rarely, chondrocalcinosis may occur in association with acromegaly, hypomagnesemia, hypophosphatasia, ochronosis, and oxalosis. When calcific tendinitis has also occurred, calcium apatite deposition disease is likely. Synovial fluid may show weakly birefringent clumps of amorphous material.

Paraneoplastic Syndromes

Cancer Arthropathy

A rheumatoid factor-negative (seronegative) asymmetric polyarthritis involving mostly the lower limb joints. Cancer presentation may occur within 3 months and can arise in any organ. If considered and searched for, the malignancy may be curable. Unfortunately, the arthritis does not always remit upon treatment of the malignancy.

Hypertrophic Pulmonary Osteoarthropathy

A triad of clubbing of the digits, periostitis of long bones, and synovitis usually of the knees. Cancer of the lung occurs in about 10% of patients.

Septic Arthritis

Two infectious arthritides that can cause a chronic pauciarticular or even a symmetrical polyarticular arthritis are Lyme disease and *Parvovirus* infections.

Lyme Disease

Just as syphilis can cause a multisystem chronic illness, this *Borrelia burgdorferi* spirochete-caused illness can lead to perplexing disease.

Diagnosis: Features necessary for diagnosis are erythema migrans and more than or equal to one of the following: Arthralgias, arthritis, myalgias, headache, palpitations, heart block, visual changes, paresthesias, cognitive problems, depression, Bell's palsy, radiculopathies, fevers, lymphadenopathy, and fatigue. Without erythema migrans, the diagnosis is tenuous. At present, serologic diagnosis is not reliable. Synovial biopsy may be unrewarding. Diagnosis will be enhanced when DNA probes or other techniques are available.

Treatment of Lyme disease before cardiac or neurologic involvement can be effected with doxycycline 100 mg bid for 2 weeks. For more severe cases or late treatment, a 2-week course of ceftriaxone 2 g/day intravenous (IV) may be necessary.

(A review article in JAMA is presented by Sanchez et al.)

Parvovirus B19 Infection

This agent has caused diverse disease ranging from erythema infectiosum to an acute symmetrical arthritis indistinguishable from rheumatoid arthritis. Serologic identification is useful only if performed within 8 weeks of onset. The arthritis is nonerosive, and patients sometimes have symptoms for up to 15 months.

Laboratory findings are nonspecific; joint fluid is less inflammatory than in Reiter's syndrome. NSAIDs are helpful.

Acquired Immunodeficiency Syndrome

Approximately 5% of patients with AIDS will develop a reactive arthritis with features of Reiter's syndrome or psoriatic arthritis. Certainly if risk factors are present, human immunodeficiency virus (HIV) testing should be done. Sulfasalazine, NSAIDs, and brief steroid use are tolerated. Methotrexate should be avoided.

Seronegative Rheumatoid Arthritis

Approximately 10% of patients with typical rheumatoid pannus and bone erosions have a seronegative pauciarticular arthritis. Sometimes, the synovitis is barely palpable. Upper-extremity joints are usually affected. Occasionally, the sheep cell agglutination test will be abnormal in the presence of a normal latex rheumatoid test. The absence of other nonrheumatoid arthritis disease features, and persistence more than 3 months, suggests rheumatoid arthritis.

Treatment: If NSAIDs are not helpful, sulfasalazine or hydroxychloroquine should be added. Most patients with this form of rheumatoid arthritis have long remissions, but attacks may last several years.

RHEUMATOID DISEASES

This is a diverse group of immunologically mediated diseases that lead to a deforming polyarthritis chiefly involving the hands and feet, often with multisystem involvement and damage. Monoarticular rheumatoid has been discussed.

Rheumatoid Arthritis

Rheumatoid arthritis is characterized by proximal, symmetric involvement of the joints of the hands and feet, with sparing of the distal interphalangeal joints, whereas in more than 50% of patients with psoriatic arthritis, the distal joints are affected (Ritchlin et al.).

Diagnosis is based on the presence of four of the following seven criteria:
1. Morning stiffness in joint areas of more than or equal to 1-hour duration.
2. Synovial swelling of more than or equal to three joint areas (excluding the spine) observed by a physician.
3. More than or equal to one of the joints must include the wrist, metacarpophalangeal (MCP), or PIP joints.
4. Simultaneous symmetrical joint swelling (the earlier features must have been present for ≥ 6 weeks).
5. Presence of rheumatoid nodules observed by a physician
6. Positive test for rheumatoid factor in high titer
7. Typical roentgenographic changes.

Features of psoriasis, spondylitis, giant cell arteritis, or other connective tissue disorders are relative exclusions for the diagnosis.

If joint destruction is to be prevented, diagnosis must be early and vigorously treated. Early diagnosis depends on the examiner's ability to palpate joint synovium (the technique was discussed in the first section). Boggy or doughy synovitis involving the MCP joints and the ulnar styloid bursa are very good evidence for rheumatoid arthritis.

Systemic features include episcleritis, carditis, pleuroparenchymal lung disease, neuropathy, leg ulcers, and digital infarcts (nail fold lesions) (Figs. 23.1 and 23.2). Persons with limited education tend to have more severe disease.

Ominous laboratory features include thrombocytosis, extreme ↑ of the Westergren sedimentation rate, marked ↑ of C1q or cryoglobulin, and depressed serum albumin.

Onset may occur at any age, usually insidiously, with variability from day to day. Acute onset often follows stress, trauma, or infection. Although spontaneous remission is frequent in the early years, for most patients

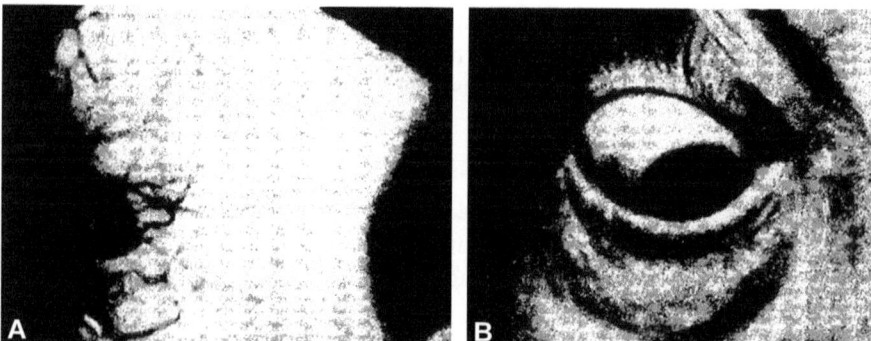

Figs. 23.1A and B: Episcleritis.
Source: McCarty DJ, Koopman WJ. Arthritis and Allied Conditions, 12th edition. Philadelphia: Lea & Febiger; 1992.

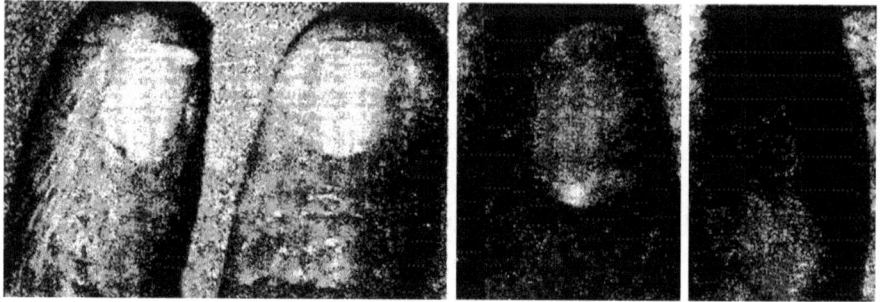

Fig. 23.2: Nail fold lesion, at edge of nail, often a finding in rheumatoid vasculitis.
Source: McCarty DJ, Koopman WJ. Arthritis and Allied Conditions, 12th edition. Philadelphia: Lea & Febiger; 1992.

the disease recurs, and in later life remissions are rare while relentless destructive polyarthritis is common.

Pathogenesis

Increasing evidence points to the short arm of chromosome 6; the α-helix of certain DR β chains within the class II region of the major histocompatibility complex has a strong relation to rheumatoid arthritis. These genes may respond to a superantigen, possibly a bacterial heat shock protein. Then, T cells invade the synovium and release cytokines, and the inflammatory pathways become activated.

Differential Diagnosis

Inflammatory polyarthritis can result from more than 100 diseases (Table 23.1). Although Raynaud's phenomenon can occur in rheumatoid arthritis, other features would suggest SLE or mixed connective tissue disease.

Rheumatic fever can be a difficult differential; look for extra-articular features and note the prompt response to therapeutic doses of salicylates. Polyarticular gout and pseudogout rarely affect the small hand joints; synovial fluid analysis from larger joints is essential. Lyme disease should be considered in areas that harbor the deer tick. In elderly patients with a seronegative symmetrical arthritis of the hands, giant cell arteritis should be considered, particularly with a significantly elevated sedimentation rate. A therapeutic trial of hydroxychloroquine may help avoid use of steroids if the temporal artery biopsy is negative. Reactive arthritis usually affects the lower limbs and has cutaneous features. Diseases that infiltrate joints include sarcoidosis, amyloid, hypothyroidism, and hemochromatosis.

Workup

Rheumatoid factor titer should be determined using an experienced laboratory. CBCs, platelet count, Westergren sedimentation rate, and baseline chemistries are necessary for assessing systemic disease severity as well as excluding other diagnoses. ANF is also helpful at baseline; some think that it is a poor prognostic finding. A baseline chest X-ray for identifying rheumatoid lung disease is important. Joint changes on roentgenography are rare before 6 months of disease duration. Most rheumatologists no longer obtain a baseline joint roentgenographic survey. Characteristic erosions are a late finding, perhaps too late. If nodules, or other features of systemic disease, are evident, a quantitative cryoglobulin, fibrinogen, and sedimentation rate can be used to monitor treatment.

If synovial effusion is present, the effusion should be aspirated fully and synovial analysis carried out (Boxes 23.3 and 23.4). If not purulent, a local steroid injection will be greatly helpful and can be instilled through the same needle following aspiration.

Treatmentt

Age, mode of presentation, serologic status, past medical history, and past drug history are all important for individualizing treatment.

Goals of treatment are to reduce pain and inflammation and prevent deformities. Absence of morning stiffness is an objective. This often requires maximum doses of salicylates or NSAIDs. If not, move on to methotrexate.

All patients with established rheumatoid arthritis benefit from detailed instructions in physical and occupational therapy if provided early in the course of disease. Only a few visits for home education are needed in most instances. Because of soft tissue inflammation and damage, these measures can greatly reduce pain and disability.

Mild disease: With morning stiffness of less than or equal to 1 hour, moderate joint swelling without effusions, no nodules, and no constitutional features, can be treated with nonacetyl salicylates or NSAIDs. But, if the disease does not improve within a few weeks, begin either hydroxychloroquine or sulfasalazine and continue the NSAID or salsalate.

Moderate disease: Patients with boggy synovium and recurrent effusion should be strongly considered for gold salt therapy, methotrexate, or both. Most rheumatologists do not like oral corticosteroids in any schedule. The osteoporosis and poor resistance to infection due to the arthritis are often compounded by steroids.

These problems are avoided by joint aspiration and steroid injections at 8–12-week intervals until remission occurs.

Long-acting drugs are often used sequentially: Gold salts or antimalarials are tried first, always in conjunction with salicylates or NSAIDs.

- Gold salt therapy by injection is preferred; save auranofin for patients who have remitted with gold salts but then develop side effects. If patient is a late failure on gold, try pumping the gold back to weekly doses for six doses; if successful, resume a q 3-week schedule (Table 23.5).

If gold and chloroquine fail, move on to sulfasalazine, then D-penicillamine, and lastly azathioprine.

Never use sulfasalazine and methotrexate together. Similarly, sulfa-based antibiotics should be avoided with methotrexate. Severe bone marrow depression can result.

Methotrexate should be considered early in older patients. It is safer than an NSAID in the very old.

Severe disease: Patients with episcleritis or vasculitis should be considered for D-penicillamine treatment. Because the drug may take several months to work, most rheumatologists would use oral prednisone beginning with 1 mg/kg in divided dose. If this fails, nitrogen mustard, bolus cyclophosphamide, or high-dose steroid or bolus steroid therapy can be considered, but should be undertaken only by an experienced physician.

Synovectomy is a consideration if joint effusion of a single joint is resistant to repeated aspiration/injection treatment. Arthroscopic synovectomy of a knee or shoulder can be helpful.

Arthroplasty of a major joint should be considered if intensive therapy both with adequate medication and physical therapy has failed. Indications for elbow or shoulder arthroplasty include inability to feed, dress, or perform toilet activity. Indications for lower extremity joints are inability to dress, walk from car through grocery store, inability to perform sexually if desired, or intractable night pain.

When patients have had severe GI or pulmonary side effects with salicylates and NSAIDs, then gold salt therapy and intra-articular steroid injections should be tried and oral medication avoided. Never inject the same joint more often than every 6 weeks.

- Patients with sinusitis, nasal polyps, or marked GI sensitivity can be tried on nonacetylated salicylates, including choline salicylate, salsalate, or magnesium salicylate. Gold salt therapy may be very helpful for such patients. Methotrexate can also aggravate pulmonary problems but can be cautiously tried.

If laryngeal involvement is a problem, particularly with hoarseness, ACTH can be helpful. Give 40 U three times a week for 2-3 weeks.

When C1-C2 subluxation occurs, with paresthesias to scalp and arms, prescribe a hard cervical collar and get prompt orthopedic consultation. Patients with severe hand deformities are likely to have moderate but silent C1-C2 subluxation. They are at risk during intubation for a general anesthetic. Such patients should have high cervical CT beforehand, and the anesthesiologist should be apprised.

Novel therapies unavailable at this time are provided in Table 23.6.

The ORAL Strategy trial by Fleischmann et al. studied patients with active rheumatoid arthritis; all responded inadequately to methotrexate, the dominant conventional disease-modifying antirheumatic drug (DMARD). The key comparison in the trial was the effects of a combination of different treatments with methotrexate. One treatment was tofacitinib. This drug is an orally active Janus kinase (JAK) inhibitor, a relatively new type of drug for rheumatoid arthritis. The other treatment was adalimumab, a biological therapy that is an established injectable tumor necrosis factor inhibitor for rheumatoid arthritis (Scott et al.).

Over 6-12 months, both combined treatments improved symptoms with disease activity decreasing by similar amounts. At 6 months, the American College of Rheumatology response criteria of at least 50% (ACR50) were achieved by 173 (46%) of 376 patients receiving tofacitinib with methotrexate and 169 (44%) of 386 patients receiving adalimumab with methotrexate, which met the criteria for noninferiority. The adverse events were similar between groups.

The ORAL Strategy trial and other studies show tofacitinib to be effective in patients with rheumatoid arthritis without major concerns about toxic effects. As a result of this and other trials, tofacitinib will be used by some patients with active rheumatoid arthritis. Another oral JAK inhibitor, baricitinib, is available for active rheumatoid arthritis, which has similar efficacy and side-effect levels. The merits of one of these JAK inhibitors over the other are uncertain but patients and clinicians benefit when there are choices between effective oral drugs. Although a combination of JAK inhibitors with methotrexate is likely to be the way they are used in clinical practice, monotherapy results in clinical and functional responses, as shown in the ORAL Strategy trial, and thus might be appropriate in some patients. The clinical use of these JAK inhibitors will show two things: (1) their risks and benefits in routine practice settings and (2) healthcare funders' views about what is affordable (Scott et al.).

Oral JAK inhibitors also increase serious infections, shown in the ORAL Strategy trial. Caution is, therefore, needed when JAK inhibitors are used

Table 23.6: Newer, novel drugs under investigation.

Agents	Mechanism	Side effects
Cyclosporine	Reduces IL-2 production	Nephrotoxic
Levamisole	–	–
Minocycline	Inhibits collagenase	Vertigo, rash, and phototoxicity; nausea
Amiprilose hydrochloride	Anti-inflammatory; reduces IL-2	Visual, nausea, and headache
Superoxide dismutase	Reduces free radical	–
Tenidap	Anti-IL-1; antioxidation	
Gamma interferon	–	Fever, headache, and GI upset
N-(fluorenyl-9-methoxy-carbonyl amino acids) (leumedins)	Stimulates leukotriene B4	–
2-cyanoaziridine	T- and B-cell inhibitor	Rash, liver enzymes increase
Anti-CD4 or CD5	T-cell modulation	Rash, fever
Monoclonal antibodies	Anti-CD4 and CD7	Anaphylaxis risk
Antithymocyte globulin	Deletion of T-cell clones	Fever, urticaria, and vasculitis

(GI, gastrointestinal; IL-1, interleukin-1)

routinely. Trials reported no specific concerns with tofacitinib. But only a few patients attain remission with any treatment strategy (Scott et al.).

Assessment of risks and benefits in routine clinical practice is difficult. When biologics were introduced, there were substantial uncertainties about their risks. Consequently, large prospective registers were established of patients with rheumatoid arthritis who were treated. Together with trials, these registers showed biologics increased serious infections. However, the balance of risks and benefits was deemed to be acceptable for patients with severe rheumatoid arthritis. Oral JAK inhibitors also increase serious infections, shown in the ORAL Strategy trial. Caution is, therefore, needed when JAK inhibitors are used routinely. Reassuringly, a systematic review of serious adverse events in 117 rheumatoid arthritis trials reported no specific concerns with tofacitinib.

Sjögren's Syndrome

Diagnosis is based on occurrence of keratoconjunctivitis sicca, xerostomia, and an autoimmune disease. Most patients can be screened with fluorescein or Rose Bengal staining. The Schirmer test is easily performed and can be used to follow the course of the disease. Sialogram, scintigraphy, and lip biopsy are only occasionally necessary. ANAs, rheumatoid factors, anti-Ro (SS-A), and Anti-La (SS-B) antibodies occur in the majority of patients; thyroglobulin antibodies, cryoglobulins, and anti-DNA may be found even in the absence of any evident connective tissue disease.

These patients are subject to focal neurologic and neuropsychiatric sequelae. Cerebral vasculitis may be seen on MRI.

These patients also may develop lymphoproliferative diseases with pseudolymphoma and malignant lymphomas. Diffuse interstitial pneumonitis, and renal diseases with glomerulosclerosis and renal tubular acidosis, can occur.

Treatment

This includes that of the underlying rheumatic disease. Shohl's citrate solution can help. Mix 1 ounce in 32 ounces of water. Ingest in divided dose daily. Prescribe 1 g ascorbic acid qd. Used for 30 days, patients claim to experience relief. Oral symptoms may be helped by sipping a glass of water containing a few drops of oil of peppermint. Sour candy also may help.

Felty's Syndrome

It consists of a triad of rheumatoid arthritis, leukopenia, and splenomegaly. Also, anemia, lymphadenopathy, and leg ulcers are common. The bone marrow is usually hyperplastic. Hypersplenism is common. Splenectomy is of variable benefit and should be considered if two serious infections have occurred. Most patients can be treated with gold salts or D-penicillamine. In this condition, the baseline WBC is used and the drug withheld if the WBC falls to 50% of the baseline, or the absolute neutrophil count drops to lower levels.

SYSTEMIC LUPUS ERYTHEMATOSUS

Features include:
- Skin and mucous membrane changes, including malar rash, discoid rash, photosensitivity, alopecia, and oral ulcers
- Arthritis (often of fingers, and intermittent)
- Serositis, including pleuritis, pericarditis, and mesenteritis
- Nephritis with persistent proteinuria or casts
- Hematologic disease, including thrombocytopenia, hemolytic anemia; often with leukopenia of less than 4,000 cells and a positive direct Coombs' test
- Evident immunologic disorder with positive LE preparation, positive test for syphilis, anti-DNA, or anti-Sm antigens
- Antinuclear antibody in significant titer.

More than or equal to four positive features are needed for diagnosis. Patients with less than four criteria can be designated as having "undifferentiated connective tissue disease".

Patients tend to have certain patterns of disease, and new flares usually follow the initial pattern.

- *Skin-joint disease*: Mild disease with any or all of the skin manifestations and significant symmetrical polyarthritis. No major organ involvement.
- *Hematologic disease*: This can occur as an isolated idiopathic thrombocytopenia or as an autoimmune hemolytic anemia.
- *Brain, heart, and kidney disease*: Convulsions, psychosis, depression, transverse myelitis, endocarditis with Libman–Sacks valvulitis, or nephrotic syndrome.

Drug lupus can present as any of the earlier, rarely with nephritis. Such patients may require steroids. The offending drugs include procainamide, hydralazine, anticonvulsants, isoniazid, levodopa, propylthiouracil, D-penicillamine, sulfasalazine, and lithium. Each year adds more to the list. Although antihistone antibodies are common in drug lupus, they are neither diagnostic nor specific. Although the clinical features ultimately clear when the offending drug has been removed, the ANA remains positive and in high titer for years.

Differential diagnosis depends on mode of presentation and duration. Consider other photosensitizing diseases, such as porphyria, bacterial endocarditis, syphilis, Lyme disease, AIDS, histoplasmosis, other systemic infections, paraneoplastic syndromes, sarcoidosis, and hematologic diseases.

Workup should initially include CBC with differential, ANA, chemistry panel, urinalysis, and chest X-ray. Then, in addition, depending on features, echocardiogram, further immunologic tests, including antidouble-stranded DNA, C3, C1q, and creatinine clearance and 24-hour urine protein.

Treatment and Follow-up

- *Skin-joint disease*: NSAIDs, nonacetylated salicylates, and hydroxychloroquine are often effective. Stubborn joint swelling can be treated with intra-articular injections of corticosteroids. Try to avoid steroids at this level of disease, but follow the patient closely for evidence of more systemic disease. Anti-DNA is not of value unless serositis or nephritis have appeared. If the patient is planning pregnancy, anticardiolipin lupus anticoagulant, SS-A and SS-B antibody tests should be obtained.
- *Hematologic disease*: Low-dose prednisone (0.5 mg/kg/day) with slow taper is necessary. These patients should be monitored as earlier.
- *Brain and transverse myelitis*: These patients should be treated with parenteral bolus corticosteroids as soon as symptoms suggest diagnosis. Do not wait for test results. As soon as the emergency spinal tap has been obtained, use more than or equal to 250 mg Solu-Medrol q 6 hours. MRI of the spinal cord can be helpful for assessing transverse

myelitis. Anticardiolipin antibodies and the lupus anticoagulant should be tested.
- Carditis usually responds to prednisone (beginning with 1 mg/kg/day in divided dose). Glomerulonephritis and nephrotic syndrome should have nephrology consultation, with renal biopsy to guide treatment. Evidence of proliferative glomerulonephritis is currently treated with bolus cyclophosphamide or nitrogen mustard and corticosteroids. This process is seen more commonly in non-Caucasians. Be more alert to nephritis in them.

ANTIPHOSPHOLIPID SYNDROME

Features include arterial and venous thrombosis, stroke, transverse myelitis, fetal loss, and thrombocytopenia. Assessment should include both anticardiolipin and lupus anticoagulant. Patients may or may not have any connective tissue disease, but features for SLE should be sought.

At the present time, patients with central nervous system (CNS) disease, or venous and arterial thrombosis, are treated with long-term anticoagulation; those also with SLE are treated additionally with steroids. Patients who have had miscarriages can often be carried to term using daily prednisone (0.5–1.0 mg/kg/day) and aspirin.

MIXED CONNECTIVE TISSUE DISEASE

Similar to SLE but with three distinguishing features:
1. Sausage-like swelling of fingers with evolution of features of rheumatoid arthritis, scleroderma, myositis, and lupus
2. Presence of anti-U1 ribonucleoprotein (RNP) in high titer RNP
3. Low incidence of cardiac or renal disease.

It may have ↑ed incidence of pulmonary fibrosis, pulmonary hypertension, Sjögren's syndrome, and Hashimoto's thyroiditis.

Treatment for most patients is corticosteroids in moderate to high doses. Those patients with a predominant arthritis manifestation can be treated with antimalarials and NSAIDs. Those patients with scleroderma features are least likely to improve. No prospective studies are available. No data is available on use of D-penicillamine for this group.

Systemic Sclerosis

A group of local or generalized connective tissue diseases with the major manifestation of fibrosis and degeneration of skin (scleroderma), synovium, and muscles; less commonly the internal organs.

Classification of Scleroderma

- *Diffuse cutaneous scleroderma:* With early appearance of pulmonary, cardiac, GI, and renal disease. Limited cutaneous scleroderma: With

skin limited to face and distal limbs; late onset of pulmonary arterial hypertension, biliary cirrhosis. Commonly known as CREST syndrome (with Calcinosis; Raynaud's phenomenon; Esophageal dysfunction; Sclerodactyly; and Telangiectasia).
- *Localized scleroderma*: Morphea: Single or multiple plaques of leathery skin with pigmentation.
- *Linear scleroderma*: Deep cutaneous fibrosis, with or without melorheostosis.

Features

Raynaud's phenomenon may precede disease by months or years. The diffuse type may begin with generalized edema; widespread dysesthesia may be very uncomfortable and last for many months.

Speckled ANAs are common but of no significance. Anti-topoisomerase I antibodies (Scl-70) tend to occur in the diffuse type of scleroderma, and pulmonary interstitial fibrosis is linked.

Anticentromere antibodies have remarkable specificity for limited cutaneous scleroderma. These patients can present with a malignant form of Raynaud's phenomenon with digital gangrene as the first manifestation of disease.

Differential Diagnosis

Environmental agents that can trigger scleroderma-like changes include silica dust, silicone, vinyl chloride, trichlorethylene, bleomycin, cisplatin, benzene, phenylenediamines, epoxy resins, carbidopa, hydroxytryptophan, toxic oil syndrome, and the graft-versus-host disease.

Treatment

No controlled data exist supporting a specific form of treatment. Dermatologists like penicillin for localized scleroderma. Anecdotal data suggest a positive outcome. For diffuse disease, most rheumatologists use D-penicillamine for more than or equal to 3 years (Table 23.5). Treatment of Raynaud's phenomenon includes local cold protection with gloves, face mask, and nifedipine (30–90 mg/day); reserpine 0.5 mg bid, dibenzyline 10 mg tid, or biofeedback training can be tried sequentially. Asymptomatic proteinuria may herald renal scleroderma and malignant hypertension. A nephrologist should be involved as soon as the condition is recognized.

Patients with systemic sclerosis should be followed with monitoring of BP and DLCO, and with attention to joint range of motion, nutrition, dentition, and renal function.

Polymyositis/Dermatomyositis

Features include:
- Symmetric weakness of neck and girdle muscles
- Elevated serum skeletal muscle enzymes [e.g. CPK, SGOT (AST)]
- Electromyographic changes consistent with an inflammatory myopathy
- Muscle biopsy findings of fiber necrosis, inflammation, phagocytosis and regeneration, and variation in fiber size.

Electron microscopy should be part of a routine workup. Diagnosis requires three of the earlier.

Skin changes for dermatomyositis include the characteristic heliotrope eyelid, Gottron's patches (red scaly patches over the MCP joints), and rose-red rash on face, trunk, or limbs. Dermatomyositis is more common in children and in patients who have an occult neoplasm.

Synovitis of hands, pulmonary interstitial infiltration, myocardiopathy, vasculitis of the intestinal tract, dysphagia, or dysphonia can occur.

Ominous features are dysphonia (aspiration pneumonia can occur), CPK ↑es more than 10,000, lack of response to prednisone within 1 month, and extensive rash (occult neoplasm).

Pathogenesis

HLA-DR3, HLA-DR52, and HLA-B8 are frequently related. Anti-Jo-1 antibodies and antisynthetase autoantibodies may be found also. Picornaviruses, coxsackievirus, and *Toxoplasma gondii* have been implicated.

Differential Diagnosis

The list of causes for dysfunction of muscle is extensive. Most are noninflammatory. Toxic myopathies from alcohol, cocaine, colchicine, clofibrate, and D-penicillamine may be difficult to differentiate and need to be excluded. Muscular dystrophies have a helpful family history. Polymyalgia and fibromyalgia do not cause weakness.

Treatment

Corticosteroid therapy is still the cornerstone of treatment. Depending upon severity at onset, prednisone dosage of 1-2 mg/kg is given with slow taper for 6 months. Divided doses at tid are necessary in the beginning. If vasculitis is present, IV delivery is necessary. Single morning maintenance dosages are determined by enzyme levels. Steroid myopathy is an insidious lower-extremity problem that requires trial-and-error care. Use of urine creatine ratios may be helpful in this situation.

Use bedrest along with passive range of motion until enzymes ↓. Then progress with graded exercises.

When more aggressive treatment is needed, methotrexate, azathioprine, or cyclophosphamide have had variable success. Cyclophosphamide 1–4 mg/kg should be seriously considered in childhood-resistant myositis. IV immune serum globulin has been reported helpful in a 15-year-old resistant to all other forms of treatment. Dosage reported was 1 g/kg/day for 2 consecutive days each month.

NECROTIZING VASCULITIS

A protean group of diseases that affect many organ systems, with ischemia resulting from inflammation and swelling of the vascular tree. Table 23.7 summarizes the histopathology and some demographic features.

Constitutional features of fever, weight loss, myalgia, and anemia are common at presentation. Limited forms are not uncommon, with less illness and greater difficulty in diagnosis. Progress has been made in identifying serologic markers specific for vasculitis.

Antineutrophil cytoplasmic antibodies can be found in systemic necrotizing vasculitis, particularly Wegener's granulomatosis. The specificity and sensitivity are not yet known.

Pathogenesis

Because of the sporadic occurrence of vasculitis, lack of familial involvement, lack of association with any specific infectious agent, and marked variability of case presentation, these diseases likely represent an immunopathogenic response to infection. Indeed, the finding of hepatitis virus in association with cryoglobulinemia and polyarteritis nodosum is suggestive of this mechanism.

Systemic vasculitis should be considered if three organ systems appear affected by a systemic inflammatory process. Electromyography for denervation may prove neurologic system involvement if needed. Most of these patients will have either articular swelling (giant cell arteritis, Wegener's granulomatosis), skin lesions, pulmonary lesions, or evidence of renal involvement as well.

Workup

Sedimentation rate, sinus and chest X-ray, and sinus biopsy if the sinus walls appear involved; abdominal visceral angiography if renal or neurologic systems appear involved; and skin and muscle biopsy if arteriogram is negative or inconclusive.

In patients with predominant CNS involvement, cerebral arteriography is often necessary; in many cases MRI is inconclusive.

Table 23.7: Features of vasculitis syndromes.

	Polyarteritis nodosa	Churg–Strauss syndrome	Wegener's granulomatosis	Hypersensitivity vasculitis	Henoch–Schönlein purpura	Giant cell (temporal) arteritis	Takayasu arteritis
Type of vessels involved	Medium and small muscular arteries, and sometimes arterioles	Small arteries and veins, often arterioles and venules	Usually small arteries and veins, sometimes larger vessels	Arterioles and venules, often small arteries and veins	Arterioles and venules, often small arteries and veins	Vessels of all sizes	Elastic arteries and selected muscular arteries
Distribution and localization	Visceral, cutaneous, and infrequently, cerebral vessels and lung	Upper and lower respiratory tract, viscera, heart, and skin	Upper and lower respiratory tract, often kidney, and infrequently skin, heart, viscera, and brain	Predominantly skin and less commonly viscera, heart, and synovium	Predominantly skin, gastrointestinal, kidney, and synovium	Predominantly temporal arteries, and less often any other large, medium, and small vessels	Aorta, arch vessels and other major branches (coronary, renal, visceral), and pulmonary arteries
Type of vasculitis and inflammatory cell infiltrate	Necrotizing, with mixed cells and few eosinophils rarely granulomatous	Necrotizing or granulomatous with mixed cells and prominent eosinophils	Necrotizing or granulomatous with fixed cells and occasional eosinophils	Leukocytoclastic or lymphocytic with variable number of eosinophils, occasionally granulomatous	Leukocytoclastic, mixed-cell, or lymphocytic, with variable number of eosinophils	Granulomatous, with variable number of giant cells, sometimes only lymphoplasmacytic	Granulomatous, with few giant cells in active phase, and sclerosing fibrosis in chronic stage with scanty infiltrate

Contd...

Contd...

	Polyarteritis nodosa	Churg–Strauss syndrome	Wegener's granulomatosis	Hypersensitivity vasculitis	Henoch–Schönlein purpura	Giant cell (temporal) arteritis	Takayasu arteritis
Special features	Focal segmental involvement of vessels, coexisting acute and healed vascular lesions, or normal and affected vessels: microaneurysms	Extravascular necrotizing granulomas with prominent eosinophils: may manifest as "limited form"	Geographic pattern of tissue necrosis and positive antineutrophil cytoplasmic antibodies: may manifest as "limited form"	May be associated with myocarditis, interstitial nephritis, or hepatitis	Immunoglobulin A (IgA) immune deposits in affected tissue	Affected extracranial large vessels indistinguishable from Takayasu arteritis: may form aneurysm or cause dissection	Aneurysmal in 20%; may be segmental, and cause rupture or dissection
Demographic and environmental predisposition	Vascular lesion of infantile polyarteritis is indistinguishable from fatal cases of Kawasaki disease	Most patients have asthma or history of allergy	Occurs in all ages with a slight male preponderance associated with HLA-DR2 may respond to antimicrobial agents	Patients may have history of drug or chemical allergy, vaccination, or occult malignancy	Predominantly children and young adults	Virtually all patients with temporal arteritis are over age 50 years; may be clinically asymptomatic	Most commonly in women of childbearing age; more prevalent in the Orient; an important cause of renovascular hypertension in adolescents

Source: Hunder GG, Arend WP, Bloch DA, et al. The American College of Rheumatology 1990 criteria for the classification of vasculitis. Introduction. Arthritis Rheum. 1990;33:1065-7.

Differential Diagnosis

Other conditions to consider include cardiac myxoma, multiple cholesterol embolization syndrome, subacute bacterial endocarditis and other systemic infections, leukemia and paraneoplastic syndromes, hypersensitivity reactions, carcinoid, and porphyria.

Treatment

Wegener's granulomatosis should be treated with cyclophosphamide and prednisone as soon as diagnosis is evident. Oliguric renal failure may occur within days of onset.

Polyarteritis nodosum may respond to corticosteroid given in daily (1–2 mg/kg) divided dose, but if not quickly responsive, cyclophosphamide is added, even when hepatitis virus is evident. Most rheumatologists would initiate treatment with combination therapy (prednisone and cyclophosphamide) because late sequelae are less likely and prolonged high-dose steroid therapy can be avoided. Late occurrence of malignancy, particularly of bladder cancer, is common. Hopefully other effective nonsteroidal treatment will be found.

Giant cell arteritis usually responds to corticosteroids, beginning with prednisone 60–80 mg/day as a single dose. After several weeks, this dose may be ↓ed by 10 mg every 2 weeks, then from 20 mg, the taper can be ↓ed 1 mg/week. Symptomatic stability is more important than sedimentation rate. If steroids are ineffective, or causing great distress, methotrexate can be substituted. Add the methotrexate (10–20 mg/week in a single dose each week) and slowly taper the steroid after the 4th week. Visual symptoms are present in some patients.

Nonsteroidal anti-inflammatory drugs have no role in these diseases, may cover up important symptoms and add to the renal injury, and should not be used.

See the previous section on use of corticosteroids and Table 23.5 for use of immunosuppressive medication.

GIANT CELL ARTERITIS

This is the most common systemic vasculitis among North Americans, causes granulomatous inflammation chiefly of the aortic arch and the extracranial portion of the carotid artery (Hellmann). The disease manifests after 50 years of age, most frequently with headache, polymyalgia rheumatica, jaw claudication, and visual loss. The laboratory hallmark of active disease is a markedly elevated ESR [or C-reactive protein (CRP) level]. The ESR is very high in many cases (use Westergren not Wintrobe) if the ESR is not more than 60, search for another diagnosis.

The most feared complication is blindness, which is usually irreversible. Early diagnosis and treatment with prednisone at a daily dose of 40-60 mg/day prevents blindness and dramatically ameliorates symptoms. The tapering of prednisone usually begins after the first 2-4 weeks of treatment. Although a minority of patients can taper off prednisone over a period of 3-6 months, the majority have repeated cycles of flares and remissions that result in a yo-yoing of prednisone therapy over a period of many months or years. Unfortunately, alternatives to glucocorticoids have not been reliably effective in randomized, controlled trials (Hellmann), the ESR and CRP levels fall with reduction of this inflammatory disease.

BIBLIOGRAPHY

1. Denton CP, Khanna D. Systemic sclerosis. Lancet. 2017;390:1685-99.
2. Fleischmann R, Mysler E, Hall S, et al. Efficacy and safety of tofacitinib monotherapy, tofacitinib with methotrexate, and adalimumab with methotrexate in patients with rheumatoid arthritis (ORAL Strategy): a phase 3b/4, double-blind, head-to-head, randomised controlled trial. Lancet. 2017;390:457-68.
3. Hellmann DB. Giant-cell arteritis—More ectasy, less agony. N Engl J Med. 2017;377:385-6.
4. Qaseem A, Harris RP, Forciea MA, et al. Management of Acute and Recurrent Gout: A Clinical Practice Guideline from the American College of Physicians. Ann Intern Med. 2017;166:58-68.
5. Ritchlin CT, Colbert RA, Gladman DD. Psoriatic arthritis. N Engl J Med. 2017;376:957-70.
6. Sanchez E, Vannier E, Wormser GP, et al. Diagnosis, Treatment, and Prevention of Lyme Disease, Human Granulocytic Anaplasmosis, and Babesiosis: A Review. JAMA. 2016;315:1767-77.
7. Scott DL, Stevenson MD. Treating active rheumatoid arthritis with Janus kinase inhibitors. Lancet. 2017;390:431-2.
8. Watts NB, Manson JE. Osteoporosis and Fracture Risk Evaluation and Management: Shared Decision Making in Clinical Practice. JAMA. 2017;317:253-4.
9. Wenger HC, Cifu AS. Treatment of Low Back Pain. JAMA. 2017;318:743-44.
10. White WB, Saag KG, Becker MA, et al. Cardiovascular Safety of Febuxostat or Allopurinol in Patients with Gout. N Engl J Med. 2018;378:1200-10.

CHAPTER 24

Sodium, Potassium, and Calcium Disturbances

HYPONATREMIA

Definition

A serum sodium (Na) less than 134 mEq (mmol)/L, after exclusion of pseudohyponatremia, usually due to severe hyperlipidemia and hyperproteinemia, or hyperglycemia, causing a shift of water from cells. Every 100 mg/dL (5.6 mmol/L) ↑ in glucose above normal causes a ↓ in serum Na of 1.5 mEq (mmol/L). *Note*: 1 mEq/L Na or K = 1 mmol/L Na or K. Hyponatremia is the most common electrolyte abnormality in patients admitted to hospitals. Hyperkalemia is life-threatening and is seen more commonly in the past decade because of the use of spironolactone, amiloride, eplerenone [potassium (K)-retaining diuretics] in patients with renal insufficiency. Hypokalemia is not uncommon in patients administered diuretics particularly, chlorthalidone, high-dose furosemide, and metolazone.

Causes

All causes are due to Na loss or water gain (Flowchart 24.1).

Sodium Loss

- *Renal loss*: Diuretics, renal salt-wasting diseases, and primary adrenal insufficiency [secondary adrenal insufficiency is not a cause since the renin–angiotensin–aldosterone system is intact and controls Na–K balance; adrenocorticotropic hormone (ACTH) has little effect].
- *Gastrointestinal (GI) loss*: Vomiting, diarrhea, and fistulas.
- *Third-space loss*: Ascites, burns.
- *Drugs*: Diuretics, antibiotics, proton-pump inhibitors, antidepressants, and antiepileptics.

These conditions are readily identifiable clinical problems that can be spotted without resort to serum and urine osmolality, urine electrolytes, or complicated algorithms that describe tonicity and volume of compartments.

Flowchart 24.1: Causes of true hyponatremia.

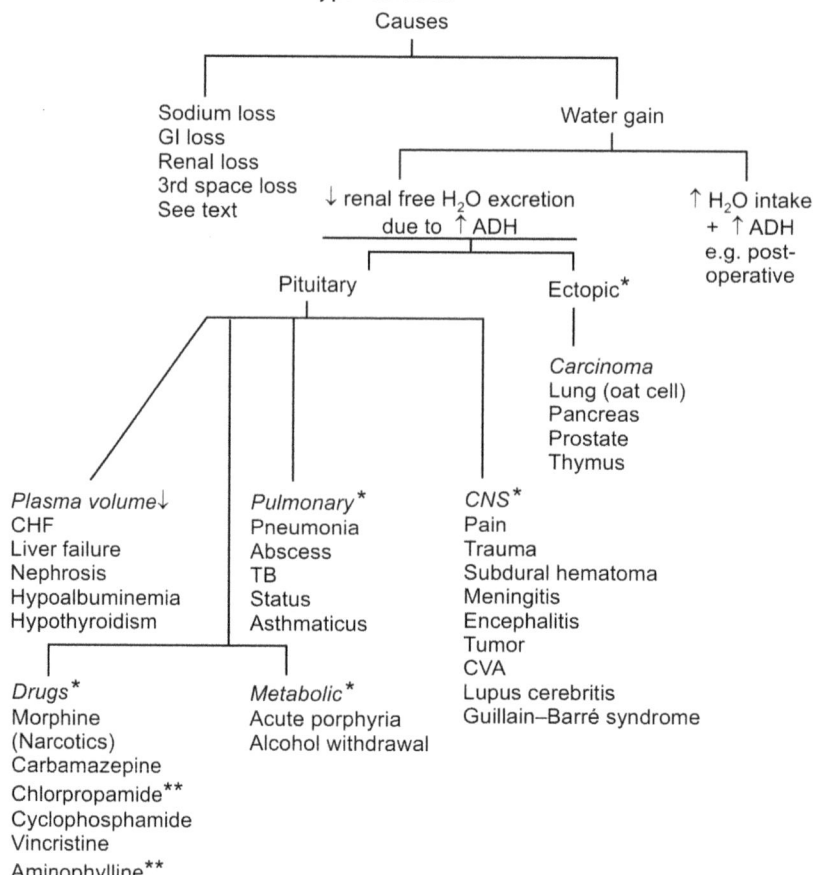

*So-called SIADH
**Potentiate ADH action
(ADH, antidiuretic hormone; CHF, congestive heart failure; CVA, cerebrovascular accident; CNS, central nervous system; GI, gastrointestinal; SIADH, syndrome of inappropriate ADH secretion; TB, tuberculosis)

Water Gain Due to Increased Antidiuretic Hormone Secretion

↑ secretion of antidiuretic hormone (ADH) causes a ↓ in renal free-water (H_2O) excretion, thus a ↓ in serum Na, ↓ serum osmolality, ↑ urine osmolality, and a urinary Na more than 25 mEq/L. In contrast, a low-effective circulating plasma volume as with congestive heart failure (CHF) produces urinary Na less than 105 mEq/L and chloride (Cl) less than 15 mEq/L in the absence of diuretic use. Serum osmolality = 2 (Na) + (glucose ± 18) + (BUN ÷ 2.8), where BUN is blood urea nitrogen; normal range: 275–295 mOsm/L.

Causes of water gain include:
- *Increased antidiuretic hormone from the pituitary or hypothalamus (Flowchart 24.1):*
    - Decreased circulating plasma volume as seen in CHF, liver failure, nephrotic syndrome, other hypoproteinemia, and severe hypothyroidism.

- Drugs (especially narcotics), tricyclics, phenothiazines, and vincristine.
- Pain, vomiting, and psychosis.
- *Central nervous system (CNS) lesions*: Trauma, subdural hematoma, meningitis, encephalitis, tumor, cerebrovascular accident (CVA), lupus cerebritis, and Guillain–Barré syndrome.
- Pulmonary infections, pneumonias, abscess, and tuberculosis (TB).
- *Metabolic*: Acute intermittent porphyria, alcohol withdrawal.

- *Ectopic antidiuretic hormone production*:
  - *From tumors*: Carcinomas, especially oat cell of lung, pancreas, prostate, and thymus.
- *Antidiuretic hormone potentiating drugs*:
  - Chlorpropamide (adenylate cyclase activation).
  - Aminophylline, caffeine (phosphodiesterase inhibition).

In some of the above-mentioned conditions (1–3), hypothalamic or posterior pituitary ADH is ↑, there is ectopic production regardless of serum osmolality, or there is enhancement of ADH action on renal tubules as with chlorpropamide. Thus, the listing of these conditions in most textbooks as the syndrome of inappropriate (SI) ADH secretion is questionable. The so-called syndrome confuses the facts and relegates clinical medicine to complicated algorithms that require determination of serum and urine osmolality and volume status.

A relevant history and physical examination usually reveal volume status and most causes listed in Flowchart 24.1 including the above-mentioned causes of ↑ ADH production or enhancement. Serum electrolytes, creatinine, if needed, and chest X-ray are assessed. At this point, if a cause is not readily identifiable, assessment of serum and urine osmolality and urine Na is advisable. If the hyponatremia is due to conditions causing ↑ ADH secretion (Flowchart 24.1), then serum osmolality is low, urine osmolality relatively higher, and urine Na more than 25 mEq/L; serum uric acid and urea are low and the hyponatremia responds to fluid restriction.

Clinical Manifestations

Acute hyponatremia, especially if associated with ↓ serum osmolality, may cause confusion, weakness, lethargy, nausea and vomiting, seizures, respiratory arrest, and coma. Chronic hyponatremia causes mild symptoms: headache, lethargy, muscle cramps, agitation, and confusion.

Treatment

Hyponatremia Due to Sodium Loss

Correct with intravenous (IV) infusion of isotonic (0.9%) saline. When urine output is adequate, potassium chloride (KCl) is added to the infusion to maintain a normal serum Na and K.

Table 24.1: Guidelines for correction of serum sodium less than 114 mEq (mmol)/L with hypertonic saline.

Presence of	Saline 1 L contains mEq/L	Infuse volume	Total mEq = mmol	Expected iodine serum Na and mEq/L/h
Central nervous system (CNS) symptoms or signs: no seizures	3% = 500	500 mL over 5 hours, then	250 50/h	7 ± 1 1.4 mEq/L/h
Seizures	5% = 850 250	300 mL over 3 hours then* slow infusion if needed**		7 ± 1 2.3 mEq/L/h

*Furosemide 20–40 mg; K replacement and fluid restriction.
**Do not increase serum Na to above 120 mEq (mmol)/L in first 24 hours. Measure serum Na 2 hourly for 6 hours, then as needed.

Severe Hyponatremia with Seizures

The hypotonic state with reduced serum osmolality causes H_2O to pass into cells, producing dangerous cerebral edema. This is a life-threatening situation and is usually seen with serum Na in the range of 95–115 mEq/L, especially where an acute ↓ in Na has occurred, e.g. a ↓ from 140 mEq/L to 120 mEq/L in 24–48 hours. Seizures may be unresponsive to diazepam or phenytoin. Table 24.1 gives guidelines for the administration of hypertonic saline. There is no advantage in calculating the deficit and trying to restore this in 12–24 hours since it is not advisable to ↑ the serum Na from the baseline beyond 10 mEq (mmol)/L in the first 24 hours, and certainly not advisable to ↑ the total serum Na to more than 120 mEq/L in the first 24 hours.

Acute Hyponatremia with Central Nervous System Symptoms and/or Signs in the Absence of Seizures

If the serum Na has fallen quickly over a period of days to less than 115 mEq/L, give 300–500 mL 3% saline over 5 hours, then 40 mg furosemide. 3% saline, 0.5–1.4 mEq/L/h infused over a few hours should suffice to raise the serum Na 10 mEq to maximum (max) 14 mEq from baseline over the first 24 hours. Thereafter, water restriction should suffice to ↑ serum Na about 5 mEq (mmol)/L daily.

Patients without Seizures and Central Nervous System Signs

They should be treated with fluid restriction 750 mL/day for 2 days, 1 L/day for 3 days, then 1.2 L/day until the serum Na reaches more than 130 mEq/L.

It is important not to correct the Na deficit too rapidly to normal levels because this may cause central pontine myelinolysis, albeit rarely. The possible role of the rate and extent of correction of hyponatremia in the development of pontine myelinolysis remain uncertain; malnutrition and alcoholism ↑ the risk of this complication. Concentrations as high as 29.2% saline have been used to ↑ serum Na 10–20 mmol from baseline in 24 hours in patients with seizures unresponsive to diazepam and phenytoin without adverse effects. This approach is not recommended, however, a formula can be used to estimate the Na deficit, volume of 3% sodium chloride (NaCl), and duration of infusion. However, such calculations often result in the use of too large an amount of Na infused. Use 120 mEq/L as a goal. Na deficit = 0.6 (or 0.5 for women; 50% lean weight = total body H_2O) × weight (kg) × (120 − measured Na). The suggested number of hours for correction by NaCl infusion = (120 − measured Na).

Give half the above-calculated deficit in the first 24 hours. See Table 24.1 for a more practical and prudent approach to the correction of severe acute hyponatremia.

Demeclocycline impedes the effect of ADH on the distal and convoluted tubules of the kidney, resulting in free H_2O excretion. Its effect may not be apparent for more than 1 week. Dosage: 300–600 mg bid in patients with chronic hyponatremia. Caution: The drug is metabolized in the liver and a ↓ in dosage is required in the presence of hepatic failure to avoid nephrotoxicity.

HYPOKALEMIA

Definition

Intracellular K concentration is approximately 30 times higher than extracellular. Fall of serum K 1 mEq represents approximately a 300-mEq deficit. The serum K level dictates an alteration of the K gradient across myocardial cell membranes that can result in severe electrical changes and cardiac arrhythmias. Serum K levels less than 3 mEq/L can produce premature atrial or ventricular beats, junctional tachycardias, ventricular tachycardia (VT), or fibrillation. A low-serum K reduces ventricular fibrillation (VF) threshold and ↑ the risk of sudden death.

Causes

The causes of serum K less than 3.5 mEq (mmol)/L include:
- *Renal loss*: Diuretics, renal diseases including renal tubular acidosis, and hyperaldosteronism.
- *Gastrointestinal loss*: Vomiting, nasogastric suction, diarrhea, laxative abuse, and villous adenoma.

- *Shift into cells*: (a) alkalosis: Every 0.1 ↑ in pH causes a ↓ of 0.5 mEq K/L; (b) insulin and glucose infusion, β-agonists, and hypokalemic periodic paralysis.

Treatment

- *Mild K depletion 3-3.5 mEq/L*: This is usually asymptomatic but requires correction in patients on digoxin or diuretics, or in the presence of ischemic heart disease (IHD), hepatic encephalopathy, or metabolic acidosis, where serum K less than 3.5 reflects severe K depletion. Give KCl orally.
- *Moderate K depletion 2.5-2.9 mEq/L*: Correction can be with oral therapy. IV is used if a line already exists or if symptoms, such as weakness, confusion, or arrhythmias and/or digitalis toxicity are present.
- *Severe depletion, K less than 2.5 mEq/L or metabolic acidosis with K less than 3.5*: IV KCl is necessary, given in 0.9% saline. In some cardiac patients, where Na load may be hazardous, the first liter given in 0.9% saline can alternate with 5% dextrose/H_2O (D5W). However, severe K depletion must not be corrected with K in dextrose solution because this ↑ the K shift into cells under the activity of insulin.
- Liquid and oral preparations containing adequate K, 20 mEq, and Cl, 20 mEq, are available.
- *Intravenous KCl*: IV for serum K 2.5-3 mEq/L: 40 mEq KCl added to 1 L 0.9% saline given q 8 hours = 125 mL q h = 5 mEq K/h (for cardiac with CHF, dilute in 1 L 5% D5W). IV KCl always should be given in saline. May need to add oral KCl to prevent fluid overload, e.g. K-Dur 20 or K-Contin 20 mEq tid. Max rate without cardiac monitor 10 mEq K/h. Above solution 250 mL/h (note the large volume required), Max K dosage: 20 mEq/h.
- *In life-threatening situations with serum K less than 2 mEq/L or less than 3 mEq/L with metabolic acidosis*: Put 60 mEq KCl/L in 0.9% saline, infuse through a large vein, run at 333 mL/h, but not in a central vein, because cardiac toxicity may result if a bolus more than 20 mEq/h is infused directly into the heart. Only extremely rarely is 30 mEq/h needed. K concentration per hour and volume of fluid per hour that can be tolerated are important considerations.

HYPERKALEMIA

Causes

If serum K more than 5 mEq (mmol)/L, quickly exclude pseudohyperkalemia (poor phlebotomy techniques, hemolyzed specimen, severe thrombocytosis, and leukocytosis), then approach systematically (Flowchart 24.2).

Flowchart 24.2: Hyperkalemia.

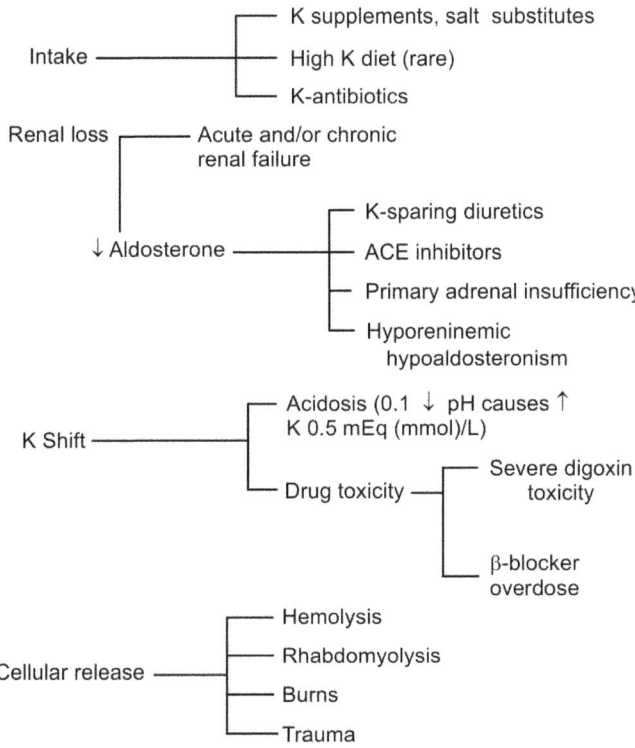

(ACE, angiotensin-converting enzyme; K, potassium)

Manifestations

Alteration in cardiac excitability is the most important sequelae, with typical electrocardiography (ECG) changes.
- Narrow-based peaked T (tented) waves occur mainly in V2–V4 when serum K is more than 6 mEq/L (Fig. 24.1), PR interval may be prolonged.
- *Potassium more than 7 mEq/L*: QRS widens. The S wave moves steeply into the T wave: There is no longer a normal isoelectric ST segment. P waves flattened or absent.
- *Potassium more than 8 mEq/L*: Absent P, wide QRS complex, and peaked T wave (sine wave).
- *Ventricular fibrillation or asystole*: VT may occur with K more than 6 mEq/L without the earlier ECG changes.

Treatment

Serum K more than 6 mEq/L and/or ECG manifestations dictate rapid correction of hyperkalemia.

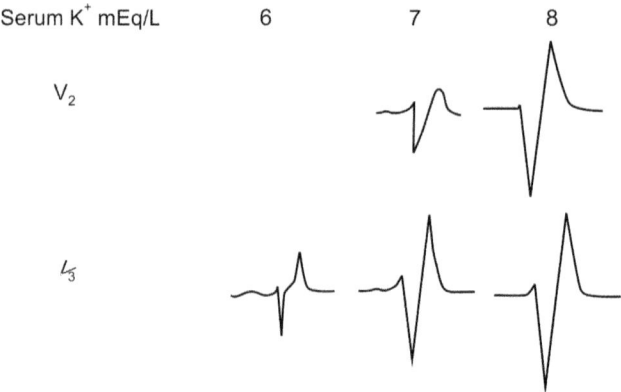

Fig. 24.1: Electrocardiographic signs of hyperkalemia.
For K⁺:
- 5.7 mEq (mmol)/L: Earliest signs; T wave peaked, narrow base ("tented"); PR interval may be prolonged.
- 7 mEq/L: P wave flat or absent; QRS widens, prominent S wave.
- 8 mEq/L: S wave becomes wider and deeper, and moves steeply into the T wave; there is virtually no isoelectric ST segment; occasionally ST segment elevation.

Restrict Intake of Potassium

Curtail dietary K, salt substitutes, K supplements, and/or K-retaining medications [K-sparing diuretics and angiotensin-converting enzyme (ACE) inhibitors].

Promote Shift into Cells

Sodium bicarbonate: IV, two ampules 88 mEq (mmol) over 15 minutes produces immediate K shift into cells. Effect lasts 1–2 hours. Repeat in 2 hours if no effect and ECG signs persist. Caution: Can precipitate CHF, tetany, or intracellular acidosis.

Insulin (regular): 10 U in 50 mL 50% dextrose, IV bolus, or 10 U in 500 mL 20% D/W over 1 hour; effect is immediate, lasts about 2 hours, and should ↓ serum K 1 mEq/L after 2 hours.

Albuterol (salbutamol) IV or fenoterol (β_2 agonists) aerosol: They have an immediate effect but short duration. This approach should be considered where sodium bicarbonate ($NaHCO_3$) is contraindicated or has had little effect.

Stabilize Cardiac Cell Membrane

For serum potassium more than 6.5 or ECG signs of hyperkalemia: Calcium chloride (CaCl) or calcium gluconate 10–20 mL, 10% IV bolus over 3 minutes; action within minutes and lasts about 30–60 minutes. If no salutary response in 5 minutes, repeat the dose.

Promote Renal Loss of Potassium

- *Furosemide*: 80-160 mg IV plus isotonic saline, depending on cause of ↑ K.
- *Fludrocortisone*: 0.5-2 mg by mouth (PO) if hypoaldosteronism is suspected.

Promote Gastrointestinal Loss

Sodium or calcium polystyrene sulfonate bind K and release Na or Ca in the colon. Enemas have a quicker onset of colonic action (within 1 hour).

Sodium polystyrene sulfonate (Kayexalate, Resonium A): 50 g powder in 200 mL of 20% sorbitol solution retained for about 1 hour and given q 4-6 hours. Orally, 15-30 g powder in H_2O, then sorbitol 50 mL 20% solution to facilitate quick transit to the colon and elimination; repeat q 4-6 hours.

Calcium polystyrene sulfonate (Resonium Calcium): Exchanges calcium (Ca) for K and is preferable in patients with CHF and severe renal failure where Na load may be hazardous. *Caution*: Conditions prone to hypercalcemia. Dosage is the same for both resins.

Dialysis: Failure to maintain K less than 7 mEq/L with the earlier measures, rapidly increasing K, increasing ECG signs (especially if due to renal failure or rhabdomyolysis) often require hemodialysis; peritoneal dialysis is less efficient.

HYPERCALCEMIA

Normally, serum Ca is controlled primarily by the action of parathyroid hormone (PTH), vitamin D, and to a lesser extent calcitonin, on bone, kidneys, and intestine. Normal serum Ca range: 8.8-10.4 mg/dL (2.2-2.6 mmol/L).

Causes

Bone Pathology

Increased bone resorption: Increased osteoclastic activity; ↑ prostaglandin E2 (PGE2) or PTH-like chemicals and mechanical erosion.
- *Carcinomas*: Breast, lung, kidney, ovary, prostate, and pancreas
- *Hematologic*: Myeloma, lymphomas
- Hyperparathyroidism
- Paget's disease.

Kidney

Increased reabsorption of Ca in the proximal tubule and ↓ Ca excretory capacity.
- Hyperparathyroidism
- Thiazide diuretics
- Familial hypocalciuric hypercalcemia.

Intestine

Increased absorption.
- Excessive intake of Ca, vitamin D
- Milk alkali syndrome
- Vitamin D effect, as with sarcoidosis.

Bone and Intestine

- Hyperparathyroidism
- Vitamin D intoxication
- *Sarcoidosis*: Increased level and sensitivity to vitamin D.

Others

- Vitamin A intoxication
- Prolonged immobilization
- Thyrotoxicosis
- Addison's disease
- Lithium therapy.

Symptoms and Signs

- *Gastrointestinal*: Anorexia, vomiting, constipation, ileus, peptic ulcer or pancreatic abdominal pain, stones, bones, and groans of hyperparathyroidism.
- *Renal*: Hypercalcemia interferes with renal mechanisms for the reabsorption of Na and H_2O: polyuria caused by osmotic diuresis and impaired concentrating ability results in volume depletion, hemodynamic deterioration, and renal insufficiency, which further ↑ serum Ca. Pain due to nephrolithiasis may occur.
- *Central nervous system*: Change in mental status: confusion, lethargy, agitation, hyporeflexia, psychosis, and coma.
- *Cardiovascular system (CVS)*: Shortened QT interval, arrhythmias.

Acute Management

Medical therapy is indicated in patients with serum Ca levels more than 12 mg/dL (3 mmol/L) and/or if symptoms are present and when the patient's underlying disease warrants treatment. Serum Ca levels are adjusted if serum albumin is low: A ↓ of 1 g/dL of albumin causes a 0.8 mg/dL ↓ in

Flowchart 24.3: Acute management of hypercalcemia.

```
Hypercalcemia
    ↓
  Causes
Ca⁺⁺ra → Diuresis            ← Corrects ←  Give isotonic saline
    ↓                                        200–500 mL/h
Dehydration ↓ GFR                                 ↓
    │                                      Causes
    │                          Decrease proximal Na⁺, Ca⁺⁺ resorption
    │                                          ↑
    │                                    Furosemide
    │                                    20–40 mg q 6–12 h
    │
    ↓
Hyperparathyroidism
    present?
    ↓
  No    Yes ─── Calcitonin
              │
  Diagnosis?  Surgery

Renal failure
phosphate↑*

Myeloma        Other              Calcitonin
Sarcoid        treatable          then either
Vitamin D ↑    malignancy    →    mithramycin or
Breast cancer  or Paget's         biphosphonates
    ↓
Calcitonin + Corticosteroids**

           Ca⁺  ≥16 mg/dL
                4 mmol/L
Calcitonin       ↓
           Consider
           dialysis
```

*Very rare   ▲ = Increase
**See test   ▼ = decrease

(Ca, calcium; GFR, glomerular filtration rate; Na, sodium)

serum Ca (a ↓ of 10 g/L of albumin causes a 0.2 mmol/L ↓ in serum Ca). In patients with Ca levels more than 14 mg/dL (3.5 mmol/L), urgent treatment is required. Suggested steps in how to manage this clinical situation are given in Flowchart 24.3. Detailed drug therapy is given in Table 24.2.

Table 24.2: Drugs used in the management of hypercalcemia.

Drug	Mechanism	Onset of action	Indications-advice	C/I	Dosage
Phosphate	• Ca^{++} ↑ deposition to bone and soft tissue • ↓ GI absorption • ↓ Bone breakdown.	2–3 days (chronic management)	• Chronic hypercalcemia • Keep serum phosphate in normal range.	Serum phosphate elevated, renal failure	Oral 250–500 mg q 6 hours. IV not recommended
Glucocorticoids	• ↑ Ca^{++} excretion • ↓ GI absorption • ↓ Osteolytic activity.	36–72 hours	Sarcoidosis, breast carcinoma, myeloma, and vitamin D intoxication	—	Prednisone 30–40 mg twice daily
Calcitonin (salmon; salcatonin)	• ↑ Renal excretion of Ca^{++} • ↓ Release of Ca^{++} from bone • ↑ Phosphate excretion in urine.	Immediate but mild ↓ Ca^{++}	Hypercalcemia unresponsive to saline and furosemide hyperparathyroidism vitamin D malignancy: with ↑ phosphate levels	Allergy positive skin test	4.8 U/kg q 6 hours or 12 hours SC or IM for 1–2 days
Plicamycin (mithramycin)	Osteoclast toxin, ↓ bone resorption	12–24 hours	Symptomatic serum Ca^{++} >3.5 mmol/L (15 mg/dL)	Hepatic and renal failure, ↓ platelets	10–25 mg/kg IV infusion over 6 hours. Repeat in 3 days only if absolutely necessary
Bisphosphonates	↓ Bone resorption by osteoclasts	2–5 days	Malignancy, Paget's disease	Severe renal failure	See text

(Ca, calcium; GI, gastrointestinal; IM, intramuscular; IV, intravenous; SC, subcutaneous)

Acute management always requires rapid volume expansion. Give 500 mL 0.9% NaCl rapidly, then 2-4 L q 24 hours.

Furosemide IV 20 mg q 6-12 hours is commenced only after volume repletion with 2-4 L isotonic saline IV. The effect of furosemide depends on the delivery of Ca to the ascending limb. Higher doses (80-100 mg) of furosemide are not usually necessary and may cause volume depletion with hemodynamic deterioration. A dose of 10-20 mg IV q 6 hours is preferable in the elderly or in patients at risk for CHF. The urinary output is measured hourly and should be replaced with IV saline, rate adjusted to match urine output.

Calcitonin is the most rapid-acting osteoclast inhibitor and is indicated for the rapid lowering of life-threatening serum Ca levels more than 16 mg/dL (4 mmol/L). However, the drug has a mild effect and should not be used as sole drug therapy.

Dosage: 2-8 IU/kg IV over 24 hours or 4-8 IU/kg subcutaneous (SC) q 6 hours. *Caution*: Do allergy test in patients with history of allergy: 1 IU intradermal prior to therapy; use plastic IV bag, not glass.

Corticosteroids enhance the activity of calcitonin and should be added, especially in patients with sarcoidosis, vitamin D intoxication, myeloma, or breast carcinoma. Alternatively, plicamycin should follow the administration of calcitonin if no contraindications exist.

Plicamycin (mithramycin) may cause significant nephrotoxicity, hepatotoxicity, and thrombocytopenia. Usually given as one dose, Max two doses. Reduce dose 50% with renal failure.

Chronic Management

- Low Ca/high Na diet.
- *High-fluid intake*: 2-4 L/day.
- Prednisone 30-40 mg bid for 3 days, then decreasing doses.
- Oral phosphate, where the serum phosphate is normal and in the absence of renal failure.
- The combination of phosphate and corticosteroids.
- *Indomethacin*: 75-150 mg once a day (qd) for PGE2-associated hypercalcemia.
- Bisphosphonates inhibit bone resorption and have a role along with saline infusion in stable patients with only moderate symptoms. These agents are more potent and have a longer duration of action than calcitonin and are far less toxic than plicamycin. Disodium etidronate or pamidronate is available.

Disodium etidronate (didronel) dosage: For Paget's or malignancy: 5 mg/kg PO once daily for less than equal to 6 months, or 10 mg/kg for 3 months. For severe hypercalcemia of malignancy: 7.5 mg/kg in 250 mL 0.9% saline IV over 4 hours qd for 3-7 days. On day of last IV dose, commence oral dose 20 mg/kg once daily for 1 month.

Pamidronate: 60–90 mg in 1 L saline or 5% D/W IV over 24 hours. *Caution:* Avoid food, especially Ca products, for 2 hours before and after bisphosphonates. Discontinue treatment if fractures occur. Reduce dose in renal impairment. CI with severe renal failure.

Gallium nitrate: Inhibits bone resorption by absorbing and reducing solubility of hydroxyapatite crystals. Lowering of serum Ca occurs in 3–5 days, i.e. a slower action than calcitonin, but causes a higher response rate. Adverse effects include nephrotoxicity. Avoid in patients with renal insufficiency. *Dosage*: 200 mg/m^2 in 1 L 0.9% saline IV over 24 hours qd for 5 days. Maintain adequate hydration with more than equal to 2 L saline IV daily.

BIBLIOGRAPHY

1. Ahmad S, Kuraganti G, Steenkamp D. Hypercalcemic crisis: a clinical review. Am J Med. 2015;128(3):239-45.
2. Bilezikian JP. Management of acute hypercalcemia. N Engl J Med. 1992;326(18):1196-203.
3. Dellay B, Groth M. Emergency management of malignancy-associated hypercalcemia. Adv Emerg Nurs J. 2016;38(1):15-25.
4. Khan GM, Bartlett JG, Chopra S, et al. Medical Diagnosis and Therapy. Philadelphia: Lea and Febiger; 1994.
5. Liamis G, Milionis H, Elisaf M. A review of drug-induced hyponatremia. Am J Kidney Dis. 2008;52(1):144-53.
6. O' Donnell JM, Nácul FE. Disorders of electrolytes. In: Nácul FE, Vieira JM (Eds). Surgical Intensive Care Medicine. New York: Springer; 2016. pp. 539-51.
7. Palmer BF, Clegg DJ. Electrolyte disturbances in patients with chronic alcohol-use disorder. N Engl J Med. 2017;377(14):1368-77.

CHAPTER 25
Type 2 Diabetes Mellitus

INTRODUCTION

Diabetes affects more than 415 million people worldwide; more than 1 million diabetics die in India annually and 1.5 in China.

A MAJOR ERROR MADE BY THE MEDICAL PROFESSION OVER 70 YEARS

- Death is mainly caused by myocardial infarction (MI) and stroke as a result of atheromatous arterial disease and thrombotic occlusions. It is important for the medical professionals to recognize errors made over the past 70 years by concentrating on strict reduction of elevated blood glucose. Hyperglycemia does not cause atheroma or thrombosis. Glucose is an innocuous lifesaving substance and does not damage cells. It is true that there are metabolic derangements caused by hyperglycemia including increase of low-density lipoprotein cholesterol (LDL-C).
- But diabetic people from India and China do not consume much meat and LDL-C is elevated in few. The majority of deaths occur in individuals with normal or borderline LDL-C. The author searched for a culprit other than glucose and discovered that sitosterol derived from vegetables-plant foods and shellfish is the most likely cause of atheromatous arterial disease causing MI and stroke in diabetics. (*see* Chapter 4: Sitosterolemia).

NEW A1c RECOMMENDATIONS

In March 2018, the American College of Physicians (ACP) called for less-intensive blood glucose control in type 2 diabetes:
- The ACP (2018) recommends that most patients with type 2 diabetes aim for a hemoglobin A1c (HbA1c) level between 7% and 8%.
- This represents a loosening of the group's 2007 recommendation, which said less than 7% was "a reasonable goal" for many patients.
- In a guideline update published in the Annals of Internal Medicine, the ACP cites evidence that treating to targets of 7% or lower rather than 8% does not reduce the risk for death or macrovascular events over 5–10 years—but does result in "substantial harms", such as hypoglycemia.

Recommendations are also adjusted further depending on age and life expectancy:
- 7–8.5% for those with established microvascular or macrovascular disease, comorbid conditions, or a life expectancy of 5–10 years.
- 8–9% for those with a life expectancy less than 5 years, significant comorbid conditions, advanced complications of diabetes, or difficulties in self-management attributable to mental status, disability, or other factors.
- All guidelines recognize that HbA1c targets can be higher in patients with comorbid conditions and limited life expectancy.
- *A fasting glucose 5–6 is too low and will stimulate glucagon production.* For more than the past 30 years, many specialists have recommended fasting levels of 5.5–6.5 mmol/L; *this is an error.* Tight control to this level provides no reduction in diabetic complications and is of no clinical value, increases glucagon and metabolites that can be culprits; in addition, hypoglycemia causes distress, deaths and emergency room (ER) visits.
- "Most important total mortality and hypoglycemic events are increased." Complications of diabetes that affect the lower extremities are common, complex, and costly. Foot ulceration is the most frequently recognized complication annually, foot ulcers develop in 9.1–26.1 million people with diabetes worldwide (Armstrong et al.). Infection of ulcers and recurrence present management problems and amputation may be required. But this is all caused mainly by atheromatous arterial obstruction; sitosterol blood elevation causes atheroma and must be lowered.
- *Peripheral vascular disease (PVD) is a root cause and sitosterol blood elevation may be implicated as a cause of atheromatous disease.*

DIAGNOSIS

- The recommended screening test for diabetes is a fasting plasma glucose (FBG) level. A FBG 126–130 mg/dL (7.0 mmol/L) indicates a need for further testing; a level greater than 7.5 mmol/L is most likely diabetes but glucose intolerance and some medications (diuretics, beta-blockers) can increase levels by 1 mmol/L. If A1c is available, it can be used but is not essential as proclaimed by American, British and European experts. The ACP cites evidence that treating to targets of 7% or lower rather than 8% does not reduce the risk for death or macrovascular events over 5–10 years—but does result in "substantial harms," such as hypoglycemia.
- Presence of classic symptoms—polyuria, polydipsia, ketonuria, and rapid weight loss—together with a random venous plasma glucose level greater than or equal to 200 mg/dL (11.1 mmol/L).
- Fasting venous plasma glucose greater than 126 mg/dL (7 mmol/L) [except in patients on medications that increase FBG (beta-blocker,

Table 25.1: Screening test for diabetes.

Test results		OGTT test ranges	
Normal	≤115 (6.4)	<200 (11.1)	<140 (7.8)
Impaired glucose tolerance	<140 (7.8)	>200 (11.1)	140–200 (7.8–11.1)
Diabetes mellitus	≥140 (7.8)	OGTT not needed	
Diabetes mellitus	<140 (7.8)	≥200 (11.1)	≥200 (11.1)

(OGTT, oral glucose tolerance test)
The test should be done
- After 3 days of a diet supplying more than 150 g of carbohydrates per day.
- In the morning after a 10–14 hours fast.
- With the patient lying down or sitting in a quiet room, without smoking.

Table 25.2: Characteristic features of the two main types of diabetes mellitus.

	Type 1 insulin-dependent diabetes mellitus (IDDM)	Type 2 noninsulin-dependent diabetes mellitus (NIDDM)
Prevalence	10%	90%
Age of onset	Typically onset <30 years but any age possible	Onset usually >40 years
Body weight	Usually thin	>80% obese
Presentation	Acute onset, with polyuria, polydipsia, weight loss, lethargy, pruritus vulvae, balanitis	Insidious onset, micro- and macrovascular complications may be present at diagnosis
Etiology	Inadequate insulin secretion due to autoimmune destruction of the pancreatic beta-cells	Impaired insulin secretion, increased hepatic glucose production and peripheral insulin resistance
Ketosis	Prone	Not prone
Genetics	HLA-DR3 and DR4 common; 50% concordance in identical twins	HLA unrelated: 100% concordance in identical twins

diuretic, or statin)] because these agents may increase FBG 1–2 mmol/L due to glucose intolerance.
- Fasting plasma glucose less than 140 mg/dL (7.8 mmol/L) and a 2-hour plasma glucose greater than 200 mg/dL (11.1 mmol/L) with 1 intervening value greater than 200 mg/dL (11.1 mmol/L) following a 75-g glucose load on more than 1 occasion. It is not convenient and expensive for most people; thus, the author does not recommend glucose tolerance tests (Table 25.1).

TYPES

The differences between type 1 and type 2 diabetes mellitus have been shown in Table 25.2.

IMPAIRED GLUCOSE TOLERANCE

Individuals with impaired glucose tolerance (IGT) have plasma glucose levels that are slightly higher than those considered diagnostic for diabetes mellitus. Of all patients with IGT, 1-5% develop overt diabetes mellitus in a year (because they are prediabetic).

HYPERSITOSTEROLEMIA

Increased blood level of sitosterol is present in ~50% of diabetics and is a major cause of atheromatous blockage of arteries leading to fatal and nonfatal MI, stroke and PVD.

- Sitosterol is harmful for diabetics (*see* Chapter 4: Sitosterolemia).

ACUTE COMPLICATIONS OF DIABETES

Diabetic Ketoacidosis

Definition

- Hyperglycemia: Glucose usually greater than 250 mg/dL (14 mmol/L).
- Hyperketonemia: Ketones present in the blood and urine.
- Acidosis: pH less than 7.2 or bicarbonate less than 15 mEq (mmol)/L.

Causes

Diabetic ketoacidosis (DKA) is always caused by insulin deficiency, either absolute (e.g. a previously undiagnosed patient or one who omitted insulin) or relative (e.g. too little insulin injected or antagonism by stress hormones) (Flowchart 25.1).

Signs and Symptoms

Diabetic ketoacidosis is characterized by nausea, vomiting, dehydration, fruity breath, Kussmaul respirations (rapid and deep) respirations, abdominal pain, and central nervous system (CNS) depression, with drowsiness progressing to coma.

Typical Laboratory Abnormalities

- Plasma glucose greater than 300 mg/dL (17 mmol/L)
- Urinary and plasma ketones
- Bicarbonate less than 15 mEq (mmol)/L
- Arterial pH less than 7.2
- ↑ed anion gap—usually greater than 16 mEq (mmol)/L

Flowchart 25.1: Pathogenesis of diabetic ketoacidosis.

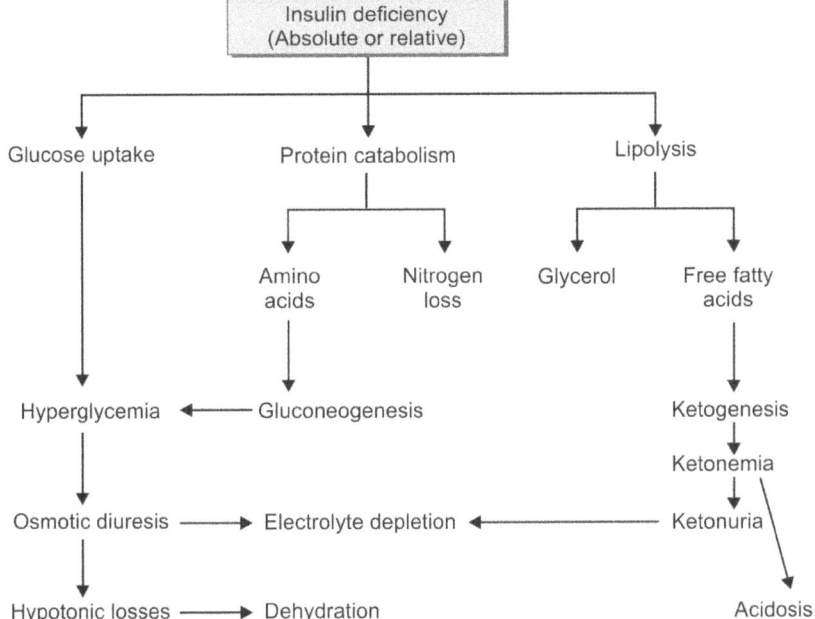

- Low plasma sodium (Na): Hyperglycemia lowers Na level by 1.6 mEq (mmol)/L for every 100 mg/dL (5.5 mmol/L) ↑ in blood glucose greater than 100 mg/dL (5.5 mmol/L).
- ↑ed urea and creatinine.
- Elevated white blood cell (WBC): May occur in the absence of infection.

Other Laboratory Abnormalities

- Elevated amylase: May be ↑ in greater than 50% of patients without evidence of pancreatitis. Salivary isoenzyme is usually responsible for the ↑.
- Mild to moderate ↑ in creatine phosphokinase (CPK): May occur in 25-40% of patients without electrocardiogram (ECG) or clinical evidence of MI.
- Mild to moderate ↑ of hepatic transaminases [aspartate transaminase (AST) and alanine transaminase (ALT)] in 25-50% of patients without clinical evidence of hepatic disease.

Management

Modifiable risk factors should be changed. Smoking must be stopped. Dyslipidemia should be treated, initially with nonpharmacologic therapy: weight ↓, a ↓ in total fat intake to less than 300% of calories with less than 100% of these coming from saturated fatty acids, and a ↓ in dietary

Table 25.3: Typical fluid and electrolyte deficits in diabetic ketoacidosis.

Fluid or electrolyte	Deficit
Water	60–100 mL/kg
Sodium	6–12 mEq (mmol)/kg
Potassium	4–6 mEq (mmol)/kg
Phosphate	2–5 mEq (mmol)/kg

Table 25.4: Potassium replacement for diabetic ketoacidosis.

Plasma potassium level [mEq (mmol)/L]	Potassium infusion [mEq (mmol)/kg/h]
<3.0	>0.5
3.0–4.0	0.4
4.0–5.0	0.3
5.0–6.0	0.1–0.2
>6.0	0 (until K⁺ <60)

cholesterol. Lipid-lowering agents should be added if nonpharmacologic therapy is not successful.

- The initial goal of therapy is to treat life-threatening emergencies, including dehydration, insulin deficiency, and potassium (K) deficiency.
- Monitor vital signs, blood glucose, Na, K, chloride, bicarbonate, and urea q 2 hours until stable. Typical fluid and electrolyte deficits are shown in Table 25.3.
- Fluid replacement: Initial goals are to restore circulating volume, reverse hypotension, and maintain cerebral, coronary, and renal perfusion. Isotonic saline (0.98% NaCl) is usually the initial choice of rehydrating fluid. For patients who are hypernatremic or at risk for congestive heart failure (CHF), a solution containing half (0.45%) isotonic saline may be preferred. The rates and volumes of administration will depend on the patient's clinical status. As a guide, give 1 L/h × 1 h, 500 mL/h × 2 h, 250 mL/h × 4 h, then 150 mL/h. Reduce fluid administration in the elderly and in patients with cardiac disease, and check cardiopulmonary status regularly. Fluid replacement should normally be completed over 12–24 hours. However, with mild cases of DKA, fluid replacement may be completed in the ER over 6–8 hours.
- K replacement: Hypokalemia is a significant cause of mortality. K levels may be normal or ↑ initially due to the metabolic acidosis. However, total body K levels are always depleted. Administer K replacement from the outset unless the initial K level is greater than 6.0 mEq (mmol)/L or oliguria is demonstrated by bladder catheterization. Guidelines for K replacement are shown in Table 25.4. ECG monitoring may be helpful in assessing K status.

- Insulin: If the blood glucose is greater than 270 mg/dL (15 mmol/L), give a bolus of short-acting insulin 0.15 U/kg intravenously (IV). Then start a continuous infusion of short-acting insulin of 0.1 U/kg/h. The blood glucose level should ↓ at an average rate of 75 mg/dL (4.0 mmol/L/h). If no response has occurred after 2-4 hours, double the infusion rate of short-acting insulin. Once the blood glucose has reached 250 mg/dL (<14 mmol/L), start 5% dextrose/H_2O at 100 mL/h in addition to the insulin infusion. This permits continued administration of insulin to abolish ketosis while protecting the patient from hypoglycemia. In addition, ↓ the insulin infusion rate to 1-2 U/h to maintain the plasma glucose at 150-250 mg/dL (8-14 mmol/L). When the acidosis is corrected and the patient able to drink and eat, give the patient's usual dose of subcutaneous (SQ) insulin and discontinue the insulin infusion 2 hours later.
- Bicarbonate: Its use in DKA is controversial. It may precipitate or worsen hypokalemia, leading to cardiac arrhythmias; cause a paradoxical ↓ of cerebrospinal fluid (CSF) pH, leading to worsening of the CNS depression; and cause a shift in the Hb O_2 disassociation curve (Bohr effect), leading to tissue hypoxia. Indications for bicarbonate therapy include: severe acidosis (pH <7.0); serum HCO_3^- less than 10 mEq (mmol)/L; acidosis accompanied by hypotension, shock, or arrhythmias; and hyperkalemia [serum K >6.5 mEq (mmol)/L]. Administer 1-2 mEq (mmol)/kg of sodium bicarbonate in 500 mL of 0.9% NaCl over 2 hours. Check the arterial pH 30 minutes after the bicarbonate infusion finishes and give further doses of bicarbonate until the pH is greater than 7.0. The amount of bicarbonate administered should generally not be greater than 3 mEq (mmol)/kg over 12 hours.
- Identify and correct the precipitating cause. It is important to teach patients proper management of sick days at home.

Hyperglycemic Hyperosmolar Coma

Hyperglycemic hyperosmolar coma usually occurs in older patients with type 2 diabetes who cannot recognize thirst or express their need for H_2O. A precipitating factor is usually present [e.g. MI, cerebrovascular accident (CVA), infection, diuretics, total parenteral nutrition, glucocorticoids, or phenytoin]. The pathogenesis of hyperosmolar coma is shown in Flowchart 25.2. Hyperglycemia results in a chronic osmotic diuresis that causes dehydration and loss of K and Na. Renal impairment from dehydration and declining creatinine clearance with aging is usually present and contributes to the hyperglycemia and hyperosmolality. Ketosis is absent, which is probably due to several reasons: A critical amount of insulin is still present and capable of suppressing lipolysis; there is less ↑ of

Flowchart 25.2: Pathogenesis of hyperosmolar state.

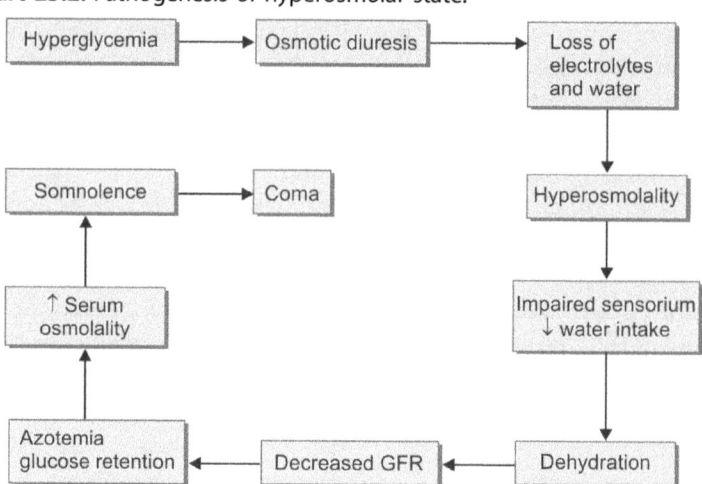

counter-regulatory hormones than in DKA; and the hyperosmolality itself may suppress lipolysis. Patients present with dehydration, often with shock, and disorientation progressing to coma.

Laboratory Findings

- Severe hyperglycemia [blood glucose >600 mg/dL (30 mmol/L)]
- Absence of, or slight, ketosis
- Calculated or measured serum hyperosmolality greater than 330 mOsm (mmol)/kg H_2O
- Profound dehydration with ↑ed urea and creatinine
- Serum Na may be normal or high due to dehydration.

Management

- Rehydration should be done more slowly than in DKA. Monitoring of central venous pressure or pulmonary capillary wedge pressure (PCWP) is often necessary to aid in the management of fluids in elderly patients with renal and cardiac failure. Serum Na less than 150 mEq (mmol)/L: use 0.9% NaCl. Serum Na greater than 150 mEq (mmol)/L and normotensive, use 0.45% NaCl.
- K replacement should be administered as in the management of DKA.
- Insulin should be given as outlined for DKA. Most patients are quite sensitive to insulin. Rehydration alone may produce a substantial ↓ in blood glucose by improving renal plasma flow and glomerular filtration.
- Identify and treat the precipitating cause.

Hypoglycemia

Most common cause of visits to the ER among patients with diabetes. The incidence ↑es as patients strive for tighter glycemic control. Adrenergic symptoms are caused by activation of the sympathetic nervous system and include diaphoresis, palpitations, tremor, anxiety, and pallor. Neuroglycopenic symptoms include cognitive impairment, visual changes, hunger, seizures, and loss of consciousness. They are produced by neuronal dysfunction secondary to glucose deprivation. Glucose is the only fuel the brain can use as an energy source. The brain cannot synthesize or store glucose and is dependent on a continuous supply from the circulation.

Management

- Conscious patient: Give 10 g rapidly absorbable glucose, i.e. one of the following: 4 oz (125 mL) juice or regular soft drink, sugar (2 cubes, 2 packets, or 2 tsp), several small candies. Wait 5–10 minutes. If the patient does not improve, repeat the treatment. After the patient recovers, give a snack equivalent to 1 starch and 1 protein exchange if the next regularly scheduled meal or snack is greater than 1 hour away. Chocolate and ice cream should be avoided due to their fat content.
- Unconscious patient: Give 25 mL of 50% dextrose/H_2O IV bolus or 1 mg of glucagon SQ or IM every 5–10 minutes until the patient awakens, then feed orally.
- Identify the precipitating cause. Patients should be taught how to adjust food and insulin for changes in diet and activity. Hypoglycemia induced by the longer-acting sulfonylureas or long-acting insulins can be prolonged. Glucose levels should be followed for 24 hours. The patient may need to be admitted to hospital for a continuous glucose infusion.

Differential Diagnosis of Coma in Patients with Diabetes

See Table 25.5.

CHRONIC COMPLICATIONS OF DIABETES

Macrovascular Disease

- Cardiovascular disease is the leading cause of death in patients with diabetes, particularly in women who lose their premenopausal protection against coronary heart disease (CHD). Atherosclerotic lesions tend to occur at an earlier age and to be more diffuse. PVD is a major factor for the increased risk of amputation in patients with diabetes.

Table 25.5: Differential diagnosis of coma in patients with diabetes.

Signs and Symptoms

Diagnosis	Ventilation	Dehydration	Pressure	Skin
DKA	+++	+++	Normal/Low	Warm
HONC	++++		Normal/Low	Normal
Hypoglycemia	0	0	Normal	Cool, clammy
Lactic acidosis	+++	0	Low	Warm
Nonmetabolic	0 to +	0 to +	Variable	Normal

Laboratory tests

Diagnosis	Glucose	Ketones
DKA	>300 mg/dL (17 mmol/L)	++ to ++++
HONC	>800 mg/dL (44 mmol/L)	0 to +
Hypoglycemia	<50 mg/dL (3.0 mmol/L)	0
Lactic acidosis	Variable	0 to +
Nonmetabolic	Variable	0 to +

- The metabolic derangement causes an increase in blood glucose that is believed to be harmful. But LDL-C also increases and is a major culprit but may not account for the rampant atherosclerotic disease found in diabetics.

  Strict treatment of hyperglycemia is not the answer, not even for nephropathy. A large well-run study enrolled 10,251 high-risk type 2 diabetics and treated hyperglycemia, which I emphasize is not the root of diabetic complications, failed: Action to Control Cardiovascular Risk in Diabetes (ACCORD) (2008).
- More patients died in the intensively treated group: 257, compared with 203 within the standard treatment group. The standard arm had a HbA1c target *between 7% and 7.9%,* and the intensive arm targeted levels under 6%.
- The trial's safety monitoring board recommended ending the intensive arm when it found increased all-cause mortality.
- Surprisingly, there was no significant effect on retinopathy; a complication that a couple of smaller trials indicate some prevent.

  The Veterans study enrolled 1,791 veterans with poorly controlled type 2 diabetes (mean HbA1c level, 9.4%) to either intensive or standard glucose control. Patients received metformin plus rosiglitazone, and those with body mass index (BMI) less than 27 initially received glimepiride plus rosiglitazone.
  - At a median long follow-up of 5.6 years, intensive glucose control had no significant effect on the rates of major cardiovascular events, death,

or microvascular complications, including retinopathies, neuropathies and nephropathies (Duckworth et al. 2009).
- Neither poor glycemic control (HbA1c ≥9.0%) nor moderately increased HbA1c (7.0–8.9%) was significantly associated with an increased rate of ischemic stroke compared with patients who had HbA1c less than 7.0%. This recent study showed that even stroke rate is not improved by moderate or strict glycemic control (Ashburner et al. 2016).

Sitosterolemia in Diabetics

Annually more than 1 million die in India (Go et al. 2013) because of diabetes mellitus. Our well-tried medical therapies that effectively control hyperglycemia do not significantly reduce the incidence of MI and stroke (Duckworth et al. 2009; ACCORD 2008) caused mainly by atheroma. Thus, the author searched for culprits other than hyperglycemia and LDL-C.

A "Holmes" deduction dictated the following thinking:
- Meat consumption causes elevation of LDL-C that is known to cause atheroma and MI.
- Carbohydrates may cause hyperglycemia in diabetics and overweight in some.
- If two of three much consumed foods cause harm, should we exempt the third large group, vegetables and plant foods? *A culprit may be lurking within.*

Diabetics, of necessity, consume much vegetables and plant foods that contain sitosterol.

This widely used plant sterol, sitosterol, is known to cause atheromatous coronary artery disease (CAD) and fatal MI in children and young adults with sitosterolemia (Salen et al. 1985; Bhattacharyya and Connor 1974).

In this genetic disease, mutations in either ABCG5 or G8 proteins cause intestinal hyperabsorption of sitosterol (Lee et al. 2001).

Most important, this intestinal genetic defect is present in diabetics and causes hyperabsorption of sitosterol as shown in a study of six diabetic and six nondiabetic control subjects (Lally et al. 2007).

Bhattacharyya and Connor (1974) reported on a newly described lipid storage disease in two sisters. Because of markedly elevated plasma and tissue sitosterol levels, premature atherosclerosis may develop.

Salen et al. (1985) described the autopsy findings from an 18-year-old white male who died suddenly of an acute MI caused by atheromatous occlusion of coronary arteries. From age 10, he had noted tendon xanthomas that began on the left elbow and back and then subsequently in the Achilles tendons, knees, and wrists. Measurements of plasma sterols 4 years prior to death revealed high concentrations of plant sterols with mild hypercholesterolemia and a diagnosis of sitosterolemia with xanthomatosis was established (Salen et al. 1985).

Fasting plasma concentrations of sitosterol above 10 mg/L are diagnostic of familial genetic sitosterolemia.

Levels of 5.2–9.5 mg/L present in diabetic individuals for more than 20 years represents significant sitosterolemia and may cause atheromatous arterial disease.

The author conducted a nonfunded study of 57 subjects and confirmed a abnormal increase in sitosterol absorption resulted in abnormally high sitosterol levels in diabetics particularly in patients with CAD.

This genetic defect in the intestine that causes hyperabsorption of sitosterol in diabetics is essentially unknown to the medical profession and the public and must be publicized.

Results of sitosterol study by Dr Khan: 75% of diabetic subjects with CAD showed elevated sitosterol 5.1–9.5 mg/L. About 45% of diabetics showed elevated sitosterol blood levels. Sitosterol was not elevated in 100% of control subjects, 1.5–3.6 mg/L and 100% of diabetics without CAD, 0.7–4.2 mg/L. This novel study shows that sitosterol levels are elevated in most diabetic patients with CAD. This report should engender large studies that can be completed within months to verify the above findings and implications.

This is the first study to show that in diabetics, 12–14 hours fasting blood sitosterol levels are abnormally increased. This increase can only occur because of hyperabsorption of sitosterol.

Sitosterolemia is a recessively inherited disorder that results from mutations in either ABCG5 or G8 proteins, with intestinal hyperabsorption of dietary sterols and decreased hepatic excretion of plant sterols and cholesterol (Lee et al. 2001).

A similar genetic defect is present in diabetics. Two independent genetic disturbances are present in most diabetics; a fact that is essentially unknown.

Mild diabetics on no drug therapy may have elevated sitosterol levels (Khan, 2017); caution is required in assessing risks.

- The study confirms that patients with type 2 diabetes mellitus hyperabsorb sitosterol because of an intestinal genetic defect similar to that of sitosterolemia (Hazard and Patel 2007; Lally et al. 2007).

  Nephropathy appears to be caused by diabetic sitosterolemia (Khan 2017).
- Retinopathy may be caused by elevated sitosterol levels and must be assessed.

  An abundance of sitosterol was found in:
  - Carotid artery atheroma plaques (Miettinen et al. 2005)
  - In aortic valve tissue of patients with CAD undergoing aortic valve replacement (Luister et al. 2015).

Foods to Minimize

Some foods with high sitosterol content should be minimized.

- All vegetable oils (corn, canola, safflower, and coconut oils are high compared with soybean, and flaxseed, margarine, avocado, nuts: pistachio, almonds, cashew.
- Canola oil and corn oil: One tablespoon contains 59 mg of beta-sitosterol.

Foods with Lower Sitosterol Levels

- Carrots, cauliflower, cabbage, bananas, apples, peaches and pears
- Soybean oil: 23 mg in a tablespoon
- Flaxseed oil: 28 mg in a tablespoon.

Ezetimibe

Drug therapy and dietary restriction are both necessary.
- Ezetimibe reduces blood sitosterol ~21% (Salen et al. 2004).
- Ezetimibe is indicated as adjunctive therapy to diet for the reduction of elevated sitosterol levels in patients with homozygous familial sitosterolemia. Thus, ezetimibe is indicated as adjunctive therapy to diet for the reduction of elevated sitosterol in diabetic patients.

Dosage: 12-13 hours fasting sitosterol blood level:
- 7-10 mg/L—20 mg daily (two 10 mg tablets)
- 4.5-6.9 mg/L—10 mg daily.

Sitosterol level not determined because of cost or unavailable.

Advice:
- 10 mg daily
- If positive family history of MI or stroke before age 75: 20 mg/day is advisable.

Gliclazide

Hypoglycemia—while gliclazide was shown to have the same efficacy as glimepiride, it has approximately 50% less hypoglycemic confirmed episodes in comparison with glimepiride or glyburide.

Dosage: 30 mg (tablets cannot be split in half) should be swallowed whole with a glass of water. The 60 mg tablets can be halved; maximum 120 mg/day. Gliclazide modified-release 60 mg tablets are advisable used once daily; the tablet is breakable.

Interacting Drugs

- Antibiotics (sulfonamides/sulfa drugs, clarithromycin), antituberculosis drugs
- Antifungal drugs (fluconazole, miconazole)
- Nonsteroidal anti-inflammatory drugs (NSAIDs).
- Acarbose inhibits alpha glucosidase, an intestinal enzyme that releases glucose from larger carbohydrates. It slows down the enzyme that turns

carbohydrates into glucose. Because acarbose prevents the digestion of complex carbohydrates, less glucose is absorbed as the carbohydrates are not broken down into glucose molecules. Thus after a carbohydrate meal a smaller rise in blood glucose occurs. It is cheap and popular in China, but not in the United States. One physician explains the use in the United States is limited because it is not potent enough to justify the side effects of diarrhea and flatulence.

Dosage: 25 mg three times daily, increasing to 100 mg three times a day.

Newer Agents

Dipeptidyl peptidase-4 (DPP-4) inhibitors: These agents lower glucagon secretion likely from pancreatic alpha cells glucose production. Pancreatitis, all be it rare, is of concern because these agents act on pancreatic cells.

Conclusion: In this first population-based study, the use of DPP-4 inhibitors was associated with an increased risk of inflammatory bowel disease. Although these findings need to be replicated, physicians should be aware of this possible association.

The glycemia reduction approaches in diabetes: A Comparative Effectiveness Study (GRADE) compared glycemic lowering of four commonly used classes of diabetes mellitus medications (sulfonylureas, DPP-4 inhibitors in combination with metformin) in 5,000 subjects with an anticipated observation period of 4–7 years.

For sitagliptin, rare pancreatitis observed, and heart failure may be precipitated as was observed for saxagliptin.

Pioglitazone: It is not advisable. When added to baseline antihyperglycemic therapy regimens in the prospective pioglitazone clinical trial in macrovascular events (PROactive), pioglitazone had no apparent benefit on the primary end point, *an increase in heart failure occurred.*

An increased prostate and pancreatic cancer risks associated with use of pioglitazone is a concern.

Rosiglitazone: It is not advisable in the SAVOR RCT saxagliptin caused heart failure ($p = 0.007$). These agents should not be used until proven to reduce outcomes in soundly run RCTs and heart failure is not caused.

Sitagliptin, A DPP-4 inhibitor, is under review for pancreatic cancer.
- Caution using sitagliptin, vildagliptin or saxagliptin.
- Newer agents linagliptin and alogliptin (DPP-4 inhibitors) have a modest effect on lowering blood glucose levels and rarely cause hypoglycemia. RCTs should clarify their role. Caution is needed because they are renally excreted and like metformin should not be used if estimated glomerular filtration rate (eGFR) is less than 45 mL/min (serum creatinine >1.5 mg/dL).

Empagliflozin: Patients with type 2 diabetes at high risk for cardiovascular events who received empagliflozin, as compared with placebo, had a slightly lower rate of the primary composite cardiovascular outcome and of death from any cause when the study drug was added to standard care. A total of 7,020 patients were treated (median observation time, 3.1 years). The primary outcome occurred in 490 of 4,687 patients (10.5%) in the pooled empagliflozin group and in 282 of 2,333 patients (12.1%) in the placebo group (HR in the empagliflozin group, 0.86; 95.02% CI, 0.74-0.99; p = 0.04 for superiority). Further studies are needed with similar agents to observe a better outcome with p value less than 0.02 to be clinically meaningful. Note there was no decrease in fatal or nonfatal MIs the main disaster caused by diabetes. But heart failure was reduced probably by volume depletion.

There were no significant between-group differences in the rates of MI or stroke, but in the empagliflozin group there were significantly lower rates of death from cardiovascular causes (3.7% vs 5.9% in the placebo group; 38% relative risk reduction), hospitalization for heart failure (2.7% and 4.1%, respectively; 35% relative risk reduction), and death from any cause (5.7% and 8.3%, respectively; 32% relative risk reduction). There was no significant between-group difference in the key secondary outcome (p = 0.08 for superiority).

Among patients receiving empagliflozin, there was an increased rate of genital infection but no increase in other serious adverse events.

The drug may increase serum creatinine and decrease eGFR. Renal function should be evaluated prior to initiating empagliflozin and periodically thereafter. More frequent monitoring is recommended with eGFR below 60 mL/min/1.73 m². The risk of impaired renal function with empagliflozin is increased in elderly patients and patients with mild to moderate renal impairment, a common finding in diabetics. Empagliflozin should be discontinued in patients with a persistent eGFR less than 45 mL/min/1.73 m².

- If eGFR is less than 50 mL/min. It is best to wait a few years for further RCTs and warnings before using these agents.
- Increases in LDL-C can occur.
- When empagliflozin was administered with insulin or sulfonylurea, the incidence of hypoglycemic events was increased.
- Caution needed coadministration of empagliflozin, with diuretics resulted in increased urine volume and frequency of voids, which might enhance the potential for volume depletion; diminished efficacy and adverse effects in elderly patients who commonly have some degree of renal dysfunction despite a normal serum creatinine.
- The incidence of volume depletion-related adverse reactions and urinary tract infections (UTIs) increased in patients more than or equal to 75 years treated with this agent.

Sodium-glucose cotransporter 2 inhibitors and gliflozins: Sodium-glucose cotransporter 2 (SGLT2) inhibitors prevent the vast amount of glucose filtered through glomeruli into the proximal tubules from being absorbed: a most intriguing strategy to abort hyperglycemia. The labels of SGLT2 inhibitors—drugs used to treat type 2 diabetes—will be updated to warn of the risks for ketoacidosis and serious UTIs.

Caution needed as coadministration of empagliflozin with diuretics resulted in increased urine volume and frequency of voids, which might enhance the potential for volume depletion; diminished efficacy and adverse effects in elderly patients who commonly have some degree of renal dysfunction despite a normal serum creatinine.

Retinopathy

- Nonproliferative (background) retinopathy (dot and blot hemorrhages, hard and soft exudates, microaneurysms) is present in 50% of patients with type 1 diabetes 10 years after onset of symptoms. Proliferative retinopathy (growth of new capillaries and fibrous tissue within the retina and into the vitreous chamber) is present in 50% of patients after 15 years.
- Refer to an ophthalmologist: All patients with type 1 diabetes who are greater than 10 years old and have had the disease for greater than 5 years; all patients with diabetes who at diagnosis are greater than 30 years old; and all female patients planning a pregnancy in the near future. Pregnant women should be reassessed early in the 1st trimester and seen each trimester thereafter unless more frequent visits are indicated for retinal disease.
- Laser therapy can halt the progression of retinal disease. Vitrectomy (surgical removal of the vitreous) may help restore vision in severely diseased eyes with a significant retinal bleed.

Nephropathy

- End-stage renal disease occurs in 30–40% of patients with type 1 diabetes. Renal disease manifests itself by the appearance of persistent proteinuria, usually after 10–15 years.
- Urinalysis and serum creatinine should be checked at least annually.
- After the patient has had diabetes for greater than 5 years, total urinary protein excretion (in the patient with proteinuria on urine dipstick) or microalbuminuria (in the patient with no detectable proteinuria on routine urinalysis) should be measured annually.
- Blood pressure (BP) should be measured at every follow-up visit.

- When persistent proteinuria or declining renal function is confirmed, the patient should be referred to a nephrologist for medical treatment and to a dietician for instruction in low-protein diets.
- Aggressive treatment of hypertension is the only therapy that slows progression of established diabetic nephropathy. Antihypertensive agents that may be used include angiotensin-converting enzyme (ACE) inhibitors, calcium (Ca) antagonists, and cardioselective beta-blockers (may mask symptoms of hypoglycemia).

Neuropathy

- The most common chronic complication of diabetes. Affects 50% of patients with long-standing diabetes.
- Distal symmetrical sensorimotor polyneuropathy: Glove and stocking loss of sensation for pinprick and light touch. Vibration sense and reflexes are diminished. Pain is typically nocturnal. It may be relieved by amitriptyline 10–150 mg/day at hs or capsaicin cream applied three to four times a day to the affected area.

Autonomic Neuropathy

- Orthostatic hypotension: It may respond to salt supplementation, fludrocortisone acetate (Florinef) 0.05–0.2 mg/day, or midodrine hydrochloride (Amatine) 2.5 mg tid.
- Gastroparesis: It may present with nausea and vomiting secondary to delayed gastric emptying. Cisapride 5–10 mg bid to qid, metoclopramide 5–10 mg tid or qid, or domperidone 10 mg tid or qid may help. All of these agents are taken 15–30 minutes before meals.
- Diabetic diarrhea: It may respond to tetracycline 250 mg qid for 7 days, loperamide hydrochloride (lmodium) 2 mg with each bowel movement up to 16 mg/day, or diphenoxylate hydrochloride (lomotil) 5 mg tid or qid.
- Diabetic cystopathy (neurogenic bladder): It results in chronic urine retention. It may respond to bethanechol 10–20 mg tid to stimulate detrusor function or intermittent self-catheterization.
- Impotence: It may be managed with penile implant, intrapenile injections of papaverine and phentolamine, or an external suction device.

Focal Neuropathies

- Cranial mononeuropathy: Unilateral 3rd nerve paresis is the most common. It presents with abrupt onset of diplopia, typically accompanied by orbital or retro-orbital pain. Ptosis may occur, but pupillary function is spared. Usually resolves in 6 weeks to 6 months.

- Mononeuropathy/mononeuropathy multiplex: It may involve more than one nerve of the extremities or trunk. It results from ischemic infarction of the nerve and is heralded by the acute onset of muscle weakness and pain in the area supplied. Spontaneous recovery occurs in 3-6 months.

Foot Care: Diabetic Foot Ulcers

- In patients with neuropathy or PVD, a minor trauma to the foot can often lead to skin ulceration, infection, and ultimately gangrene. Feet should be examined at each follow-up visit. Patients must be taught preventive foot care.
- The risk of death at 5 years for a patient with a diabetic foot ulcer is 2.5 times as high as the risk for a patient with diabetes who does not have a foot ulcer. More than half of diabetic ulcers become infected.
- Approximately 20% of moderate or severe diabetic foot infections lead to some level of amputation.
- Peripheral artery disease independently increases the risk of nonhealing ulcers, infection, and amputation.
- Despite the best care given for diabetics in the United Kingdom over 50 years, partial amputation of the foot continues. High glucose is not the causative problem. Ulcers begin because of PVD caused by atheromatous occlusion. High glucose allows bacterial invasion and increases the problems.
- High sitosterol blood level is a root cause of atheromatous PVD along with LDL-C.
- *Sitosterol dietary restriction and ezetimibe are required at first sign of PVD prior to foot ulceration.*

MANAGEMENT OF DIABETES MELLITUS

Diabetic Way of Eating

- Decrease carbohydrates and also vegetables/plant foods and shellfish—containing high concentration of sitosterol.
- A new plan of action has been advanced by the author: Sitosterol is elevated in greater than 50% of diabetics and causes vascular disease (Khan, 2017), see list of sitosterol foods to restrict.
- In the obese patient with type 2 diabetes, weight ↓ is the most important goal. In the patient with type 1 diabetes, proper timing of meals and snacks, and consistency of food quantities, are important to good glycemic control.
- Energy: Individual energy needs are difficult to predict accurately. An approximation can be obtained.
- Carbohydrates: Approximately 55-60% of total calories. Unrefined, high-fiber, complex carbohydrates are preferred.

- Protein: Less than or equal to 15% of total calories (0.8 g/kg desirable body weight).
- Fat: Less than 35% of total calories. Fat should be reduced through restriction of saturated fat to less than 10% of total calories. Polyunsaturated fat should contribute less than 10% of calories, with monounsaturated fat supplying the remainder of energy needs.
- Alcohol: Consumption should be restricted in patients with obesity, hypertension, or hypertriglyceridemia. Alcohol may also impair recognition and recovery from hypoglycemia.
- Noncaloric sweeteners (e.g. aspartame, sucralose) may be used in moderation. Nutritive sweeteners (e.g. sorbitol, fructose, and sucrose) may be included as a free food when the total serving provides less than or equal to 60 kJ (15 kcal).
- Sodium: Intake should be restricted to less than 90 mEq (mmol)/day in hypertensive patients.

Exercise

- A physical activity plan should be developed for each patient. Aerobic exercise is preferred.
- Capillary blood glucose should be checked before and after exercise so that the patient can learn to adjust diet and/or hypoglycemic medications to activity. Mild exercise of short duration may require little change other than extra carbohydrates. More prolonged exercise may require a ↓ in the insulin dose. Patients should avoid injecting into an exercising limb, as exercise may ↑ the rate of absorption.
- The major risk of exercise in patients taking insulin or oral hypoglycemic agents is hypoglycemia. This may occur during or less than or equal to 20 hours after exercise.
- *Caution* is required not to give hypoglycemic drugs if the urine is always glucose-free or one with minimal glycosuria the urine must be positive otherwise hypoglycemia is high common and falls occur particularly in the elderly.
- Exercise should be prescribed with caution in patients with cardiovascular disease, neuropathy, proliferative retinopathy, or hypoglycemia unawareness. An exercise stress test may be indicated in certain patients before starting an exercise program.

Hypoglycemic Medications

Oral Hypoglycemic Agents

Oral hypoglycemic agents should be used in patients with type 2 diabetes when diet and exercise have failed to achieve individual treatment goals. Sulfonylureas are the first-line drugs. The biguanide, metformin, may be useful first-line drugs in the very obese. Combination therapy with metformin and a sulfonylurea may be tried when target glycemic control is not achieved with either agent alone.

Monitoring

- Second voided urine glucose testing: Easy and inexpensive; however, there is poor correlation between simultaneous blood and urine glucose measurements. In addition, the renal threshold for glucose varies greatly from patient to patient, and in the same patient from time to time.
- Self-monitoring of blood glucose: Mandatory for patients on insulin therapy and desirable for patients on oral hypoglycemic agents. More frequent tests are performed on sick days, with changes in exercise or meal patterns, on travel days, or when hypoglycemia is suspected. Allows daily glucose patterns to be visualized and correlated with insulin, food, and activity.
- Urine ketone testing: It should be performed during illness or when blood glucose greater than 360 mg/dL (20 mmol/L).
- Glycated Hb (glycosylated Hb, HbA1c), nonfasting: Created by glycation of the amino-terminal valine of the beta-subunit of Hb. Reflects blood glucose control over the preceding 3 months (the lifespan of RBCs). The normal value depends on the method used and the laboratory.

Glycated Hemoglobin

Several conditions interfere with the interpretation of results: Sickle cell is not uncommon in individuals of Asian Indian origin and Africans, alterations in red cell turnover (e.g. hemolytic anemia) recent transfusion, pregnancy, blood loss; lack of assay standardization, cost and lack of availability in many countries.

- HbA1c is expensive and not a necessary test; it is overused in the United States of America.
- Fructosamine: Measures glycated albumin and reflects glucose control over the previous 2-3 weeks. May be useful in pregnancy and other states when changes in glycemic control over weeks rather than months is important. Test may be interfered by hypoproteinemia, hemolysis of the blood sample, hypertriglyceridemia, and hyperbilirubinemia.

Metformin

Supplied: Tablets 500 mg. Dosage: 500 mg bid with meals; to minimize gastrointestinal (GI) upset.

Maximum 1,000 mg bid. Excreted by the kidney.

Advised to use urine testing: Blood test a few times annually if blood facility available. Fingertip blood test only useful for insulin treated to

prevent hypoglycemia. Urine testing was used in 1950-1995 successfully. Tight control to achieve FBG greater than 6.5 is not advisable because it does not prevent complications. A goal of 8-9 mmol/L is recommended if blood is done once/month.
- Urine testing should suffice.
- Metformin 500 mg twice daily; if FBG more than 9 mmol/L; HbA1c more than 9%.

Caution: Avoid with renal problem. Duration of action: 7-19 hours. Do not use if eGFR is less than 45 mL/min; for 46-60 years, use half dose 500 mg bid maximum dose.

Avoid if liver impairment, or illness that may lead to hypoxia.

Metformin, surprisingly, was never adequately tested in a large RCT with adequate follow-up.

See discussion under "Newer Agents" for gliptins and others.

Glyburide

Supplied: Tablets 2.5, 5 mg. Dosage: 2.5-5 mg qd or bid, maximum 20 mg/day (elderly 1.25 mg qd bid, max. 10 mg/day). Metabolized by the liver. Duration of action: 12-24 hours.

Glipizide

Supplied: Tablets 5, 10 mg. Dosage: 5 mg once daily, maximum 20 mg bid. Metabolized by the liver. Duration of action: 10-24 hours.

Gliclazide

Supplied: 80 mg. Dosage: 80 mg bid, maximum 160 mg/day (elderly less than age 80, 40 mg bid). Duration of action: 10-24 hours.
Gliclazide modified release (MR): 30 mg, 60 mg: Take 30 mg once daily, increase to maximum 60 mg if needed at the same time every day. (Manufacturer's maximum = 120 mg/day). Gliclazide has the same efficacy as newer sulfonylureas, such as glimepiride; a European Guide study has shown that it has approximately 50% less hypoglycemic confirmed episodes in comparison with glimepiride.
Caution: Do not use sulfonylureas if allergic to sulfur or take some forms of miconazole, or have renal failure.

Beta-blocker: A New Indication for Type 2 Diabetes

All diabetics at high risk (*see* earlier section on risk for CVD events) should be given a small to medium dose of, preferably a noncardioselective beta-blocker, timolol (propranolol in nonsmokers), but bisoprolol or metoprolol are also first-choice beta-blockers recommended for the treatment of diabetic patients. These drugs are not usually advised because of hypoglycemia may be prolonged but with my strategy, keeping blood glucose fasting much higher (8-8.5) than conventional advice, hypoglycemia is avoided and cardioprotective drugs can be used to save lives and prevent sudden cardiac deaths. Atenolol is not recommended. Diabetics are at high risk, similar to post-MI patients, so the experts should be more logical.

Physicians are afraid to use nonselective agents because they are more dangerous if hypoglycemia occurs. *But beta-1 and beta-2 blockers are needed to more effectively prevent fatal MI and sudden deaths.*

Statins

Statins to maintain LDL-C less than 2 mmol/L (<77 mg/dL) in all diabetics. 1.4-1.8 mmol/L in those with a parent or family member with a history of MI. This strict control of lipids, maintenance of normal blood sitosterol, systolic BP (SBP) ~130-139 mm Hg, cessation of smoking and avoiding exhaust fumes from motor vehicles on probabilities would prevent further atheroma formation and progression, the cause of CAD.

Advice for Diabetics to Reduce Sitosterol Blood Levels

About 50% of diabetic patients are expected to have sitosterolemia, 5-10 mg/L (Khan, 2017) and levels should be reduced to less than 4.4 mg/L.

Foods to minimize: Some foods with high sitosterol content should be minimized.
- All vegetable oils (corn, canola, safflower, and coconut oils are high compared with soybean, and flaxseed.
- Canola oil and corn oil: One tablespoon of contains 59-80 mg of beta-sitosterol.
- Avocado, nuts: Pistachio, almonds, cashew chocolates.
- Shellfish: Including shrimp, clams, scallops, lobsters, crabs and abalones.
- Margarines and other foods may have sitosterol added by manufacturers.

Foods with lower sitosterol levels:
- Carrots, cauliflower, cabbage, bananas, apples, peaches and pears, many others.
- Soybean oil: 23 mg in a tablespoon
- Flaxseed oil: 28 mg in a tablespoon.

Ezetimibe

Drug therapy and dietary restriction are both necessary.
- Ezetimibe reduces blood sitosterol ~21% (Salen et al. 2004)
- Ezetimibe is indicated as adjunctive therapy to diet for the reduction of elevated sitosterol levels in patients with homozygous familial

sitosterolemia. Thus, I advise that ezetimibe is indicated as adjunctive therapy to diet for the reduction of elevated sitosterol in diabetic patients.
Dosage: 12-13 hours fasting sitosterol blood level:
- 7-10 mg/L 20 mg daily (two 10 mg tablets)
- 4.5-6.9 mg/L 10 mg daily.
Sitosterol level not determined because of cost or unavailable.
Advise:
- 10 mg daily
- If positive family history of MI or stroke.

Blood Pressure Goal

Goal is 130-140 mm Hg. Cardiovascular mortality is reduced if baseline SBP is greater than 150 mm Hg and reduced to 130-140 mm Hg. When baseline SBP was 140-150 mm Hg, the effect of treatment on cardiovascular mortality was not significant. If the initial baseline is 130-140 mm Hg, do not give an antihypertensive agent, particularly ACE inhibitor or angiotensin receptor blocker (ARB) as it increases mortality and events. Beta-blockers are safest to use as they do not lower BP much if already low, and they do prevent deaths contrary to popular medical belief.

Education

Patient education is essential for compliance with a management regimen. All patients should be offered an education program covering the important aspects of self-care, knowledge, and skills. Ongoing counseling is necessary to achieve long-term compliance. Table 25.6 outlines guidelines for the goals of therapy in diabetes.

Surgery

Patients with diabetes who require surgery must be adequately controlled to avoid hypoglycemia, hyperglycemia, and ketosis during surgery. With elective surgery, the patient should be under as good metabolic control as possible and free of ketosis. With emergency surgery, any acidosis and dehydration should be corrected before the procedure.

Minor Procedure without a General Anesthetic

Patients treated with oral hypoglycemic agents:
- Hold morning dose of oral hypoglycemic agents.
- Monitor blood glucose before, during, and after surgery.
- Give IV fluids to provide hydration and prevent hypoglycemia.
- Give supplemental short-acting insulin SC if blood glucose greater than 250 mg/dL (14 mmol/L).

Table 25.6: Targets for control of diabetes.

	Optimal	Acceptable	Compromised
Blood glucose • Fasting • After eating	80–120 mg/dL (4–7 mmol/L) 90–180 mg/dL (5–10 mmol/L)	<180 mg/dL (10 mmol/L) <220 mg/dL (12 mmol/L)	>180 mg/dL (10 mmol/L) >220 mg/dL (12 mmol/L)
Glycated hemoglobin (% of upper limit)	<110	<140	>140
Total cholesterol	<160 mg/dL (4.2 mmol/L)*	<180 mg/dL (4.7 mmol/L)*	>200 mg/dL (>5 mmol/L)
LDL cholesterol	< 62 mg/dL (1.6 mmol/L)*	<77 mg/dL (2 mmol/L)*	>120 mg/dL (>3 mmol/L)
HDL cholesterol	Not important	Outcomes not clinically affected by increasing levels	-
Triglycerides	<150 mg/dL (1.7 mmol/L)*	<220 mg/dL (2.5 mmol/L)	>300 mg/dL (3.4 mmol/L)‡
Body mass index • Male <65 years • Female <65 years	<25 <24	<27 <26	>27 >26
Blood pressure (mm Hg)†	<140/90	<160/95	>160/95

*Should be adjusted for other risk factors. Less strict targets may be appropriate for older patients with limited life expectancy.
†For patients with diabetic nephropathy, it has been suggested that optimal BP should be 130/80–135/85 mm Hg; however, conclusive evidence is lacking.
‡Always responds to weight reduction, increased exercise, and restriction of carbohydrates and most important beer and other alcohol.

Patients treated with insulin:
- Administer one-half to two-thirds of the usual morning dose of intermediate-acting insulin SQ.
- Hold the usual morning dose of short-acting insulin.
- Infuse 5% dextrose/water at 100 mL/h while the patient is nil per os (NPO).t
- Monitor the blood glucose immediately after the operation and q 4 hours thereafter.
- Give extra short-acting insulin SC in small amounts for blood glucose greater than 200 mg/dL (12 mmol/L).
- If the patient is drinking and eating well, give the usual evening dose of insulin.

Table 25.7: Insulin–Glucose infusion for surgery.			
Blood glucose (mg/dL) (mmol/L)	Insulin infusion (mL/hr)	Insulin infusion (units/hr)	D5W infusion (mL/hr)
<70 (4)	2	0.4	150
71–100 (4–6)	5	1.0	125
101–150 (6.1–8)	7	1.4	100
151–200 (8.1–10)	10	2.0	100
201–250 (10.1–14)	15	3.0	100
251–300 (14–16)	20	4.0	75
>300 (16)	25	60	50

Major Procedure with a General Anesthetic

Patients not well controlled on oral hypoglycemic agents:
- Discontinue oral hypoglycemic agents the night before surgery.
- On the morning of surgery, start an infusion of 5% dextrose/water at 100 mL/h.
- Also, start an insulin drip by diluting 100 U of short-acting insulin in 500 mL of 0.9% NaCl.
- Check the blood glucose q 2 hours preoperatively, q 1 hour during surgery, and q 2 hours postoperatively, and adjust each infusion as outlined in Table 25.7.
- When patient is eating and drinking well, resume oral hypoglycemic agents if changes will be made to the patient's meal plan and exercise program; otherwise, switch the patient to a SQ insulin regimen.

Patients well controlled on insulin:
- Hold the usual SQ insulin on the morning of surgery.
- Start an infusion of 5% dextrose/water at 100 mL/h.
- Also, start an insulin drip by diluting 100 U of short-acting insulin in 500 mL of 0.9% NaCl.
- Check the blood glucose q 2 hours preoperatively, q 1 hour during surgery, and q 2 hours postoperatively and adjust each infusion as outlined in Table 25.7.
- Continue the insulin and glucose infusions until the patient is able to take food, and then restart the usual dose of SQ insulin.
- Continue both the insulin and glucose infusions for 1–2 hours after the SQ insulin has been given to prevent the blood glucose level from rising before the SQ insulin has begun to work.

Patients not well controlled on insulin:
- Start insulin drip and glucose infusion as outlined above the day before surgery.

BIBLIOGRAPHY

1. A randomized trial of propranolol in patients with acute myocardial infarction. I. Mortality results. JAMA. 1982;247:1707-14.
2. Abrahami D, Douros A, Yin H, et al. Dipeptidyl peptidase-4 inhibitors and incidence of inflammatory bowel disease among patients with type 2 diabetes: population based cohort study. BMJ. 2018;360:k872.
3. ACCORD Study Group, Cushman WC, Evans GW, et al. Effects of intensive blood-pressure control in type 2 diabetes mellitus. N Engl J Med. 2010;362(17):1575-85.
4. ACCORD Study Group, Ginsberg HN, Elam MB, et al. Effects of combination lipid therapy in type 2 diabetes mellitus. N Engl J Med. 2010;362(17):1563-74.
5. Action to Control Cardiovascular Risk in Diabetes Study Group, Gerstein HC, Miller ME, et al. Effects of intensive glucose lowering in type 2 diabetes. N Engl J Med. 2008;358:2545-59.
6. ADVANCE Collaborative Group, Patel A, MacMahon S, et al. Intensive blood glucose control and vascular outcomes in patients with type 2 diabetes. N Engl J Med. 2008;358(24):2560-72.
7. American Diabetes Association. (2018). Statistics about diabetes. [online] Available from www.diabetes.org/diabetes-basics/statistics/. [Accessed September, 2018].
8. Armstrong DG, Boulton AJ, Bus SA. Diabetic foot ulcers and their recurrence. N Engl J Med. 2017;376:2367-75.
9. Ashburner JM, Go AS, Chang Y, et al. Effect of diabetes and glycemic control on ischemic stroke risk in AF patients; ATRIA Study. J Am Coll Cardiol. 2016;67(3):239-47.
10. Assmann G, Cullen P, Erbey J, et al. Plasma sitosterol elevations are associated with an increased incidence of coronary events in men: results of a nested case-control analysis of the Prospective Cardiovascular Munster (PROCAM) study. Nutr Metab Cardiovasc Dis. 2006;16:13-21.
11. Beaser R, Houlden R. Diabetes mellitus. In: Khan MG, Bartlett JG, Chopra S, Topol EJ (Eds). Medical Diagnosis and Therapy. Pennsylvania: Lea and Febiger; 1994.
12. Bhattacharyya AK, Connor WE. Beta-sitosterolemia and xanthomatosis. A newly described lipid storage disease in two sisters. J Clin Invest. 1974;53:1033-43.
13. Cannon CP, Blazing MA, Giugliano RP, et al. Ezetimibe added to statin therapy after acute coronary syndromes. N Engl J Med. 2015;372:2387-97.
14. DREAM Trial Investigators. Bosch J, Yusuf S, et al. Effect of ramipril on the incidence of diabetes. N Engl J Med. 2006;355(15):1551-62.
15. Duckworth W, Abraira C, Moritz T, et al. Glucose control and vascular complications in veterans with type 2 diabetes. N Engl J Med. 2009;360(2):129-39.
16. Hart T, Milner R, Cifu A. Management of a diabetic foot. JAMA. 2017;318(14):1387-8.
17. Hazard SE, Patel SB. Sterolins ABCG5 and ABCG8: regulators of whole body dietary sterols. Pflugers Arch. 2007;453:745-52.
18. Hingorani A, LaMuraglia GM, Henke P, et al. The management of diabetic foot: a clinical practice guideline by the Society for Vascular Surgery in Collaboration with the American Podiatric Medical Association and the Society for Vascular Medicine. J Vasc Surg. 2016;63(2 Suppl):3S-21S.

19. Intensive blood-glucose control with sulphonylureas or insulin compared with conventional treatment and risk of complications in patients with type 2 diabetes (UKPDS 33). UK Prospective Diabetes Study (UKPDS) Group. Lancet. 1998;352(9131):837-53.
20. International Diabetes Federation. (2015). IDF Diabetes Atlas, 7th edition. [online] Available from http://www.diabetesatlas.org. [Accessed September, 2018].
21. Khan GM. Sitosterol blood levels are elevated in diabetics and may be the cause of coronary artery disease and stroke. J Med Sci. 2017;3:89-94.
22. Lally SE, Owens D, Tomkin GH. Sitosterol and cholesterol in chylomicrons of type 2 diabetic and non-diabetic subjects: the relationship with ATP binding cassette proteins G5 and G8 and Niemann-Pick C1-like 1 mRNA. Diabetologia. 2007;50(1):217-9.
23. Lee M, Lu K, Patel SB. Genetic basis of sitosterolemia. Curr Opin Lipidol. 2001;12(2):141-9.
24. Luister A, Schött HF, Husche C, et al. Increased plant sterol deposition in vascular tissue characterizes patients with severe aortic stenosis and concomitant coronary artery disease. Steroids. 2015;99(Pt B):272-80.
25. Miettinen TA, Railo M, Lepäntalo M, et al. Plant sterols in serum and in atherosclerotic plaques of patients undergoing carotid endarterectomy. J Am Coll Cardiol. 2005;45(11):1794-801.
26. Nicolas A, Fatima S, Lamri A, et al. ABCG8 polymorphisms and renal disease in type 2 diabetic patients. Metabolism. 2015;64(6):713-9.
27. Nilsson PM. ACCORD risk-factor control in type 2 diabetes. N Engl J Med. 2010;362(17):1628-30.
28. Norwegian Multicenter Study Group. Timolol-induced reduction in mortality and reinfarction in patients surviving acute myocardial infarction. N Engl J Med. 1981;304:801-7.
29. Qaseem A, Wilt TJ, Kansagara D, et al. Hemoglobin A1c targets for glycemic control with pharmacologic therapy for nonpregnant adults with type 2 diabetes mellitus: a guidance statement update from the American College of Physicians. Ann Intern Med. 2018;168(8):569-76.
30. Salen G, Horak I, Rothkopf M, et al. Lethal atherosclerosis associated with abnormal plasma and tissue sterol composition in sitosterolemia with xanthomatosis. J Lipid Res. 1985;26:1126-33.
31. Salen G, von Bergmann K, Lutjohann D, et al. Ezetimibe effectively reduces plasma plant sterols in patients with sitosterolemia. Circulation. 2004;109: 966-71.
32. Singh N, Armstrong DG, Lipsky BA. Preventing foot ulcers in patients with diabetes. JAMA. 2005;293(2):217-28.
33. Vergès B, Fumeron F. Potential risks associated with increased plasma plant-sterol levels. Diabetes Metab. 2015;41(1):76-81.
34. Zinman B, Lachin JM, Inzucchi SE. Empagliflozin, cardiovascular outcomes, and mortality in type 2 diabetes. N Engl J Med. 2016;374(11):1094.

CHAPTER 26

Endocrine Disorders

THYROID DISEASES

Thyroid Tests

Serum total thyroxine (TT4) reflects the total T4 concentration (both free and bound). Used for screening and follow-up of hyper- and hypothyroidism. The disadvantage of TT4 as a screening test is that it is affected by changes in the concentration of thyroxine-binding globulin (TBG).

Serum total triiodothyronine (T3) is used for diagnosis and follow-up hyperthyroidism. May be useful in certain hyperthyroid states where the serum T4 is normal (*T3 toxicosis*). Like TT4, it is affected by changes in TBG.

T3 resin uptake (T3RU) is used to distinguish hyper- and hypothyroidism from ↑ and ↓ TBG concentrations. The test measures indirectly the unoccupied binding sites for T4 and T3 on TBG. It is performed by mixing radiolabeled T3 with the patient's serum, adding a resin, and then determining the amount of radiolabeled T3 bound to the resin.

Causes of a high T3RU include:
- Hyperthyroidism (more binding sites occupied with T4).
- Salicylates, dilantin, and clofibrate (compete with T4 for binding to TBG).
- Decreased TBG production secondary to androgen therapy, severe hypoproteinemia, glucocorticoid excess, or hereditary TBG deficiency.

Causes of a low T3RU include:
- Hypothyroidism (fewer binding sites occupied with T4)
- Increased TBG production secondary to estrogen therapy, pregnancy, acute hepatitis, acute intermittent porphyria, or hereditary TBG excess.

Free thyroxine index (FT4I) is used to correct changes in TBG by normalizing discordant serum T4 and T3RU values. It is calculated by multiplying T4 by the T3 ratio (T3RU of patient ÷ T3RU for normal subjects).

Free T4 and free T3 are currently used to diagnose thyroid disease because the serum total T4 and T3 may be altered by changes in protein binding.

Thyroid-stimulating hormone (TSH) is the screening test of choice for hypo- and hyperthyroidism (Flowchart 26.1). It is also used to evaluate thyroid hormone replacement for hypothyroidism and suppression therapy for thyroid cancer. Conventional TSH assays were not sensitive enough to differentiate between hyperthyroid and euthyroid individuals at the lower

Flowchart 26.1: Screening for thyroid disease.

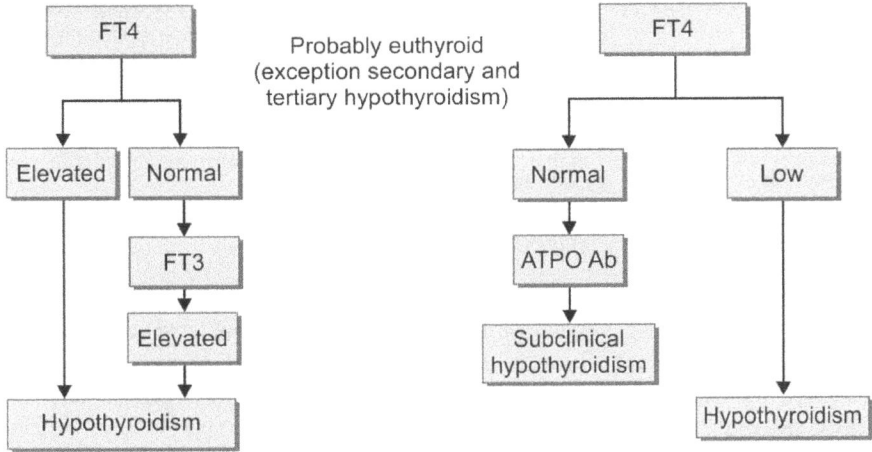

(ATPO Ab, antithyroid peroxidase antibody; FT3, free triiodothyronine; FT4, free thyroxine)

range. The newer third-generation immunometric assays (*sensitive* TSH) are able to distinguish normal from hyperthyroid patients (Houlden).

Thyrotropin-releasing hormone (TRH) stimulation test is used in patients with suspected hyperthyroidism in whom thyroid function tests are equivocal. TRH 200 µg is injected intravenous (IV) over 15–30 seconds. Serum TSH levels are drawn at 0, 30, and 60 minutes. Side effects are brief (1–2 minutes) and include nausea, facial flushing, metallic taste, and the urge to micturate. The normal response is a tenfold ↑ relative to the basal level. Blunted or absent responses are seen in hyperthyroidism, pituitary hypothyroidism, acromegaly, glucocorticoid therapy, chronic renal failure, severe systemic illness, depression, and normal elderly subjects. This test has become less useful since the availability of "sensitive" TSH assays.

Antithyroid peroxidase (microsomal) and antithyroglobulin antibodies are used primarily in making a diagnosis of Hashimoto's thyroiditis. Antithyroid peroxidase antibodies are more sensitive than antithyroglobulin antibodies.

Thyroglobulin indicates the presence of functioning thyroid tissue. Used primarily in thyroid cancer for follow-up of patients who have had thyroid gland ablation. Best measured of thyroid hormone suppression therapy. Levels ↑ with the occurrence of metastases. It may also be useful in distinguishing factitious hyperthyroidism from thyroiditis.

Thyroidal radioactive iodine uptake (RAIU) test: Radioactive iodine (RAI) is administered by mouth (PO) and the uptake is measured over the thyroid with a scintillation counter. The count is usually done at 24 hours, when the uptake plateaus. A measurement is frequently done at 6 hours as well, as the RAIU may reach a maximum earlier with severe hyperthyroidism. The RAIU is useful in the differential diagnosis of hyperthyroidism and in calculating the dose of ^{131}I needed for RAI therapy (Table 26.1).

Table 26.1: Thyroid scanning and RAIU findings in hyperthyroidism.		
Disease	Thyroid scan	Radioactive iodine uptake (RAIU)
Graves' disease	Diffuse goiter	Increased
Toxic multinodular goiter	Patchy uptake	High normal to elevated
Thyroiditis	Little uptake	Low

Euthyroid Sick Syndrome

It refers to patients with nonthyroidal illness and abnormal thyroid tests. Primary thyroid disease is not present. The abnormal thyroid function tests are the result of abnormalities in serum thyroid hormone binding and extrathyroidal thyroid hormone metabolism. The syndrome can be classified into the following categories:

- Low T3 syndrome is most common. Characterized by normal or slightly ↑ TT4, low T3, ↑ reverse T3 (rT3), and normal TSH levels, due to ↓ed extrathyroidal conversion of T4 to T3. Occurs with severe systemic illnesses and following the administration of some drugs (dexamethasone, cholecystographic dyes, amiodarone, and high doses of propranolol).
- Low T3 and low TT4 syndrome is characterized by low TT4, low T3, high rT3, normal or slightly ↓ TSH, and an impaired TSH response to TRH stimulation. Postulated to be due to a circulating inhibitor of T4 binding to thyroid-binding proteins. The normal or low TSH may reflect hypothalamic adaptation to severe illness. This occurs in severely ill patients. There is no evidence that treatment with levothyroxine helps. The low T4 and T3 may be an adaptive mechanism to spare protein catabolism.
- High TT4 syndrome is characterized by a high TT4 and normal T3. Causes include thromboelastography (TEG) excess inherited or secondary to liver disease (acute viral hepatitis, chronic active hepatitis, and primary biliary cirrhosis), estrogen therapy, or acute intermittent porphyria; familial dysalbuminemic hyperthyroxinemia (abnormal binding of T4 by albumin); ↑ triethylene phosphoramide (TEPA); drug-related from amiodarone, oral cholecystographic contrast agents [iopanoic acid (Telepaque) or ipodate (Oragrafin)], and high doses of propranolol (Houlden).

Hypothyroidism

Chaker et al. provide an excellent review article.

Causes of Hypothyroidism

Primary: It is due to thyroid hormone deficiency.
- Chronic autoimmune thyroiditis (Hashimoto's thyroiditis) is the most common cause. High concentrations of antithyroid antibodies (predominantly thyroid peroxidase antibodies and antithyroglobulin antibodies) are present in most patients with autoimmune thyroiditis.

- *Iodine*: Severe iodine deficiency, mild and severe iodine excess, post-RAI treatment, and external radiation.
- *Drugs*: Amiodarone, lithium, tyrosine kinase inhibitors, interferon-α, thalidomide, monoclonal antibodies (e.g. ipilimumab and nivolumab), antiepileptic drugs (e.g. valproate), and drugs for second-line treatment of multidrug-resistant tuberculosis.
- *Transient thyroiditis*: Viral (de Quervain's syndrome), postpartum, silent thyroiditis, and destructive thyroiditis.
- *Rare causes of primary hypothyroidism*: Infectious (e.g. mycoplasma), malignant (e.g. thyroid malignancy, lymphoma, and metastasis of malignancy elsewhere), autoimmune (e.g. sarcoidosis), and inflammatory (e.g. Riedel's thyroiditis).

Central hypothyroidism (rare)
- Pituitary tumors (secreting or nonsecreting).
- Pituitary dysfunction (e.g. Sheehan's syndrome), hypothalamic dysfunction (e.g. posttraumatic).
- Resistance to TSH or TRH.
- *Secondary (TSH deficiency)*: Disease of the pituitary gland.
- *Tertiary (TRH deficiency)*: Disease of the hypothalamus.

Clinical Manifestations

The onset may be slow and unnoticed. The most important symptoms diagnostically are generalized weakness, tiredness, and lethargy, cold intolerance, dry skin and hair loss, and memory impairment. Other symptoms and signs include weight gain, constipation, muscle cramps, aching and stiffness, facial and peripheral edema, heavy, prolonged menstrual periods, deepening of the voice, hearing loss, bradycardia, pseudomyotonia (delay in the relaxation phase of the deep tendon reflexes), and carpal tunnel syndrome. But clinical presentation can differ with age and sex, among other factors.
- Clinical primary hypothyroidism is defined as TSH concentrations above the reference range and FT4 concentrations below the reference range.
- Mild or subclinical hypothyroidism, which is commonly regarded as a sign of early thyroid failure, is defined by TSH concentrations above the reference range and FT4 concentrations within the normal range.
- Differences in iodine status affect the prevalence of hypothyroidism; this occurs more frequently both in populations with a relatively high-iodine intake and in severely iodine-deficient populations.
- Hypothyroidism occurs more frequently in women, in individuals over age 65 years.
- Hypothyroidism is more common in patients with autoimmune diseases, such as type 1 diabetes, autoimmune gastric atrophy, and celiac disease.
- It can occur as a part of multiple autoimmune endocrinopathies.
- Individuals with Downs' syndrome or Turners' syndrome have an increased risk of hypothyroidism.

Diagnosis

Primary hypothyroidism is defined by TSH concentrations above the laboratory reference range and FT4 concentrations below the reference range.

The upper limit of TSH reference ranges typically increases with age in adults.

Treatment

Levothyroxine monotherapy, taken on an empty stomach, is the treatment of choice each morning.
Sodium L-thyroxine (Eltroxin, Synthroid): *Supplied*: Tablets 25, 50, 75, 88, 100, 112, 125, 150, 175, 200, and 300 µg. *Dosage*: Less than 60 years with no cardiac disease start with 100 µg/day. Assess adequacy of dose with sensitive TSH in 6–8 weeks (elderly start with 25 µg/day and ↑ every 6–8 weeks). The recommended daily dose in overt hypothyroidism is 1.5–1.8 µg/kg of body weight.

- For elderly commence with 1.5–1.8 µg/kg of body weight.
- In patients with coronary artery disease, the starting dose is generally 12.5–25.0 µg/day and should be gradually increased on the basis of symptoms and TSH concentrations.
- Warn the patient that initiation of thyroid hormone replacement may precipitate angina or palpitations.
- A proportion of patients treated with levothyroxine have persistent complaints despite reaching the biochemical therapy targets.
- The question of whether levothyroxine treatment is sufficient for all patients or whether alternative therapies (e.g. combination with liothyronine preparations) could be adopted is debatable.

Myxedema Coma

- Severe hypothyroidism with unresponsiveness, hypothermia, hypotension, hypoventilation, hyponatremia, and bradycardia.
- Precipitating illness or event is usually present.
- Treat promptly without waiting for laboratory confirmation.

Management
- *Thyroid hormone replacement*: 500 µg of sodium levothyroxine IV bolus, then 50–100 µg IV bolus qd until oral therapy can be substituted.
- *Respiratory support*: Hypoventilation may lead to carbon dioxide (CO_2) retention and central nervous system (CNS) unresponsiveness. Monitor arterial blood gases (ABGs) and provide intubation and mechanical ventilation if indicated.
- Hypotension may respond poorly to pressor agents until thyroid hormone is replaced. Carry out volume replacement cautiously with isotonic fluids.
- *Hypothermia*: Warm passively with blankets.

- Hyponatremia is caused by impaired free water clearance. Usually corrected by L-thyroxine therapy and fluid restriction. If severe, may require partial correction with hypertonic saline.
- Hypoglycemia is rare. Correct with 5% dextrose/water IV.
- Glucocorticoids are given to cover the possibility of concomitant adrenocorticotropic hormone (ACTH) or adrenal insufficiency. Give hydrocortisone sodium succinate (Solu-Cortef) 100 mg IV q 8 hours.
- Identify and treat any precipitating illnesses.

Hyperthyroidism

- Thyrotoxicosis is a clinical syndrome caused by excess circulating thyroid hormones. A review article by De Leo et al. provides useful information. Hyperthyroidism is characterized by increased thyroid hormone synthesis and secretion from the thyroid gland.

Causes

- Graves' disease
- *Thyroiditis*: Subacute (pseudogranulomatous, de Quervain's), silent (painless), and radiation-induced
- Toxic nodular goiter and multinodular goiter
- Toxic solitary thyroid adenoma (Plummer's disease)
- *Exogenous thyroid hormone ingestion*: Iatrogenic, factitious
- *Excess TSH production*: Pituitary adenoma, trophoblastic tumors
- *Ectopic T4 production*: Struma ovarii, metastatic follicular thyroid cancer
- Factitious ingestion of excess thyroid hormones.

Symptoms

- Heat intolerance, excessive sweating
- Nervousness, irritability
- Weight loss with normal or ↑ed appetite
- Palpitations
- Tiredness, tremulousness
- Proximal muscle weakness
- Diarrhea
- Scanty or absent periods
- Dyspnea on exertion
- Elderly patients often present differently with lethargy, atrial fibrillation, congestive heart failure (CHF), weight loss with anorexia, muscle weakness, and wasting. The absence of adrenergic and hyperkinetic symptoms is sometimes called apathetic or masked hyperthyroidism.

- Tachycardia, hyperkinesis, agitation, goiter, fine tremor, brisk reflexes, warm-moist skin, proximal muscle wasting, and onycholysis (separation of the nail from its bed distally).
- *Noninfiltrative eye signs*: Lid lag, lid retraction, and stare can occur in all hyperthyroid patients. Infiltrative signs: Periorbital edema, chemosis, conjunctivitis, exophthalmos, and ophthalmoplegia usually occur only in Graves' disease.
- Pretibial myxedema is a less common feature of Graves' disease; the skin appears brown and indurated.

Management of Graves' Disease

Graves' disease is the most common cause of hyperthyroidism, with a female to male ratio of 8 to 1. It is distinguished from other forms of hyperthyroidism by the presence of diffuse thyroid enlargement, ophthalmopathy, and occasionally pretibial myxedema. Ophthalmopathy is present in 20-40% of patients with recent onset Graves' disease and may develop before hyperthyroidism, at the onset of hyperthyroidism, or years later, after the patient's hyperthyroidism has been treated. Graves' disease is an autoimmune disease mediated by thyroid-stimulating immunoglobulins (TSAb or TSI). These antibodies recognize the TSH receptor as antigen, attach to the receptor, and activate the thyroid follicular cell. At present the treatment of Graves' disease is directed at the thyroid gland rather than at the basic immunologic process (Houlden).

- Antithyroid drugs remain useful. They are not generally used long term in toxic nodular goiter, because of the high relapse rate of thyrotoxicosis after discontinuation.
- Radioactive iodine therapy, surgery.
- Beta-blockers are used in symptomatic thyrotoxicosis, and might be the only treatment needed for thyrotoxicosis not caused by excessive production and release of the thyroid hormones.
- Thyroid storm and hyperthyroidism in pregnancy and during the postpartum period are special circumstances that need careful assessment and treatment.

Radioactive iodine therapy: It is the treatment of choice for most adults with Graves' disease. The most commonly used isotope is ^{131}I in a dose of 4-10 mCi (150-370 megaBq). The dose is determined by the size of the thyroid and the RAIU. The response to RAI is slow and patients may remain hyperthyroid for 3 months. Occasionally, patients require a second or third treatment if they are still hyperthyroid 6-12 months after RAI. Patients with severe hyperthyroidism, a cardiac condition, or an elderly age should be rendered euthyroid with antithyroid drugs and beta-blockers before treatment with RAI, as radiation thyroiditis may occur with leakage of stored hormone and exacerbation of the hyperthyroidism. Antithyroid drugs should be stopped 4-7 days before RAI and may be restarted 3 days afterward.

There is no ↑ed incidence of thyroid cancer, leukemia, or birth defects after doses of RAI used to treat hyperthyroidism. The most common complication of RAI is the development of hypothyroidism. Patients must be monitored lifelong and started on thyroid hormone replacement as soon as they become biochemically hypothyroid.

Propylthiouracil (PTU) and methimazole (tapazole): They block thyroid peroxidase and inhibit thyroid hormone synthesis. Both agents have weak immunosuppressive effects. PTU also inhibits the extrathyroidal conversion of T4 to T3. The half-life of PTU is 1-2 hours whereas methimazole is 6-8 hours. The major reason to choose antithyroid drug therapy is that a spontaneous remission of Graves' may occur, allowing drug therapy to be discontinued and leaving the patient with normal thyroid function. Remissions occur in 30-50% of patients treated for 1 year. Factors believed to favor the probability of a remission include female sex, recent onset of symptoms, mild or moderate severity of symptoms, and modest thyroid enlargement.

Propylthiouracil: Supplied: Tablet 50, 100, and 250 mg. *Dosage*: Initial dose is 100-200 mg 3-4 times a day. The larger doses are given to patient with more severe clinical hyperthyroidism and/or a large goiter. After the patient becomes euthyroid (usually 6-8 weeks), taper dose by one-third every 4-6 weeks to a maintenance dose of 50 mg once daily.

Methimazole (tapazole): Supplied: Tablets 5, 10 mg. *Dosage*: Initial dose is 5-10 mg tid. Maintenance dose is 5-15 mg once daily.

Carbimazole (Neo-Mercazole) (UK): *Supplied*: Tablets 5 mg. *Dosage*: Initial dose is 30-60 mg once daily. Maintenance dose is 5-15 mg once daily.

Continue therapy for 12-18 months, then discontinue. The vast majority of relapses occur with 3-6 months of cessation of therapy, at which time alternative treatment is recommended.

Adverse effects: Most common complications are dermatologic (pruritus, urticaria). It may subside with no treatment. Generally do not require discontinuation of drug therapy. Agranulocytosis is the most serious side effect. It occurs in 0.2% of patients, usually within the first 3 months. It is an idiosyncratic reaction and not dose-related. Patients should be instructed to report immediately any symptoms suggestive of agranulocytosis, such as fever or sore throat. The drug should be stopped immediately and the white blood cell (WBC) checked. Routine blood counts are not helpful.

Surgery: Subtotal thyroidectomy is reserved for children who are noncompliant or cannot be controlled with antithyroid drugs, and patients with large goiters with pressure symptoms. The patient should be made euthyroid preoperatively with an antithyroid drug. Potassium iodide (SSKI) 1-2 drops (PO tid) is usually added for 2 weeks before surgery. This ensures that the patient is euthyroid and also reduces the vascularity of the gland. Patients who cannot tolerate antithyroid drugs can be managed preoperatively with high doses of propranolol.

Beta-blockers are useful in controlling the adrenergic manifestations of hyperthyroidism such as tachycardia.

Dosage: Propranolol 20–40 mg qid. The dose should be titrated to produce the desired symptoms.

If blockers are contraindicated, verapamil has a role; the drug is more effective than dihydropyridine calcium (Ca) antagonists because it has a bradycardic effect; also diltiazem may prove useful to reduce heart rates.

Management of Toxic Multinodular Goiter

Durante et al. provide an excellent JAMA review article.

Antithyroid drugs have no role in the long-term treatment of a multinodular goiter, as spontaneous remissions rarely occur. The treatment of choice is RAI. As with Graves' disease, elderly patients and patients with heart disease should be rendered euthyroid with antithyroid drugs before RAI. Large doses of RAI 10–30 mCi (370–1,110 megaBq) are given because the thyroid uptake of ^{131}I is usually only moderately ↑ed Occasionally, with a large gland causing tracheal compression, surgery is the treatment of choice.

Management of Toxic Solitary Adenoma

Lobectomy is the treatment of choice in a younger patient. In an older person, RAI may be indicated. The dose used should be large [20–30 mCi (740–1,110 megaBq)] to destroy the nodule.

Thyroid Storm

- Severe, life-threatening hyperthyroidism.
- Usually develops in an undiagnosed hyperthyroid patient who has another major stress or illness (i.e. infection, injury, or surgery).
- Clinical manifestations include fever, tachycardia, nausea, vomiting, abdominal pain, and cardiac failure.
- Features of the precipitating illness (i.e. fever, tachycardia) may be difficult to distinguish from thyroid storm.
- Free T4 and T3 are ↑ed, but no more so than in "ordinary" hyperthyroidism.

Management includes general supportive measures (IV fluids, glucose for hypoglycemia, acetaminophen, and cooling blanket for fever—avoid aspirin as it displaces thyroid hormones from their binding proteins) and antithyroid drugs, which may be given PO or by nasogastric tube. PTU is theoretically preferable to methimazole as it also inhibits extrathyroidal production of T3.

Propylthiouracil: Dosage: 300–400 mg PO initially followed by 250 mg q 6 hours.

Methimazole: Dosage: 30–40 mg PO initially followed by 20–30 mg PO q 8 hours. After stabilization, the dosages of either preparation should be ↓ed to the usual ones used for treatment of hyperthyroidism.

Iodide is the most effective agent for lowering serum T4 acutely. It inhibits release of thyroid hormones. Iodide therapy should be initiated 1–2 hours after starting antithyroid medications as the iodide could theoretically be used to synthesize additional thyroid hormone, thereby worsening the clinical state. If the patient is unable to take oral medications, 1 g of sodium iodide can be administered as a continuous infusion over 12 hours q 12 hours.

Lugol's solution: 10 drops PO q 8 hours or SSKI 5 drops PO q 8 hours can also be used.

Propranolol: 40–80 mg PO q 6 hours can be used to block the catecholamine effects. If the patient is nauseated, may give 1–2 mg IV over 5 minutes q 4–6 hours with cardiac monitoring.

Dexamethasone: 2 mg IV q 6 hours is recommended for 24–48 hours as high doses of glucocorticoids block the peripheral conversion of T4 to T3.

Sodium ipodate: It is an iodide-containing oral cholecystographic agent that impairs the conversion of T4 to T3. It may be given instead of iodide in a dosage of 1 g PO once daily.

Subacute Thyroiditis

It is also called pseudogranulomatous, de Quervain's, or giant-cell thyroiditis. The most common cause is thyroid pain. It is believed to be viral in etiology although the exact causative agent is unknown. A history of preceding upper respiratory infection is common. It presents with abrupt onset of neck pain, malaise, myalgias, and fever. Clinical manifestations of hyperthyroidism occur in 50% of patients. Serum T4 and T3 levels may be ↑ed due to release of preformed hormone. The erythrocyte sedimentation rate (ESR) is usually ↑ed. RAIU is low in the acute stage due to follicular cell destruction. In most patients, symptoms subside over 2–6 weeks. Transient hypothyroidism occurs in 15–25% of cases. Permanent hypothyroidism occurs in less than 10%.

Treatment: Salicylates (650 mg qid) or other nonsteroidal agents can be used for pain relief. Prednisone (30–40 mg once daily) can be used for severe pain in patients unresponsive to salicylates. Treatment should be continued for 2–3 weeks and then tapered. Propranolol (20–40 mg tid to qid) may be used for relief of symptoms of hyperthyroidism. Antithyroid drugs are not indicated and do not work. Transient hypothyroidism may be treated with temporary thyroid hormone replacement.

Silent Thyroiditis (Painless Thyroiditis)

Inflammatory disorder characterized by abrupt onset of hyperthyroid symptoms and a painless, nontender goiter. The etiology is uncertain but is probably a form of autoimmune thyroid disease. Treatment is the same as subacute thyroiditis except that salicylates are omitted. Silent thyroiditis occurs in 3-5% of women in the postpartum period and may recur with subsequent pregnancies.

Solitary Thyroid Nodules

Most thyroid nodules are benign. The goal is to select for surgery those patients whose nodules are at risk for malignancy, and to avoid unnecessary operations on nodules that are likely to be benign. In some clinical situations, carcinoma is more likely to be present and a more aggressive approach is justified. These include:
- History of therapeutic irradiation to the head, neck, or chest
- Age less than 40 years
- Male sex
- Family history of thyroid carcinoma [i.e. medullary thyroid carcinoma with multiple endocrine neoplasia (MEN) type II]
- Compression of adjacent structures (i.e. trachea, esophagus, vocal cord or sympathetic nerves, superior vena cava)
- Palpable regional lymph nodes and/or abnormalities in distant sites (i.e. lung, bone).

Investigation:
- Fine-needle aspiration (FNA) biopsy is the initial procedure in the evaluation of thyroid nodules in many centers. Requires persons skilled in the technique and in cytopathology. Follicular lesions pose a problem as it is difficult to distinguish benign from malignant ones. Flowchart 26.2 outlines management of the solitary thyroid nodule based on FNA biopsy as the initial diagnostic test.
- *Thyroid radioisotope scan*: The most commonly used isotopes are ^{123}I, ^{131}I, and 99m-technetium. Nodules appear hypofunctioning (*cold* or *cool*), isofunctioning (*warm*), or hyperfunctioning (*hot*). Thyroid cancer cells do not trap radionuclides as well as normal thyroid cells and appear hypofunctioning on scanning. However, most cold nodules are still benign (only 10-15% are malignant).
- *Thyroid ultrasound*: Nodules are classified as solid, cystic, or mixed solid/cystic. Malignancy is three- to fourfold more frequent in solid compared to cystic nodules.

Flowchart 26.2: Investigation of the solitary thyroid nodule.

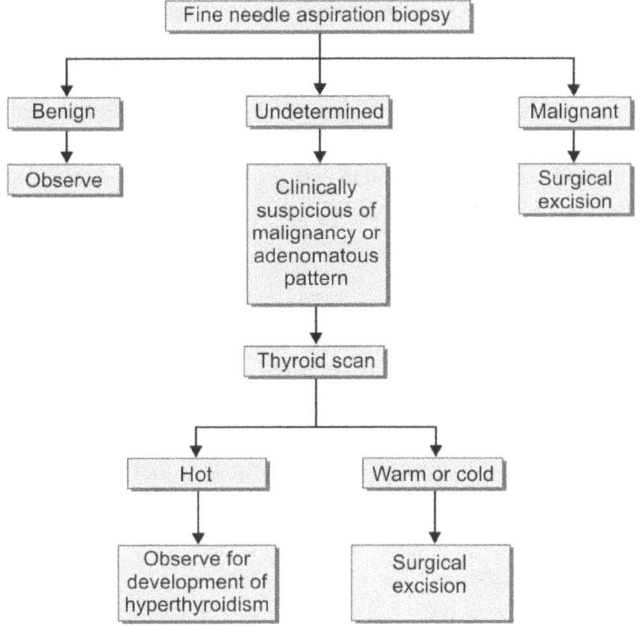

ADRENAL DISEASES

Adrenal Insufficiency

Causes

- *Primary (Addison's disease)*: Autoimmune (most common cause); infectious [tuberculosis, fungal, cytomegalovirus, and acquired immunodeficiency syndrome (AIDS)]; infiltrative (amyloidosis, sarcoidosis, metastatic carcinoma, and hemochromatosis); hemorrhage [anticoagulants, disseminated intravascular coagulation (DIC)]; iatrogenic: drugs that block steroid hormone synthesis (ketoconazole, mitotane, metyrapone, and aminoglutethimide).
- *Secondary*: Hypothalamic–pituitary–adrenal axis suppression following exogenous glucocorticoids; pituitary and hypothalamic lesions.

Clinical Manifestations

- Weight loss, fatigue, anorexia, nausea, vomiting, and postural hypotension.
- Hyperpigmentation with primary adrenal insufficiency (particularly in the creases of the hand, over the knuckles, in the axillae, over the gingival and buccal mucosa, in the areola of the breasts, and in the perineum). Scars formed after the onset of adrenal insufficiency may also be pigmented.

- Autoimmune Addison's disease may be associated with other autoimmune diseases, such as Hashimoto's thyroiditis, pernicious anemia, vitiligo, hypoparathyroidism, premature ovarian or testicular failure, and diabetes mellitus.
- Symptoms and signs of other pituitary hormone deficiencies may be present [e.g. luteinizing hormone (LH), diabetes-stimulating hormone (FSH), growth hormone (GH), and TSH] with secondary adrenal insufficiency.

Laboratory Findings

- Hyponatremia, hyperkalemia (usually in the range of 5.4–5.9 mEq (mmol)/L), and mild metabolic acidosis.
- Increased blood urea or blood urea nitrogen (BUN).
- Low or normal blood glucose.
- Normocytic normochromic anemia, lymphocytosis, and eosinophilia.
- Hypercalcemia (infrequently).

Diagnostic Procedures

- Treatment should not be delayed in the seriously ill patient with acute adrenal insufficiency. A plasma cortisol and ACTH level should be drawn for future interpretation. A low plasma cortisol and an ↑ed plasma ACTH level are diagnostic of primary adrenal insufficiency.
- Short ACTH test is a useful screening test if the index of suspicion is low (i.e. weak, tired, and normally pigmented subject in whom one wishes to rule out Addison's disease). Administer 250 μg of synthetic ACTH (Cosyntropin, Cortrosyn) IV and draw plasma cortisol levels at 0, 30, and 60 minutes. The normal increment in plasma cortisol is more than 7 μg/dL (200 nmol/L), and the absolute level achieved should be more than 20 μg/dL (500 nmol/L). A normal response rules out primary adrenal insufficiency. Most patients with secondary adrenal insufficiency do not respond normally because of secondary atrophy of the adrenal cortex.
- Plasma ACTH levels, if available, are an easy way to differentiate primary and secondary adrenal insufficiency. Levels are ↑ed in primary and low in secondary adrenal insufficiency.
- Prolonged ACTH stimulation test is useful for differentiating primary and secondary adrenal insufficiency when an assay for plasma ACTH is not available or cause is uncertain. Collect a baseline 24-hour urine free cortisol and creatinine. Infuse synthetic ACTH 250 μg in 500 mL of 0.9% sodium chloride (NaCl) over 8 hours (8 AM to 4 PM) on 3 consecutive days with concomitant 24-hour urine collections for free cortisol and creatinine. Also, draw serum cortisol levels at 8 AM and 8 PM daily. When adrenal insufficiency is strongly suspected, the patient should receive coverage with dexamethasone 0.5 mg bid during the test. Patients

with primary adrenal insufficiency have no ↑ in their serum and urinary cortisol levels. Patients with secondary adrenal insufficiency exhibit a gradual, usually stepwise, ↑ in their plasma and urinary cortisol levels due to reactivation of their anatomically intact adrenal glands. Levels ↑ed 2-3 times baseline by the 3rd day. The daily urinary creatinine should be ± 10% to ensure complete and consistent urine collections.
- Insulin tolerance test is useful for confirming the diagnosis of suspected secondary adrenal insufficiency; assessing the functioning of the hypothalamic-pituitary-adrenal axis following long-term glucocorticoid therapy to determine whether glucocorticoids can be stopped safely (glucocorticoid therapy should be held for 36 hours prior to the insulin tolerance test). After overnight fasting, the patient is injected with 0.15 U of short-acting insulin/kg IV bolus. Plasma cortisol levels are collected at 0, 30, 60, and 90 minutes. A physician should be in attendance and glucose must be available for IV administration if severe symptoms of hypoglycemia occur. An adequate degree of hypoglycemia must be obtained [blood glucose ≤40 mg/dL (2.2 mmol/L)]. A normal cortisol response is an ↑ of more than or equal to 7 μg/dL (200 nmol/L) with a peak level of more than 20 μg/dL (550 nmol/L). An inadequate response is seen with primary and secondary adrenal insufficiency.
- Adrenal calcifications may be seen on plain films of the abdomen in patients with primary adrenal insufficiency from tuberculosis.

Treatment of Acute Adrenal Insufficiency

- Therapy should be instituted immediately. Diagnostic investigations, with the exception of a serum cortisol and plasma ACTH, should be postponed until the patient is completely well.
- *Volume repletion*: Give 1-2 L 0.9% NaCl over the first 2 hours, followed by 3-5 L over the following 24 hours.
- *Glucocorticoid therapy*: 100 mg hydrocortisone sodium succinate (Solu-Cortef) IV bolus followed by 100 mg IV q 8 hours. The dosage should be ↓ed by 50% each day thereafter until the maintenance dosage is achieved, assuming the patient's course is uncomplicated.
- Mineralocorticoid therapy is not required initially since cortisol in large doses (>100 mg/day) has enough salt-retaining activity. However, when the dose is ↓ed below this level, treatment with fludrocortisone (Florinef) should be started in patients with primary adrenal insufficiency.
- Precipitating factors should be corrected, such as infection, trauma, surgery, myocardial infarction, or noncompliance with glucocorticoid therapy.
- General supportive measures should be provided, such as treatment of persistent electrolyte abnormalities, hypoglycemia, hypothermia, and hypotension refractory to IV fluids and glucocorticoids (Houlden).

Management of Chronic Adrenal Insufficiency

- Maintenance of glucocorticoid replacement may be given with one of the following:
  - Hydrocortisone 20 mg on waking and 10 mg at 4–6 PM.
  - Prednisone 5 mg on waking and 2.5 mg at 4–6 PM.
  - Cortisone acetate 25 mg on waking and 12.5 mg at 4–6 PM.

  Patients should be told to double their dose of glucocorticoid with a mild illness. If they cannot take their steroid by mouth, it should be given parenterally. Patients should wear a medical identification bracelet or necklace giving details of their condition.
- Maintenance mineralocorticoid replacement is usually given with fludrocortisone acetate (Florinef) in doses of 0.05–0.2 mg qd in patient with primary adrenal insufficiency. If the dose is excessive, edema, hypokalemia, and hypertension may result.
- *Minor surgery*: 100 mg of hydrocortisone hemisuccinate intramuscular (IM) or 100 mg of hydrocortisone sodium succinate IV should be given with the premedication.
- *Major surgery*: The steroid regimen outlined for acute adrenal crisis should be adopted.

Cushing's Syndrome

A review by Longo and editor Loriaux in the N Engl J Med focuses on the problems introduced into the diagnosis and differential diagnosis of Cushing's syndrome by the obesity epidemic (approximately 10% worldwide) and uses the antianabolic changes of excess cortisol to separate patients with Cushing's syndrome from obese patients with the insulin-resistant metabolic syndrome.

- Cushing's syndrome is indeed rare and caution is needed in differentiating from metabolic syndrome among obese persons to avoid expensive investigations and traumatic unnecessary surgery.
- The metabolic syndrome caused by glucocorticoid hypersecretion can be differentiated from the obesity-associated metabolic syndrome with the use of a careful assessment of Albright's antianabolic effects of cortisol. These effects are:
  - Osteopenia
  - Thin skin, and
  - *Ecchymoses*—Present in patients with Cushing's syndrome but not in patients with simple obesity (Loriaux).

Clinical depression increases urinary free cortisol excretion, levels may reach 60 µg/day (healthy adults 8–51 µg/day) in a patient presenting with obesity, hypertension, type 2 diabetes mellitus hirsutism, thin skin, osteopenia, and ecchymoses. Elevated urinary free cortisol level more than or equal to 62 µg/day, the probability of Cushing's syndrome is 100% (Loriaux).

- The commonly used dexamethasone-suppression test, no longer has a role in the evaluation and treatment of patients with Cushing's syndrome (Loriaux). Three biochemical tests are needed:
  - Urinary free cortisol is the test that confirms the clinical diagnosis of Cushing's syndrome (Loriaux).
  - *Plasma corticotropin*: To separate corticotropin-dependent from corticotropin-independent causes of Cushing's syndrome and to separate eutopic from ectopic secretion of corticotropin (Loriaux).
  - *Plasma cortisol measurements have one use*: Determining the success or failure of transsphenoidal microadenomectomy or adrenalectomy (Loriaux).

Urinary free cortisol excretion is the test that confirms the clinical diagnosis of Cushing's syndrome.

Causes

- *Adrenocorticotropic hormone dependent*: Pituitary adenoma (Cushing's disease) (70%); ectopic ACTH syndrome (10%); and ectopic corticotropin releasing hormone (rare).
- *Adrenocorticotropic hormone independent*: Adrenal adenoma (10%); adrenal carcinoma (10%); micronodular adrenal disease (rare); and iatrogenic (exogenous glucocorticoids).

Clinical Manifestations

- Truncal obesity, facial rounding (moon facies)
- Proximal muscle weakness
- Thin skin with purple striae, ecchymoses, and facial plethora
- Osteoporosis
- Hypertension
- Glucose intolerance or diabetes mellitus
- Nephrolithiasis
- Oligomenorrhea, acne, hirsutism, and loss of libido
- Psychologic disturbances (depression, emotional lability).

Treatment

- *Cushing's disease*: Transsphenoidal surgery.
- *Ectopic ACTH syndrome*: Treatment of the underlying tumor if possible; correction of hypokalemia with potassium (K) replacement and spironolactone; drugs that block steroid synthesis: ketoconazole, metyrapone, and aminoglutethimide, and o,p'-DDD (mitotane).
- *Adrenal tumors*: Adrenalectomy.

Primary Hyperaldosteronism

Autonomous overproduction of aldosterone occurs in about 2% of patients with hypertension.

Causes

- Aldosterone-producing adenoma (85%).
- Bilateral adrenocortical hyperplasia (15%).
- Dexamethasone-suppressible hyperaldosteronism (rare).
- Adrenocortical carcinoma (rare).

Clinical Manifestations

- Hypertension may be resistant to usual antihypertensive medications. It is rarely malignant.
- Potassium depletion may produce muscle weakness, easy fatigability, polyuria, and polydipsia.

Investigations

- Serum K less than 3.5 mEq (mmol)/L after the patient has remained off diuretics for 3 weeks and adhered to a high Na diet [>120 mEq (mmol)/day] for more than or equal to 3 days merits further investigation.
- Twenty four-hour urinary aldosterone excretion is usually ↑ed in primary hyperaldosteronism.
- *Captopril suppression test*: 25 mg of captopril is given PO. The patient remains seated, and plasma renin activity (PRA) and plasma aldosterone are drawn 2 hours later. Plasma aldosterone does not suppress less than 15 ng/dL (415 pmol/L) in patients with primary hyperaldosteronism.
- *Saline suppression test*: 2 L of 0.9% NaCl are infused over 4 hours with the patient recumbent. Plasma aldosterone does not suppress less than 8.5–10 ng/dL (235–275 pmol/L) with primary hyperaldosteronism.
- *Furosemide stimulation test*: 40 mg of furosemide is given IV and the patient lies down for 1 hour to promote diuresis, followed by standing for 2 hours. PRA fails to rise and remains less than 1.7 ng/mL/h (0.47 ng/L/s).

Differentiating Adrenal Adenoma from Bilateral Hyperplasia

- *Eight AM plasma 18-hydroxycorticosterone levels on a high-sodium (Na) diet*: More than 100 ng/dL are usually found with an adenoma and less than 100 ng/dL with hyperplasia.
- *Plasma aldosterone levels after 4 hours of upright posture*: ↓ with an aldosterone-producing adenoma and ↑ with bilateral hyperplasia.

Procedures to Localize an Adrenal Adenoma

- Computed tomography (CT) or magnetic resonance imaging (MRI) scan of the adrenals.
- Adrenal vein catheterization with aldosterone and cortisol sampling.
- ^{131}I-iodocholesterol scanning.

Treatment

- *Bilateral adrenal hyperplasia*: Spironolactone (Aldactone) 100–400 mg qd or amiloride 10–20 mg qd restores K balance. Hypertension may be treated with Ca channel-blocking agents or angiotensin-converting enzyme inhibitors.
- *Aldosterone-producing adenoma*: Unilateral adrenalectomy.

Pheochromocytoma

It is a tumor of chromaffin tissue that produces excessive catecholamines. 90% are found in the adrenals. Ten percent are extra-adrenal, usually in the organ of Zuckerkandl, located at the bifurcation of the abdominal aorta. Ten percent are familial and may be part of type II MEN syndrome. Ten percent are bilateral and 10% are malignant (see Chapter 1).

ANTERIOR PITUITARY DISEASES

Hyperprolactinemia

Clinical Manifestations

- *Women*: Amenorrhea, galactorrhea, and infertility.
- *Men*: Decreased libido, impotence, and infertility.

Differential Diagnosis

- *Physiologic*: Pregnancy, postpartum, newborn, and stress.
- *Pituitary disorders*: Prolactin-secreting pituitary tumor, acromegaly, and empty sella syndrome.
- *Hypothalamic disorders*: Craniopharyngioma, metastatic disease, pituitary stalk section, or compression.
- Hypothyroidism.
- Chronic renal failure.
- Liver disease.
- Chest wall or spinal cord lesions.
- *Drugs*: Phenothiazines, tricyclic antidepressants, reserpine, α-methyldopa, estrogen therapy, oral contraceptives, metoclopramide, H_2 blockers, opiates, and verapamil.

Workup

- *Serum prolactin*: Values more than 150 ng/mL (µg/L) suggests a pituitary tumor. Modest elevations [30–100 ng/mL (µg/L)] often present a diagnostic challenge.
- Exclude pregnancy, estrogen administration, hypothyroidism, and drug-induced hyperprolactinemia.
- *Computed tomography or MRI scan*: Perform if no cause is identified. Indicated even with mild hyperprolactinemia since tumors may be poorly functioning.
- Assess estrogen status in amenorrheic women with serum estradiol or response to medroxyprogesterone acetate (Provera) 10 mg qd for 5 days. Assess gonadal status in men by clinical history and serum testosterone.

Therapy of Prolactinomas

- *Women with hyperprolactinemia without evidence of an adenoma, or with a microprolactinoma (<10 mm) and not desiring pregnancy*: Less than 10% of microadenomas grow the size of macroadenomas; less than or equal to 30% disappear spontaneously. Close follow-up with no drug treatment is an option. Many patients are started on bromocriptine to reduce the risk of osteoporosis associated with estrogen deficiency.
- *Women with hyperprolactinemia or a microprolactinoma desiring pregnancy or restoration of menstruation*: Bromocriptine (Parlodel), a dopamine agonist, restores prolactin to normal in 80–85% of patients with microadenomas. Galactorrhea usually ceases in a few weeks, and ovulatory menses are established within the first 2 months of treatment. *Supplied*: Tablets 2.5, 5 mg. *Dosage*: Start with 1.25 mg given with food at bedtime to minimize the side effects of nausea, vomiting, and postural hypotension. Gradually ↑ the dose until milk secretion has ceased, or in the case of menstrual dysfunction until the menstrual cycle has returned to normal. *Transsphenoidal surgery*: Initial cure rate of 70–80% with a late recurrence rate of less than or equal to 20–30%.
- *Pregnant women with a microprolactinoma*: Discontinue bromocriptine once pregnancy is confirmed. Follow patient clinically throughout pregnancy. Complications occur in less than 5% of patients and may be safely treated by reinstitution of bromocriptine.
- *Women with a macroprolactinoma (>10 mm)*: Bromocriptine reduces prolactin to normal in 70–80% and causes tumor ↓ to less than one-half of the original size in 50%. Surgery cure rate less than 50% with a late recurrence rate of 20–50%. Generally reserved for patients unresponsive to bromocriptine or needing tumor debulking. Radiotherapy or proton beam therapy is usually reserved for bromocriptine nonresponders not cured by surgery.

- Pregnant women with a macroprolactinoma have a 15% risk of tumor enlargement. Monitor visual fields monthly. Reinstitute bromocriptine if tumor enlarges. Surgery may be used for nonresponders.
- *Men with a microprolactinoma or a macroprolactinoma*: Management is similar to that for women. With bromocriptine therapy, testosterone levels ↑ as prolactin ↓. It may take 3-6 months for restoration of normal sexual function.

Acromegaly

The clinical syndrome caused by excess secretion of GH.

Clinical Manifestations

- Headache, visual field defects (bitemporal hemianopsia).
- Growth of hands, feet, and head. Increase in ring, glove, or shoe size. Ask for old photographs for comparison.
- Coarsening of facial features, skin tags (fibroma moluscum), ↑ed perspiration.
- Hepatomegaly, cardiomegaly, and thyromegaly.
- Arthralgias and arthritis, carpal tunnel syndrome.
- Glucose intolerance, hypertension.
- Amenorrhea, ↓ libido.

Diagnosis

The diagnostic workup of acromegaly is outlined in Flowchart 26.3.
- *Insulin-like growth factor-1 (IGF-1; somatomedin-C) level*: ↑ in acromegaly. Acts as a mediator of some of the effects of GH and integrates GH secretion.
- *Glucose suppression test with GH levels*: 100 g PO glucose load is given, and GH levels are measured at baseline, 1 and 2 hours. Normally, administration of glucose suppresses GH secretion. In acromegaly, the tumor is autonomous and does not respond to hyperglycemia. About 20-30% shows no change in GH levels, 20-40% show a paradoxical ↑, and 5-7% show suppression but not to normal levels.
- *Thyrotropin-releasing hormone stimulation test*: Increase in GH in response to TRH 200 µg IV bolus is seen in 80-90% of patients.
- Computed tomography scan or MRI of sella turcica.
- *Prolactin*: Excess secretion is found in 30% of patients with acromegaly.
- *Plasma growth hormone-releasing hormone (GHRH) levels*: Occasionally needed to identify the very rare case of acromegaly caused by excess GHRH secretion.

Flowchart 26.3: Diagnosis of acromegaly.

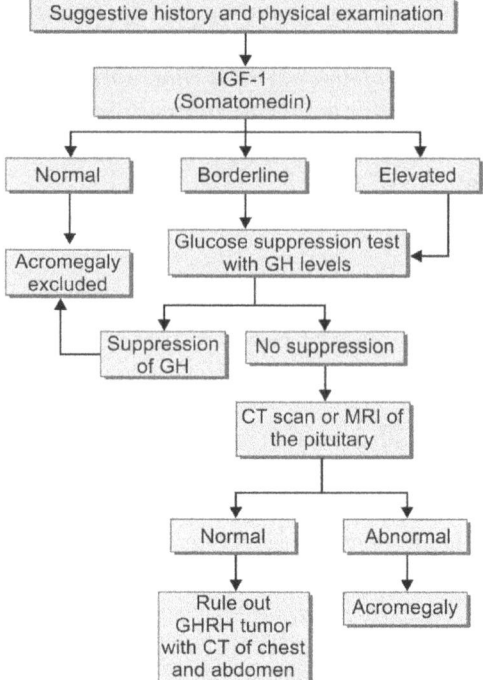

(CT, computed tomography; GHRH, growth hormone-releasing hormone; IGF, insulin-like growth factor; MRI, magnetic resonance imaging)

Management

- Surgery results in improvement in less than or equal to 90%. In patients whose GH levels return to normal, recurrence occurs in 5%. With incomplete tumor removal, the recurrence rate is more than 50%. Patients must be followed indefinitely after treatment to assess the efficacy of control of GH secretion and tumor growth. Typically, patients are evaluated 3 months postoperatively with measurement of IGF-1 levels and performance of a glucose suppression test. TRH testing may also be performed if it was abnormal before treatment. CT scanning or MRI is used to follow tumor size. Visual field should be followed, particularly in patients who had abnormalities on baseline studies.
- External irradiation is used to treat residual tumor from surgery and for inoperable patients. Annual assessment is necessary as late hypopituitarism can occur.
- Bromocriptine is useful for cases resistant to surgery and radiotherapy. Used in doses of 10–20 mg qd with meals.

POSTERIOR PITUITARY DISORDERS

Polyuria

It is defined as a persistent 24-hour urinary volume more than 2.5 L.

Causes

- Osmotic diuresis secondary to excessive solute secretion (i.e. hyperglycemia) or other agents (i.e. mannitol, loop diuretics).
- Primary polydipsia with suppression of arginine vasopressin (AVP) [antidiuretic hormone (ADH)] by excessive water intake.
- Central (neurogenic) diabetes insipidus with absolute or partial deficiency of AVP.
  - *Idiopathic*: Familial, sporadic.
  - *Secondary*: Trauma (head injury, surgery to hypothalamic-pituitary region), neoplasms (hypothalamic, pituitary, craniopharyngioma, and metastatic), granulomas (sarcoid, histiocytosis), infection (meningitis, encephalitis), and external radiation.
- Nephrogenic diabetes insipidus with resistance to AVP in the kidney.
  - *Idiopathic*: Familial, sporadic.
  - *Secondary*: Metabolic (hypercalcemia, hypokalemia), toxic (lithium, demeclocycline, methoxyflurane, colchicine, amphotericin, vinblastine, gentamicin, and methicillin), vascular (sickle cell disease or trait), infectious (pyelonephritis), postobstructive, and other (sarcoidosis, polycystic kidney, and amyloidosis).

Differential Diagnosis

In principle, it should be easy to differentiate the various causes of polyuria. A comparison of urinary osmolality during dehydration and after the administration of aqueous vasopressin should reveal a rapid ↑ in osmolality only in patients with central diabetes insipidus. In patients with primary polydipsia, urinary osmolality should ↑ normally in response to dehydration. However, these distinctions are not always clear because of a number of factors:

- Chronic polyuria of any etiology interferes with the maintenance of the renal medullary concentration gradient. This washout effect diminishes the maximal concentrating ability of the kidney.
- Most patients with central diabetes insipidus maintain a small capacity to secrete AVP during severe dehydration.
- Many patients with acquired nephrogenic diabetes insipidus have an incomplete deficit in AVP action and will concentrate their urine during severe dehydration.

Indirect Testing

Arginine vasopressin secretion is indirectly assessed through changes in urinary osmolality during dehydration and after vasopressin administration.
- The patient is maintained on complete fluid restriction. Testing is performed during the working day rather than overnight so that the patient is adequately supervised and severe dehydration is avoided. The patient is weighed every hour and the test is stopped if more than 3% of the initial body weight is lost.
- Urinary volume and osmolality are measured every hour. When the urinary osmolality reaches a plateau, as indicated by an hourly ↑ of less than 30 mOsm/kg (mmol/kg) for 3 successive hours, 5 U of aqueous vasopressin are administered SQ. Urinary osmolality is measured 30 minutes and 60 minutes later. The last urinary osmolality obtained before the administration of vasopressin and the highest value obtained after the injection are compared.
- In subjects with normal pituitary function, urinary osmolality does not ↑ by more than 9% after the injection of vasopressin. In central diabetes insipidus, the ↑ in urinary osmolality after vasopressin is more than 9%. Patients with nephrogenic diabetes insipidus usually show little ↑ in urinary osmolality with dehydration and no further ↑ after vasopressin injection. Patients with primary polydipsia often require prolonged water deprivation before a plateau in urinary osmolality is reached and urinary osmolality fails to rise by more than 9% after the administration of vasopressin.

Direct Testing

- Plasma vasopressin levels are measured at the end of the dehydration test. The results are plotted on a nomogram depicting the normal relationship between plasma Na or osmolality and plasma AVP in normal subjects. If the relationship between plasma AVP and osmolality ↓ below the normal range, a diagnosis of central diabetes insipidus is made.
- Partial nephrogenic diabetes insipidus and primary polydipsia can be differentiated by analyzing the relationship between plasma AVP and urinary osmolality at the end of the dehydration period.

Chronic Treatment of Neurogenic Diabetes Insipidus

- Desmopressin (DDAVP) is a synthetic vasopressin analog. *Supplied*: Metered dose intranasal spray pump delivering 10 µg per depression. *Dose*: Must be individualized. Average daily dose for adults is 10–40 µg qd. Initially, start with a single evening dose to control nocturia. May add a morning dose if required to control daytime polyuria.
- Chlorpropamide (Diabinese) ↑ renal tubular sensitivity to circulating endogenous AVP. Effective in less than or equal to 80% of patients. *Dose*: 250–500 mg bid. *Adverse effects*: May cause hypoglycemia.

Treatment of Nephrogenic Diabetes Insipidus
- Correct any underlying disorder.
- Thiazide diuretics (i.e. hydrochlorothiazide 50 mg qd) with Na restriction may ↑ urinary concentration by a vasopressin-independent mechanism.
- Amiloride may be useful in patients with nephrogenic diabetes insipidus from lithium therapy as it prevents the uptake of lithium in the collecting ducts.

Hirsutism

Hirsutism is defined as the excessive growth of terminal hair (coarse and pigmented) in androgen-sensitive regions (e.g. beard area, trunk, and inner upper thighs).

Causes
- *Adrenal*: Cushing's syndrome, androgen-producing tumors, and congenital adrenal hyperplasia (CAH).
- *Ovarian*: Polycystic ovarian disease (PCOD), insulin resistance, and ovarian tumors.
- *Combined ovarian and adrenal*: Idiopathic hirsutism (mostly ovarian).
- *Medication*: Androgens, anabolic steroids.
- Most common causes are PCOD and idiopathic hirsutism.

Investigations
- *History*: Inquire concerning
  - Age of onset: Prepubertal hirsutism suggests CAH; peripubertal onset is compatible with PCOD and idiopathic hirsutism.
  - Mode of onset: Abrupt onset and rapid progression suggest an androgen-secreting tumor.
  - Menstrual abnormalities: Common in PCOD.
  - Galactorrhea: Hyperprolactinemia is a rare cause of hirsutism.
  - Medications: Inquire about the use of anabolic steroids.
  - Family history: Frequently positive for hirsutism with PCOD and idiopathic hirsutism.
- *Physical*: Document
  - Amount and distribution of hair: Facial, periareolar, and lower abdominal hair is common; hair over the upper chest, upper abdomen, and upper back suggests more severe androgen excess.
  - Signs of virilization (clitoromegaly, balding, deepening of voice, and ↑ed muscle mass) suggest an androgen-secreting tumor.
  - Features of Cushing's syndrome.
  - Presence of ovarian or adrenal masses.

- *Serum testosterone*: A level less than 2 ng/mL (7 nmol/L) suggests an ovarian tumor. Often mildly ↑ in PCOD.
- *Serum dehydroepiandrosterone sulfate (DHEA-S)*: A level more than 6,630 ng/mL (18 μgmol/L) suggests an adrenal tumor. May be mildly ↑ed PCOD.
- *Serum gonadotropins*: An ↑ ratio of LH/FSH (>2.5) may be seen in the early follicular phase with PCOD.
- *Plasma 17-hydroxyprogesterone*: ↑ed suggests late-onset CAH. ACTH stimulation test may be needed to confirm this diagnosis.
- *Serum prolactin*: Useful to rule out hyperprolactinemia.
- *Overnight dexamethasone suppression test*: Perform if Cushing's syndrome is suspected.
- *Adrenal CT scan*: Perform if adrenal tumor is suspected.
- *Pelvic and vaginal ultrasound*: Ovaries may be enlarged with multiple cysts in PCOD.

Polycystic Ovarian Disease

Exact pathophysiology is not known but is probably multifactorial, involving disorders of the adrenals, ovaries, and hypothalamus. Diagnosis is made after excluding other causes of hirsutism. The ultrasound finding of polycystic ovaries is nonspecific and can occur in a variety of hyperandrogenic anovulatory states. Clinical manifestations vary. Classic signs and symptoms consist of chronic anovulation, amenorrhea/oligomenorrhea, and slowly progressive hirsutism on setting just after menarche. Obesity, acne, and infertility are common. Family history is often positive for similar complaints.

Idiopathic Hirsutism

Menstrual cycles are usually regular and ovulatory. The hirsutism tends to start in the late teens or early 20s. Family history is common. Most women have ↑ed ovarian production and bioavailability of androgens.

Management

- Local measures (electrolysis, shaving, bleaching, and waxing) are often useful by themselves or while awaiting the full benefits of drug therapy.
- Weight loss may improve hirsutism by increasing hepatic production of sex hormone-binding globulin (SHBG) and thereby reducing bioavailable testosterone.
- Oral contraceptive agents ↓ed ovarian androgen secretion by suppressing gonadotropin secretion and ↑ed SHBG levels decreasing the levels of free testosterone. Avoid agents containing desogestrel, as this progestin has enhanced androgenic activity. Agents containing

desogestrel, norethindrone, or ethynodiol diacetate are generally preferred. Maximum therapeutic effect takes 9-12 months.
- *Antiandrogens*: Spironolactone (aldactone). *Supplied*: Tablets 25, 100 mg. *Dosage*: Usual initial dose is 50 mg bid. Maximum therapeutic effect takes 9-12 months. *Adverse effects*: Nausea, irregular menses or amenorrhea, fatigue, and headache. Spironolactone must not be given during pregnancy because it interferes with normal masculinization of a male fetus. Cyproterone acetate (Androcur; Canada). *Supplied*: Tablets 50 mg. *Dosage*: Initial dose with severe hirsutism is 25-50 mg days 5-14 of each calendar month. In mild hirsutism or with maintenance therapy, 2 mg days 5-14 may be sufficient. An estrogen (ethinyl estradiol 25 μg days 5-25) is given to induce regular menstrual bleeding. *Adverse effects*: Nausea, fatigue, and ↓ed libido.

Late-onset Congenital Adrenal Hyperplasia

It may be present in 1-5% of hirsute women. Most commonly caused by a partial block in 21-hydroxylase activity, which leads to ↑ed serum levels of 17-hydroxyprogesterone (17-OHP). Diagnosed by ACTH stimulation: Inject ACTH 250 μg IM or IV and draw 17-OHP levels at 0, 30, and 60 minutes. Patients with a partial enzymatic defect demonstrate ↑ed 17-OHP levels (>2,000 ng/dL) after ACTH. Treatment consists of dexamethasone (Decadron) 0.25-0.50 mg at bedtime.

BIBLIOGRAPHY

1. Chaker L, Bianco AC, Jonklaas J, et al. Hypothyroidism. Lancet. 2017; 390(10101):1550-62.
2. De Leo S, Lee SY, Braverman LE. Hyperthyroidism. Lancet. 2016;388(10047): 906-18.
3. Durante C, Grani G, Lamartina L, et al. The diagnosis and management of thyroid nodules: A review. JAMA. 2018;319(9):914-24.
4. Houlden RL. ??? In: Khan GM, Bartlett JG, Chopra S, Topol EJ (Eds). Medical Diagnosis and Therapy. Philadelphia: Lea and Febiger; 1994.
5. Husebye ES, Anderson MS, Kämpe O. Autoimmune polyendocrine syndromes. N Engl J Med. 2018;378(12):1132-41.
6. Loriaux DL, Longo DL. Diagnosis and differential diagnosis of Cushing's syndrome. N Engl J Med. 2017;376(15):1451-9.
7. Selmer C, Faber J. Mild thyroid dysfunction. A potential target in prevention of atrial fibrillation. Circulation. 2017;136(22):2117-8.
8. Stott DJ, Rodondi N, Kearney PM, et al. Thyroid hormone therapy for older adults with subclinical hypothyroidism. N Engl J Med. 2017;376(26):2534-44.

CHAPTER 27

Miscellaneous Disorders

INTRODUCTION

In this chapter, relatively uncommon cardiac disorders are discussed, these include amyloidosis, atrial myxoma, Brugada syndrome, Chagas disease, Ehlers–Danlos syndrome, hemochromatosis, Marfan syndrome, Kawasaki syndrome, Lyme carditis, Takayasu arteritis (TA), and Turner syndrome.

AMYLOID

Cardiac involvement caused by primary amyloidosis, amyloid light-chain (AL) amyloidosis, is not uncommon. Benign monoclonal gammopathies, myeloma, macroglobulinemia, and lymphomas are the main causes of AL amyloidosis. Senile amyloidosis occurs mainly after age 80 years. Amyloid infiltration of the myocardium results in a very slow, progressive, often mild, restrictive cardiomyopathy; extensive ventricular involvement leads to severe heart failure (HF).

Diagnosis

Severe distress, shortness of breath, edema, elevated jugular venous but absent orthopnea, or paroxysmal nocturnal dyspnea should suggest restrictive pathology causing mainly right HF.

Electrocardiogram (ECG) findings are helpful:
- Approximately 60% show low voltage less than 0.05 mV in all limb leads or less than 1 mV in chest leads. Poor R-wave progression in the precordial leads or pseudoinfarct pattern (Rahman et al., 2004) but no history of myocardial infarction (MI), left anterior fascicular block, or intraventricular conduction delay (IVCD).

Echocardiography

- Nonspecific granular sparkling is shown in Figures 27.1A to D. Small pericardial effusion supporting the diagnosis. Evidence of left ventricular wall thickening, biatrial enlargement, and increased echogenicity in

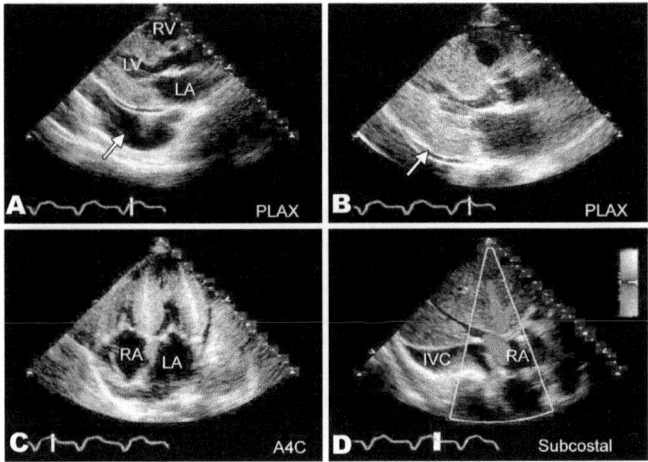

Figs. 27.1A to D: Amyloid heart disease, restrictive cardiomyopathy. (A and B) Concentric left ventricular hypertrophy with reduction in left ventricular cavity size, dilated left atrium, left-sided pleural effusion (arrow), and smaller pericardial effusion (arrow) are features consistent with cardiac amyloidosis. *Note*: Thickened right ventricular wall and interatrial septum with moderate increase in right ventricular cavity size; (C) A distinctive, but not specific sign of cardiac amyloidosis is the "ground-glass" or "sparkling" appearance of the myocardium; and (D) Right heart failure with increased right-sided pressures is evident in this patient. *Note:* The markedly dilated inferior vena cava (IVC).
Source: Reproduced with permission from Solomon SD. Amyloid heart disease. In: Solomon SD, Bulwer BE (Eds). Essential Echocardiography: A Practical Handbook. Totowa: Humana Press; 2007. p. 167.

conjunction with reduced electrocardiographic voltages is strongly suggestive of cardiac amyloidosis (CA) (Selvanayagam et al., 2007).
- Newly diagnosed patients with CA showed a median survival of 6 months in patients with detectable troponin I/T compared with 22 months in those without any detectable troponin I/T (Dispenzieri et al., 2003).

Therapy

- Chlorthalidone 12.5 mg plus amiloride 5 mg (or spironolactone 50 mg, eplerenone 50 mg). Loop diuretics are not generally recommended in patients with restrictive pathology.
- Angiotensin-converting enzyme (ACE) inhibitors and angiotensin receptor blockers (ARBs) are poorly tolerated in subjects with AL amyloidosis. Small doses may result in severe hypotension (Falk, 2005).
- *Beta-blockers*: Nebivolol [2.5–10 mg in elderly patients with HF with preserved ejection fraction (HFpEF)] proved sufficiently useful (Flather et al., 2005; van Veldhuisen et al., 2009), and should be tried because all other HF therapies have not proved useful. Recently, isosorbide dinitrate was shown not useful for HFpEF (Redfield et al., 2015).

- Digoxin is of no value in amyloidosis; these patients may be at increased risk of digoxin toxicity.

Cardiac amyloidosis is part of a systemic disease characterized by the deposition of amyloid in multiple tissues. In familial amyloidosis, CA may accompany a painful neuropathy; in AL amyloidosis, it may be found when a patient presents with nephrotic syndrome, whereas in senile systemic amyloidosis, it is almost invariably responsible for the presenting symptom.

ATRIAL MYXOMA

A left atrial myxoma is the most common cardiac tumor and is usually symptomatic.
- Symptoms include fever, weakness, malaise, Raynaud's phenomenon, finger clubbing, and symptoms of embolization.
- Diagnosis may be missed because of nonspecific findings.
- Shortness of breath on exertion, cough, orthopnea, paroxysmal nocturnal dyspnea, syncope, and palpitations may fluctuate causing missed diagnosis. Embolization of tumor fragments may cause transient cerebral ischemia attacks or small strokes. Embolization may occur to the limbs causing limb ischemia. Multiple embolization may mimic vasculitis or infective endocarditis.
- Mobile pedunculated left atrial myxomas may prolapse into the mitral valve orifice, causing obstruction to blood flow that results in syncope or cardiogenic shock. Symptoms and signs may mimic mitral stenosis.
- Arrhythmias such as supraventricular tachycardia, ventricular premature beats, and occasionally ventricular tachycardia may occur.
- Sedimentation rate is usually markedly elevated.
- Transesophageal echocardiography is diagnostic.
- Magnetic resonance imaging (MRI) can confirm the diagnosis.

Figures 27.2A and B show a large left atrial myxoma.

Treatment

Surgical removal of the lesion usually produces a complete cure.

BRUGADA SYNDROME

The Brugada syndrome is a congenital disorder of sodium cardiac channel function (Antzelevitch et al., 2003, 2005; Antzelevitch, 2007).
- The first known case brought to the attention of the Brugada brothers involved a 3-year-old boy from Poland who presented in 1986 following multiple episodes of syncope (Antzelevitch et al., 2003).
- Most patients have a family history of syncope, sudden death, or abnormal ECG changes.

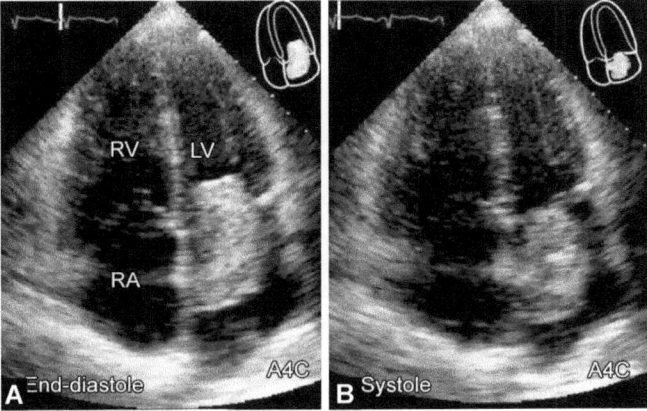

Fig. 27.2: This large atrial myxoma caused functional mitral stenosis and constitutional symptoms. They are usually solitary, mobile masses that are heterogeneously hyperechoic. They arise most commonly from the interatrial septum and have predilection for the left atrium.
Source: Reproduced with permission from Wu JC. Atrial myxoma. In: Solomon SD, Bulwer BE (Eds). Essential Echocardiography: A Practical Handbook. Totowa: Humana Press; 2007. p. 348.

Diagnosis

- Atrial fibrillation (AF) is the most common atrial arrhythmia found in Brugada syndrome (Francis and Antzelevitch, 2008). Sudden cardiac death is often preceded by several episodes of syncope that often occur without warning. Brugada syndrome is a major cause (approximately 30%) of all cases of ventricular fibrillation (VF) of unknown cause.
- The vast majority of patients show no evidence of structural heart disease but the electrical system has a minor derangement, probably in the "bundle of His-Purkinje electrical conducting system" that in some individuals can trigger VF and death (Remme et al., 2001).
- About 60% of affected individuals are of Asian origin particularly Southeast Asia. Sudden unexpected death particularly during sleep sometimes associated with nightmares in East Asia and Southeast Asia is a major cause of death, approximately 80% in young men (age 40–50 years) without known underlying cardiac diseases (Nademanee et al., 1997). In Thailand, unexplained sudden cardiac death (Lai Tai in Thailand, *death during sleep*), Bangungut (scream followed by sudden death) in the Philippines is the leading cause of death in young men, and approximately 40% of these patients have a family history of sudden deaths.
- Epidemiological studies in Japan for Pokkuri (unexpected death at night) showed the prevalence of Brugada syndrome to be from 0.12% to 0.14% in the general population (Matsuo et al., 2001; Miyasaka et al., 2001). Abnormal ECG findings may be intermittent, found in 0.15% of

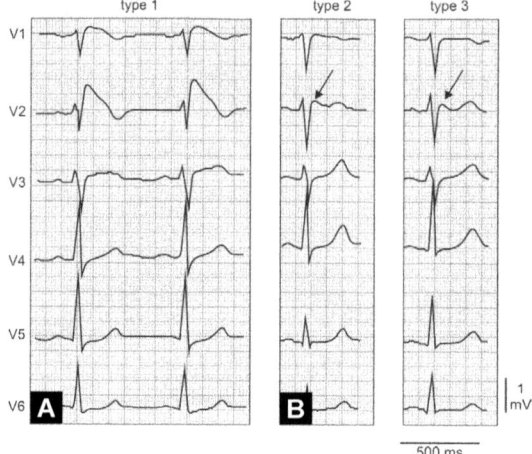

Figs. 27.3A and B: (A) ECG tracing in a patient during sinus rhythm: ST-segment elevation of the coved-type in V1 and V2, characteristic of Brugada syndrome; and (B) ECG tracing in a patient with Brugada syndrome. Atypical RBBB: the ST segment is elevated and reveals a typical saddleback deformity in V1 and V2. (ECG, electrocardiogram; RBBB, right bundle branch block).

Japanese adults associated with a greater than 50-fold increase in the risk of unexpected death in Japanese men. Although much less common than in Southeast Asia, this syndrome is not rare in Western countries and in North America (Chen and Priori, 2008).

- Syncope or AF may be a presenting problem.

Electrocardiography Features

- A distinctive type of atypical right bundle branch block. The ST segment is elevated in chest leads V1, V2, and V3 where the atypical right bundle branch pattern is usually seen as shown in Figures 27.3 and 27.4. The elevated ST segment has a curious convex curve or a coved and saddleback shape.

Therapy

- Junttila et al. (2008) observed that patients who are in an acute situation and who present with a Brugada-type ECG are at a considerably higher risk of sudden cardiac death and should be considered a medical emergency.
- Antiarrhythmic agents are not sufficiently effective in preventing VF in these patients and implantation of a cardioverter defibrillator is advisable to prevent sudden death. Zipes et al. (2006), particularly in patients with a previous history of cardiac arrest and who are receiving optimal medical therapy. This is supported by a randomized trial carried out by

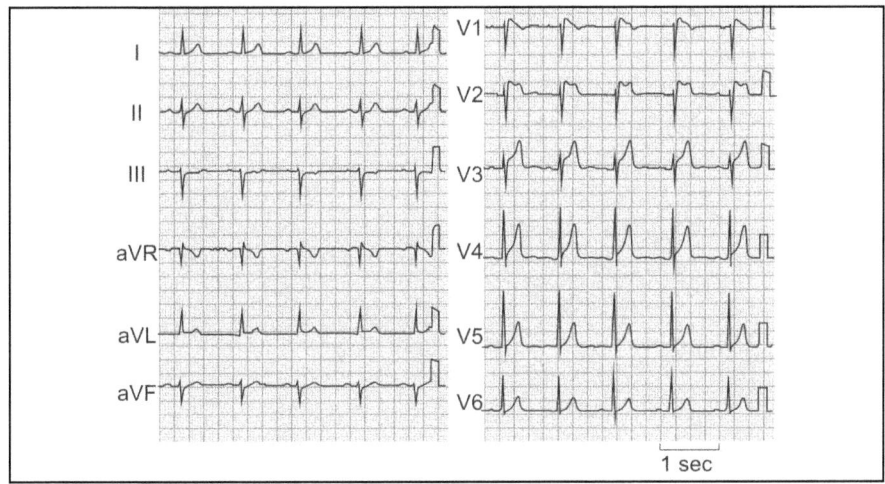

Fig. 27.4: Brugada syndrome.

Nademanee et al. (2003) (for DEBUT—Defibrillator versus Beta-blockers for Unexplained Death in Thailand) that showed effective prevention of sudden death by the implantable cardioverter defibrillator (ICD). Sacher et al. (2006) have described findings after implantation of a cardioverter defibrillator in patients with Brugada syndrome.

Quinidine

- High-dose quinidine administration appears to have a probable role (Belhassen et al., 2004). A study suggests that a much lower dosage of quinidine (300–600 mg a day) may be effective in preventing VF (Mizusawa et al., 2006). Viskin et al. (2007) emphasized that for patients with short QT syndrome, Brugada syndrome, and idiopathic VF, the sudden unavailability of quinidine supplies, because of a halt in production, is potentially life-threatening. Investigators appear convinced that quinidine is the most effective, and in many cases the only effective antiarrhythmic therapy, for patients suffering from unique malignant ventricular arrhythmias, including the short QT syndrome, Brugada syndrome, and idiopathic VF (Kaufman, 2007; Belhassen et al., 2004).
- Individuals with Brugada syndrome and their family members who are genetic carriers of a sodium channelopathy should be aware that some substances or medications (such as cocaine, methadone, procainamide, propofol, antidepressants, and antihistamines), may increase their risk of arrhythmias. Certain foods consumed at night by men age 40–50 years with this disease particularly in Thailand may be precipitants and deserve investigations.

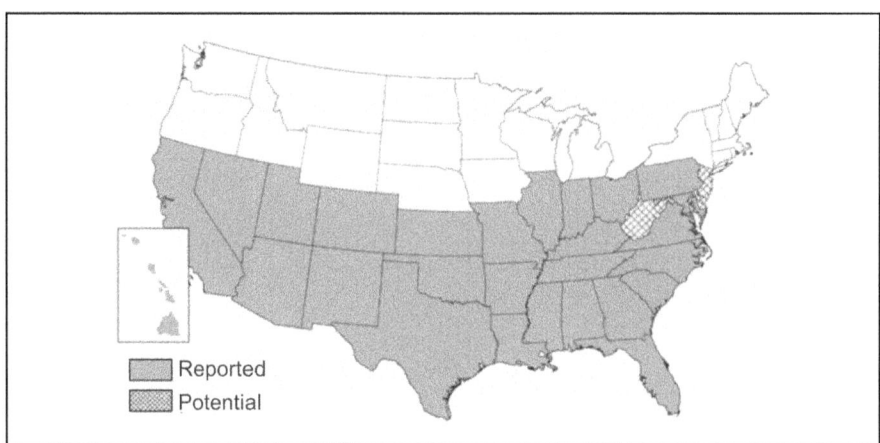

Fig. 27.5: Distribution of Chagas disease in Americans.
Source: Acquatella H. Cardiomyopathies, myocarditis and pericardial diseases. In: Abelmann WH, Braunwald E (Eds). Atlas of Heart Diseases. Philadelphia: Springer; 2007. pp. 811-8.

- Propranolol should be tried for any of these individuals who present with syncope or recurrence. The drug prevents VF and sudden death (*see* Chapter 13: Syncope).

CHAGAS DISEASE

Trypanosoma cruzi causes Chagas disease. More than 30 million individuals are affected with more than 50,000 deaths annually. Chagas disease is prevalent in Central and South America, particularly in Argentina, Chile, Bolivia, Paraguay, Southern Peru, Uruguay, and parts of Brazil and Mexico (Fig. 27.5). It is seen in the southern USA, where Latin Americans are believed to be infected.

- Transmission to children and young adults less than age 20 years is through the bite of a bug (reduviid, subfamily Triatominae). The bug becomes infected by feeding on infected animals such as the armadillo, opossum, raccoon, and skunks. Dogs and cats provide an extensive reduviid reservoir for infecting entire families. The bug dwells in the roofs and walls of mud and straw houses. The disease is transmitted to humans through the feces of infected bloodsucking insects in endemic areas. During the night, the bug drops onto the sleeping individual and inflicts bites around the eyes. Infection is transferred when the trypanosomes in the animals excrement enters the wounded skin or penetrates the conjunctiva.
- The protozoa multiply and then migrate through most organs of the body including the myocardium, pericardium, liver, spleen, and brain. The disease can be transmitted from mother to child and through blood transfusions.

- If the entry is through the skin, a one-sided swelling around the eye (periorbital edema) and swelling of the eyelid, a chagoma may occur (Romana sign). In about 10% of infected individuals, acute symptoms, such as muscle aches and pains, fever, sweating, and enlargement of the liver and spleen occur. If the parasitic infection involves the cardiac muscle, an acute myocarditis, and HF may supervene. Spread to involve the endocardium with clot formation and embolization. The pericardium may be involved causing pericardial effusion. Children become more seriously ill than young adults, and rarely the acute disease is fatal.
- Many patients recover, however, and symptoms disappear over 1-2 years. Symptoms may only appear after about 20 years when about 25% of those infected go on to develop the chronic form of the disease most commonly affecting the heart (Dias 1995; Maguire et al., 1987). Cardiac involvement develops in approximately 40% of infections manifested as cardiomyopathy, HF, and arrhythmias. About 70-80% of infected individuals remain in the indeterminate form throughout their lives, but in approximately 25% the heart muscle is uniformly destroyed and replaced by fibrous tissue and mainly right HF symptoms and signs become obvious.

Investigations

Chest X-ray

It confirms dilation of the heart and presence of HF.

Echocardiography

It is virtually always abnormal and reveals hypokinesis, poor contractility of the left ventricular posterior wall, relatively preserved intraventricular septal wall motion, and poor movement of the apical segment of the heart with dilatation and in some aneurysmal formation.

It is often abnormal revealing: intraventricular conduction defect (IVCD), right bundle branch block (RBBB) + left anterior fascicular (hemiblock) block, ventricular premature complex (VPBs), ventricular tachycardia (VT) and grades of heart block.

Therapy

- The only available drugs are the triazole derivatives, nifurtimox, and benznidazole. Naturally resistant *Trypanosoma cruzi* strains pose further problems with available drug treatment. These agents are not effective in the chronic phase, and have serious side effects, including neurotoxicity. Trypanocidal therapy with benznidazole in patients with established Chagas' cardiomyopathy significantly reduced serum parasite detection

but did not significantly reduce cardiac clinical deterioration through 5 years of follow-up (Morillo et al., 2015). But the drug is helpful in some at earlier stages. Building better homes, nets for sleeping, and screening cats and dogs would prevent the majority of infections in poorer rural areas.
- Rassi Junior and colleagues provided an informative review and indicate that in patients with established chronic disease, several pharmacological and nonpharmacological interventions are available, and have been increasingly used with the intention of preventing or delaying complications of the disease (tertiary prevention) (Rassi et al., 2009).

EHLERS-DANLOS SYNDROME

- Defects of type III collagen dictate skin, joint and cardiovascular manifestations associated with spontaneous rupture of medium- and large-caliber arteries.
- The eyes may show a blue coloring of the sclerae, seen also with osteogenesis imperfecta.
- Rupture of an artery without aneurysm formation or dissection may occur. The abdominal aorta or medium-sized branches of aorta, for example the subclavian or large arteries of the limbs, may rupture, but true aneurysms rarely form. Aortic root dilatation is rare. Mitral valve prolapse occurs.

HEMOCHROMATOSIS

The genetic mutation C282Y produces a mutant HFE protein that is not associated with the transferrin receptor and does not act as a brake on iron uptake into cells.
- The precise mechanism by which C282Y HFE protein, ferroportin, and hepcidin interact is unclear (Pietrangelo, 2004). Deficiency of hepcidin is the reason for increased iron absorption and iron overload that are seen in many hereditary forms of hemochromatosis. The exact reason why iron absorption in the intestine is markedly increased has not been clarified.
- Iron-saturated transferrin attaches to cell transferrin receptors and excess iron gains entry into the cell. Free iron catalyzes the formation of reactive oxygen species and the hydroxyl radical causes damage to cells. With damage and destruction of cells, there is replacement by collagen and fibrous tissue that weakens the muscular wall of the heart. Severe damage and weakness primarily to heart muscles occur with symptoms and signs of HF.
- Emerging details of the physiology of hepcidin, the key hormone in iron recycling, suggest a resolution of the apparent paradox of an important

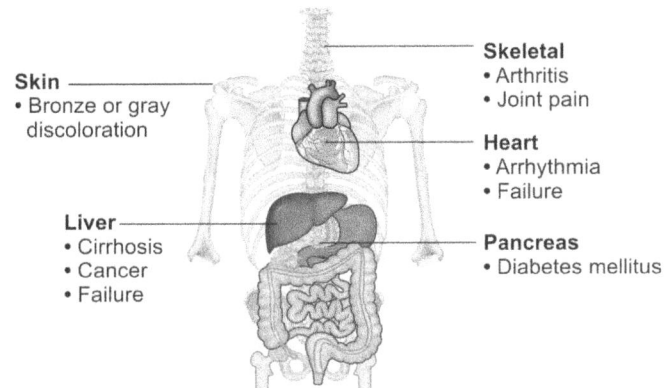

Fig. 27.6: Complications of hemochromatosis.

role for iron in atherogenesis in the possible absence of increased plaque burden in most types of hereditary hemochromatosis (Mascitelli and Goldstein, 2014).

Diagnosis

- Palpitations caused by arrhythmias may be bothersome and serious arrhythmias including complete heart block can cause death. Other signs and symptoms due to other organ involvement include enlargement of the liver; cirrhosis and cancer of the liver may be a terminal event. Arthritis may be severe with iron replacing the cartilage of the hip and destroying the hip or knee joint. Hypogonadism causes erectile dysfunction. Diabetes occurs in some because of involvement of the pancreas. A bronze pigmentation of the skin is present with advanced disease (Fig. 27.6).
- Although serum ferritin levels are usually elevated, these levels are unsatisfactory as a diagnostic tool to detect organ overload such as cardiac iron. The level of serum ferritin at which iron deposition is detected in the heart has not been defined. Heavy cardiac iron deposition occurs despite the presence of low-serum ferritin levels (Brownell et al., 1986; Fischer et al., 2003).

Magnetic Resonance Imaging

- This is noninvasive and is recommended to assess quantitative cardiac iron load. Biochemical markers and tissue biopsy, used to diagnose and guide therapy, are not sensitive enough to detect early cardiac iron deposition (Gujja et al., 2010).

Echocardiography

It can identify early pathophysiology due to iron overload, and has been successfully employed to evaluate iron-depleting therapy in idiopathic hemochromatosis as it demonstrated a decrease in the left ventricular (LV) mass and wall thickness, that correlated with the reversal of myocardial iron infiltration (Cecchetti et al., 1991).

Therapy

- Venesection with removal of 500 mL of blood every 2–3 weeks for several months followed by monthly venesection for a year usually results in a reduction of serum ferritin level to less than 50 mg/L. Phlebotomies are continued every 3–4 months to maintain a ferritin level 20–50 mg/L range. If the serum iron is kept within the normal range, hematocrit approximately 45% before serious cardiac involvement has occurred, the prognosis is good. If cardiomyopathy resulting in HF has occurred, the prognosis is poor.
- Gujja et al. (2010) indicate that phlebotomy and chelating drugs are suboptimal therapy. The roles of gene therapy, hepcidin, and calcium antagonists are being actively investigated. L-type Ca^{2+} channels provide a major pathway for iron entry into cardiomyocytes in iron-overload cardiomyopathy, thus dihydropyridine calcium antagonists may prove of some value (Gujja et al., 2010). Verapamil should not be used because HF can be precipitated.

LYME CARDITIS

Lyme disease is an immune-mediated disease secondary to exposure to *Borrelia burgdorferi*. Infection of individuals by the bite of the *Ixodes scapularis* tick, with the spirochete *Borrelia burgdorferi* causes a multisystem disease.

Diagnosis

- The disease begins in approximately 80% with erythema migrans. In 20%, erythema migrans is absent; lymphadenopathy, fever and arthralgia, and other manifestation should be assessed if a tick is removed. Less than 6% of patients develop cardiac, neurologic and/or arthritic complication.
- In less than 5% of patients the heart is involved. The most common cardiac abnormality caused by this tick-borne infection is myocarditis and varying degrees of transient atrioventricular (AV) nodal block (Steere, 2001).
- Less than 50% of infected individuals recall a history of the tick bite because the deer tick nymphs are small and often go unnoticed.

- Lyme titers are positive for both immunoglobulin M (IgM) and IgG antibodies, but are insensitive during the first several weeks of infection (Wilske, 2005). The clinical diagnosis is based on appropriate serology and clinical manifestations. It is critical that the serologic features be interpreted correctly to avoid a false diagnosis of Lyme disease. The serologic features are often misinterpreted and may have false positives if confirmatory laboratory testing is not performed (Borchers et al., 2015).

Electrocardiography Findings

In the presence of cardiac involvement shows diffuse ST-segment and T-wave abnormalities that may be mild, nonspecific, and transient, accompanied by varying degrees of AV block (first degree, second degree, and rarely complete heart block) (Van der Linde et al., 1990). Lyme carditis is an important cause of reversible heart block (McAllister et al., 1989).

Magnetic Resonance Imaging

Gadolinium-enhanced cardiac magnetic resonance (CMR) appears useful in the evaluation of myocarditis (Munk et al., 2007). Significantly diminished extent of late gadolinium enhancement at 6 weeks follow-up, which correlated with significant improvement of AV block after antibiotic treatment has been observed (Naik et al., 2008).

Therapy

- Treatment with doxycycline, amoxicillin, or cefuroxime is safe and highly efficacious for early Lyme disease. A single 200-mg dose of doxycycline reduces the risk of Lyme disease in persons bitten by *Ixodes scapularis* ticks (Shapiro, 2014).
- Doxycycline 100 mg orally twice daily after meal (with 8 oz of water to minimize nausea and vomiting) or amoxicillin 500 mg orally three times daily for 2–3 weeks. If allergic to these agents, 500 mg of cefuroxime orally for 2–3 weeks.
- Reversible complete AV block may occur (McAllister et al., 1989). If bradycardia caused by complete heart block develops, temporary pacing may be required for 1–2 weeks and rarely permanent pacing is needed for complete heart block. In patients with AV block without clinical or laboratory evidence of Lyme disease, gadolinium-enhanced CMR may aid in suggesting the diagnosis of Lyme carditis (Naik et al., 2008).
- The study in 2016 showed that longer-term therapy does not improve quality of life in patients with Lyme disease symptoms months or years after diagnosis (Berende et al., 2016).
- Investigators conducted a multicenter, randomized, double-blind, placebo-controlled trial involving 280 Lyme disease patients with

persistent musculoskeletal pain, arthritis, arthralgia, neuralgia, sensory disturbances, dysesthesia, neuropsychological disorders, or cognitive disorders, with or without persistent fatigue. The median duration of symptoms was longer than 2 years (Berende et al., 2016).
- Patients received initial intravenous (IV) ceftriaxone for 2 weeks followed by one of three oral regimens: doxycycline, clarithromycin plus hydroxychloroquine, or placebo for 12 weeks. The primary outcome was health-related quality of life at the end of treatment; a secondary outcome was fatigue.
- Health-related quality of life and fatigue scores were similar across the groups, as was the rate of treatment discontinuation (5%). Four serious adverse events occurred, none of which were drug-related (Berende et al., 2016).

MARFAN SYNDROME

Drug treatment remains poorly effective to prevent and manage progression of complication in patients with Marfan syndrome. Pyeritz (2007) states that beta-blocker administration remains the "standard of care", for all patients, with Marfan syndrome even in the presence or absence of aortic dilatation. These experts state that "atenolol administered twice daily is the drug of choice because it has fewer central nervous system and other side effects". It appears that experts including those at the National Institutes of Health (NIH) do not know that atenolol is a most ineffective beta-blocker. The choice of atenolol by Lacro et al. for a well-run NIH randomized controlled trial (RCT) in patients with Marfan syndrome is unfortunate (Khan, 2011). In 2014, the NIH reported that atenolol administration resulted in a result similar to that observed with angiotensin-receptor blocker (ARB) therapy. The use of a more effective beta-blocker (bisoprolol, propranolol, and timolol) may have produced a difference.
- Marfan syndrome is an autosomal dominant disorder that occurs in all races and ethnic groups. The abnormalities causing aortic root dilatation in Marfan syndrome is a degeneration of the medial layer, with fragmentation, disarray, and loss of elastic lamina and replacement by basophilic-staining proteoglycan (Schlatmann and Becker, 1977). Death is usually caused by aortic dissection, rupture, and pericardial tamponade.

Diagnostic Symptoms and Signs

- Aorta, the heart, eye, and skeleton show features that are diagnostic.
- Clinical variability and a high rate of new mutation make diagnosis of mildly affected young sporadic patients difficult leading to failures to diagnose Marfan syndrome.

- Mitral valve prolapse, dilatation of the sinuses of Valsalva, and aortic valve regurgitation are common findings.
- Dilatation of the aortic root and ascending aorta leads to aneurysm formation and aortic dissection and mortality at age 40–50 years.
- Eyes show a tremulous iris, dislocation of the lens (ectopia lentis), myopia, and retinal detachment and occasionally a blue sclera.
- *Skeletal changes*: Joint hypermobility, long extremities and fingers, typical arachnodactyly (spider finger); the thumb protrudes beyond the little finger when the fist is clenched, tall stature, pectus excavatum or pectus carinatum, a high-arched palate, and scoliosis.

Treatment

- The use of beta-adrenergic blocking drugs has been shown to delay the rate of aortic dilatation and the risk of aortic dissection.
- Pyeritz (2007) states that beta-blocker administration remains the "standard of care", for all patients, even in the presence or absence of aortic dilatation.
- These experts state that "atenolol administered twice daily is the drug of choice because it has fewer central nervous system and other side effects". It appears that experts including those at NIH do not know that atenolol is a most ineffective beta-blocker. In the 90s and up to 2010, worldwide atenolol was the most prescribed beta-blocker.
- The choice of atenolol by Lacro et al. for a well-run NIH RCT in patients with Marfan syndrome is unfortunate (Khan, 2011). In 2014, the NIH reported that atenolol administration resulted in a result similar to that observed with ARB therapy.
- The use of a more effective beta-blocker (bisoprolol, propranolol, timolol, and carvedilol) may have produced a difference.
- It must be emphasized that atenolol is a poorly effective beta-blocker because it is nonlipophilic and thus gains low-brain concentration. The drug is not advisable and its use for all cardiac indications should be curtailed (Khan, 2003).
- The subtle differences in beta-blockers may provide the solution for the apparent lack of cardioprotection of some beta-blockers (Khan, 2005).
- Atenolol is a hydrophilic beta-blocker that attains low-brain concentration. Increased brain concentration and elevation of central vagal tone confer cardiovascular protection (Pitt, 1992). Lipid-soluble beta-blockers (bisoprolol, carvedilol, metoprolol, propranolol, and timolol) with high-brain concentration block sympathetic discharge in the hypothalamus better than water-soluble agents (atenolol, nadolol, and sotalol).
- Angiotensin-receptor blockers and ACE inhibitors affect transforming growth factor-beta (TGF-β) metabolism. These findings suggest that

pathways that block angiotensin II might help to prevent aortic dissection and perhaps aneurysmal dilation.
- In a small cohort study of 19 patients followed or in 12–47 months, the use of ARB therapy in patients with Marfan syndrome significantly slowed the rate of progressive aortic-root dilation (Brooke et al., 2008; Lacro et al., 2007).
- van Dijk et al. raised the following important question: "First, are ARBs beneficial in Marfan syndrome irrespective of the underlying FBN1 mutation? Second, are ARBs beneficial in cases of Marfan syndrome that are caused by mutations in other genes?" Decreased TGF-β signaling in Marfan syndrome due to mutations in the gene encoding TGF-β receptor 2 has been reported (Mizuguchi et al., 2004), suggesting a possible adverse effect of ARBs (van Dijk et al., 2008).
- Endocarditis prophylaxis is necessary for valvular involvement. Advice on restriction of severe exertional activity including weight lifting and contact sports should be given.
Surgical intervention in patients with Marfan syndrome, timing of surgical intervention is crucial to prevent the morbidity and mortality associated with ascending aortic dissection. The risk of type A dissection is proportional to the overall size of the proximal aorta. Replacement of the aortic root and ascending aorta with a composite graft (valved conduit) is recommended when the greatest diameter of the proximal aorta reaches 5 cm in adults. (Kouchoukos and Dougenis, 1997; Gott et al., 1999). When the rate of change of aortic diameter is rapid (Legget et al., 1996), or when the patient has had relatives suffer aortic dissection (Silverman et al., 1995), elective surgery should be considered at a maximal diameter of 4.5 cm (Karck et al., 2004; Ates, 2007).
- Hydralazine is contraindicated in all patients with Marfan syndrome because the drug may cause expansion of aneurysms. This drug is commonly used appropriately for hypertension in pregnancy but should not be used in patients with Marfan syndrome.

TURNER SYNDROME

Diagnosis

This anomaly is manifested in females who lack an X chromosome (45, X karyotype).
- Body habitus includes low hairline, low-set ears, deafness, small jaw, short-webbed neck, short stature, broad chest with widely spaced nipples, hypertelorism, epicanthal folds, ptosis, and a shortened fifth finger. Cardiovascular lesions include coarctation of the aorta, bicuspid aortic valve, aortic stenosis, and dilatation of the ascending aorta with the risk of aortic dissection may occur in the absence of a coarctation.
- *Assess echocardiography, CT chest, aorta; ECG.*

Treatment

- A beta-blocker is advisable if dilation of the aorta is observed: bisoprolol 5–10 mg, not atenolol.
- For coarctation of the aorta prior to interventional therapy, an ACE inhibitor is advisable because coarctation causes activation of the renin-angiotensin-aldosterone system.

KAWASAKI SYNDROME

The condition is seen worldwide but in Japan, children with a mean age of 12 months are affected; and in the USA, the mean age is closer to 3 years.

Approximately, 25% of untreated children with Kawasaki develop coronary artery aneurysms. The risk of developing coronary artery aneurysms is greatest for children younger than 6 months of age.

Diagnosis

The diagnosis of Kawasaki should be considered in any infant with prolonged, unexplained fever, and there should be a low threshold for performing echocardiography in this age group (Son MB et al., 2015). The fever has no identifiable cause (fever of unknown origin) and occurs without the common manifestation of an upper respiratory tract viral infection or flulike illness. The diagnosis is entertained if fever of an unknown origin is accompanied by at least four of the following:

1. Bilateral conjunctival redness, injection, and iritis.
2. Inflamed throat, redness of the tongue (strawberry tongue), and fissuring of the lips.
3. Redness of the palms and soles of the feet, swelling, and edema of the hands and feet.
4. Body rash is an early manifestation, desquamation, and peeling around the nails, the palms, and the soles.
5. Enlargement of lymph nodes around neck (cervical lymphadenopathy); usually one large node measuring at least 1.5 cm or larger and arthralgia.

Infants with three or more of the earlier symptoms with unexplained fever for more than 2 weeks should have an echocardiographic evaluation to exclude coronary artery aneurysms. Damage to the coronary arteries by vasculitis occurs in more than 25% of infants and in about 10% of children aged 2–5 years.

A review by Newburger et al. states: Kawasaki disease is an acute, self-limited vasculitis of unknown etiology that occurs in infants and children. If not treated early with high-dose intravenous immunoglobulin (IVIG), one in five children develop coronary artery aneurysms; this risk is reduced fivefold if IV immunoglobulin is administered within 10 days of fever onset. Aneurysms evolve dynamically over time, reaching a peak dimension by 6 weeks after onset. Almost all the morbidity and mortality occur in patients with giant aneurysms. Risk of MI is greatest in the first 2 years after illness onset. The disease is no longer a rare cause of acute coronary syndrome presenting in young adults. Despite 4 decades of research, the etiology of Kawasaki remains elusive, and a traditional pathogen seems unlikely as the trigger for the disease (Newburger et al., 2016).

Therapy

Intravenous gamma globulin 2 g/kg in a single infusion over 10-22 hours given within the first 10 days of illness. The prevalence of aneurysms is reduced to approximately 4% for patients treated with the IVIG infusion within 10 days of illness onset (McCrindle, 2009). Half of aneurysms heal to a normal size after 1-2 years, although healing may cause the wall of the artery to become thicker than usual (Baker and Newburger, 2008). The incidences of retreatment and coronary artery abnormalities within 1 month after the start of treatment were less frequent in the corticosteroid group than in the group receiving immune globulin alone (Inoue et al., 2006).

New initiatives must seek to understand the mechanisms of IVIG in order to replace it one day with more affordable and more targeted therapies (Burns JC et al., 2015).

Aspirin: The anti-inflammatory actions of moderate doses of aspirin are useful in controlling fever; the dose is then reduced to approximately 5 mg/kg/day for 8 weeks. This small dose inhibits platelet aggregation and may prevent thrombosis.

The variation by nationality in incidence, clinical characteristics, and female/male ratio suggests a genetic component to the disease, but no reliable marker has been identified. The most common time of diagnosis is the 2nd and 3rd decades of life. In the United States, the age of the patient is important, for it is one method of distinguishing TA from giant-cell arteritis, which is commonly diagnosed in the 8th decade of life but has many signs and symptoms overlapping those of TA (Beckman, 2015).

TAKAYASU ARTERITIS

Takayasu arteritis is a nonspecific panarteritis that affects the intima and the adventitia, mainly of the aorta and many of its main branches. The disorder is seen mainly Asian females, about age approximately (20-55 years) and is now seen in Africa, Europe, Latin America, and North America. It is extremely rare in white people; fortunately it is an uncommon disease, even in Asian countries.

Diagnosis

The disease onset is insidious, and prominent symptoms are nonspecific or absent in two-thirds of the patients in the early stage; diagnosis is then delayed (Ogino, 2008). Patients present with stenotic or occlusive lesions of the aortic arch hence the term pulseless disease (Shimizu, 1948). Affected arteries include: the descending thoracic or abdominal aorta, renal arteries (Inada, 1975), coronary arteries (Cipriano, 1977), and pulmonary artery. Aortic regurgitation and aortic aneurysm with ascending aortic dilatation may develop (Ogino et al., 2008).

- Watanabe and colleagues (2015) reported among the 7,779 patients, 1,372 newly registered patients with TA were enrolled; 83.8% were female. The median age at onset was 35 years, but higher in male patients (median 43.5 years). Local symptoms and findings were most commonly observed in the cervicobrachial area, with more complaints in the head or neck than in the upper limbs. Approximately 85% of the patients had vascular involvements in the aortic arch or its major branches.
- In Japanese patients, the ascending aorta and aortic arch with its branches are more frequently involved, whereas in patients from Korea, India, and Western countries, the abdominal aorta and renal arteries are most frequently affected. Aortic regurgitation used to be the main cause of mortality of Japanese patients, and cerebrovascular accidents relating to hypertension have been the cause of death in other countries.
- Its cause remains uncertain. 10 pairs of identical twins having TA have been reported. Clinical features indicate an important role of genetic factors in its pathogenesis.
- The age of the patient is important, for it is one method of distinguishing TA from giant-cell arteritis, which is commonly diagnosed in the eighth decade of life but has many signs and symptoms overlapping those of TA (Beckman, 2015).
- Clues for the diagnosis are hypertension, vascular bruits, asymmetrical arm blood pressure, and other ischemic symptoms. The criteria of Ishikawa, 1988, have been widely applied, which consist of:
    - Obligatory criterion (age < 40 years)
    - Major criteria (left and right mid-subclavian artery lesions)
    - Nine minor criteria [high erythrocyte sedimentation rate (ESR), common carotid artery tenderness, hypertension, aortic regurgitation or annuloaortic ectasia, lesions of the pulmonary artery, left mid common carotid artery, distal brachiocephalic trunk, thoracic aorta, and abdominal aorta].

Investigations

Computed tomography scanning and magnetic resonance angiography have replaced angiography; ESR and C-reactive protein (CRP) are elevated.

Therapy

- Pharmacological treatment with corticosteroids is usually the initial treatment. Corticosteroids are still used in the active phase of TA. There is evidence that adequate, long-term prednisolone therapy contributes to an angiographic improvement. 30 mg/day of adrenocorticosteroids as the initial dose for adult patients with active TA. The initial dose is tapered at a rate of 5 mg every 2 weeks down to 10 mg and thereafter at a rate of 2.5 mg every 2 weeks until withdrawal or to the minimum required dose to control inflammation, while the ESR and serum CRP concentration are monitored.
- Mekinian et al. (2015) reported on a nationwide study that showed a high efficacy of biological-targeted treatments treated by tumor necrosis factor-α antagonists (80%) or tocilizumab (20%) in refractory patients with TA with an acceptable safety.
- Antihypertensive agents are frequently used because more than 70% of the patients have hypertension related to atypical coarctation or renovascular hypertension.
- Aspirin and antiplatelet agents are advisable.
- Some patients require surgical treatment such as bypass grafting and graft replacement or endovascular repair including percutaneous transluminal angioplasty (PTA) and stent grafting, even in the active phase or in the inactive chronic phase with adequate control of the inflammation. The indication for PTA was symptomatic stenosis of more than 70% or a peak systolic gradient of more than 50 mm Hg.
- Surgery has been associated with low mortality and morbidity except for surgery of aortic aneurysm, especially a ruptured aneurysm. Although less than 20% of adult patients require surgical treatment, in the pediatric field, 80% of the patients need surgery for stenotic/occlusive lesions because 70% are in the active phase and on steroid therapy.

BIBLIOGRAPHY

1. Ablad B, Bjuro T, Bjorkman JA, et al. Role of central nervous beta-adrenoceptors in the prevention of ventricular fibrillation through augmentation of cardiac vagal tone. J Am Coll Cardiol. 1991;17:165A.
2. Acquatella H. Echocardiography in Chagas heart disease. Circulation. 2007;115(9):1124-31.
3. Ates M. When should we replace the ascending aorta in Marfan syndrome? Eur J Cardiothorac Surg. 2007;31(2):331-3.
4. Baker AL, Newburger JW. Kawasaki disease. Circulation. 2008;118(7):e110-2.
5. Beckman JA. Takayasu arteritis: it is time to work together. Circulation. 2015;132(18):1685-6.
6. Berende A, ter Hofstede HJ, van Middendorp H, et al. Randomized trial of longer-term therapy for symptoms attributed to Lyme disease. N Engl J Med. 2016;374(13):1209-20.

7. Bern C, Montgomery SP, Herwaldt BL, et al. Evaluation and treatment of Chagas disease in the United States: a systemic review. JAMA. 2007;298(18):2171-81.
8. Beta-Blocker Heart Attack Trial Research Group. A randomized trial of propranolol in patients with acute myocardial infarction. I. Mortality results. JAMA. 1982;247(12):1707-14.
9. Borchers AT, Keen CL, Huntley AC, et al. Lyme disease: a rigorous review of diagnostic criteria and treatment. J Autoimmun. 2015;57:82-115.
10. Brooke BS, Habashi JP, Judge DP, et al. Angiotensin II blockade and aortic-root dilation in Marfan's syndrome. N Engl J Med. 2008;358(26):2787-95.
11. Burns JC, Franco A. The immunomodulatory effects of intravenous immunoglobulin therapy in Kawasaki disease. Expert Rev Clin Immunol. 2015;11(7):819-25.
12. Burns JC. The riddle of Kawasaki disease. N Engl J Med. 2007;356(7):659-61.
13. Campbell DA, Westenberger SJ, Sturm NR. The determinants of Chagas disease: connecting parasite and host genetics. Curr Mol Med. 2004;4(6):549-6.
14. Cipriano PR, Silverman JF, Perlroth MG, et al. Coronary arterial narrowing in Takayasu's arteritis. Am J Cardiol. 1977;39(5):744-50.
15. Dias JC, Silveira AC, Schofield CJ. The impact of Chagas disease control in Latin America: a review. Mem Inst Oswaldo Cruz. 2002;97(5):603-12.
16. Falk RH. Pondering the prognosis and pathology of cardiac amyloidosis. J Am Coll Cardiol. 2016;9(2):139-41.
17. Gott VL, Greene PS, Alejo DE, et al. Replacement of the aortic root in patients with Marfan's syndrome. N Engl J Med. 1999;340(17):1307-13.
18. Gujja P, Rosing DR, Tripodi DJ, et al. Iron overload cardiomyopathy: better understanding of an increasing disorder. J Am Coll Cardiol. 2010;56(13):1001-12.
19. Hagar JM, Rahimtoola SH. Chagas' heart disease. Curr Probl Cardiol. 1995;20(12):825-924.
20. Inada K, Yokoyama T, Nakaya R. Atypical coarctation of the aorta. Angiology. 1963;14(10):506-17.
21. Inoue Y, Okada Y, Shinohara M, et al. A multicenter prospective randomized trial of corticosteroids in primary therapy for Kawasaki disease: clinical course and coronary artery outcome. J Pediatr. 2006;149(3):336-41.
22. Karck M, Kallenbach K, Hagl C, et al. Aortic root surgery in Marfan syndrome: comparison of aortic valve-sparing reimplantation versus composite grafting. J Thorac Cardiovasc Surg. 2004;127(2):391-8.
23. Keane MG, Pyeritz RE. Medical management of Marfan syndrome. Circulation. 2008;117(21):2802-13.
24. Khan MG. Angina, which beta-blocker to choose. In: Khan MG (Ed). Heart Disease Diagnosis and Therapy: A Practical Approach, 2nd edition. Totowa: Humana Press; 2005. pp. 150-2.
25. Khan MG. Marfan syndrome: Encyclopedia of Heart Diseases, 2nd edition. New York: Springer; 2011.
26. Khan MG. Results of recent clinical trials: Cardiac Drug Therapy, 6th edition. Philadelphia: Saunders/Elsevier; 2003. p. 502.
27. Kokkinos P, Chrysohoou C, Panagiotakos D, et al. Beta-blockade mitigates exercise blood pressure in hypertensive male patients. J Am Coll Cardiol. 2006;47(4):794-8.
28. Kouchoukos NT, Dougenis D. Surgery of the thoracic aorta. N Engl J Med. 1997;336(26):1876-88.

29. Lacro RV, Dietz HC, Wruck LM, et al. Rationale and design of a randomized clinical trial of beta-blocker therapy (atenolol) versus angiotensin II receptor blocker therapy (losartan) in individuals with Marfan syndrome. Am Heart J. 2007;154(4):624-31.
30. Legget ME, Unger TA, O'Sullivan CK, et al. Aortic root complications in Marfan's syndrome: identification of a lower risk group. Heart. 1996;75(4):389-95.
31. Maguire JH, Hoff R, Sherlock I, et al. Cardiac morbidity and mortality due to Chagas disease: prospective electrocardiographic study of a Brazilian community. Circulation. 1987;75(6):1140-5.
32. Marin-Neto JA, Cunha-Neto E, Maciel BC, et al. Pathogenesis of chronic Chagas heart disease. Circulation. 2007;115(9):1109-23.
33. Mascitelli L, Goldstein MR. Hereditary hemochromatosis, iron, hepcidin, and coronary heart disease. Medical Hypotheses. 2014;82(3):402-3.
34. McAllister HF, Klementowicz PT, Andrews C, et al. Lyme carditis: an important cause of reversible heart block. Ann Intern Med. 1989;110(5):339-45.
35. McCrindle BW. Kawasaki disease: a childhood disease with important consequences into adulthood. Circulation. 2009;120(1):6-8.
36. Mekinian A, Comarmond C, Resche-Rigon M, et al. Efficacy of biological-targeted treatments in takayasu arteritis: multicenter, retrospective study of 49 patients. Circulation. 2015;132(18):1693-700.
37. Melia MT, Auwaerter PG. Time for a different approach to Lyme disease and long-term symptoms. N Engl J Med. 2016;374(13):1277-8.
38. Miles MA, Feliciangeli MD, de Arias AR. American trypanosomiasis (Chagas' disease) and the role of molecular epidemiology in guiding control strategies. BMJ. 2003;326(7404):1444-8.
39. Morillo CA, Marin-Neto JA, Avezum A, et al. Randomized trial of benznidazole for chronic Chagas' cardiomyopathy. N Engl J Med. 2015;373(14):1295-306.
40. Munk PS, Ørn S, Larsen AI. Lyme carditis: persistent local delayed enhancement by cardiac magnetic resonance imaging. Int J Cardiol. 2007;115(3):e108-10.
41. Naik M, Kim D, O'Brien F, et al. Images in cardiovascular medicine. Lyme carditis. Circulation. 2008;118(18):1881-4.
42. Newburger JW, Sleeper LA, McCrindle BW, et al. Randomized trial of pulsed corticosteroid therapy for primary treatment of Kawasaki disease. N Engl J Med. 2007;356(7):663-75.
43. Newburger JW, Takahashi M, Burns JC. Kawasaki disease. J Am Coll Cardiol. 2016;67(14):1738-49.
44. Norwegian Multicenter Group. Timolol-induced reduction in mortality and reinfarction in patients surviving acute myocardial infarction. N Engl J Med. 1981;304(14):801-7.
45. Ogino H, Matsuda H, Minatoya K, et al. Overview of late outcome of medical and surgical treatment for takayasu arteritis. Circulation. 2008;118(25):2738-47.
46. Peters RW, Muller JE, Goldstein S, et al. Propranolol and the morning increase in the frequency of sudden cardiac deaths (BHAT Study). Am J Cardiol. 1989;63(20):1518-20.
47. Petty R, Laxer R, Lindsley C, et al. Kawasaki disease. In: Son MB, Sundel RP (Eds). Textbook of Pediatric Rheumatology, 7th edition. Philadelphia: Elsevier; 2016. pp. 467-83.
48. Pietrangelo A. Hereditary hemochromatosis: a new look at an old disease. N Engl J Med. 2004;350(23):2383-97.

49. Pinto Dias JC. Natural history of Chagas' disease. Arq Bras Cardiol. 1995; 65(4):359-66.
50. Pitt B. The role of beta-adrenergic blocking agents in preventing sudden cardiac death. Circulation. 1992;85(1 Suppl):107-11.
51. Rassi A, Dias JC, Marin-Neto JA, et al. Challenges and opportunities for primary, secondary, and tertiary prevention of Chagas' disease. Heart. 2009;95(7):524-34.
52. Rassi A, Rassi A, Rassi SG. Predictors of mortality in chronic Chagas disease: A systematic review of observational studies. Circulation. 2007;115(9):1101-8.
53. Schlatmann TJ, Becker AE. Pathogenesis of dissecting aneurysm of aorta. Comparative histopathologic study of significance of medial changes. Am J Cardiol. 1977;39(1):21-6.
54. Shapiro ED. Clinical practice. Lyme disease. New Engl J Med. 2014;370(18): 1724-31.
55. Shimizu K, Sano K. Pulseless disease. Clin Surg (Tokyo). 1948;3:377-96.
56. Shores J, Berger KR, Murphy EA, et al. Progression of aortic dilatation and the benefit of long-term beta-adrenergic blockade in Marfan's syndrome. N Engl J Med. 1994;330(19):1335-41.
57. Steere AC, Sikand VK. The presenting manifestations of Lyme disease and the outcomes of treatment. N Engl J Med. 2003;348(24):2472-4.
58. Steere AC. Lyme disease. N Engl J Med. 2001;345(2):115-25.
59. Takayasu M. A case with peculiar changes of the central retinal vessels. Acta Soc Opthal Jpn. 1908;12:554-5.
60. Tuncer M, Fettser DV, Gunes Y, et al. Comparison of effects of nebivolol and atenolol on P-wave dispersion in patients with hypertension. Kardiologiia. 2008;48(4):42-5.
61. Utz G, Simon B, Mickisch R, et al. Giant-cell (Takayasu) arteritis as a cause of renovascular hypertension. Z Kardiol. 1975;64(5):482-8.
62. van Dijk FS, Meijers-Heijboer H, Pals G. Angiotensin II blockade in Marfan's syndrome. N Engl J Med. 2008;359(16):1732-4.
63. Watanabe Y, Miyata T, Tanemoto K. Current clinical features of new patients with takayasu arteritis observed from cross-country research in Japan: age and sex specificity. Circulation. 2015;132(18):1701-9.

CHAPTER 28

Superior Quality Electrocardiograms Produced by Electrode Placements

INTRODUCTION

The author conducted a large novel study; this showed that placement of the wrist electrode on the mid-arm and the ankle electrode on the lower abdomen produces better quality electrocardiograms (ECGs). The procedure is faultless and can replace the old wrist–ankle method. The ECG, a frequently used diagnostic test, is made more reliable. Physicians can provide more precise interpretation for all ECGs. Patients obtain better care.

The standard placement of electrodes on the ankle and wrist used since 1944 produces poor quality ECGs due to several factors, e.g. limb movement, tremors, anxiety, pain, and dry skin particularly above the ankles. In cold climates, cold extremities certainly cause distortion of the baseline and ECG waveforms; this leads to inaccurate ECG interpretation and diagnostic delays. It is established that placing the ankle–wrist electrodes on the torso (modified leads) provides rapid acquisition of better quality ECGs, but causes major changes in R-wave amplitude and thus erroneous ECG (Khan, 2015).

- Rapid diagnosis is needed for timely coronary interventions or thrombolytic therapy.
- Lives can be saved by rapid acquisition of better quality ECGs.
- 1,112 patients received standard and new electrode placement (NEP) recordings. ECG parameters were assessed by the author and a blinded interpreter.
- Electrodes positioned on the mid-arm and lower abdomen (Fig. 28.1) revealed ECGs identical with the standard without artifacts or loss of inferior infarction or appearance of lateral infarcts.

Not having to remove leg garments is convenient and allows more rapid acquisition of ECGs. The forearms are freed for, intravenous, radial access, and ECGs needed during procedures.

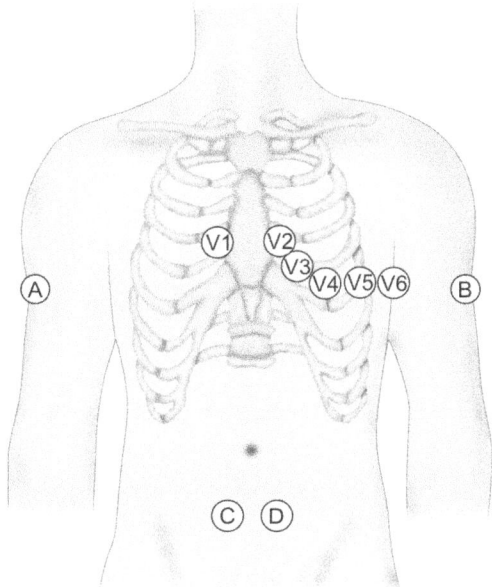

Fig. 28.1: The arm electrodes (A and B) are placed on the mid-arm, on the lateral aspect of the biceps, immediately below the V4 horizontal line. The abdominal electrodes (C and D) placed 7.6 cm (approximately 3 inches) below the umbilical horizontal line, and 5 cm (approximately 2 inches) on either side of the umbilical vertical line. The distance between these two electrodes to be 10 cm (approximately 4 inches).
Source: Khan GM. A new electrode placement method for obtaining 12-lead ECGs. Open Heart. 2015;2:e000226.

Placing the limb electrodes on the torso (modified leads) as done for exercise stress testing (Sevilla et al., 1989) or variations in placements cause an increase in R-wave amplitude in inferior leads that can result in disappearance of inferior myocardial infarction (MI), and a more than 2 mm decrease in leads 1 and aVL that may simulate a lateral infarct (2005). The author hypothesized that finding electrode placements, that do not cause alterations in R-wave amplitude, should correct the problems.

The lower limb electrodes were moved to the lower abdomen 7.6 cm (3 inches) below a horizontal line running across the umbilicus. This position, well below the umbilicus, was maintained for all 1,112 subjects tested in a pilot study (Fig. 28.1).

Figures 28.2A and B show a standard wrist–ankle ECG: artifacts prevent ECG interpretation. An ECG done after 30 seconds using the new placement method (NEP) shows no artifacts. Examples of inferior infarcts and other diagnoses are shown in Figures 28.3 to 28.5.

Figures 28.2 to 28.5 show that the five major problems observed with torso leads are not observed with recordings done using the new placements.

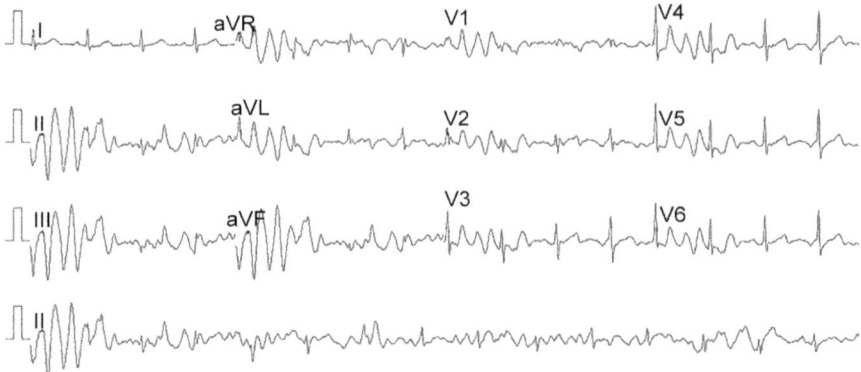

Fig. 28.2A: Standard 12-lead electrocardiogram (ECG) showing artifacts.

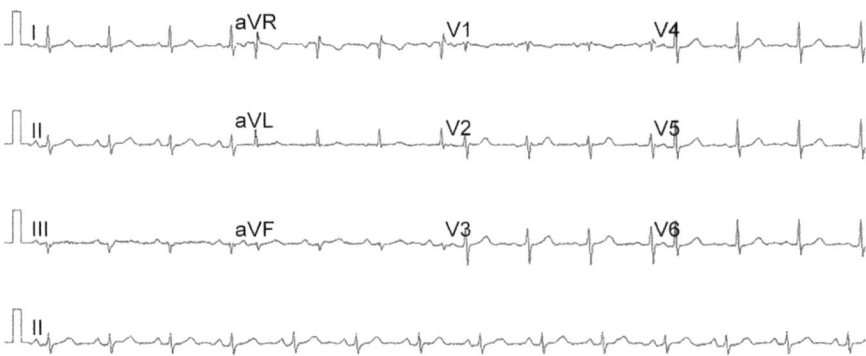

Fig. 28.2B: New electrode placement ECG done within 30 seconds of the standard tracing reveals no artifacts.
Source: Khan GM. A new electrode placement method for obtaining 12-lead ECGs. Open Heart. 2015;2:e000226.

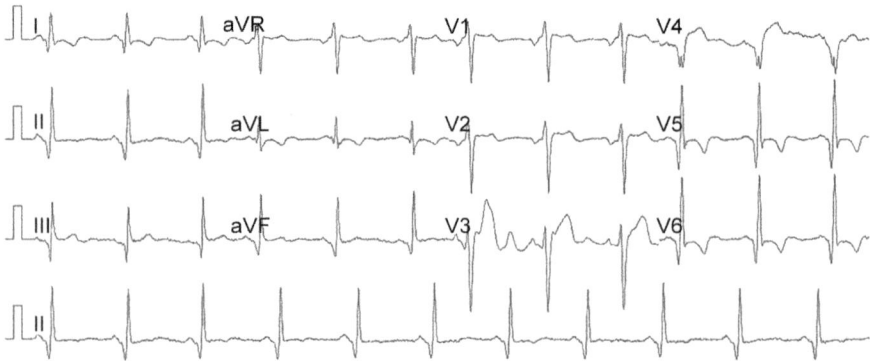

Fig. 28.3A: Standard lead ECG: deep wide Q waves in leads II, III, aVF: old inferior, and anterolateral MI, artifacts in V3, V4. (ECG, electrocardiogram; MI, myocardial infarction)

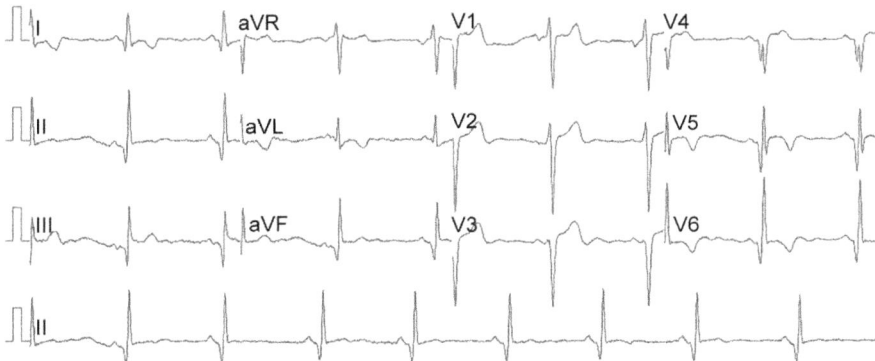

Fig. 28.3B: New electrode placement ECG, old inferolateral infarct; the tracing is similar to the standard recording, but with clearing of artifacts in V3 and V4. The R-wave amplitude in all 12 leads is the same in the standard and NEP ECG.
Source: Khan GM. A new electrode placement method for obtaining 12-lead ECGs. Open Heart. 2015;2:e000226.

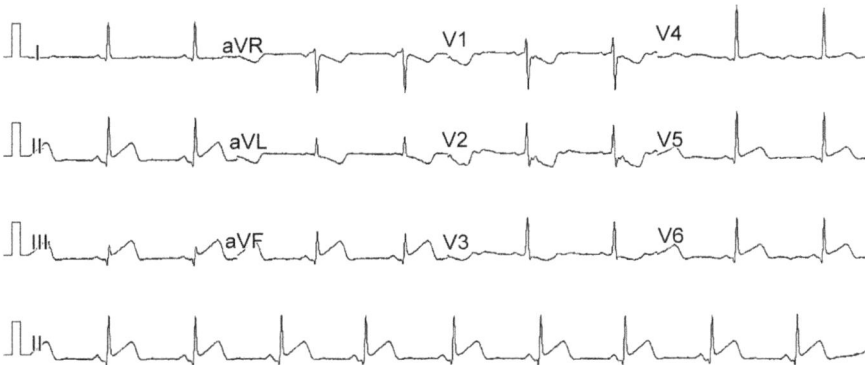

Fig. 28.4: New electrode placement ECG from a female, age 57 years, shows abnormal ST elevation in leads II, III, aVF, V5, and V6: typical findings of acute inferior MI with lateral involvement, ST-segment elevation MI. Reciprocal depression V1–V3, aVL is not diagnostic but helps confirm the diagnosis of acute MI. (ECG, electrocardiogram; MI, myocardial infarction)
Source: Khan GM. A new electrode placement method for obtaining 12-lead ECGs. Open Heart. 2015;2:e000226.

Figures 28.3A and B shows the ECG of a patient with a proven old inferior and anterolateral MI. Diagnostic wide Q waves are seen in leads II, III, aVF: (a) standard ECG, and (b) NEP ECG.

The NEP ECG of a 57-year-old female patient, with acute chest pain and acute inferior MI, is shown in Figure 28.4. No standard ECG was done in order to avoid delays to percutaneous coronary intervention (PCI).

The 2007 American Heart Association (AHA)/American College of Cardiology (ACC) guidelines on ECG Part 1 recommends studies to look at

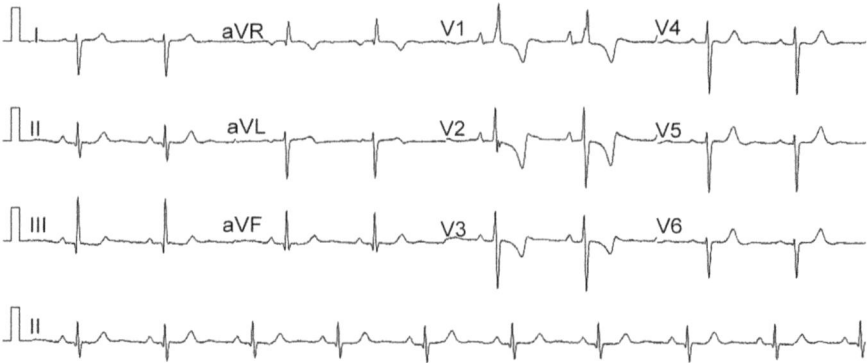

Fig. 28.5A: It shows the standard 12-lead electrocardiogram (ECG) from a patient with Eisenmenger syndrome, marked right ventricular hypertrophy: R >1 mV in V1, R/S >1 in V1, R/S <1 in V4, V5, V6, right atrial hypertrophy, and right axis deviation 153. The NEP ECG shown in Figure 28.5B reveals virtually the same waveforms and QRS axis of 155.

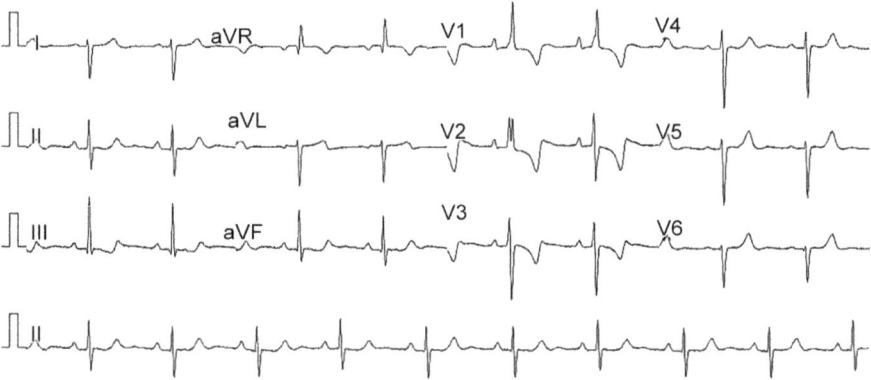

Fig. 28.5B: NEP ECG from the patient shown in Figure 28.5A, QRS axis 155; findings are identical to the standard.
Source: Khan GM. A new electrode placement method for obtaining 12-lead ECGs. Open Heart. 2015;2:e000226.

modified leads (Kligfield et al., 2007). Studies by Jowett et al. (2005), Sevilla and colleagues (1989), Papouchado (1987) and our pilot study indicate that modified leads (all torso) cause serious errors.

CONCLUSION

This large study showed that our new method provides better quality ECGs than the old wrist–ankle placements, with no recalls and without risk for misinterpretations. See Khan 2015 for tables and further information.

BIBLIOGRAPHY

1. Diamond D, Griffith DH, Greenberg ML, et al. Torso mounted electrocardiographic electrodes for routine clinical electrocardiography. J Electrocardiol. 1979;12(4):403-6.
2. Jowett NI, Turner AM, Cole A, et al. Modified electrode placement must be recorded when performing 12-lead electrocardiograms. Postgrad Med J. 2005;81(952):122-5.
3. Khan GM. A new electrode placement method for obtaining 12-lead ECGs. Open Heart. 2015;2(1):e000226.
4. Kligfield P, Gettes LS, Bailey JJ, et al. Recommendations for the standardization and interpretation of the ECG: part I: The electrocardiogram and its technology: a scientific statement from the American Heart Association Electrocardiography and Arrhythmias Committee, Council on Clinical Cardiology; the American College of Cardiology Foundation; and the Heart Rhythm Society: endorsed by the International Society for Computerized Electrocardiology. Circulation. 2007:115(10):1306-24.
5. Papouchado M, Walker PR, James MA, et al. Fundamental differences between the standard 12-lead electrocardiograph and the modified (Mason-Likar) exercise lead system. Eur Heart J. 1987;8(7):725-33.
6. Sevilla DC, Dohrmann ML, Somelofski CA, et al. Invalidation of the resting electrocardiogram obtained via exercise electrode sites as a standard 12-lead recording. Am J Cardiol. 1989;63(1):35-9.
7. Takuma K, Hori S, Sasaki J, et al. An alternative limb lead system for electrocardiographs in emergency patients. Am J Emerg Med. 1995;13(5):514-7.
8. Wilson FN, Johnston FD, Rosenbaum FF, et al. The precordial electrocardiogram. Am Heart J. 1944;27(1):19-85.

Index

Page numbers followed by *b* refer to box, *f* refer to figure, *fc* refer to flow chart, and *t* refer to table.

A

Abscess
    intra-abdominal 378, 397
    perivalvular 184
Acalculous cholecystitis 442, 443
Acebutolol 17, 58
Acetylcholine 134
Acid hypersecretion 406
Acidemia 308
Acidosis 119, 500
    severe 258
Acinetobacter 337, 338
    calcoaceticus 339, 348
    species 336, 350, 353, 356, 364
Acquired disorders 517
Acquired immunodeficiency syndrome 166, 275, 396, 410, 439, 442, 481, 586, 594, 663
Acromegaly 671
    clinical manifestations 671
    diagnosis of 671, 672*fc*
    management 672
Activated partial thromboplastin time 534
Adalimumab 416
Addison's disease 282, 663
Adenosine 135, 136*t*, 137
    deaminase 386
    monophosphate 292
    thallium scintigraphy 52
    triphosphate 514
Adizem 16, 61
Adrenal adenoma 669
Adrenal diseases 663
Adrenal hyperplasia
    bilateral 669
    late-onset congenital 677
Adrenal insufficiency 663
    causes 663

    clinical manifestations 663
    diagnostic procedures 664
    management of chronic 666
    treatment of acute 665
Adrenal tumors 667
Adrenocorticotropic hormone 583, 657
    dependent 667
    independent 667
Adriamycin 275
    toxicity 274
Aerobic gram-positive organisms 336
Aeromonas species 409
Aerosol metered dose inhaler 306*t*
Aeruginosa 480
Agnogenic myeloid metaplasia 519
Agranulocytosis 19
Air pollution 302, 310
Airflow obstruction 314
    expiratory 309
    severe 314
Airway inflammation 299
Akinetic seizures 283
Alanine aminotransferase 436
Albumin-creatinine ratio 1, 99*t*, 496
Albuterol 294, 315, 618
Alcohol
    abuse 140
    consumption 234
    excess 212
Alcoholism 232
Aldosterone 497
    antagonists 118
Aldosterone-producing adenoma 669
Alirocumab 210
Alkaline diuresis 494
Allergic pulmonary edema 108
Allergic purpuras 543
Allopurinol 300, 494
Alopecia 232
Alosetron 401

Alpha-adrenergic antagonists 16
Alpha-antitrypsin deficiency 310
Alpha-blockers 9, 282
Alpha-thalassemia major 526
Aluminum-containing antacids 407
Alveolar proteinosis 108
Alveolar pulmonary edema 107
  diffuse 107f
Amebicide 485
Ameliorate
  bothersome 116
  cardiogenic shock 3
American College of Cardiology 3, 207, 703
American Heart Association 3, 703
  guidelines 207
Amikacin 355, 356, 441, 481, 547
Amiloride 14, 157, 434
Aminoglycosides 355, 493, 547
Aminopenicillins 344
Aminophylline 138, 613
Amiodarone 134, 153, 154, 157-160, 257, 270, 286, 379, 399, 655
  blocks 157
Amiprilose hydrochloride 600
Amlodipine 16, 23, 61
Amniotic fluid leak 493
Amoebic abscesses, treatment of 485
Amoxicillin 245-247, 289, 328, 344, 345, 583
Amphetamine 451
Amphotericin B 482
Ampicillin 242, 243, 245, 246, 344, 345, 347, 481, 583
  susceptible strains 348
Ampullary stenosis 443
Amylase 386
Amyloid 678
  diagnosis 678
  heart disease 275, 679f
  therapy 679
Amyloidosis 505, 587, 678
Anaerobic pleuropulmonary infections 340
  clinical features 341
  epidemiology 340
  microbiology 341
  therapy 342
Ancillary therapy 82
Androgen-producing tumors 675

Anemia 500, 511, 515, 517, 549
  classification of 511, 511b
  mild 526
  secondary 511, 518
  with marrow disruption 511, 519
Anesthesia, general 247, 341
Anesthetics, injection of 476
Angina 43, 175, 263
  classification 43
  diagnosis of 43
  management of 45
  pathophysiology of 45fc
  severe 49f
Angiography, selective 426
Angiotensin-converting enzyme 94, 169, 505, 583
  inhibitors 15, 16, 59, 125, 197, 267, 269, 273, 679
    dosages of 19t
Angiotensin-receptor blockers 3, 21, 126, 691
Anistreplase 81
Ankylosing spondylitis 564, 578, 587
  treatment of 590
Annulus 196
Anserine bursitis 579
Antacids 121, 406
Antagonists 3
Antiarrhythmic agent 129, 133t, 152, 286
Antiarrhythmic drugs 133, 155t, 399
  action 154f
  dosage 154t
Antiatheroma drugs 207
Antibacterials 418
Antibiotic 228, 445, 486, 493
  combined with needle aspiration 445, 486
  policy 547
  selection 486
  therapy 342, 590
Antibody, incomplete 523
Anticancer agents 517
Anticardiolipin antibodies 376
Anticholinergic agents 315
Anticholinergic bronchodilators 294, 295
Anticholinesterase inhibitors 471
Anticonvulsant
  agents 460, 461
  tricyclic 293, 460

Antidiuretic hormone 497
  ectopic 613
  potentiating drugs 613
  secretion of 612
  secretion, increased 612
Antidromic tachycardia 146
Antifungal agents 228
Antiglobulin
  absence of 523
  test 523
Antihistamines 683
Antihypertensive agents 461
Antihypertensive drugs, daily dosage of 16t
Anti-inflammatory drugs 314
Antimicrobial agents 342
Antimicrobial resistance 343
Antimicrobial spectrum 343, 344, 345, 346, 347, 350, 353
Antimicrobial therapy 547
  modification of 338
Antimigraine drug 399
Antineoplastic agents 583
Antineoplastic drug 399
Antinuclear antibody 386, 592
Anti-Parkinson's drug 399
Antiphospholipid syndrome 603
Antipseudomonal penicillins 342, 346, 347, 481
Antiretroviral therapy 212
Antirheumatic drugs, disease-modifying 591t
Antistaphylococcal penicillins 343, 481
Antithrombin deficiency 543
Antithrombotic regimens 181
Antithymocyte globulin 600
Antithyroglobulin antibodies 653, 654
Antithyroid
  agents 517
  drugs 660
  peroxidase 653
    antibody 653
Antrum syndrome 406
Anxiety 200, 369
Aorta
  abdominal 695
  coarctation of 40
Aortic arch syndrome 285
Aortic balloon valvuloplasty 182
Aortic diastolic murmurs 272

Aortic dilatation
  absence of 10
  presence of 10
Aortic dissection 26, 182, 251, 280
Aortic prosthetic valve surgery 178t
Aortic regurgitation 181
  causes of 182t
  diagnostic hallmarks 182
  management of chronic 184
  moderate 185
  severe 185
Aortic root dilatation 182
Aortic stenosis 108, 174, 177, 280, 286
  causes of 174
  diagnosis 174
  moderate 175t, 176, 178
  physical signs 174
  severe 143, 175t, 176, 176t, 178, 181
  signs of 174
  surgical therapy 177
Aortic systolic murmur 183, 272
Aortic valve
  bioprosthesis 181
  replacement 181
    surgical 186
  types of 184
Aortic valvular stenosis, causes of 174t
Apical hypertrophic cardiomyopathy 266f
Apical pansystolic murmur 205
Aplasia 518
Aplastic anemia 511, 517
  severe 517
Aplastic disorders 517
Apresoline 34
Areflexia 472
Arizona strategy 253
Aromatic hydrocarbons 517
Arrhythmia 129, 134, 136, 148, 204, 290, 463
  benign 151
  life-threatening 124
  malignant 151
  management of 129
  non-life-threatening 124
  termination of 136
Arterial blood gas 114, 304, 305t, 372, 557
Arterial pressure, diastolic 182
Arteriography 426

Arteriosclerosis 182
Arteriovenous fistula 111, 265f
Arteriovenous shunts 336
Artery
    infarct-related 65
    intercostal 382
Arthralgias 398
Arthritides 215
    infectious 593
Arthritis 52, 205, 206, 329, 398, 585, 588
    migratory 586
    pauciarticular 587
    treatment of reactive 590
Arthropod venoms 493
Asbestos exposure 379
Ascites 167, 379, 431, 432, 490
    causes of 432b
    clinical features 433
    complications of 433
    management 434
Ascitic fluid, analysis of 433
Aspiration 453, 457
    pneumonia 341, 361
        causes of 341
Aspirin 54, 65, 79t, 206
    enteric-coated 166
    maintenance of 206
Astemizole 133, 159
Asthma 289, 290, 294, 299
    causes of 303
    chronic stable 293
    clinical trial 305
    controlled 305, 306
    etiology of 292
    leukotriene receptor antagonists 305
    mechanical ventilation of 308
    severe 304
    therapy of 305
    treatment of 293
        chronic 306t
        stable 306t
    triggers 301
        allergens 301
        exercise and stress 302
        infections 302
    uncontrolled 291
    underestimation of 303
Asymmetric hypertrophy 261
Asymptomatic proteinuria 501

Ataxia 472
Atelectasis 336, 372
Atenolol 9, 10, 17, 32, 58, 120, 791
    therapy, chronic 32
Atheroma 67, 207, 249
    development 214
    formation 258
        pathophysiology of 67fc
    percentage of 209
    rupture 207
Atheromatous arterial disease 625, 636
Atheromatous coronary stenosis 55, 177
Atheromatous disease 222
    cause of 626
Atherosclerotic renovascular disease 36
Atopy 311
Atorvastatin 227, 228, 232
Atrial fibrillation 22, 91, 131, 140, 143, 145, 147, 194, 263, 264, 280, 298, 465, 681
    causes of 140
    quick ventricular response 143f
Atrial flutter 131, 140, 147
Atrial myxoma 280, 678, 680
    treatment 680
Atrial natriuretic hormone 497
Atrial rate 131
Atrial septal defect 111
Atrial tachycardia, multifocal 137, 139, 298
Atrioventricular block 287
    first-degree 205
Atrioventricular nodal reentrant tachycardia 131, 132f, 134, 135fc, 136, 147, 148
Atropine 255, 315
Audible sound, generate 312
Autohemolytic anemia 523
Autoimmune thyroiditis, chronic 654
Autonomic disturbances, treatment of 81
Azalides 358
Azathioprine 414, 421
Azithromycin 228, 289, 290, 328, 358
    resistant bacteria 290
Azlocillin 342, 346, 347, 481, 547
Azotemia 501
Aztreonam 354, 355

B

Bacampicillin 344
Bacillus cereus 408, 409
Bacteria 237
Bacterial endocarditis 182, 239, 586
   acute 237
   prevention of 241*b*, 244, 244*b*, 246*t*
   prophylaxis 244
   subacute 237
Bacterial infections 378, 393, 409, 586
Bacterial pneumonias 330
Bacteriologic stains 388
Bacteroides fragilis 340
   species 353
Bacteroides gragilis 340, 347, 350, 357, 358
   group 351
Bacteroides melaninogenicus 340, 351, 358
Bacteroides species 341
Balloon
   aortic valvuloplasty 180
   flotation catheter 136, 138
   tamponade 427
Barbiturate 300
   withdrawal 451
Barrett's esophagus 404
Basal membrane 503
Basilar artery migraine 282
Basilar reticulonodular disease 382*f*
Beclomethasone 306
Behçet's disease 564
Behçet's syndrome 182
Benazepril 16, 20
Bendrofluazide 14, 18
Bendroflumethiazide 18
Bentiromide test 423
Benzathine penicillin G 206
Benzene 517
Benzthiazide 18
Benzylpenicillin 343
   molecule 344
Berry aneurysms 40
Beta-adrenergic
   agonists 291
   blockade, salutary effects of 68*fc*
   blockers 273, 461
Beta-agonist
   long-acting 289
   preparation 294*t*
   subcutaneous 307

Beta-blockade results 56
Beta-blockers 9, 17, 31, 35, 39, 81, 89, 118, 140, 153, 156, 250*t*, 267, 285, 459, 460, 645, 660, 679
   combination 60
   drugs 7*t*
   effects 55
   first choice 54
   for angina, dosage of 55*t*
   heart attack trial 251
   randomized control trials 57*t*, 66*t*
   therapy 89
   use 268
Beta-lactams 342, 355
Bezafibrate 233
Bicarbonate 631
Bicuspid valve 181
Biguanide 643
Bile ascites 432
Bile duct lymphoma 442
Biliary cirrhosis 212
   primary 233, 654
Biliary pain 420
Biliary pseudolithiasis 351
Biliary system 442, 442*b*
Bioprosthetic valve 180
Biopsy, open 390
Bisoprolol 4, 9, 10, 11, 118
Bisphosphonates 622
Bitolterol tomalate 294
Bladder 491
   neck 491
      obstruction 492
   rupture 492
Blastocystis hominis 588
Bleeding diathesis 538
Bleeding disorder 196
Bleeding episode, treatment of acute 536
Blocadren 18
Blood
   brain barrier 469
   cells 489
   cholesterol 210, 216
   coagulation
      factors, characteristics of 531*t*
      systems 532*fc*
   cultures 443
      collection of 242
      from ears 448

glucose 648
  less-intensive 625
  Gram's stain of 239
  leukocytes 531
  levels 215
    campesterol 99t
    essential 215
    sitosterol 99t
  lymphocytes 553
  platelets 531
  pressure 3, 5fc, 33, 65, 168, 272, 369, 453, 498
    control of 28
    goal 647
    low 490
    systolic 1, 4fc, 6fc
  sitosterol, elevated 98
  urea nitrogen 1, 239, 436, 489
  vessel, major 251
Bloody fluid 386
Bone
  and intestine 620
  pathology 619
  resorption, increased 619
Bone marrow 547
  autologous 551
  biopsy 556
  colony growth 556
  generalized disorders of 546
  transplantation 518, 551
Borrelia burgdorferi 588, 594
Botulinum toxin 460
Bowel X-rays, small 416
Brachial pulse 175
Brachiocephalic trunk, distal 695
Bradyarrhythmia 161, 257, 280, 286
Bradycardia 70, 283, 285, 288
  severe 161, 286
  symptomatic 287
Brain 602
  abscess, causes of 484t
  concentration 10, 89
  parenchyma 476
Brainstem 462
Branhamella catarrhalis 328
Breast cancer 476
Breath
  mild shortness of 175
  severe shortness of 175
Bromocriptine 282, 379, 399, 469, 670

Bronchial hyperresponsiveness 305
Bronchial smooth muscle 309
Bronchitis 330
  chronic 309, 311
Bronchoconstriction 305
Bronchodilators 289, 292t, 315t
Bronchodilatory capabilities 291
Bronchopneumonia 330
Bronchoscopy 390
Bronchospasm, treatment of 313
Brucella 588
Brudzinski's sign 476
Brugada syndrome 252, 253, 678, 680, 683, 683f
  characteristic of 682f
  diagnosis 681
  therapy 682
Bruising 538
Budd-Chiari syndrome 432, 433
Budesonide 306
Bumetanide 18
Burkholderia cepacia 360, 364
Bursitis 563, 575

C

Caffeine 138, 459, 613
Calcitonin 622, 623
  gene-related peptide 461
Calcium 3, 106, 498, 499
  antagonists 16, 22, 23t, 35, 60, 93, 270
    for angina, dosages of 61t
  carbonate, mobilization of 497
  chloride 134, 255, 256
    dosage 256
  disturbances 611
  gluconate 256
  phosphate 498
  polystyrene sulfonate 619
Calorie control 499
Campylobacter 409, 410, 442
  jejuni 473, 588
  species 408
Canadian cardiovascular classification 44
Cancer 207
  arthropathy 593
  chemotherapy 481
Candesartan 460, 461

Candida 442
   albicans 587
Capillary blood glucose 643
Captopril 16, 20, 27, 126
Carbachol 295
Carbamazepine 300, 450
Carbapenems 342, 353
Carbenicillin 346
Carbidopa 469
   treatment 469
Carbimazole 659
Carbohydrates
   decrease 642
   diabetic restrict 94
Carbon dioxide, partial pressure of 305
Carbon monoxide 313
   poisoning 140
Carbon tetrachloride 493, 517
Carboxylic acid 20
Carboxypenicillins 346
Carcinoid syndrome 304
Carcinoma 492
Cardene 17
Cardiac amyloidosis 680
Cardiac arrest 249, 465
   causes 250
   drug 255t
      therapy 254
   prevention of 249
Cardiac arrhythmia
   malignant 298
   suppression trial 150
Cardiac catheterization 171, 185
Cardiac deaths 251
   preventing 11
Cardiac decompensation 129
Cardiac disease 630, 681
Cardiac disorders 250
Cardiac dysfunction 490
Cardiac erythrocytosis 557
Cardiac failure 660
Cardiac impulse, abnormal 262
Cardiac insufficiency bisoprolol study 251
Cardiac medications 279
Cardiac muscle 275
Cardiac output, low 490
Cardiac protection 10
Cardiac regional tamponade 169
Cardiac risk 249

Cardiac sympathetic overstimulation 284
Cardiac syncope 278
   diagnosis of 286
Cardiac tamponade 111, 112, 163, 167, 168, 251, 280, 490
   diagnostic hallmarks 168
   therapy 169
Cardiogenic shock 168, 249, 367
   causes of 490
Cardioinhibitory response 288
Cardiomyopathy 18, 261
Cardiopulmonary failure 457
Cardiopulmonary resuscitation studies 252
Cardiovascular
   deaths 226
   disease 125, 207, 231, 643
   events, prevention of 226
   surgery 494
   system 497, 620
Carditis 206
   signs of 206
Cardizem 16, 61
Carotid artery, common 695
Carotid disease 134
Carotid endarterectomy 464
Carotid sinus
   massage 134
   syncope 280
Carotid upstroke, rapid 262
Carotidynia 576
Carpal tunnel syndrome 577
Carvedilol 119
Casts 492
Catapress 17
Cataracts 207, 226, 229
Catastrophic deterioration, managing 467
Catecholamine 38, 252
   crisis 26
   metabolic pathway 37*fc*
   release 46
Catheterization data 172t
Cefamandole 348
Cefazolin 348
Cefixime 353
Cefonicid 349
Cefoperazone 350, 352
Cefotaxime 350-353

Cefotetan 342, 348, 349
Cefoxitin 348
Ceftazidime 338, 347, 350, 351, 353, 481
Ceftizoxime 350-353
Ceftriaxone 335, 347, 350-353
Cefuroxime 329, 347-349
   axetil 328, 349
Cells 492
   membranes 529
   promote shift into 618
Central hypothyroidism 655
Central nervous system 10, 124, 360, 407, 497, 520, 592, 613, 614, 620
   infections of 475
Central venous pressure 491
Centriacinar emphysema 310
Cephalosporins 342, 347, 350, 361, 481
   first-generation 348
   second-generation 348
   third-generation 350, 352, 353
Cephalothin 348
Cephapirin 348
Cephradine 348
Cerebral abscess 483
Cerebral blood flow 278
Cerebral hemorrhage, risk of 544
Cerebral ischemia 30
Cerebral pyogenic abscess 483
   diagnosis 483
   treatment 484
Cerebrospinal fluid 476, 483
   analysis 477t
Cerebrovascular
   accident 631
   disease 282
Certolizumab pegol 416
Cervical
   arthritis 282
   lymphadenopathy 330
Chagas disease 678, 684
   distribution of 684f
   echocardiography 685
   investigations 685
   therapy 685
Charcot joint 581
Chemosis 658
Chemotherapeutic agents 476
Chest
   compressions, continuous 252
   discomfort 185
   illness, acute 311
   infections 193
   normal posteroanterior radiograph of 321f
   tightness 311
   trauma 167, 169
Chest pain 51, 65, 69, 163, 188, 200
   atypical 47
Chest X-ray 106, 264, 272, 372
   hallmarks 175, 189
Childhood cancer 550
Chlamydia 237, 321, 325, 329, 331, 333, 343, 344, 348, 356-363, 588
   pneumoniae 329, 331
   species 320, 330, 334
Chloramphenicol 363, 481, 517
Chlorothiazide 18
Chlorpromazine 398
Chlorpropamide 613, 674
Chlortetracycline 359
Chlorthalidone 13, 18, 679
Cholecystitis 445, 486
   acute 420
   diagnosis 445, 486
   surgery 487
   treatment 445, 486
Choledocholithiasis 420, 421
Cholera 408
Cholesterol 223, 227, 230
   absorption 102, 230
   gallstones 420
Cholestyramine 121
Chondroitin sulfate 575
Chordae 196
Chordal rupture 201
Christmas disease 540
Churg-Strauss syndrome 379, 386, 388
Churg-Strauss vascular syndrome 564
Chylous ascites 433
   causes of 433
Cilastatin 338, 353
   plus 338
Cilazapril 20
Cimetidine 300, 407
Ciprofloxacin 360-362, 441
Cirrhosis 378, 379, 430
   causes of 430
Citric acid 514
Citrobacter 336, 348
   freundii 350
   species 350, 358

Clarithromycin 228, 328, 356, 357
Clavulanate 328, 338
Clindamycin 206, 246, 247, 343, 355, 364, 445, 450
Clonidine 17
Clostridium
   difficile 405, 588
   species 446, 487
Clots 492
Cloudy fluid 386
Cloxacillin 344
Coagulase-negative staphylococci 340
Coagulation, acquired inhibitors of 542
Cocaine 451, 683
Colestipol 121
Collagen vascular disease 379, 398
Collapsing bounding pulse, causes of 183*t*
Collapsing pulse, typical 182
Colonic cancer 415
Colorectal carcinoma 414
Coma 317, 447
   differential diagnosis of 633, 634*t*
Community-acquired pneumonia 320
   antibiotic therapy for 334*fc*
Complete blood count 1, 592
Computed tomography pulmonary
   angiogram 373
   angiography 371
Congestive heart failure 1, 55, 68, 119, 165, 174, 203, 251, 285, 293, 336, 378-380, 383, 432, 589, 657
   risk for 630
   signs of 129, 262
   symptoms of 262
Conjunctivitis 658
Connective tissue
   disease 169, 566, 603
      mixed 603
   disorders 595
   mixed 564
Consciousness 447
   loss of 288, 447
Consolidation, sharp inferior margination of 322*f*
Constipation 228, 438
Constrictive pericarditis 111, 112, 169, 170, 170*t*, 432
   diagnostic hallmarks 170

investigations 171
therapy 172
Cor pulmonale
   acute 367
   signs of 312
Cordarone 157
Coronary angiography 65
Coronary artery 65-67, 67*fc*, 215
   anatomy 276
   bypass grafting 62
   disease 97, 210, 250, 635
      severe 52
   spasm 43, 253, 280
Coronary atheroma, result of 252
Coronary care unit 78
Coronary heart disease 1, 8, 102, 140, 211, 231, 263, 285, 633
Coronary insufficiency, acute 26
Coronary occlusion, acute 89
Coronary revascularization 230
Coronary syndrome, acute 210
Coronary thrombosis 65
Corrigan's pulse 182
Corticosteroid 165, 212, 289, 290, 300, 307, 315*t*, 623
   high-dose 475
   therapy 167, 481, 605
      chronic 314
Costochondral joints 578
Costochondritis 578
Costophrenic sulcus, posterior 377
Cough 166, 188, 311
Coumarins 300
Coxiella 237
Craniospinal irradiation 552
C-reactive protein 206, 215, 695
Creatine kinase 228
Creatine phosphokinase, elevated 457
Creatinine 239, 489, 491
Creeping fat 416
Crescendo-decrescendo starts 262
Crest syndrome 382*f*
Critical care unit 457
Crohn's disease 415, 418, 564
   clinical manifestations 416
   complications 418
   diagnosis 416
   treatment 416
Crushing trauma 493
Cryoglobulinemia, mixed 564

Cryptococcal meningitis 481
  diagnosis 482
  treatment 482
Cryptococcus neoformans 481
Cryptosporidiosis 442
Crystal-induced arthropathies 565, 593
Crystalloids 491
Cushing's disease 667
Cushing's syndrome 666, 667, 675, 676
  causes 667
  clinical manifestations 667
  treatment 667
Cutaneous allodynia 458
Cutaneous lupus erythematosus 405
Cutaneous scleroderma, diffuse 603
Cyanotic heart disease 484
Cyclobenzaprine 576
Cyclophosphamide 276
Cyclosporine 227, 228, 600
Cystic fibrosis 347
Cytogenetic abnormalities 551
Cytology 387
Cytomegalovirus 410, 441, 473, 547
  infection 323*f*, 324*f*
Cytotoxic
  chemotherapy 548
  drugs 227

D

Dantrolene 379
Daunorubicin 276
de Quervain's syndrome 655
Decubitus, bilateral 377
Deficiency disorders 275
Dehydration 631
Dental extractions 247, 538
Denver shunt 434
Deoxygenation, abrupt severe 521
Deoxyribonucleic acid 526
Depression 360
Derivatives tetracycline hydrochloride 359
Dermatomyositis 493, 564, 605
Desacetyl cefotaxime 351
Desmopressin 674
Dexamethasone 165, 315, 661
Diabetes 508, 634*t*
  acute complications of 628
  causation of 207
  chronic complications of 633
  complications of 626
  control of 648*t*
  heart attacks 94
  indication for type 2 645
  screening test for 627*t*
  stimulating hormone 664
  type 2 625, 634
Diabetes mellitus 97, 212, 231, 465
  management of 642
  type 2 625
    diagnosis 626
    types 627
    types of 627*t*
Diabetic cystopathy 641
Diabetic diarrhea 641
Diabetic foot ulcers 642
Diabetic glomerulosclerosis 496, 504
Diabetic ketoacidosis 628, 630*t*
  causes 628
  management 629
  pathogenesis of 629*fc*
  signs 628
  symptoms 628
Diabetic sitosterolemia 69, 94
Diabetic way of eating 642
Diabinese 674
Diagnostic hallmarks 37, 105, 168
  signs 105
  symptoms 105
Dialysis, types of 500
Diaphoresis 633
Diaphragmatic fatigue, sign of 312
Diarrhea 228, 307, 357, 406, 410
  acute 408
  bloody 409
  chewing gum 408
  chronic 409
  infectious 409
  nocturnal 409
  severe 405
  warning 359
Diastolic
  dysfunction 112, 273
  hypertension 3
  pressure 172
  stiffness, ventricular 112
Diazepam 454
Diazoxide 27

Dibenzyline 38
Dichlorodiphenyltrichloroethane 517
Dicloxacillin 344
Dietary
    cholesterol 216
    management 216
    modification 216
    protein, excess 438
    restriction 95
Digitalis 160, 286
    intoxication
        signs of 123
        symptoms of 123
    toxicity 134
Digoxin 119t, 120, 139, 140, 267, 273, 285
    interactions 123b
Digoxin toxicity 123, 124
    major manifestations of 124t
    management of 125
Dihydropyridine 60
    calcium 46, 660
Dihydroxyphenylalanine 516
Dilated cardiomyopathy 271
    clinical hallmarks 271
    diagnosis of 271
    echocardiography 272
    therapy 272
Diltiazem 16, 23, 35, 36, 61, 141, 285, 286, 300
Dipeptidyl peptidase-4 638
Dipyridamole 52, 297
    thallium scintigraphy 52
Dirithromycin 356
Disaccharides 400, 401
Disease groups, six major 564t
Disodium etidronate dosage 623
Disopyramide 134, 151, 153-155, 159, 267
Distal joints, palpation of 584
Diuretics 13, 18, 59, 116, 267
Divalproex sodium 461
Diverticular disease 419
    clinical manifestations 419
    treatment 419
Diverticulitis 419
Dizziness 146, 199, 281fc, 361
    causes of 462
Dizziness vertigo 461
    diagnosis 461
    pathophysiology 461
    therapy 462

Dopamine 469
    agonists 469
Dopaminergic drugs, alternative 469
Dopaquinone 516
Doppler echocardiography 171
    two-dimensional 240
Doppler peak systolic pressure 175
Downs' syndrome 655
Doxazosin 9
Doxorubicin 276
Doxycycline 335, 359, 360
Dressler's syndrome 166
Drug
    abuse 341
    exposure 508
    nephrotoxicity 492
    resistant organisms 314
    therapy 40, 221
        previous 1
Drug-combination choice 115
Drug-related seizures 450
    diagnosis 450
    pathophysiology 451
    therapy 451
Duodenal ulcer
    active 405
    disease 404
Dysautonomia 456
Dysgammaglobulinemia 212
Dyslipidemia 207
    causes of primary 211
    primary 210
    secondary 212
Dyspnea 166, 187, 311
    progressive 188
    severe 383
    signs of 263
    symptoms 263
Dystonia 462

E

Earache 330
Early life-threatening arrhythmias, control of 81
Eaton-Lambert syndrome 470
Ebstein's anomaly 145
Ecchymoses 666
Echocardiography 109, 240t, 276, 374
    ejection fraction 129

Eclampsia 26
Edema 301
Edrophonium 280
Effusion, malignant 386
Ehlers-Danlos syndrome 199, 678, 686
Ejection fraction 133t, 272
Electrical disease, primary 253
Electrocardiogram 1, 498
    abnormalities, stages of 163
    superior quality 700
Electrocardiography 109, 266, 276
    findings 264
Electrode placements 700
Electromechanical dissociation 257
    management of 258
Electron microscopy 507
Electrophysiologic study 287
Embden-Meyerhof pathway 516
Embolism, acute 490
Emergency medical services 252
Emesis 359
Empagliflozin 639
Emphysema 296, 310, 311
    predominant 313
    signs of 318
Empiric antibiotic therapy 435
Empiric therapy 241, 333, 338
Empyema 324f
Enalapril 16, 20, 126
Encainide 151, 153, 155
Encephalitis 476
Encephalopathy 456
End diastolic dimensions 272
Endocarditis 181, 484
    acute 238, 242
    infective 237, 240, 242
        diagnosis of 237
        division of 237
        echocardiography 240
        investigations 238
        physical signs 238
        therapy 241
    prophylaxis 241, 244, 247b
    right-sided acute 239
Endocrine
    disorders 652
    function 498
    system, abnormalities of 431
Endogenous prostaglandins 407
Endomyocardial biopsy 272, 275
Endomyocardial fibrosis 171, 275

Endomyocardial level 273
Endoscopic variceal sclerotherapy 378
Endotracheal intubation 308, 317
End-systolic pressure 113
Enflurane 493
Enoxacin 360
Entamoeba histolytica 445
Enteritis 410
Enterobacter 344, 345, 348, 358, 486
    cloacae 350, 364
    species 336, 338, 339, 345, 350, 356
Enterobacteriaceae 320, 352, 357, 362
Enterococcus 357, 446, 478, 486
    faecalis 351
    faecium 351, 353
    species 343
Enteropathic arthritis 590
Enzyme plasma lipoprotein lipase 232
Eosinophilia 495
Eosinophilic gastroenteritis 432
Eosinophilic syndromes 274
Epigastric distress 357
Epilepsy 449
    diagnosis 449
    pathophysiology 450
    therapy 450
Epinephrine 254, 255, 315
    indications 254
    salutary effects of 254
Episcleritis 596b
Epistaxis 538
Epithelial injury 492
Epstein-Barr virus 473
Erosions 207
Erythema 232
    nodosum 588
Erythrocyte sedimentation rate, high 695
Erythroleukemia 549
Erythromycin 133, 206, 227, 228, 246, 300, 333, 335, 356-358
    estolate 357
    gluceptate 357
    lactobionate 357
    sensitive strains 358
    stearate 247, 357
Erythropoietin 518
    levels 556
Escherichia coli 321, 338, 339, 344, 348-351, 358, 408, 409, 435, 445, 480, 486
    strains 408

Esmolol 138
Esophageal
 disease 341, 350
 perforation 378, 386, 397
 rupture 388
 varices 431
Esophagus 404
Estrogens 212, 300
Ethambutol 167, 441, 481
Ethanol withdrawal 451
Ethosuximide 450
Ethylene glycol 493
Eubacterium lentum 121
Euro-alcohol septal ablation 271
Euthyroid sick syndrome 654
Evans syndrome 544
Exacerbations, acute 315
Exercise 643
 stress testing 47
Exocrine insufficiency 423
Exogenous thyroid hormone ingestion 657
Exogenous toxins 493
Exophthalmos 658
Extracorporeal biliary lithotripsy 421
Extrapyramidal reactions 462
Exudative pleural effusions 378, 382, 385
Eyelids 211
Ezetimibe 53, 100, 101, 209, 230, 232, 637, 646

F

Fabry's disease 275
Fallot's tetralogy 237, 280
Familial dysalbuminemic hyperthyroxinemia 654
Familial hypercholesterolemia 211
Familial mediterranean fever 379
Familiar erythrocytosis 520
Famotidine 300, 407
Fastidious organisms 239
Fasting glucose 626
Fasting plasma glucose 626
Fasting venous plasma glucose 626
Fat and cholesterol content of foods
 saturated 217t, 219t
 unsaturated 219t
Febrile encephalopathy, acute 479

Febrile seizures 452
 causes of simple 452
 complex 452, 453
 diagnosis 452
 pathophysiology 452
 simple 453
 therapy 453
Felcainide 153
Felodipine 17
Felty's syndrome 564, 601
Fenofibrate 232
Fermentable oligosaccharides 400, 401
Ferritin 513
Ferrous sulfate 514
Fibrates 227-229, 232
Fibrinogen levels 227
Fibromyalgia 575, 580
Fibrosing alveolitis 106
Fine-needle aspiration 662
Fistulae 418
Flatulence 228
Flecainide 151, 154, 155
Floxin 362
Flucloxacillin 242
Fluconazole 637
Fluid, redistribution of 490
Flunisolide 306
Fluorescent antibody, direct 331
Fluoroquinolones 328, 360
Flurithromycin 356
Focal neuropathies 641
Focal oligemia 372
Focal segmental glomerulosclerosis 504
Folate deficiency 544
Folic acid 376
 deficiency 528
 intermediates 528
Fontan procedure 378, 385
Food and Drug Administration 360
Foods with comparative sodium content, list of 2t
Foods with lower sitosterol levels 637, 646
Foot care 642
Formiminoglutamic acid 528
Fosinopril 16, 20
Fossa ovale 203
Free thyroxine index 652
Fungal infections 378
Fungal peritonitis 432

Fungal precipitins 239
Fungi 237, 325
Furosemide 18, 27, 35, 116, 623
Fusobacterium nucleatum 340, 341

G

Gallbladder
    disease 233
    mucosa 442
Gallium nitrate 624
Gallop sounds 262
Gallstones 232, 420
    diagnosis 420
    epidemiology 420
    pancreatitis 420
    treatment 420
Gamma interferon 600
Gamma-glutamyl transferase 273
Ganglion blockers 282
Gastric acid secretion 298
Gastric symptoms 165
Gastric ulcer 403
Gastrin production 529
Gastrinoma 404, 406
Gastritis, erosive 426
Gastrointestinal absorption 292
Gastrointestinal bleeding 424, 438
    lower 428
    upper 426
Gastrointestinal diseases 378, 379, 400
Gastrointestinal disturbances 19, 232
Gastrointestinal loss 611, 615
    promote 619
Gastrointestinal procedures 246t, 248
Gastrointestinal symptoms 329
Gastrointestinal system 497
Gastrointestinal tract 396
Gastroparesis 641
Generation cephalosporins 487
Genetic counseling 522
Genetic disease 98, 635
Genetic intestinal defect 97
Genitourinary
    instrumentation 248
    procedures 246t
    surgery 248
Gentamicin 245, 246, 355, 356, 445, 481, 487, 493, 547
Geriatric endocarditis 242
Giant cell arteritis 182, 564, 595, 609

Giardia 410
    lamblia 409
Giardiasis 409
Glasgow coma scale 447
Gliclazide 637, 645
    modified release 645
Glioblastomas 476
Glipizide 645
Glomerular basement membrane 503, 505
Glomerular disease 489, 496, 501
    prognosis 508
    treatment 508
    types of 501
Glomerular filtration rate 489
Glomerular hyperfiltration 500
Glomerular injury, characteristics of 505t
Glomerulonephritis, types of mixed 502t
Glomerulopathy, minimal change 504
Glucocorticoid 413, 417, 622, 657
    replacement, maintenance of 666
    therapy 665
Glucose 386
    insulin infusion 494
    low 476
    suppression test 671
    tolerance, impaired 628
Glucose-6-phosphate dehydrogenase 513, 516
Glyburide 645
Glycated hemoglobin 644, 648
Glycemia reduction 638
Glycogen storage disorders 212
Glycolytic enzymopathy 516
Goblet cells 309
Gonadal hormonal function 518
Goodpasture syndrome 508
Gout 582
Gouty arthritis attacks 585
Graft-versus-host disease 518
Gram's stain 334, 337, 341, 388
Gram-negative
    bacillary infections 350
    bacilli 320, 478
    organisms 354
Gram-positive
    bacilli 352
    bacteria 350
    organisms 354

Granulocyte 529
    colony-stimulating factor 518
    macrophage 518
Granulocytopenia 517
Granulomatous colitis 564
Graves' disease 654, 657, 658, 660
    management of 658
Growth hormone 664
Guanabenz 17
Guillain-Barré syndrome 472, 473

H

Haemophilus influenzae 240, 320, 321, 325-328, 333-335, 344-346, 348-350, 352, 356-362, 473, 478, 480, 515, 521
    pneumonia 328
    therapy 328
Haemophilus parainfluenzae 350
Haemophilus species 350
Hairy cell leukemia 555
Hampton's hump 372
Hashimoto's thyroiditis 654
Headache 233, 329, 361, 556
Head-up tilt testing 288
Heart 602
    atonic 257
    block, complete 251
    border, blurring of right 322*f*
    muscle disease 111, 261, 275
    rate 46
    valves 515
    weight 203
Heart disease 50*f*, 74*f*
    acquired 205
    congenital 237
    history of 307
    hypertensive 112
Heart failure 7*fc*, 57*t*, 66*t*, 105, 108, 110, 115, 120, 268*t*
    causes 110
    management of 105
    pathophysiology 111
    precipitating factors 111
    therapy 114
Heart sound
    fourth 263
    third 171, 263
Heavy chain disease 562

Helicobacter pylori 402, 403
Hemagglutination 523
Hemarthrosis 581
Hematologic disease 602
Hematologic disorders 511
Hematomas 538
Hematuria 501, 544
Hemochromatosis 274, 678, 686
    complications of 687*f*
    diagnosis 687
    therapy 688
Hemodialysis shunts 336
Hemodynamic status 129
Hemoglobin 46, 498
Hemoglobinuria 493, 516, 524
    causes of 493*b*
Hemoglobinuric losses 516
Hemolysis, complement-mediated 524
Hemolytic
    anemia 493, 544
    uremic syndrome 492, 506, 540, 541
Hemophilia 534, 537
    A 534, 536
    B 540
Hemophiliac, treatment of 537
Hemoptysis 188
Hemorrhage 490
    canoe-shaped 238
    intracerebellar 468
    intracranial 535
        caution of 83
    subarachnoid 26
Hemorrhagic strokes 465
Hemostasis 431
    disorders of 530
Hemostatic balance, natural 542
Hemothorax 382, 386, 388
Heparin 375
Hepatic dysfunction 228, 232
Hepatic encephalopathy 431, 437
    causes of 438*t*
    pathogenesis 437
    stages of 439*t*
    treatment 438
Hepatic failure 540
Hepatic hydrothorax 383
Hepatic necrosis, acute 32
Hepatic vein 171
Hepatitis 232
    B 439

bacterial agents 517
C 440
  new drug 440
  chronic active 654
Hepatobiliary
  iminodiacetic acid 443
  manifestations of 439
Hepatocellular carcinoma, primary 431
Hepatojugular reflux 312
Hepatorenal syndrome 431, 433, 435, 436
  diagnosis 436
  management 436
Hereditary disorders 496
Hereditary elliptocytosis 515
Hereditary enzyme defects 493
Hereditary spherocytosis 515
Hernia, diaphragmatic 378
Hexose monophosphate pathway 516
Hickman catheters 336
Hip
  bursitis of 579
  osteoarthritis of 574
Hirsutism 675
  causes 675
  investigations 675
Histamine 295, 529
  H2 receptor antagonists 407
Hoarseness 188
Holosystolic murmur 246
Holter monitor 149f, 267, 278
Homozygous
  disease 525
  thalassemia 526
Hoover's sign 312
Hospital-acquired pneumonias 361
Human immunodeficiency virus 275, 410, 545, 594
Human leukocyte antigen 518
Hydralazine 27, 30, 31, 33, 34, 36, 398
  intravenous infusion 25
Hydraulic stress, reduces 65
Hydrochlorothiazide 14, 18, 462, 509
Hydroflumethiazide 18
Hydrogen atoms 516
Hydrogen potassium ATPase inhibitors 405
Hydrolyze cephalosporins 350
Hydronephrosis 492
Hydrophilic agents 89, 227

Hydroxy-methylglutaryl-coenzyme A reductase inhibitors 222
Hydroxyurea treatment 521
Hyperaldosteronism, primary 39, 668
Hyperbilirubinemia 436
Hypercalcemia 421, 559, 619
  acute management of 620, 621fc
  causes 619
  chronic management 623
  management of 622t
  reduction of 560
  symptoms and signs 620
Hypercapnia 313
  absence of 317
  signs of 312
  worsening 317
Hypercholesterolemia 208, 465, 501
Hyperglycemia 97, 314, 500, 611, 631
Hyperglycemic hyperosmolar coma 631
  management 632
Hyperkalemia 119, 258, 494, 616, 617fc
  causes 616
  electrocardiographic signs of 618f
  manifestations 617
  treatment 617
Hyperlipemia 421
Hyperlipidemia 225
  familial combined 212
  moderate 224
  primary combined 212
  severe 211, 611
Hyperlipoproteinemia 211
Hypermobility syndrome 575, 579, 580
Hyperosmolar state, pathogenesis of 632fc
Hyperperfusion 498
Hyperplasia, smooth muscle 309
Hyperprolactinemia 669
  women with 670
Hyperproteinemia 611
Hypersitosterolemia 628
Hypertension 1, 25, 140, 182, 225, 465, 489, 500
  accelerated 24
    malignant 26
  in elderly 23
  in pregnancy 31
    malignant 24
  mild-to-moderate 4fc, 6fc
  moderate 224

primary 1
  drug therapy 3
  nondrug therapy 1
secondary 25, 35
severe 25
treatment of 15
Hypertensive crisis 25, 34
Hypertensive emergency 25
  treatment of 27t
  types of 26
Hypertensive encephalopathy 26
Hypertensive urgencies 25
Hyperthermia 453, 456, 493
Hyperthyroidism 657
  causes 657
  differential diagnosis of 653
  symptoms 657
Hypertriglyceridemia
  primary 212
  treatment of 233
Hypertrophic cardiomyopathy 251, 261, 263, 267t, 280, 282, 286
  clinical hallmarks of 262, 263t
  echocardiography 266
    findings 264
    hallmarks of 266b
  mild 265f
  pathophysiology 261
  therapy 267
Hypertrophic pulmonary osteoarthropathy 593
Hypertrophy 49f
Hypoalbuminemia 233, 408, 501
Hypocapnia 372
Hypochromia 526
Hypoglycemia 282, 633, 637, 657
  management 633
  unawareness 643
Hypoglycemic medications 643
Hypokalemia 14, 119, 252, 611, 615
  causes 615
  hypomagnesemia, severe 159
  treatment 616
Hypomagnesemia 119
Hyponatremia 611, 657
  acute 614
  causes 611
    of true 612fc
  clinical manifestations 613
  to sodium loss 613

  treatment 613
  with seizures, severe 614
Hypotension 137, 164, 288
  mild 134
  postural 282, 284
Hypothermia 493, 656
Hypothyroidism 159, 212, 654
  causes of 654
    primary 655
  clinical manifestations 655
  diagnosis 656
  treatment 656
Hypoventilation 282
Hypovolemia 258
Hypovolemic shock 424
Hypoxemia 119, 139, 282, 313, 317, 372

I

Ibuprofen 165, 166
Idiopathic endocardial fibrosis 274
Idiopathic hirsutism 676
  management 676
Idiopathic pericarditis 164
Imipenem 338, 342, 353, 354
Immune
  dysfunction 554
  mediated hemolytic anemia 517
  neutropenias 546
  purpuras 545
  thrombocytopenic purpura 544
Immunoblastic lymphadenopathy 379
Immunofluorescence microscopy 507
Immunoglobulin G disorders 524
Immunohemolytic anemia 522
  classification of 523
Immunohemolytic diseases 522
Immunosuppressive
  agents 212
  drugs 228
Impotence 232, 641
Indapamide 14, 18, 509
Indomethacin 165, 166
Infarction
  sites, location of 76
  size of 76
Infection 438, 441, 493, 508
  induced marrow hypoplasia 516
  multitude of 443
  purulent 167

Infectious agents 274
Infectious disease 275, 378
Infectious tubulointerstitial nephritis, acute 495
Inferolateral infarction, acute 73f
Inflammation 493
Inflammatory bowel disease 400, 411, 587
  risk of 638
Inflammatory disease 578
Inflammatory disorders 215
Inflammatory mediators 295
Inflammatory monoarthritis 582
Inflammatory nonseptic arthritis 588
Inflammatory rheumatic diseases 563
Infliximab 416
Influenza 320
  A virus 473
  vaccine 300
Inhaled corticosteroids 306t
Inherited coagulation defects 534, 536
Inherited disorders 517
Inorganic poisons 517
Insecticides 517
Insulin 618, 631, 648, 649
  glucose infusion for surgery 649t
Interacting drugs 637
Interferon 300
Interferon-α, thalidomide 655
Interlobar fissure 107
Intermittent porphyria, acute 527, 654
International normalized ratio 270, 534
Interphalangeal joints, proximal 573
Interstitial pulmonary edema 106, 107f
Interventional therapy 82
Intestinal disease, mild-to-moderate 409
Intestinal obstruction 418
Intestinal shunt 587
Intestine 620
Intracranial vasculitis 465
Intractable itching 497
Intraduodenal segment 443
Intraluminal digestion, impaired 410
Intramuscular iron 514
Intrapleural streptokinase 395
Intratubular pressure 492
Intravascular devices 336
Intravascular ultrasound 209

Intravascular volume, maintenance of 494
Intravenous
  immunoglobulin 545
  theophylline 299t
Iodide 661
Iodine 655
Ionizing radiation 517
Ipilimumab 655
Ipratropium 296
Ipratropium bromide 294, 296, 315
  effect of 296
Iritis 585
Iron
  absorption 514
  deficiency 511, 513
  insoluble 514
Irritable bowel syndrome 400, 580
Ischemia 110, 134, 252, 468
  changes 51
  risk of 10
Ischemic cardiomyopathy 229
Ischemic disease 51
Ischemic heart disease 194, 286, 293
  diagnosis of 272
  history of 252
  severe 280
Isoniazid 167, 300, 398
Isoproterenol 300
Isoptin 17
Isospora belli 410
Isotonic saline 491
Isradipine 17
Ixekizumab 584

J

Joint
  aspiration and injection, principles for 571b
  motion, range of 574
  pain, symmetrical 580
  protection guide 572b
  swelling, sensation of 579
Jugular venous
  distension 312
  elevated 70
  pressure 164, 258, 271
Juvenile arthritis 564

Juvenile monoarthritis 585
  treatment 585
Juvenile spondyloarthropathy 586
  treatment 586

K

K depletion
  mild 616
  moderate 616
Kaposi's sarcoma 410, 441
Kawasaki syndrome 678, 693
  diagnosis 693
  therapy 694
Kawasaki's disease 564
Kayexalate 619
Kerley B lines 107f
Kernig's sign 476
Ketoconazole 133
Ketosis 631
Kidney 489, 620
  disease 602
    chronic 110, 495
    end-stage 489
  function 495
  injury, progressive acute 510
  size 498
Klebsiella 321, 325, 336, 338, 344, 349, 351, 352, 358, 486
  aerogenes 350
  oxytoca 350
  pneumoniae 339, 344, 345, 348, 349, 350
  species 346, 350, 352
Knee
  bursitis of 579
  osteoarthritis of 574
Kussmaul's sign 168

L

Labetalol 17, 26-28, 30, 32, 33
Lactate dehydrogenase 383, 386, 443
Lactobacillus
  casei systems 528
  plantarum 402
Lansoprazole 405
Laparoscopic cholecystectomy 420
Left atrial
  beat 263
  enlargement 189
  myxoma 110
Left bundle branch block 51, 145, 287
Left ventricular
  dysfunction 129, 136
    moderate 105
    severe 105
  ejection fraction 229
  end-diastolic pressure 172
  failure 168, 175
  hypertrophy 109, 145, 175, 282, 465, 498
  thrust 263
Leg cramps 497
Legionella 320, 330, 334, 357, 361, 362
  infections 360
  pneumoniae 332
  species 321, 326, 332, 333, 343, 348, 356-359, 361, 363
Lethal arrhythmias 68, 150, 157
Lethal ventricular arrhythmias 158
Leuconostoc citrovorum 528
Leukemia 476, 548, 549, 560
  late-occurring 517
Leukocytes 489, 546
Leukocytosis 524, 547
Leukopenia 546
Leukotriene receptor antagonists 305
Levamisole 600
Leveen shunt 434
Levofloxacin 360
Levothyroxine monotherapy 656
Libman-Sacks valvulitis 602
Lidocaine 81, 92, 152, 155, 160, 255, 256
  dosage 84t
Light microscopy 507
Lignocaine 81, 155, 255, 256
  dosage 84t
Limb electrodes 701
Lipid-lowering trial 224
Lipodystrophy 212
Lipophilic agents 227
Lipoprotein
  cholesterol, high-density 214
  high-density 518
Liquid and oral preparations 616
Lisinopril 20
Listeria monocytogenes 478, 480
Lisuride 469
Lithium 300, 655

Liver 216, 230
   cirrhosis of 432
   function 232
Liver abscess 444, 485
   diagnosis 444, 485
Liver disease 430, 654
   chronic 212
   complications of 431b
   severe end-stage 435
Lomefloxacin 360
Lorazepam 454
Lorcainide 155
Loriaux 667
Losartan 116
Lovastatin 227
Low-density lipoprotein 208, 209, 216
   cholesterol 1, 97, 207, 208, 213,
      213t, 228, 625
      blood testing centers 209, 221
Lower lobe vessels, constriction of 106
Lugol's solution 661
Lung
   infection 108
   interstitial spaces of 377
   scan 374
      non-diagnostic 371
      trapped 379
      ultrasound 108
Lupus anticoagulant 376
Lupus erythematosus 379, 398, 564
Lupus nephritis 507
Lupus pleuritis 398
Luteinizing hormone 664
Lyme carditis 678, 688
   diagnosis 688
   therapy 689
Lyme disease 594
   diagnosis 594
   treatment of 594
Lymphangitic carcinomatosis 105, 108
Lymphatic leukemia, acute 550
Lymphoblastic leukemia, acute 549-551
Lymphocytic leukemia, chronic 553, 554
Lymphoma 410, 476, 481, 655
Lymphoplasmacytoid cells 561, 562
Lyonization hypothesis 535

M

Macrocytic anemia 527
Macroglobulinemia 561

Macrolides 356
   penetrate 356
Macroprolactinoma, women with 670
Macrovascular disease 633
Maculopapular rash, diffuse 330
Magnesium sulfate 34, 160, 257
Malabsorption syndromes 121, 410
   chronic 540
   diagnosis 411
   pathophysiologic mechanisms 410
Malabsorptive disorders 528
Mallory-Weiss tear 426, 428
Mammary artery, internal 178
Mannitol 401
Marfan's syndrome 10, 184, 199, 678,
   690
   diagnostic symptoms 690
   signs 690
   treatment 691
Marrow aplasia 517
Mask pulsus paradoxus 164
Massive pulmonary embolism 168, 373f
Mastocytosis 285
Mastoiditis 483
Match-unrelated donors 518
McConnell's sign 374
Mechanical obstruction, acute 251
Mechanical ventilation 308, 317, 347
Mediastinal irradiation 169
Mediterranean linolenic acid-rich diet
   221
Mediterranean population 516
Megakaryocytes 527
Megaloblastic anemia 527
Meigs' syndrome 379, 432
Membrane disorders 514
Membranoproliferative
      glomerulonephritis 503, 506
Membranous glomerulopathy 504
Meniere's syndrome 462
Meningeal inflammation 476
Meningeal leukemia 552
Meningismus 476
Meningococcal meningitidis 478
Menorrhagia 538, 539
Meropenem 354
Mesalamine 413, 417
Mesangial cells 507
Mesothelioma 378, 379
Metabolic bone disease 497

Metabolic disorders 516
Metamucil 121
Metastatic disease 378
Metastatic nodules 381f
Metastatic peritoneal carcinomatosis 432
Metered-dose inhaler 291
Metformin 643-645
Methacholine 295
Methacholine 529
Methadone 683
Methaqualone 451
Methicillin-resistant *Staphylococcus*
 aureus 340
 epidermidis 353
Methicillin-sensitive strains 243
Methimazole 661
Methionine-methyl synthesis 529
Methonitrate salts 294
Methotrexate 552
Methoxyflurane 493
Methyl tert-butyl 421
Methylclothiazide 18
Methyldopa 17, 27, 31, 34
Methylprednisolone 315
Methylxanthine 138, 296, 307, 315
 therapy 307
Methysergide 379, 399
Meticulous fluid 494
Metoclopramide 121
Metolazone 18, 118
Metoprolol 4, 10, 11, 17, 119, 139, 255
Metronidazole 342, 409, 481, 485
Metyrosine 39
Mexiletine 153-156, 300
Mexitil 156
Mezlocillin 342, 347, 481
Miconazole 637
Microcytic anemia 513t
 causes of 511
Microcytic hypochromic anemia 511, 526
Microprolactinoma, women with 670
Midodrine 285
Migraine 458, 461
 acute 459
 attack 458
 chronic 460
 diagnosis 458
 exacerbate 458
 headache 580
 pathophysiology 458
 therapy 459
 treatment of 461
Miller-fisher variant 472
Milwaukee shoulder and knee 585
Mineralocorticoid therapy 665
Minocycline 359, 600
Miscellaneous disorders 678
Mithramycin 622, 623
Mitral annular calcification 203
Mitral balloon valvuloplasty 195
 complications of 195t
Mitral commissurotomy 195
Mitral leaflet
 anterior 203
 posterior 203
Mitral regurgitation 190, 196, 246, 262
 acute 197
 causes of 197fc
 chronic 197
 surgical treatment 197
Mitral ring, normal 198
Mitral stenosis 108, 187, 189, 198
 diagnosis 187
 echocardiographic assessment for 189, 191f
 electrocardiographic hallmarks 189
 interventional management 194
 medical therapy 193
 mild 187, 193, 194
 moderate 193
 physical signs 188
 severe 187, 193, 196
Mitral systolic murmur 263
Mitral valve
 area 196
 orifice area, excellent quantification of 192f
 replacement 196
 surgery 270
Mitral valve prolapse 198, 199, 202t, 203, 280
 causes 199
 complications 201
 prophylaxis for 246
 signs 200
 symptoms 199
 therapy 204
Mitral vein 171

Monoarticular arthritis 565t, 581, 585
Monobactams 354
Monoclonal antibodies 600, 655
Monoclonal gammopathy 212, 559, 561
Monosaccharides 400
Moraxella catarrhalis 320, 325, 328, 335, 344, 349, 350, 355, 356, 357, 358, 360, 361
   therapy 329
Morganella 336, 345, 346
   morganii 350
Moricizine 155
Morphine 80
Motor response 447
Mouth ulcers 19
Moxalactam 351
Mucosal absorption 411
Mucosal inflammation 313, 412
Mucous gland
   enlargement 309
   hypertrophy 310
Mucous secretion 309
Murmur 238
Muscarinic antagonist, long-acting 289, 290
Muscarinic receptors 295
Muscle tremors 293
Muscular ischemia 493
Muscular overexertion 493
Musculoskeletal pain 369
Myalgia 228, 329
Myasthenia gravis 470
   diagnosis 470
   pathophysiology 471
   therapy 471
Mycobacteria 325
Mycobacterium avium-intracellulare 441, 587
Mycobacterium tuberculosis 166, 410, 441
Mycoplasma 321, 325, 330, 334, 343, 348, 356, 358, 359, 362, 363, 655
   legionella 358
   pneumoniae 320, 326, 329-331, 333, 335, 344, 473
      therapy 331
   species 325, 335, 357, 360
Myelitis, transverse 602
Myelofibrosis 558
Myelogenous leukemia, chronic 552

Myeloid leukemia
   acute 541, 548, 549
   management of acute 550
Myeloma 558, 559, 562
   assessment 560
   clinical presentation 559
   management strategy 560
   multiple 493
   prognosis 560
   treatment 560
Myelomatosis 559
Myeloproliferative disorders 548, 555
Myeloproliferative syndromes 558
Myocardial contractility 113
Myocardial damage 111
Myocardial infarction 67fc, 79t, 97, 163, 207, 225, 251, 280, 490, 556, 625
   acute 65, 73, 90, 108, 119, 463
   inferior 71f, 72f
   inferior 144f, 145, 145f
Myocardial involvement 275
Myocardial ischemia 30, 44
   syndromes 138
Myocardial necrosis 68
Myocardial rupture 251
Myocarditis, hypersensitivity 276
Myocardium 45, 90, 157
Myofascial chest wall pain syndrome 578
Myofascial low back pain 578
Myofascial pain 563
   syndromes 575
Myoglobinuria 457, 494
   causes of 493b
Myopathy 232
Myositis 207, 233
Myxedema 378, 385
   ascites 432
   coma 656
   management 656
Myxomatous degeneration 182

N

Nadolol 17, 58, 691
Nafcillin 242, 481
Nail fold lesion 596f
Naproxen 166
Narcotic analgesics 422

Nasal cannula 316
  flow rate 317
Nasal polyps 302
Nasogastric aspirate 425
Nausea 228, 233, 359, 660
Nebivolol 679
Necrotic renal papilla 492
Necrotic tissue 90
Necrotizing vasculitis 606
  differential diagnosis 609
  pathogenesis 606
  treatment 609
  workup 606
Needle biopsy 389
Neisseria 350, 362
  catarrhalis 328
  gonorrhoeae 588
  meningitidis 343, 480
  species 358, 360
Neomycin 121
Neoplasm 325, 508
Neoplastic diseases 378
Neoplastic involvement 167
Neoplastic lesions 441
Neoplastic pericarditis 167
Nephritic syndrome 501
Nephritis 507
Nephrogenic ascites 432
Nephrogenic diabetes insipidus,
  treatment of 675
Nephron population decreases 496
Nephropathy 640
Nephrotic syndrome 212, 233, 378,
  384, 501
Nephrotoxic acute tubular necrosis 493*b*
Nephrotoxicity 355
Nerve entrapment disorders 563
Neuroendocrine tumors 408
Neurogenic bladder 641
Neurogenic diabetes insipidus, chronic
  treatment of 674
Neuroleptic malignant syndrome 456
  diagnosis 456
  pathophysiology 457
  therapy 457
Neurologic disorders 447
Neurologic dysfunction 19
Neuropathy 641, 643
Neurosurgery 476
Neutropenia 19
  severe 547

Neutropenic fever 547
  prevention of 547
New biological drugs 417
New Drug Class and New Therapies
  230
New York Heart Association 114
  functional class 115
Niacin 228, 233
  use of 233
Nicardipine 17
Nicorette 300
Nicotinic acid 227, 229
Nifedipine 8, 16, 23, 27, 30, 31, 35, 39,
  61, 282
Nitrates 58
  high-dose 59
Nitrendipine 17, 23
Nitric oxide 433
Nitrofurantoin 379
Nitroglycerin 27, 31, 59, 91, 94
Nitroprusside 26, 27, 29, 31, 38
  infusion pump chart 29*t*
Nivolumab 655
Nodal osteoarthritis 573
  differential diagnosis 574
  initial treatment 574
  pathogenesis 574
Nonarticular disorders 566
Nonarticular rheumatic
  disorders 575, 576
  pain disorders 563
Noncardiogenic pulmonary edema,
  causes of 105
Nondrug therapy 1
Nonfatal stroke 230
Non-Hodgkin's lymphoma 441
Noninfiltrative eye signs 658
Noninflammatory monoarthritis 581
Nonproliferative glomerular disorders,
  characteristics of 504*t*
Nonsteroidal anti-inflammatory drugs
  106, 436, 460, 491, 494, 570, 592
Norfloxacin 360
Normocytic normochromic anemias
  514
Normodyne 17
Norovirus 408
Nosocomial acquisition 332
Nosocomial pneumonia 335, 336, 339*t*
  diagnosis 336

microbiology 335
pathogenesis 335
therapy of 337, 347
N-terminal probrain natriuretic peptide 110
Nuclear cholescintigraphy 420
Nucleated red cells 512
Nutrition 414, 418

O

Obesity 110, 212
Obstructive airway disease 293, 294, 296, 311
Obstructive cardiomyopathy 47, 143
Obstructive jaundice 212
Obstructive lesion 44
Obstructive pulmonary disease 296
   chronic 12, 52, 106, 258, 289, 292, 309, 326, 367
   severe chronic 168
Ofloxacin 360, 362
Oliguria 490, 492
Olmesartan 116
Olsalazine 413
Omeprazole 405, 406
Ominous disease 578
Ondansetron 402
Ophthalmoplegia 658
Oral
   anticoagulants 375
Oral anti-inflammatory treatment 585
Oral ciprofloxacin 361
Oral contraceptives 300
Oral dissolution therapy 420
Oral hypoglycemic agents 643, 649
Oral therapy, chronic 156
Oropharynx 238
Orthodromic arrhythmia, common 146
Orthodromic tachycardia 146
Orthopnea 188
   occasionally 166
Orthostatic hypotension 284, 641
Osteoarthritis 573, 581
Osteogenesis imperfecta 182, 199
Osteomyelitis 362, 578
Osteonecrosis 581
Osteoporosis 314
Otitis 484
Ototoxicity 355

Overnight dexamethasone suppression test 676
Oxacillin 481
Oxidant-induced membrane stress 516
Oxidase inhibitors 293
Oxygen 82
   conservation devices 317
   masks 316
   partial pressure of 305
   therapy 316
Oxytetracycline 359

P

Pacemaker syndrome 280
Paget's disease 582, 587
Pain
   abdominal 233, 660
   management of 165, 574
Painless thyroiditis 662
Palla's sign 372
Palpate joint synovium 595
Palpitations 200, 293
Pamidronate 624
Panacinar emphysema 310
Pancreatic ascites 432, 433
Pancreatic cancer 476
Pancreatic pleural effusion, chronic 378, 397
Pancreatitis 212, 232, 396, 421, 490
   acute 216, 378, 421
   chronic 423
Pancuronium 300
Pancytopenia, severe 519
Panic disorders 200
Pantoprazole 405
Papilla 492
Papillary muscle 196
   dysfunction 271
Papillary stenosis 442, 443
Paracentesis, large-volume 434
Paragonimiasis 386
Parainfluenza 320
Paraneoplastic syndromes 593
Parapneumonic effusion 386, 393
   complicated 393, 394
Paraproteinemia 558, 561, 562
Parasitic infections 378, 409
Parathyroid hormone 497
Paravertebral soft-tissue swelling 380*f*

Parenteral thiamine administration 456
Paresthesia 580
Parietal cell 406
Parietal pleura 377
Parkinson's disease 468
  diagnosis 468
  pathophysiology 469
  therapy 469
Paromomycin 409
Paroxysmal atrial tachycardia 139
Paroxysmal nocturnal dyspnea 270
Paroxysmal supraventricular tachycardia
  management of 136t
  termination of 121
Parvovirus
  B19 infection 594
  infections 593
Patent ductus 237
Patent foramen ovale 203
Pedal edema 312
Pefloxacin 360
Peliosis hepatis 441
Pelvic and vaginal ultrasound 676
Penbutolol 17
Penicillin 206, 242, 245, 289, 327, 342, 356, 361, 589
  binding proteins 342
  G 343, 344, 347, 481
  replace 246
  susceptible organisms 343
  susceptible viridans group 242
Pentamidine 159, 421
Peptic ulcer 402, 426
  chronic 404
Peptic ulcer disease 402-404
  complications 404
  diagnosis 403
  diagnostic investigations 404
  etiology 402
  therapy 404
Percutaneous coronary intervention 68, 82, 231, 259
Perfusion 374
Pergolide mesylate 469
Perianal disease 418
Pericardial adherence 171
Pericardial disease 379
Pericardial fat 321*f*
Pericardial fluid 166
Pericardial resection 167

Pericardial tamponade 369
Pericardial tissue 166
Pericardiocentesis 167
Pericarditis 163, 164, 164t, 166, 206, 589
  acute 74, 74f, 75, 165f, 166
  causes of 163, 164fc
  nonspecific 166, 167
  purulent 166
Perindopril 16
Periodontal disease 341
Perioperative hypertension 26
Periorbital edema 658
Peripheral artery disease 642
Peripheral blood
  film 519
  morphology 512t
Peripheral systolic pressure 113
Peripheral vascular disease 52, 95, 213, 556, 626
Peripheral vasodilation 490
Peripheral vein, dosage using 135
Periprocedural stroke, lower 181
Perisplenitis 557
Peritoneal dialysis 378, 384
Peritoneal mesothelioma 432
Peritoneovenous shunts 434
Peritonitis 490, 500
Periumbilical pain 410
Perplexing disorder, common 400
Persantine nuclear myocardial perfusion 52
Pharmacologic agents 529
Phenobarbital 121, 450, 455
Phenoxybenzamine 38
Phentolamine 27, 38
Phenylephrine 139, 262
Phenylhydantoin 517
Phenytoin 121, 300, 398, 450, 454
Pheochromocytoma 37, 39, 285, 669
  diagnostic hallmarks 37
  therapy 38
Phosphate 622
Phosphodiesterase inhibition 613
Pigment gallstones 420
Pindolol 17, 32
Pioglitazone 638
Piperacillin 338, 342, 347, 481
Pirbuterol 294
Pituitary adenoma 667
Pituitary diseases, anterior 669

Pituitary disorders, posterior 673
Plant sterol 97
Plasma
    17-hydroxyprogesterone 676
    catecholamines 38
    corticotropin 667
    cortisol measurements 667
    growth hormone-releasing
        hormone levels 671
Platelet 547
    aggregation 65
    defects 534
    disorders 543
        functional 535
        numbers 534
Plethora 556
Pleural disease 377
    drug-induced 379
    malignant 388
Pleural effusion 106, 377, 383, 390,
        392, 396, 398, 421
    differential diagnosis of 378b
    malignant 390
    signs of 378
    symptoms of 378
Pleural fluid
    accumulates 377
    cytology 387
    formation 377
    lipid analysis 389
    presence of 377
Pleural tuberculosis 389
Pleurodesis 392
Pleuroscopy 390
Plicamycin 622, 623
Pneumocystis carinii 323f, 324f, 441
    infection 396
Pneumocystis infection 105, 547
Pneumonia 105, 320, 321, 333, 370,
        379, 457
    atypical 329
    complicates 336
    massive 522
    treatment of 355
    typical 326
Pneumothorax 168, 316, 369
Poikilocytosis 526
Polyarteritis
    microscopic 507
    pauciarticular 565b

Polyarticular arthritis 565t
Polychondritis 182
Polycystic kidney 40
    disease, adult 496
Polycystic ovarian disease 676
Polycythemia 317
    secondary 557
    vera 368, 555, 556
Polygenic hypercholesterolemia 209
Polymorphonuclear leukocytes 360
Polymyositis 564, 605
    differential diagnosis 605
    pathogenesis 605
    Toxoplasma gondii 605
    treatment 605
Polyneuropathy 559
    acute 472
        diagnosis 472
        pathophysiology 473
        therapy 473
Polyols 401
Polythiazide 18
Polyuria 673
    causes 673
    differential diagnosis 673
    direct testing 674
    indirect testing 674
Porcine valve replacement 180
Porphyria 227, 526
    treatment 527
Postabdominal surgery 378
Postbulbar duodenum 404
Postcardiac injury syndrome 379
Postcardiac surgery 169
Postcoronary artery bypass surgery 379
Postinfarction pericarditis 166
Postinfectious disorder, typical 473
Postmyocardial infarction 9, 57t, 66t,
        268t
Postrenal obstruction 492
Postsplenectomy penicillin 515
Post-thoracotomy 140
Potassium 499, 611
    replacement for diabetic
        ketoacidosis 630t
    restrict intake of 618
    sparing diuretics 14
Pramipexole 469
Pravastatin 227
Prazosin 16

Prednisolone 315
Prednisone 165, 315, 471, 495, 554
Pregnancy, hypertensive crisis of 34
Pregnant women with
    microprolactinoma 670
Prerenal acute renal failure 490
    causes of 490b
Presyncope 200, 263
Primidone 450
Procainamide 148, 151, 153-156, 159, 398, 683
Procarbazine 379, 399
Progesterone 212
Prolactin 671
Prolactinomas, therapy of 670
Proliferative glomerulonephritis, types of 502t
Proliferative retinopathy 643
Prolongation syndrome 160
Prolymphocytic leukemia 555
Propafenone 151, 153, 155
Propionic acid, metabolism of 529
Propofol 683
Proprandolol 17
Propranolol 4, 27, 33, 66, 138, 255, 269, 460, 661
Propylthiouracil 659, 661
Prostate, enlarged 492
Prosthetic valve
    choice 179
    complications 181t
    dysfunction 280
    endocarditis 242
    implant 196
    surgery 182
Protease inhibitors, deficiency of 310
Protein 489, 499
    abnormal 492
    loss 500
Proteinuria 19, 501
    presence of 496
Proteus 344, 346
    mirabilis 344, 345, 348, 350
    species 338, 344, 346, 349, 350
    vulgaris 348
Prothrombin 540
Proton pump inhibitors 405
Providencia 336, 346, 348, 350
Pruritus 232, 557
Pseudocysts 422

Pseudogout 582, 584, 593
    treatment 585
Pseudomembranous colitis 418
    clinical manifestations 418
    diagnosis 419
    treatment 419
Pseudomonas 239, 314, 346
    aeruginosa 240, 337-339, 345, 346, 347, 348, 350, 351, 352, 353, 354, 355, 360, 361, 362
    cepacia 240, 339, 350, 353, 354
    infections 586
    species 344, 353, 356, 358
Pseudomyxoma peritonei 432
Psoriasis 587, 595
Psoriatic arthritis 182, 564, 584
Psoriatic monoarthritis 584
Psychosis 360
Pulmonary angiography 370, 375
Pulmonary arterial hypertension 510
Pulmonary artery
    right descending 372
    transverse diameter of 373f
Pulmonary complications 422
Pulmonary congestion 168, 187
Pulmonary edema 28, 369
    acute 26
Pulmonary emboli 378
Pulmonary embolism 280, 336, 367, 371
    diagnosis 367
    management 375
Pulmonary embolization 378, 379, 396
Pulmonary fibrosis 469
Pulmonary function
    disorders of 431
    testing 313
Pulmonary hypertension 280, 317
Pulmonary infections 360
Pulmonary stenosis 280
Pulmonary thromboembolism 316
Pulmonary venous pressures 194
Pulseless disease 285
Pulsus paradoxus 164, 168
Putrid odor 386
Pyelonephritis
    acute 495
    chronic 495, 496
Pyogenic abscesses, treatment of 485
Pyogenic meningitis 478, 478t, 479t
    diagnosis 478
    treatment of 478, 480t

Pyrazinamide 481
Pyridostigmine bromide 471
Pyridoxine 167
Pyruvate kinase deficiency 516

Q

QT syndrome
   long 280
   prolonged 251, 287
   short 683
Quinapril 16, 20, 21
Quinethazone 18
Quinidine 121, 133, 151, 153-155, 159, 683
Quinolones 300, 355

R

Radiation 370
Radioactive iodine 653
Radionuclide
   evaluation 109
   scintigraphy 51
Ramipril 16, 20, 21
Rampant atherosclerotic disease 634
Ranitidine 300, 407
Rash 232
Raynaud's phenomenon 12, 580, 596, 604
Reactive arthritis 565, 588
Red blood cell 238, 491, 513, 515
   aplasia, pure 511
Red cell 547
   deformation 518
   hypoplasia 518
   membrane 514, 524
Reflex dystrophy 581
Refractory epilepsy, cannabidiol for 451
Refractory hypoxemia 308
Reiter's syndrome 182, 587, 588
Renal acute renal failure 492
Renal artery disease, acute 490
Renal disease 355, 489, 640
   end-stage 489, 640
   non-end-stage 110
   preexisting 493
Renal dysfunction
   acute 26
   mild 227

Renal failure 20, 28, 122, 285, 457, 489
   acute 457, 489, 498t
      diagnosis of 491t
      major causes of 489b
   chronic 169, 489, 495, 496, 498t
      diagnosis 498
      management 498
      natural history 497
      signs and symptoms 497
   index 491
   postrenal acute 491
   prerenal acute 490
      diagnosis 490
      management 490
Renal function 489
   impaired 355
Renal impairment 631
Renal insufficiency 422
Renal loss 611, 615
   of potassium, promote 619
Renal parenchymal disease 35
Renal pelvis 492
Renal stones 508
Renin angiotensin system 113
Renovascular hypertension 36
Resistant hypertension 24
Resonium calcium 619
Respiratory 557
   acidosis 317
   arrest 466
   drive depression 316
   embarrassment 500
   infections 302
   support 656
   tract infections, treatment of lower 360
Respiratory distress syndrome
   acute 108, 336, 421
   neonatal 32
Restrictive cardiomyopathy 109, 111, 170t, 273
   clinical hallmarks 274
   therapy 274
Restrictive lung disease 105
Restrictive syndrome 170
Resuscitation 424
Reticulocytopenia 517
Reticulocytosis 515, 524
Reticuloendothelial system 516
Retinal disease 640
   progression of 640

Retinitis 443
Retinoic acid 548
Retinoids 212
Retinopathy 640
Retrograde pyelogram 492
Reye's syndrome 589
Rhabdomyolysis 228, 234
  risk of 228
Rheumatic diseases 570, 575
Rheumatic disorders 563
  investigations 569
Rheumatic fever 174, 182, 205, 206, 597
  acute 187, 564, 589
  attack of 206
  clinical features 205
  secondary 206
  therapy 206
Rheumatic heart disease 199
Rheumatic pain disorders 563
Rheumatoid arthritis 564, 578, 582, 595
  differential diagnosis 596
  pathogenesis 596
  seronegative 565, 594
  treatment 582, 597
  workup 597
Rheumatoid diseases 595
Rheumatoid effusion 386
Rheumatoid pleuritis 379, 388, 398
Rheumatoid test 594
Rheumatoid vasculitis 596f
Rhinorrhea 302, 330
Rhonchi 312
Rickettsia 441
  like organism 443
  species 359
Riedel's thyroiditis 655
Rifabutin 441
Rifampin 167, 441, 481
Right bundle branch block 146, 287
Right ventricular
  collapse 169
  end-diastolic pressure 172
  hypokinesis 374
  infarction 111, 143
  strain pattern 373
Rochalimaea quintana 441
Ropinirole 469
Rosiglitazone 638
Rosuvastatin 227
Roth's spots 238

Roxithromycin 356
Ruptured esophagus 133

S

Sacroiliitis, differential diagnosis of 587
Salbutamol 289, 293, 294, 618
Salicylates 582
Salmonella 408-410
Sarcoid 274
Sarcoidosis 379, 476, 655
Scandinavian simvastatin survival study 222
Scapulothoracic syndromes 576
Schistosoma mansoni 475
Scleroderma 274, 509, 603
  classification of 603
  linear 604
  localized 604
Sclerosing cholangitis 442, 443
Sedation 462
  mild 82
Sedatives 438
Seizures 308, 464, 465
Selenium deficiency 275
Sensory nerves 459
Septal defects 40
Septic arthritis 565, 586, 593
Serratia 344, 345, 348, 350, 356
  marcescens 239, 339
  species 337, 345, 353
Serum
  albumin, low 436
  aspartate aminotransferase 436
  complement fixation 331
  concentration 298
  dehydroepiandrosterone sulfate 676
  gonadotropins 676
  iron 513
  potassium caution 117
  prolactin 676
  sodium 611
  testosterone 676
  theophylline concentrations, lower 297
  triglycerides, management of elevated 233
Serum creatinine 1
  abnormal 122
  normal 122, 639

Serum total
 thyroxine 652
 triiodothyronine 652
Sexual dysfunction 22
Sexually transmitted disease 585
Shigella 408-410
 flexneri 588
 sonnei 588
Shockable rhythm 259
Shoulder impingement syndrome 577
Shunt surgery, emergent 428
Sick sinus syndrome 280, 286
Sickle cell 522
 disease 519, 525
 treatment 521
Simvastatin 227, 228, 230
 monotherapy 230
Single photon emission computed
 tomography 374
 ventilation/perfusion 371
Sinoatrial disease 251
Sinus
 bradycardia 60, 74f
 node dysfunction 280, 286
 rhythm 140, 143
 tachycardia 90, 163, 273
Sinusitis 484
Sinusoidal 431
Sitosterol 97, 99t, 102, 214, 215
 blood levels, diabetic to reduce 646
Sitosterolemia 97, 98, 100, 101, 207, 647
 in diabetics 635
Sjögren's syndrome 564, 600
 primary 506
 treatment 601
Skin-joint disease 602
Sleep disturbance 361
Snake venoms 493
Sodium 491, 611
 bicarbonate 255, 256, 618
 channel 155
  blockers 155
 ipodate 661
 loss 611
 polystyrene sulfonate 619
Soft tissue
 disorders, regional 576
 injection, principles for 571b
 rheumatic pain, generalized 579
Solitary plasmacytoma 561

Solitary thyroid nodule 662
 investigation of 663fc
Somnolence 317
Sorbitol 401
Sotalol 17, 154, 159, 691
Spastic diverticular disease 419
Spinal cord compression, acute 474
Spine 582
 osteoarthritis of 574
Spironolactone 8, 434
Spondylitis 585, 595
Spondyloarthropathy 587
Spontaneous bacterial peritonitis 430,
  431, 434
 treatment 435
Spontaneous pneumothorax 316
Sputum culture 314
Sputum production 311
Stabilize cardiac cell membrane 618
Stable angina 43, 44
 drug therapy 53
 electrocardiograms 47
 interventional therapy 62
 investigative evaluation 46
 pathophysiology 44
 therapy 53
Stable disease 293
Staphylococcus
 aureus 239, 240, 243, 320, 325, 334,
  335, 340, 345, 349, 350, 351,
  357, 361, 362, 478
 epidermidis 242, 340, 351, 357, 363
 marcescens 240
 species 336, 478
Starling's equation 377
Statins 53, 222
 adverse effects of 228
 contraindications 227
 dose of 228
Status asthmaticus 168, 299, 306
Status epilepticus 453, 454b, 455b
 diagnosis 453
 pathophysiology 453
 therapy 453
Steatorrhea 406
Stenosis, acute 490
Steroid 570, 577, 579
 inhaler 289
 puffer 289
Stimulate glucagon production 626

Stokes-Adams attacks 287
Stomach pain 228
Streptococcal pneumonia 324f
Streptococci 340, 478
Streptococcus 435, 446, 486
   anginosus 240
   bovis 237, 242, 243, 351
   durans 243
   faecalis 243
   faecium 243
   gallolyticus 242
   milleri milleri 351
   mitis 240, 351
   mutans 351
   pyogenes 343, 351
   sanguis 351
   species 359
   viridans 243
Streptococcus pneumoniae 239, 243, 320, 321, 325-327, 334, 335, 343, 344, 347, 349, 351, 352, 355-361, 393, 478, 480
   therapy 327
Streptokinase 79t, 81, 87
Streptomyces species 359
Streptomycin 481
Stroke 97, 464, 556
   diagnosis 464
   investigations 466
   pathophysiology 465
   therapy 466
      acute 466
   volume 280
ST-segment elevation myocardial infarction 70, 163, 225
Subepithelial tracheobronchial mucous glands 309
Sucralfate 407
Sudden cardiac death 4, 7t, 65, 67fc, 250t, 252, 263, 264
   prevention of 125
Sudden dyspnea 367
Sulbactam 242, 243, 347
Sulfamethoxazole 340, 363, 481, 547
Sulfasalazine 412, 417
Sulfhydryl agent 20
Sulfonamides 206
Sulfonylureas 643
Superoxide dismutase 600
Supplemental oxygen 308

Supraventricular arrhythmias 134
Supraventricular tachycardia 94, 129, 130, 132f, 193, 280
Sydenham's chorea 205
Sympathetic system, activation of 113
Symptomatic bradycardia, severe 257
Syncope 175, 200, 263, 278
   assessment of 279fc
   cardiac causes of 280t
   causes of 177, 283
   entails, management of 280
   history 281
   noncardiac causes of 282t
   physical examination 281
Synovial fluid 583
Synovianalysis 571b
Synovium 603
Synthetic penicillin 547
Syphilis 182
Systemic acidosis 388
Systemic diseases, characteristics of 505t
Systemic endotoxemia 433
Systemic illness 409
Systemic lupus erythematosus 388, 405, 465, 503, 505, 508, 542, 601
   treatment 602
Systemic rheumatic diseases 563
Systemic sclerosis 509, 564, 603
Systemic vasculitis 507, 606
Systolic
   crescendo-decrescendo murmur 174
   function, reduced 271
   hypertension, mild-to-moderate 5fc
   murmur 263
Systolic dysfunction 112
   ventricular 115, 120

T

Tachyarrhythmias 147f, 147t, 280, 286
   types of 146
Tachycardia 147, 148, 168, 187, 293, 589, 658, 660
Tachyphylaxis 296
Takayasu's arteritis 182, 564, 678, 694
   diagnosis 695
   investigations 695
   therapy 696

Takayasu's disease 285
Takotsubo stress cardiomyopathy 75, 276, 277f
Takotsubo syndrome 276
Tapazole 517
Tarsal tunnel syndrome 579
Tartrate-resistant acid phosphatase 555
Telmisartan 116
Temporomandibular myofascial pain 576
Tendinitis 563, 575
Tenecteplase 88
Tenesmus 409
Tenidap 600
Tenormin 17
Terazosin 16
Terbutaline 293, 294
Terfenadine 133
Tetracyclines 359, 360
Thalassemia 513, 525
    treatment 526
Theophylline 297, 315
    interactions 300t
    preparations 297
    toxicity 139
Therapeutic decisions 478
Therapeutic endoscopy 426
Thermal injury 515
Thiazide 34, 421
    diuretics 31
Thoracic aorta 208, 695
Throat 330
Thrombocythemia 368, 534
    essential 558
Thrombocytopenia 534, 543, 544
Thromboembolic disease, history of 368
Thromboembolism 179
Thrombolytic agent 82
    dosage of 81t
Thrombolytic therapy 77, 83
    complications of 87
    contraindications 85
    indications for 85
    timing of 80t
Thrombopathy 543
Thrombosis, acute 490
Thrombotic disorders 542
Thrombotic thrombocytopenic purpura 492, 506, 541

Thyroid 518
    binding proteins 654
    cancer, therapy for 652
    deficiency 518
    disease 652
        screening for 653fc
    hormone replacement 656
    malignancy 655
    nodules 662
    radioisotope scan 662
    stimulating hormone 652
    storm 660
    tests 652
    ultrasound 662
Thyroidal radioactive iodine uptake test 653
Thyroiditis 654, 657
    silent 662
    subacute 661
Thyrotoxicosis 285
Thyrotropin-releasing hormone stimulation test 653, 671
Ticarcillin 338, 345-347, 481
Tight mitral stenosis 280
Tildiem 61
Timolol 4, 18, 269
Tissue
    hypoxia 631
    plasminogen activator 77, 88
Tobramycin 355, 356, 445, 481, 487, 493
Tocainide 153, 155
Tocilizumab 696
Topiramate 461
Torsades de pointes 133, 159
Torsades depends, prevention of 160
Total cholesterol 209, 214
Total colectomy 414
Toxic megacolon, severe 414
Toxic multinodular goiter 654
    management of 660
Toxic solitary adenoma, management of 660
Toxicity 344, 347, 354
Tracheal irritation 295
Tracheal tug 312
Trandate 17
Tranexamic acid 539
Tranquilizers 438
Transabdominal incision 39

Transcatheter aortic valve 186
  replacement 181
Transcobalamins 529
Transdermal nitrate preparations and
  dosage 55*t*
Transesophageal echocardiography
  196, 240
Trans-fatty acids 221
Transfusion reactions 493
Transient autonomic disturbances 472
Transient ischemia 464
Transient ischemic attacks 204, 282,
  462, 557
  diagnosis 462
  pathophysiology 463
  therapy 463
Transient myocardial stunning 276
Transient thyroiditis 655
Transsphenoidal surgery 670
Transthoracic echocardiography 240
Transudative pleural effusions 378, 383
Transvenous pacing, temporary 160
Trauma 182, 421
Trichlormethiazide 18
Tricuspid regurgitation 168
Triglyceride 216
Trimethaphan 27
Trimethoprim 328, 340, 363, 481, 547
Troleandomycin 301
Trypanosoma cruzi 275, 684
Tubercle bacillus 517
Tuberculosis 169, 274, 378, 379, 492
  peritonitis 432
Tuberculous
  effusion 386
  meningitis 478
  pericarditis 166
  pleural effusions 395
  pleuritis 388, 389
  pneumonia, acute 323*f*
Tubular necrosis, acute 490-492
Tubulointerstitial nephritis, acute
  hypersensitivity 492, 495
Tumors 441
Turners' syndrome 655, 678, 692
  diagnosis 692
  treatment 693
Tyrosine kinase inhibitors 655

U

Ulcer
  disease, symptomatic 403
  healing of 406
  pain 403
Ulcerative colitis 182, 411, 412
  chronic 564
  complications 415
  diagnosis 412
  mild-to-moderate 414
  therapy 412
  treatment 415
Umbilical cord 531
Underfill hypothesis 432
Unstable angina 44, 49*f*, 63
  cases of 63
  pathophysiology 63
  therapy 63
Upper lobe pneumonia, acute right 322*f*
Upper respiratory infection 472
Upper respiratory tract
  instrumentation of 248
  procedures 245*t*
  surgery of 248
Urea 239
Ureaplasma 588
Uremia 108, 167, 379, 438
  signs of 495
Uremic pericarditis 167
Ureter 491
Ureterocele 491
Ureteropelvic junction 492
Urethra 491
Uric acid levels 556
Urinary bladder 492
Urinary calcium, lower 509
Urinary excretion, abnormal 489
Urinary indices 491*t*
Urinary red blood cells 496
Urinary retention 285
Urinary tract
  infections 639
  obstruction 491
    acute 489
Urine
  plasma ratio 491
  sodium concentration 491
  testing 645
Urinothorax 378, 385

Urokinase 395
Urticaria 18, 232, 233
Ustekinumab 418
Uterine prolapse 491

V

Vagotomy 406
Valproate 450, 655
Valproic acid 421, 450
Valve
   endocarditis, native 241
   failure, primary 180
   leaflets 196
   prosthesis, choice of 179t
   replacement
      complications of 180
      timing of 184
Valvular abnormalities 109
Valvular heart disease 174, 237, 463, 465
Vancomycin 245, 246, 355, 356, 365, 366, 481
Variceal bleeding 427, 430, 431
Vascular collapse, signs of 421
Vascular congestion 301
Vasculitis syndromes, features of 607t
Vasodepressor syncope 278, 283
Vasopressin 255
   single dose of 255
Vasovagal syncope 278, 283, 288
Vasovagal syndrome, malignant 282
Vedolizumab 414, 416, 417
Vein
   graft 178
   intercostal 382
Vena cava
   obstruction, superior 378
   syndrome, superior 385
Veno-occlusive disease 432, 433
Venous thrombosis, deep 106
Venous ultrasonography 375
Ventilation 374
Ventricular arrhythmias 153t
   management of 151t
Ventricular fibrillation 249, 255
   management of 253
Ventricular premature
   beats 124, 148, 150f
      management of 148
      multifocal 149f
   contractions 92, 152, 298

Ventricular tachycardia 129, 131, 147f, 148, 152fc, 250, 286
   nonsustained 149f
Verapamil 23, 36, 60, 61, 94, 134, 136t, 137, 139, 140, 267, 285, 286, 301
   intravenous 134
Verelan 17
Vertigo 458, 556
   causes of 462
Vessel wall, problems of 543
Vibramycin 360
Vibrio cholerae 409
Vibrio parahaemolyticus 408
Vidarabine 301
Villonodular synovitis, pigmented 586
Viral
   arthritis 587
   hepatitis, acute 654
   infections 378, 409
   pericarditis 164, 169
   pneumonias 330
Viral encephalitis 483
   diagnosis 483
   treatment 483
Virus 320
Visceral pleura 377
Visual hallucinations 124
Vitamin 376
   B_{12} 529, 544
      deficiency 529, 530
      deficiency, treatment 530
      levels 529
      source of 529
   C, dietary deficiency of 528
   K 533
Vomiting 357, 660
von Willebrand's disease 538
   characteristics of 539t
   classification of 539t
   diagnosis 538
   management 539
von Willebrand's factor 539

W

Waldenström's cells 561
Waldenström's disease 561
   management 562
   treatment 562
Warfarin 375

Waring blender syndrome defects 515
Warm autoantibody disease 524
Water gain 612
    causes of 612
Wegener's granulomatosis 507, 564, 609
Weight loss 166, 232, 234, 409
Weight reduction diet 234
Wenckebach phenomenon 161*f*
Wernicke's encephalopathy 455
    diagnosis 455
    pathophysiology 456
    therapy 456
Westermark's sign 372
Wheezes 312
Whipple's disease 182, 564, 587
White blood cell 495
    count 387
Wolff-Parkinson-White syndrome 140, 144, 145*f*, 146, 251, 280, 286
World Health Organization 506
Wounds, minor 538
Wytensin 17

X

Xanthelasma 211
Xanthoma tendinosum, absence of 211
Xanthomonas maltophilia 340, 350, 353, 354, 358, 360, 364
Xylocaine 577
    injection 579
    mixture 577

Y

Yellow nail syndrome 379
Yersinia strains 588

Z

Zollinger-Ellison syndrome 404, 406

EU GSPR Authorised Reprsentative
Logos Europe, 9 rue Nicolas Poussin
1700, La Rochelle, France
Phone: +33 (0) 6 67 93 73 78
E-mail: contact@logoseurope.eu

www.ingramcontent.com/pod-product-compliance
Ingram Content Group UK Ltd.
Pitfield, Milton Keynes, MK11 3LW, UK
UKHW050455150426
5217IPUK00025B/1700